General Practice Medicine

General Practice Medicine

EDITED BY

J.H. Barber
MD FRCGP FRCP(G) DObstRCOG

Professor of General Practice, Norie-Miller Chair, University of Glasgow

SECOND EDITION

CHURCHILL LIVINGSTONE
EDINBURGH LONDON MELBOURNE AND NEW YORK 1984

CHURCHILL LIVINGSTONE
Medical Division of Longman Group Limited

Distributed in the United States of America by Churchill
Livingstone Inc., 1560 Broadway, New York, N. Y. 10036, and
by associated companies, branches and representatives
throughout the world.

First edition 1975
Second edition 1984

ISBN 0 443 02693 9

British Library Cataloguing in Publication Data
General practice medicine — 2nd ed.
1. Pathology
I. Barber, J.H.
616   RB111

Library of Congress Cataloging in Publication Data
Main entry under title:

General practice medicine.

Includes bibliographies and index.
1. Family medicine.   I. Barber, J.H. (James Hill)
[DNLM: 1. Family Practice. W 89 G326]
RC46.G4   1984   610   84–12120

Printed in Singapore by Selector Printing Co (Pte) Ltd

Preface

When the first edition of this textbook was published, in 1975, it was one of very few books written for and about general practice by general practitioner authors. During the last 9 years the scope of general practice has steadily widened and with a greater knowledge and awareness of the extent of medicine in the discipline, there has been an increasing number of textbooks written for established general practitioners and trainees alike. General practice is a wide and far ranging discipline and consequently while the need for textbooks on different aspects of the practitioner's work has largely been met there is a relative paucity of textbooks which attempt to cover the wide canvas of medicine in the community.

While this second edition of General Practice Medicine has been almost completely rewritten it has retained some of what I felt were important features of the first edition. With the exception of one author all who have contributed to the book are active general practitioners who not only are experienced writers but have special skills and practical experience of their particular subject. This has enabled each chapter to deal particularly with those aspects of clinical medicine that are relevant to and important for the general practitioner in his day by day work.

As with the first edition this book has been written principally for the vocational trainee. I hope it will help to provide an appropriate background of knowledge upon which the new entrant to general practice can, with experience, achieve confidence in this demanding and satisfying branch of medicine.

My special thanks are due to Miss Margaret Hagan upon whom lay the very onerous responsibility for typing and preparing the manuscript.

Glasgow
1984

J.H. Barber

Contributors

J.H. Barber MD FRCGP FRCP(G) DObstRCOG
Professor of General Practice, Norie-Miller Chair, University of Glasgow

William J. Bassett MB ChB MRCGP
General Practitioner, Craigshill Health Centre, Livingston, West Lothian; Medical Assistant in Paediatrics, Bangour Hospital, West Lothian

I. Cunningham MB ChB DObst RCOG
General Practitioner, Dufftown, Keith, Banffshire

Gordon Currie OBE MB ChB DTM&H FRCGP
General Practitioner, Glasgow; Medical Assistant in Geriatrics, Southern General Hospital, Glasgow

Derek Doyle MB ChB FRCGP
Medical Director, St Columba's Hospice, Edinburgh

C.K. Drinkwater BA MB BChir (Cantab) MRCGP DCH DObstRCOG
Senior Lecturer in Family Medicine, Department of Family and Community Medicine, University of Newcastle-upon-Tyne

Iain C. Gilchrist MB ChB MRCGP
General Practitioner, Bishop's Stortford, Herts

P.A. Greig MB ChB
General Practitioner, Sheffield

David R. Hannay MA MD PhD FFCM MRCGP DCH
Senior Lecturer, Department of General Practice, University of Glasgow

Gordon Hickish VRD MB ChB MRCGP DCH
General Practitioner, Bransgore, Hampshire;
Hospital Practitioner, ENT Department, St Bartholomew's Hospital, London

John G.R. Howie MD PhD FRCGP
Professor of General Practice, James MacKenzie Chair, University of Edinburgh

Geoffrey T. Millar MB ChB FRCS(E)
Consultant Ophthalmologist, Bangour General Hospital, Broxburn, West Lothian

H.D.R. Munro MB ChB MRCOG, MRCGP
General Practitioner, Craigshill Health Centre, Livingston, West Lothian

T.S. Murray PhD FRCGP FRCP DObstRCOG
Senior Lecturer, Department of General Practice, University of Glasgow

E.A. Neville MB ChB FRCP(G) MRCGP DObstRCOG
General Practitioner, Kirkintilloch

N.W. Poole MB ChB MRCGP
General Practitioner, Govanhill Health Centre, Glasgow

I.H. Redhead MD FRCGP
General Practitioner, Yaxley, Peterborough; Clinical Assistant in Genito-Urinary Medicine, Peterborough District Hospital

E.T. Robinson TD MB ChB FRCGP DObstRCOG
General Practitioner, Woodside Health Centre, Glasgow

R.J. Simpson MB ChB DPM MRCPsych
General Practitioner, The Health Centre, Bridge of Allan

Thomas C.G. Smith MB ChB DPharmMed
Medical Writer and General Practitioner, Pinwherry, Ayrshire

M.P. Taylor MB ChB FRCGP
Senior Associate in General Practice, University of Sheffield

Joyce M. Watson MD MFCM MRCGP DA DPH
Senior Research Fellow (Astra), Department of General Practice, University of Glasgow

Stuart F. Wood MB ChB MRCGP
General Practitioner, Glasgow

Contents

J.H. Barber

General practice medicine

INTRODUCTION

To say that general medicine differs in almost all its aspects from medical practice in the hospital is perhaps an obvious statement but an appreciation of these differences is an important first step in understanding the range and diversity of the general practitioner's work. Without this understanding, the doctor who attempts to interpret the 'facts' of general practice — whether these concern the nature and presentation of illness or the organisation of the work of the practice — is likely to find himself frustrated and confused.

The process of diagnosis, both in terms of its pathological precision and the doctor's therapeutic response to particular illnesses is not only different from the accepted norms of hospital practice but may also differ between patients in the same practice. Many of the illnesses that are seen in general practice are of a minor, self-limiting nature and frequently do not conform to accounts of specific clinical syndromes. This is particularly true, for example of upper respiratory infections in which the diagnostic 'label' and the treatment prescribed for the same syndrome will vary from doctor to doctor. The nature of many of these illnesses is such that extensive investigation in the search for a definitive diagnosis cannot be justified; symptomatic treatment, prescribed in the expectation of recovery, thus becomes a more rational approach to therapy.

The most significant factor of all is that of continuity of care; the doctor in general practice cannot simply be concerned with single episodes of illness. He will continue to see his patients and must plan his care of them to take account of social, psychological and environmental circumstances which may have an influence on the progress or outcome of the illness. He cannot readily 'discharge' his patient to the care of someone else and must broaden his therapeutic objectives beyond the management of defined diagnostic categories in order to include a concern for the lifestyle of the patient and his ability to lead a constructive independent life in the community.

It is easy to leave the impression that these wider and less precise aspects of diagnosis and therapy somehow lack the exactness that medical technology provides for the clinician in hospital. Contemporary developments mean that while this may have been true a decade ago it need no longer be so today. The diagnostic process in general practice is based on somewhat different premises and is concerned with rather different issues but this does not mean that its standards are lower or, within its own terms, that it is less precise.

A further important difference is that, when encountering a patient for the first time, the general practitioner is faced with a wide range of diagnostic possibilities; in contrast, the hospital clinician's patient is usually referred to him by another doctor who has already made two important decisions — that the patient has a 'significant' illness, and, even if it is not precisely diagnosed in pathological terms, that the illness is appropriate to that clinician's specialty. The general practitioner, on the other hand, must determined whether or not a presenting complaint is of pathological significance and must also be prepared to interpret that complaint in the context of his earlier knowledge of the patient and his circumstances.

These decisions are not simply a question of deciding whether a symptom is 'trivial' or 'serious'. An episode of upper respiratory tract infection may be of little significance in an otherwise healthy young man; as the third or fourth such episode during one winter in a heavy smoker of 50 years it may suggest that onset of chronic bronchitis, and in an elderly man with barely controlled congestive cardiac failure it may signal the end of his independent existence and his entry into some form of institutional care.

There are other ways in which the simple diagnostic answer may not be the right one and it is only by appraising presenting symptoms and signs in the context of a continuing knowledge of the patients that diagnostic insight can be achieved:

> A middle-aged professional man consulted his general practitioner with the complaint of a painful knee; later he complained of conjunctivitis and later still of a urethral discharge. These complaints were separated by intervals of about a month and each appeared to the general practitioner to be relatively

trivial. It was only when the doctor reviewed the patient's record that he realised that, taken together, these complaints resembled Reiter's syndrome. Further inquiry revealed marital disharmony and considerable psychological stress; the patient feared that he had acquired a venereal disease and had obtained his 'symptoms' from reading a medical textbook. He hoped that the doctor would recognise the nature of his problem and would investigate further

This example illustrates more than just the complexity of the diagnostic process in general practice. It is also an example of the way in which the social and cultural attitudes of patients may influence the way in which they think about illness and the complaints that are 'proper' to take to the doctor. The example above is somewhat esoteric but the presentation of a physical complaint as a mask for a psychological problem is a not uncommon strategy. The way in which symptoms are presented and the frequency with which the doctor encounters complaints of different kinds are also dependent on the personality of both patient and doctor. There are patients who, because of inadequacies of personality or the chronic nature of their inadequate social circumstances, make heavy demands on the doctor's time. The response of different doctors to these patients varies greatly between sympathy and hostility.

It is inevitable that, on occasions, the doctor will lose his patience and accuse the patient of wasting his time. This is more likely to happen when the basic problem is outwith the ability of the doctor to effect treatment and, as such, is more likely to occur when the cause is social or psychological. Most doctors are at their most confident when faced with complaints of an organic nature, when the management and prognosis can be predicted with assurance. The patient may recognise this and thus express his problem in terms of physical symptoms. If these are accepted at their face value, and treated in isolation, the fundamental complaint will remain untouched, and the situation will be perpetuated.

Similar patients may cause frustration and anxiety because, in their frequent calls for help it is difficult to know which of a series of cries of 'wolf' is a genuinely serious episode. There are also patients of another kind; those who prefer 'not to trouble the doctor' can cause concern over whether or not serious pathology may be developing and the opportunity for early treatment is being lost. This can be a particular problem in elderly people who value their independence and, in any case, consider that deterioration of mental or physical capacity is a normal result of aging.

These are frustrations and difficulties that may be brought about by the attitudes of patients, but it is also important to recognise that barriers to the correct care of patients may be created by the (often unconscious) attitudes of the doctor himself. Impatience or a lack of sympathy with particular grouups or types of patients

can lead to them being rejected or failing to get the care that they need. Such patients then devise alternative and time-wasting strategies in their attempts to have their problems recognised. The general practitioner is exposed to all sorts and conditions of men and must develop an insight into his own attitudes and the effect that they may have on the way in which he reacts to his patients.

There are a number of formal ways of describing these relationships — much of medical education is concerned with 'biological' descriptions of health and disease in which the causation, treatment and outcome of an illness are described in terms of the pathological process that is occurring; such accounts are as true in general practice as they are in the hospital. The difference is the additional significance of a social and psychological understanding of health-related problems. One useful concept developed by sociologists is that of the 'sick-role'; at its simplest, this says that people who feel themselves to be ill (or who are deemed to be ill by others) behave differently and according to their own ideas about sickness behaviour. Amongst other things, sickness provides an acceptable reason for withdrawing from social responsibilities. Different patients 'use' the sick role in various ways; some as a means of escape from other problems or inadequacies, some as a means of social manipulation and some — the great majority — in its ordinary sense. An important feature of this concept in general practice is that the doctor is to a large extent influential in determining whether a person is 'sick' or not and thus in reinforcing or changing the patient's own interpretation. The doctor's own definition of sickness and his reactions to the sickness behaviour of his patients inevitably form an important part of his management of a patient's illness.

A similar and equally important concept concerns the 'transactions' or 'negotiations' that go on between the doctor and his patient. Consultations are not rarely confined to simple organic illness and the less this is so, the more they become a process of one party attempting to influence or persuade the other. The doctor cannot simply 'tell' the patient what is right or not — his method of telling will obviously be tempered by the patient's ability to understånd, but it will also relate to other aspects of the patient's personality which affect his willingness to accept or reject the advice. Patients, on the other hand, will often present problems in a way that they hope will influence the outcome of the consultation. Failure to appreciate the nature and content of this process of negotiation can often lead to frustration and impatience; conversely, an awareness of the process provides a therapeutic advantage that can lead to a clearer understanding of the patient's real problem. Finally, it is worthy remembering that things that doctors say are often quoted as a part of other negotiations and that the way of saying them can often be more important than their content.

These various aspects of general practice concern the doctor's relationships with individual patients but there are two other features of medical practice in the community which have an important influence on the doctor's work. The first concerns the need to take account of the great variety of problems he encounters in his daily and thus to plan the organisation of his practice to provide a service for a 'population' of patients in contrast to simply responding to the *ad hoc* demands of individual patients as they present themselves. The second has to do with the doctor's relationships with various other professional and services — with the hospital, with health visitors and nurses, with social work services and, less directly, with such other agencies as the housing department and local industry.

The average general practitioner in Britain has about 2000 to 2500 people registered with him; Table 1.1 lists several other features of such an average practice although it is important to interpret numbers of this kind with caution. Practices vary widely in terms of the proportions of patients in different age groups and social circumstances and in the patterns of morbidity they experience. With this proviso, Table 1.1 affords a basis for considering the organisational problem further.

Clearly, some age groups are likely to require the doctor's services more often than others and for more complex problems. These groups will include old people (about 350 in the 'average' practice) who are not only more likely to experience chronic disease but who are also more likely to encounter social difficulties. Chronic illnesses account for only about 22% of all consultations but their importance as a cause of disability and their continuing nature means that they are a more significant part of the doctor's work than this single percentage suggests. Similar arguments apply to mothers and young children so that the 500 women between the ages of 16 and 44 years of age will also contribute significantly to the doctor's workload either on their own account or on behalf of their children.

It is easy to categorise a high proportion of the illness episodes of this group of patients as 'trivial' or 'minor' and thus to underemphasise their needs. As with any other group of patients, the doctor must see these illnesses in the context of the family and the various relationships within it and his care must take account of these factors. Seen in this way, a succession of minor illnesses in a young child may have an effect in some families that is as disturbing as a continuing illness. Similarly, anxieties and feelings of inadequacy on the part of the young mother may be made worse simply because they provide an opportunity for a grandmother to assume a dominant role. The doctor's introduction to situations of this kind is likely to be through the too frequent presentation of minor illness; this will continue — with increasing dissatisfaction on both sides — until the doctor is able to take more positive action by planning his response to individual episodes in the context of

Table 1.1 Selected data concerning an 'average' general practice of 2500 patients in Britain*

About 350 patients will be more than 65 years old
100 will be more than 75 years old
About 150 will be less than 5 years old
About 500 will be women aged between 16 and 44

60% of consultations are for 'minor' illnesses
18% are for 'major' illnesses
22% are for chronic illness

The number of people consulting for 'minor' illnesses in a year will include:
500 for upper respiratory infections
300 for emotional disorders
250 for gastro-intestinal disorders
225 for skin disorders

The number of people consulting for 'major' illnesses in a year will include:
50 for acute bronchitis and pneumonia
12 for severe depression
7 for acute myocardial infarction
5 for acute appendicitis
5 for acute strokes
5 for 'new' cancers

The number of people consulting for chronic illness will include:
100 for chronic rheumatism
55 for chronic rheumatism
50 for chronic bronchitis
43 for anaemia
30 for chronic heart failure
25 for high blood pressure
25 for asthma
25 for peptic ulcer

There will be about 40 pregnancies and about 26 deaths in a year

150 patients will be in receipt of supplementary social security benefits.
There will be 60 one-parent families with children under age 15.
There will be 70 patients with severe physical handicap and 10 with severe mental handicap
300 families will experience social problems associated with mental illness
There will be 130 families with marital problems

The consultation rate will vary both geographically and according to the type of area; it is higher in Scotland than in England and higher in urban than in rural practices. Reports vary between three and seven consultations per person per year.

The average consultation time is about 6 minutes.

Night calls between midnight and 7 a.m. (for which claims for payment were made) averaged 9 per general practitioner in 1971. The actual number of night calls may be higher.

In a year, 780 patients in an average practice will use hospital therapeutic services:
275 will be in-patients
420 will be 'new' out-patients
420 will be 'new' accidents or emergencies
15 will have domiciliary visits

*The data in this table derive from many different studies; collectively, they are taken from *Present State and Future Needs of General Practice*. London: Royal College of General Practitioners, 1973.

his knowledge of the family and the social dynamics that occur within it.

All of these factors argue in favour of a planned approach to the work of the practice which will allow the doctor to deal with these various needs in an organised way. One of the advantages of analysing the workload of an individual practice is that it allows the assembly of information (comparable to that of Table 1.1) which permits this kind of planning to proceed. One of the disadvantages of not having these data is that it then becomes easy to be over-impressed with the varying demands of traditional consulting sessions and thus to argue that setting aside time for particular purposes is impractical because of the pressure of work.

If one accepts the numbers in Table 1.1 as a basis for planning it is then reasonably easy to estimate the time that would be needed for the 'special' clinics that are discussed more fully in Chapter 3. The estimated number of patients with hypertension or chronic bronchitis, for example, can be linked to estimates of the frequency of review consultations and thus to the time needed for each patient in a planned approach to the care of that particular disease. (The ante-natal clinic is an established precedent for this approach.) Sessions of this kind, however, do not need to be based on specific disease; there are similar advantages in setting aside time during the week for the more comprehensive discussion of other kinds of problems. Such arranged sessions have the additional benefit of enabling the health visitor or social worker to be present and thus to participate.

One of the most important developments in the health care of the community in recent years has been the realisation of the idea of the health care *team*. This essentially simple concept recognises that a range of different skills is required to meet the various needs of patients and that it is sensible to bring the professions who provide these skills together so that they may complement each other. The basic team is usually formed by attaching health visitors and community nursing sisters to groups of general practitioners but this arrangement should not give the impression that the nurse and health visitor 'work for' the doctor; successful health care teams are those in which each member recognises the skills and abilities of the other members in contributing to the total care of the patient. In some cases it may be that the doctor's contribution is the most significant but, in others, the counsel of the health visitor or the practical procedures of the nurse may be the more important features of the patient's management.

It is difficult to be prescriptive about the nature of team relationships — much will obviously depend on the personalities that are involved — but there are, perhaps, two simple aspects of the team that are necessary for its success. The first is that it is important not to place too much stress on formal job divisions — on the status and position of the doctor *vis-a-vis* that of the nurse. These distinctions are relatively clear-cut in hospital practice but they are more difficult to define in the community and serve much less purpose. An approach that is based on the sharing of problems and the appreciation of patient's needs is more likely to succeed. The second aspect, from the doctor's point of view, is a corollary of the first. This is the need to understand in some depth the contribution that other professionals can make. Again, in hospital practice it is relatively easy to be detached and to 'prescribe' other services without a close involvement in their content. In general practice an understanding of the methods and objectives of other disciplines leads to an understanding of their value in particular situations and avoids the dissatisfactions and frustrations that can arise when expectations are not met. This is particularly true of social workers whose methods of 'diagnosis' and 'therapy' are often different and viewed on a longer time-scale than the more immediate problems that are perceived by the doctor (see pp. 15–16).

Apart from these more general features of the team relationship it is, of course, also necessary to make practical arrangements for its effective working. Most health care teams are based in the premises of the general practitioner and there is an obvious need to provide suitable accommodation, but other aspects of practice such as the organisation of the records and appointment systems are equally important. The doctor must arrange his work in a way that allows proper consultation and discussion between members of the team; *ad hoc* encounters and requests for visits or services are less likely to be effective and can limit the benefits that arise from collaboration.

The general practitioner is also a part of a wider system of health care and, to a large extent, controls the patient's access to other more specialised facilities. In considering the nature and organisation of his work, he must establish good relationships with the specialist services and have a critical knowledge of the contribution that they can make to the care of his patients. This contribution breaks down into three main components: firstly, the need for specialist consultation and advice on diagnosis or therapy, secondly, the need for technical procedures (such as surgery), and, thirdly, the need for patient management facilities (such as in-patient care) that are not ordinarily available to the doctor. In practice, of course, these three components are not always so easily distinguished and many patients have need of all three. But, at the same time, the doctor must try to define the purpose of his referral and the benefits the patient will obtain. The increasing technological sophistication of hospitals and the increasing number of specialist departments means that patients can sometimes get 'lost' in the hospital system; one of the general practitioner's responsibilities is to safeguard his patient from this possibility by continuing to play an active part in his care.

The role of the general practitioner

In 1972 an attempt was made to define a job description for the general practitioner which would be commensurate with the emerging specialist nature of the discipline. The role description was further amended in 1977 by the Second European Conference on the Teaching of General Practice (usually called the Leeuwenhorst Group). Although the role description is clearly idealistic and in many respects lip service only is paid to it, it forms a useful tool in attempting to describe the unique contribution that the general practitioner can give to the comprehensive health care services available to the population.

The provision of health care is constantly changing as a consequence of public and professional aspirations and demands, the spread of medical knowledge and technology, and the changing relative importance of institutional and community medical resources both in general and as applied to specific areas of medical care. The demands of a developing and changing profession had created this role definition: it has already changed and will need to be continually updated as time passes. It does however present a valuable statement of intent and provides a useful framework within which to discuss some of the more important facets of the work and responsibilities of the general practitioner. In this chapter the role definition will be taken sentence by sentence and a number of themes — thought by the author to be particularly important — will be developed. It is hoped that this more critical discussion of the role of the general practitioner will allow the reader to appreciate more fully the relevance of the clinical chapters that follow.

'THE GENERAL PRACTITIONER IS A LICENCED MEDICAL GRADUATE WHO GIVES PERSONAL, PRIMARY AND CONTINUING CARE TO INDIVIDUALS AND FAMILIES IRRESPECTIVE OF AGE, SEX AND ILLNESSES. IT IS THE SYNTHESIS OF THESE FUNCTIONS THAT IS UNIQUE.'

Key words — Personal, Primary, Continuing Care, Individuals and Families.

PERSONAL CARE

The need for a personal physician was ably described in 1960 by Fox who stated 'a person in difficulties wants .... the help of another person on whom he can rely as a friend — someone with knowledge of what is feasible but also with good judgement of what is desirable in the particular circumstances. The more complex medicine becomes the stronger are the reasons why everyone should have a personal doctor who will take continuous responsibility for him, and knowing how he lives will keep things in proportion — protecting him, if need be, from the zealous specialist'.

Clearly the personal care of the individual patient by his doctor seems an ideal objective but as is so usually the case there are potential advantages and drawbacks for both parties.

Continuity of care within an individual episode of illness is what the majority of patients, and doctors, prefer and frequently achieve. Almost as important however is continuity through the different or recurrent illnesses with which some patients will be faced. This longitudinal continuity allows for the development of strong bonds between doctor and patient which in turn can permit degrees of honesty and frankness that may in certain circumstances be not only of value to both but of considerable importance in the investigation and management of ill-health. This degree of personal doctoring however, if carried to its logical conclusion requires the full-time dedication of the doctor to his patients that has been one of the most potent pressures towards the formation of group practices. Without doubt continual personal care can result in both intellectual and physical fatigue, and to the doctor being protected from any professional review of his work, either from his own self-evaluation or from the constructive opinions of a colleague. This form of personal care is now seen only in a few remaining rural single-handed practices and the profession as a whole has judged that the risks of professional isolation far outweigh the potential benefits to the patient. Indeed trends to the United Kingdom have moved rapidly towards the formation of group practices: in 1973 approximately 20%

of general practitioners were single-handed, a figure that had dropped to below 5% in 1980 (Social Trends).

Other trends are moving the profession away from personal family doctoring and many would see the move as progressing too far and too fast. The use of rota systems for out-of-hours cover has been accepted by doctors and patients alike as a humane method of ensuring that the doctor has adequate offduty for both familial and professional pursuits. There is a realisation that with fatigue — emotional or physical — can come errors of judgement. The rota system within a group practice appears to be the best compromise between the wishes of patients for personal care and the need for the doctor for relaxation. The more widespread and growing tendency in big cities towards commercial deputising services carries the potential risk to professional identity and standards of care in the appearance of a 9 to 5 doctor who subsequently locks up his surgery and hands over a significant part of his work to someone who not only does not know the patient or, importantly, have access to his medical records, but may have only a superficial knowledge of and interest in general practice. As always when there are extremes of view or of action the most acceptable course is to combine the advantages of personal doctoring with the fewest disadvantages of the alternative system in the knowledge that what is of essence is the general wellbeing of the patient.

PRIMARY CARE

The general practitioner may provide primary medical care but primary care frequently precedes the patient's consultation through a multitude of familial, cultural and lay community agencies. Hannay (1976) in a study of medicine-taking in a 2-week period in Glasgow found that one-third of the patients interviewed were taking drugs or medicines bought from the chemist or retail shops, one-third were not taking any medicines and the remaining third were in receipt of prescribed drugs. It has been estimated that of all ill-health in the community only one-quarter is presented as a formal complaint to a general practitioner. Of this fraction of all prevalent ill-health only between 6 and 8% is referred to hospital either for in-patient or for out-patient care (Fry 1979).

A strong and responsible primary care service is of importance to the patient and, through its fiscal effects and professional satisfaction, to the general practitioner. For the patient it combines a convenient and readily available source of help for the great majority of illnesses with a professional and controlled route of access to the more sophisticated and less personal hospital service. Hospital medicine is high expense medicine — approximately 65% of the National Health Service budget is devoted to institutional care — and increases in hospital

needs and costs that would inevitably follow any reduction in the effectiveness of primary care could only be achieved at the expense of the community services. Much of the malaise in general practice that was so prevalent 15 to 20 years ago was the result of a self-perception of an inferior status. The education and training of general practitioners today together with the facilities to which they have access have had a profound effect on the development of general practice from cottage industry to specialist discipline and consequently on professional pride and satisfaction.

CONTINUING CARE

Continuity of care, as in personal care, is a concept that should be achieved in theory but has the same potential drawbacks as has personal care. The objective is to achieve a balance between the needs of the patient and the restraints imposed by a group practice system. Thus continuity of care throughout individual illnesses is in general a worthwhile objective as, apart from the emergency situation, is continuity during chronic and recurrent illness. There are a number of distinct advantages to continuity of care. Every new illness consultation begins from a base of existing knowledge about the patient and the information that the doctor has of his patient is likely to be more comprehensive and varied. Repeated illness contact between patient and doctor will have allowed the latter to witness the patient's response to a variety of stresses — illnesses of different kinds and emotional or environmental problems. This knowledge may be of value in helping the doctor to anticipate his patient's reaction to a stress as severe as bereavement.

It can be argued that the adoption by general practice of the appointment system, of group practice and of rota systems for off-duty cover has resulted in a significant reduction in continuity of care. Two other factors have however also played an important part: the tendency in inner city areas for patients to 'self-refer' to hospital accident and emergency departments and the all too common habit of the hospital retaining patient care in out-patient follow-up clinics long after there is a real need for specialist skills or knowledge.

INDIVIDUALS AND FAMILIES

The interaction that occurs in ill-health between the individual and the family or environmental factors is too well appreciated to need much elaboration. It is perhaps best described by Bain (1981) who showed the consulting patterns of individual members of a family in the 6 months before and after the birth of a severely handicapped child (Fig. 2.1). In his study not only did the number

Months	1	2	3	4	5	6	7	8	9	10	11	12
Mr A		*			**		**	*	** **		**	*** **
Mrs A	**	** **	** *	** **	** **	** ** **	*** *** **	***	*** *** **	** **	** *	** ** *
Son (5 Yrs)	*		**	*		** *		** **			** *	*
Son (3 Yrs)		*			*		**		*	** *	**	** **

* = Consultation or Visit

Fig. 2.1 Individuals and families

of consultations with the husband and wife increase dramatically following the retarded child's birth but so also did the consultation rates for the child's siblings. While it can be readily appreciated that such a dramatic and tragic event can produce increased ill-health in other family members, it must also be appreciated that an apparent illness in one member of the family may represent ill-health in another or in the family as a whole.

'HE WILL ATTEND HIS PATIENTS IN HIS CONSULTING ROOM AND IN THEIR HOMES AND SOMETIMES IN A CLINIC OR IN A HOSPITAL'

Key words — Consulting room, Home.

CONSULTING ROOM

Most people feel at ease and confident when in a familiar and stress-free environment. This security is reflected in the ease and flow of conversation and the later recall of what was said and discussed. In the context of the medical consultation the patient's security is perhaps least disturbed if he or she is visited at home and most if admitted to hospital. The general practitioner's consulting room and the hospital out-patient department represent intermediate steps and are thus associated with increasing degrees of insecurity. The changing dis-ease of the patient is one of the determinants of how the patient tells his story to the doctor and of how much of the doctor's explanation and therapeutic instructions are understood and retained. A knowledge and appreciation of patient

insecurity with the need for careful and repeated communication on the part of the doctor can greatly influence patient understanding and thus treatment compliance.

It is also worth remembering that the patient may consider that the organisation and appearance of the consulting room may reflect the doctor who works in it: the austere and clinical consulting room may therefore seem threatening; the face to face arrangement of the doctor's and patient's chairs separated by the official medical desk may suggest confrontation, and by emphasising the roles of both parties, may influence the pattern of consultation.

HOME VISITS

In the United Kingdom the number of home visits done by the general practitioner has fallen steadily over the past 20 years and except during times of epidemic illness the home visit rate can be expected to be at about two and four per 1000 patients at risk. It has been long expected, usually by medical journalists, that United Kingdom general practice will in time follow the North American pattern where home visits are only made in exceptional circumstances. There are good reasons why patients, whenever possible, should attend the surgery or health centre rather than expect a house call — the availability of the medical record and the equipment in the modern surgery are only two of many. Equally there are a number of important justifications for the preservation of home visiting. The visit to a patient at home allows the doctor to determine the patient's physical resources, the emotional climate in the home and the interaction between family members. The patient is on secure home territory where communication between him and the doctor can be both more complete and more meaningful. Additionally there are other, mainly domestic, reasons why the patient's request for a house can be justified: the patient may be old and housebound or young with a young family; the weather too inclement or distances from home to surgery too difficult when relying on public transport. It is always wise to consider other possible factors in addition to the patient's illness when deciding on the 'correctness' of a request for a house call.

'HIS AIM IS TO MAKE EARLY DIAGNOSIS'

Key words — Early diagnosis.

Figure 2.2 shows the traditional hospital — and medical school — clinical decision-making pathway. The process differs in general practice in its structure and in the content of the four steps of cues, hypotheses, search stratagems and management decisions (Fig. 2.3).

CUES

The interpretation of the many cues given by the patient is affected by the amount of background 'noise'. This can be exemplified more succinctly by the need to be aware of significant social and psychological factors being of possible importance in the aetiology of some vague physical complaint. In general practice, illnesses present at an early stage of their natural history and as such the important cues may be fewer and less precise than is usually the case in hospital medicine. The ability to detect cues to life-threatening illnesss is a major responsibility of the general practitioner. In a population of 2500 approximately 700 patients will present each year with a respiratory tract infection of which cough is likely to be a major symptom. The general practitioner must be able to identify the two patients each year in whom cough is a symptom of a bronchogenic neoplasm. It is also important for the general practitioner to be aware of how the patient is communicating — using verbal, or non-verbal,

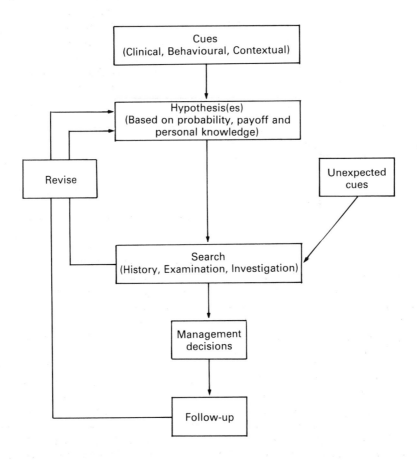

Fig. 2.2 Model of the diagnostic process

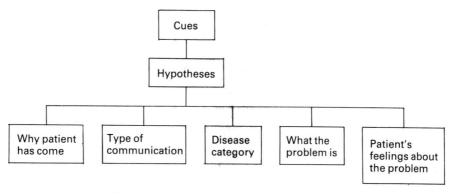

Fig. 2.3 Variety of hypotheses formed by the family physician

cues which can be the sign of a behavioural or psychological problem.

HYPOTHESES

Whereas the patient referred to a hospital specialty can be assumed likely to be suffering from an illness covered by that discipline, the consultation in general practice begins with the need to find out why the patient has presented, the principal problem as perceived by the patient and the broad disease group within which it is likely to lie. Thereafter the possibilities are decided upon in the light of the prevalence of different diseases within the community. Hypotheses relating to the reasons why the patient presented and the relative importance of social and psychological factors on the presenting complaint are influenced by the doctor's knowledge of the patient and on his reaction to previous ill-health.

SEARCH STRATAGEMS

In hospital medicine search stratagems are synonymous with one or many differing laboratory or operative investigations. From what has been said above it is clear that the search stratagems used in general practice must be more wide ranging — towards social, psychological or behavioural diagnoses — and more flexible as regards the number and timing of any investigations that may be thought necessary.

The predictive value of any laboratory test is influenced not only by its sensitivity and its specificity but also by the prevalence of the condition in the population — hospital or general practice — from which the patient comes (Kreig et al 1975). The predictive value of a pregnancy diagnostic test for instance is different when used with patients attending a gynaecological clinic where a high proportion of patients with amenorrhoea will have

pregnancy as its cause — and when used in general practice where the numbers of patients with amenorrhoea due to this cause may be much less (Robinson & Barber 1977). Some care thus needs to be taken of the real value of many laboratory tests when used in general practice where the number of false positives and negatives can be higher than in a hospital population where, and for whom, the test was first developed.

The further difference between hospital and general practice clinical decision making lies in the greater frequency with which the objective in the community may be to eliminate rather than to confirm an organic diagnosis. Thus the greater proportion of normal X-ray reports in direct referrals to X-ray departments from general practice compared with hospital reflects the different use to which the X-ray investigation can be put. Time is frequently at a premium during the general practice consultation and can again influence the path of history-taking and of clinical decision-making. In many ways the clinical problem can be less complex in general practice and short consultations may be all that are required, but few consultations do not begin from a base of considerable existing knowledge of the patient. Time can also be used to advantage in the early stages of illness — when the clinical problem may seem to be more of a syndrome than a precise diagnostic entity — to allow more definitive symptoms and signs to become apparent during the natural evolution of the condition.

MANAGEMENT DECISIONS

After the cues have been presented, a hypothesis formed and supported or rejected by search stratagems come the management decisions. Mention has been made that many illnesses appear in their early developing stages more as syndromes than as recognisable diseases. In a minority of instances this continues to hold true so that a diagnostic label cannot be given, and indeed should not be given, since a specific and perhaps erroneous treatment regime may thus be implied. In many instances therefore management decisions will have to be made in a climate of insecurity. The decisions that are made must be tailored to the particular needs of the individual patient and time must be used in a planned fashion to permit further symptoms or signs to develop, or conversely to allow the patient's illness to resolve.

'HE WILL INCLUDE AN INTEGRATE PHYSICAL, PSYCHOLOGICAL AND SOCIAL FACTORS IN HIS CONSIDERATION OF HEALTH AND ILLNESS. THIS WILL BE EXPRESSED IN THE CARE OF HIS PATIENTS.'

Key words — Physical, psychological, social.

Illness in general practice has been described as being in three broad groups; self-limiting illness (60%), acute life-threatening illness (18%) and chronic or recurrent illness (22%).

Over the last 15 to 20 years there has been increasing awareness of the need to consider psychological and social or environmental factors in the diagnosis and treatment of ill-health in general practice. To illustrate the importance of this more comprehensive approach to disease three examples will be given.

1. Self limiting illness — sore throat. Howie (1976) reported on the declared management policies of general practitioners towards patients presenting with a sore throat. A set of photographs of sore throats together with summary histories was distributed to approximately 1000 Scottish general practitioners. In one instance the photograph was accompanied by the following history: 'your patient — a woman of 28 years of age — complains of sore throat of 48 hours duration. She has no other symptoms. She is the mother of four young children. Would you prescribe an antibiotic?'. 30% of the general practitioners contacted indicated that they would prescribe an antibiotic in this instance. The photograph was reissued with the same history but with the added words: 'the two youngest of whom are twins of 18 months with whom she is not coping'. 51% of the general practitioners — drawn from the same group as previously — now indicated that they would prescribe an antibiotic ($P < 0.01$). Rightly or wrongly the addition of social information significantly altered the general practitioner's therapeutic approach to the illness.

2. Acute life-threatening illness — myocardial infarction. On the face of it the only important consideration in connection with a patient admitted to hospital with a myocardial infarction might seem to be his physical health. Expressed as a score out of 10 the relative values for physical, psychological and social considerations might on admission be 7, 4 and 1 (Fig. 2.4). The patient

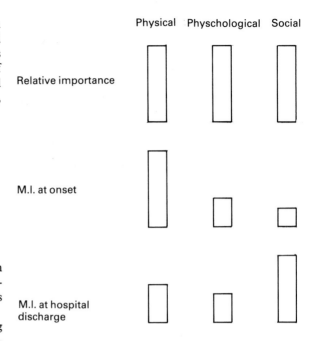

Fig. 2.4   Schematic representation of problem importance in a patient with a myocardial infarction

makes a good recovery and is discharged home. The general practitioner might now consider that the relative values would read: physical — 3, psychological — 2, and social — 5. At intervals during the patient's convalescence these relative values might have to be reassessed if his management and progress is to be at an optimum level.

3. Chronic illness — a male patient aged 70 years. Williamson (1964) has described the multi-problem states so commonly found in elderly patients. A typical problem summary list for a patient of 70 might read:

Physical	— Osteoarthritis
	Angina
	Prostatism
	Excess alcohol consumption
Psychological	— Depressive symptoms
	Loneliness
Social	— Widower
	Housebound
	Few social contacts
	Poor hygiene
	Diet suspect
Drug list	— An analgesic with a non-steroidal anti-inflammatory drug
	Trinitrini
	Nitrazepam

Interactions are known to occur between different drugs. It is as likely that interactions occur between different problems: depression may be the result of the patient being housebound and having few social contacts, and can in turn be the cause of poor hygiene and an inadequate diet. An excessive intake of alcohol may also be related to these problems. Clearly to think only in terms of drug treatments for organic diagnoses is to seriously fail to manage the patient's problems adequately.

'HE WILL MAKE AN INITIAL DECISION ABOUT EVERY PROBLEM WHICH IS PRESENTED TO HIM AS A DOCTOR'

Key words — Initial decision.

Although the key words are: 'shall make an initial decision' it is also of great importance that consideration should be given to every problem perceived to be so by the patient. In addition to the presenting symptoms of illness the patient is liable to show one or more of the following:

1. Confusion about how the illness has developed.
2. Statements of apparently logical cause and effect.
3. Concern or obvious distress at the effects of being ill.
4. Apprehension, anxiety or frank fear about future health.

The general practitioner should identify these perhaps peripheral consequences of illness and make some initial decision as to the way in which these problems are to be managed.

At the first consultation for a new illness the patient will, after the usual preliminaries, make an opening statement. This will give information about the symptoms suffered and their relative importance in the patient's eyes, the aforementioned cause and effect and perhaps the reason for consultation on that day and not on some other.

In response the doctor's initial decisions will include some estimate of the 'degree of illness' of the patient and thus the priorities of any therapeutic steps to be taken. If the condition is in an early stage some decision will be required on the advantage or disadvantage of delay in initiating treatment: treatment itself can have hazards and any alternatives to drug therapy should be explored when this would be an appropriate step to take.

'HE WILL UNDERTAKE THE CONTINUING MANAGEMENT OF HIS PATIENT WITH CHRONIC, RECURRENT OR TERMINAL ILLNESS'

Key words — Chronic, recurrent illness.

CONTINUING CARE

The continuing care of a patient with chronic illness requires a planned approach that anticipates the likely course of the condition and the changing needs of the patient. Problems and priorities will need to be continually reassessed in the light of the patient's current condition. This changing scene can be illuminated by considering the problems to be faced by both doctor and patient in the diagnosis and follow-up of a lorry driver of 50 years of age found to have a blood pressure of 160/110. At the time that the diagnosis was made the problems to be faced might include:

1. The risks of untreated hypertension and the presence of other risk factors for ischaemic heart disease.
2. The methods to be adopted in ensuring treatment compliance in an otherwise symptomless condition.
3. The possible consequences for the patient of the drug therapy itself and the illness 'label'.

Many patients with treated hypertension show less than ideal blood pressure control. Thus by the age of 60 this patient's problems might change to include:

1. Mild congestive cardiac failure.
2. Angina of effort.
3. Unemployment due to early retirement.

These problems and their management require a different strategy from those appropriate at the time of diagnosis. Between the two ages mentioned there will have been no dramatic changes, instead the consequences of poor blood pressure control — in part related to his employment — should be anticipated rather than only considered once the full clinical picture has appeared.

RECURRENT ILLNESS

Much the same approach can be as appropriate in considering recurrent ill-health. The patient with established chronic bronchitis will have spells of relative normality punctuated by exacerbations: the nature of both of which change with the passage of time. In the early stages of the condition management objectives will relate to the effective, early and complete treatment of the exacerbation while in the later stages as much attention will need to be placed on the day by day management of developing corpulmonalae and right ventricular failure.

'PROLONGED CONTACT MEANS THAT HE CAN USE REPEATED OPPORTUNITIES TO GATHER INFORMATION THAT APPEARS APPROPRIATE TO EACH PATIENT AND BUILD UP A RELATIONSHIP OF TRUST THAT HE CAN USE PROFESSIONALLY'

The key phrase in this sentence is that related to information. The types of information to be gathered and the method of storage retrieval in the medical record will be considered in more detail in Chapter 3.

'HE WILL PRACTISE IN CO-OPERATION WITH OTHER COLLEAGUES, MEDICAL AND NON-MEDICAL'

The potential hazards of single-handed practice — and of a single-handed attitude — have been mentioned but are worth restating.

1. Professional and intellectual isolation encouraged by the absence of critical review by others.
2. The persistence of knowledge that may be static or even the persistence of incorrect knowledge.
3. Physical and intellectual fatigue — or the potential hazards of delegation to largely unselected deputies.

Group practice is now the norm in the United Kingdom and despite its undoubted financial and leisure advantages it can allow the individual doctor to benefit from the special interests and knowledge of his colleagues both through the occasional use of a partner as a second opinion and through more formal and planned education. Standards of medical care can be identified and where necessary improved through such activities as research, audit and the development of practice policies. Larger groups of doctors can afford to make better use of both diagnostic and office equipment: a particularly important advantage in view of the current advances being made in medical and office technology. On the other side of the coin there must be some reduction in the degree of personal and continuing care and there is always the possibility of problems of an administrative or interpersonal nature. As has been stated the best compromise is one that retains as much that is good of single-handed doctoring to which are added the very real advantages — to both patient and doctor — of group medical practice.

THE PRACTICE TEAM

The need to consider psychological and social issues in the management of a patient with a physical complaint implies the use of skills not normally possessed by doctors. Undergraduate and, later, hospital experience has primarily been towards the diagnosis and treatment of a physical disease. The concept of the primary health care team has been developed as a response to the need for a variety of skills for patient care in general practice. District nurses were first attached to specific practices, rather than as was usual geographic areas, in the 1960s. The success of the early experimental attachments in Oxfordshire was such that by 1973 77% of all nurses were attached to general practices. It is now the norm rather than the exception for a practice to have both an attached district nurse and a health visitor. Social work split away from medicine — and from their almoner status — with the Social Service and Social Work Acts of the late 1960s and very few practices have an attached social worker despite the generally accepted view that social work is an integral part of primary care.

There seem to be two fundamental requirements for successful team care. The first is an acknowledgement that each team member is a professional with the skills and responsibilities that this implies. Acceptance of this principle means that each contributes in a specialised manner appropriate to the overall care of the patient: it does not mean that the doctor can simply delegate to another work that he considers too trivial for him — the doctor — to be burdened with. The second criterion is that each participant understands the training that the others have received, knows the responsibilities and priorities of the other disciplines and appreciates their approach to their work.

The receptionist

The receptionist is a key member of the practice team in many ways. She is often the first member of the team with whom the patient comes in contact and, therefore, plays an important part in the 'public relations' of the practice. In an equally significant way she is responsible for the day-to-day operation of many aspects of practice organisation so that her efficiency can relieve (or add to) the routine chores of the doctor. The time spent in the careful selection of a receptionist and in making sure that she has a clear understanding of her various duties — together with the reasons for particular arrangements — is a worthwhile part of practice management.

Depending upon the organisation of the practice, about a fifth of the receptionist's time is spent in talking to patients — either in the surgery or on the telephone. Her attitude and manner can mean that she may be seen by patients as a barrier between themselves and the doctor who must continue to satisfy himself that such a situation is not allowed to develop. It usually arises because of a lack of clear instructions about the actions she is to take in particular circumstances — for example, in dealing with argumentative or dissatisfied patients or those who arrive either early or late for appointments. The most difficult problem are requests for house calls or urgent appointments when, in clinical terms, the receptionist is the least qualified member of the team and the least able to judge the patient's needs. It is important for the receptionist to understand the limits of her discretion in these matters but it is equally important for the doctor to make these limits clear.

One way of recording requests for home visits which

Date		/ /		VISIT REQUEST					
No.	Time Rcd.	Name, Address, Tel. No.	Age	Reason for Visit SYMPTOMS	Origin of call	Time passed to Dr.	Dr's Intls	Urgency rating
1								
2								
3								
4								
5								

Fig. 2.5 Visit request sheet

helps this problem is the use of a specially prepared visit book (Fig. 2.5) which includes a check-list of items of information which the doctor considers necessary. This provides the receptionist with an outline of the information she should try to obtain on the telephone and also enables the doctor to make some assessment of the urgency of the call. The check-list will contain such items as the name, age, and sex and address of the patient, the nature of the complaint and its duration. Each doctor will, of course, add other items which might include specific questions relating to particular types of illness. The visit sheet should have columns for the time the visit request was received, the time it was passed to the doctor and the initials of the doctor taking the call. The experienced receptionist will be able to judge the likely urgency of the request from the way the illness has been described. This information is of additional help to the doctor and the receptionist should be encouraged to add her own assessment of urgency to the visit request sheet.

The receptionist's understanding of the scope of her responsibilities is an equally important part of the clerical and secretarial aspects of her job. She must be given flexibility and discretion in the working of the appointment system so that she knows what action to take when the demand for appointments exceeds the available time and must also have a regular routine for dealing with the receipt and filing of letters and laboratory reports. A rubber stamp comprising the date and a space for the doctor's initials is a useful method of ensuring that such documents are not overlooked: all incoming letters and reports should be date-stamped by the receptionist but not filed until the doctor has initialled them as 'read'. Similar arguments apply — although perhaps with greater force — to arrangements for the issue of repeat prescriptions; if the preparation of prescription forms is delegated to the receptionist, it is important to make sure that she is given clear instructions about procedure and is not left to deal with importuning patients on her own.

The physical lay-out of the practice premises has an important influence on the efficiency and job-satisfaction of the receptionist. In one study of comparable practices, different arrangements of the record-filing system produced an 11% difference in the receptionist's record filing and retrieval time. Other aspects are also significant: receptionists deal with confidential information and must also have conversations with patients (either face-to-face or on the telephone) which should also be private. She needs space and proper desk accommodation in which to keep the various forms and other documents she is concerned with and, ideally, should not be too exposed to the patients who are sitting waiting for appointments. All these factors mean that the working environment of the receptionist will repay careful attention.

The community nursing sister

The community nursing sister is a state registered nurse who has undertaken further training in community nursing; as such she is able to make a skilled professional contribution to the work of the team and should not be seen simply as a person who is useful for carrying out technical nursing procedures. As a nurse she will set her own objectives for the care of her patients and it is important that the doctor makes his own therapeutic objectives clear so that the two can be constructively co-ordinated. The simple 'prescription' of nursing procedures will lead to mutual frustration and a less profitable relationship.

The range of duties the nurse undertakes will depend to some extent on the nature of the practice and the particular problems it presents. Obviously, she will be able to perform a variety of treatments and procedures which will include such specific activities as the treatment of varicose ulcers, the dressing of wounds and the giving of injections. These are important activities but an increasing part of the domiciliary nurse's role should be in the on-going nursing care and rehabilitation of chronically ill or elderly patients, many of whose needs are nursing rather than medical. This can mean that it is the nurse rather than the doctor who undertakes the day-to-day supervision of the patient with the doctor seeing the patient at less frequent intervals and relying on the nurse to report significant alterations in the patient's condition. The joint approach to the care of the patient is dependent on two factors if it is to be successful; firstly, there must be clearly agreed clinical policies — both doctor and nurse must agree on the objectives of care and the methods that will be employed. It will include, for example, making sure that the nurse knows what drugs have been prescribed and the reasons for their prescription: although this may seem to be a very obvious point it is one that is not always observed in practice and yet, without such knowledge, the nurse is handicapped in her own management of the patient. The second important factor is related to this need. It is that the doctor must define those variations in the patient's condition of which he wishes to be informed, and must satisfy himself that the nurse has the appropriate skills to detect these variations. This does not mean that he should expect the nurse to be a skilled diagnostician; there are many simple tests of 'abnormality' which can be performed by nurses just as well as by doctors.

In addition to the on-going care of the chronically ill, there are other areas where the nurse can complement the doctor in patient care. It is possible, for instance, for the nurse to undertake second, or follow-up, visits or consultations in the case of illnesses which are expected to resolve themselves but where complications are a possibility. One example is measles in an otherwise healthy child. Having visited to diagnose the condition, the doctor may ask the nurse to visit a week later to check that the child is recovering and that upper respiratory complications have not occurred. This example requires that the nurse is capable of inspecting throats and ear drums properly and the doctor would either need to satisfy himself on this point or provide the necessary training. The arrangement has the advantage that it provides an opportunity for offering nursing rather than medical advice. A similar example concerns patients who are discharged from hospital. Although it is important for the doctor to satisfy himself about the medical needs of these patients, many are in need of advice about convalescent nursing and will have questions or worries that can be talked over with the nurse just as well as with the doctor. One of the problems of discharging patients from hospital is that they often move from the skilled nursing environment of the hospital ward to home circumstances that are less than ideal. Continuity of nursing care is as important as the continuity of medical care; practical advice from the nurse and a prompt assessment of the patient's needs (even in such simple matters as toilet arrangements) can make a great deal of difference[*].

In all of these activities the nurse does not *replace* the doctor and it will be necessary to ensure that the nurse does not come to be seen as another barrier in the patient's attempts to see the doctor. The nurse's role should be explained to patients and a situation created in which patients develop an understanding of the way the team works and of the part played by its different members. The converse to the risk of the nurse acting as a barrier to the doctor is also relevant: many patients will feel more at ease discussing their problems with the nurse and will often volunteer relevant information that they would withhold or feel diffident about reporting to the doctor. There is a good case for providing an opportunity for patients to choose to consult the nurse rather than the doctor and for making arrangements in the practice for the nurse to have her own consulting and treatment sessions. Apart from immediate referrals for specific procedures, sessions of this kind allow the doctor to refer patients to the nurse for the management of problems that are more appropriate to her skills.

The health visitor

A health visitor is a state registered nurse who has undertaken full or partial midwifery training and a further 12 months full-time study which includes the organisation of health and welfare services, the methods of preventive medicine, social and psychological factors in illness, health education and other fields relevant to her role as a 'medico-social worker playing a full part in both preventive medicine and social action'. Although these activities may seem to be somewhat indefinite when compared to the more practical activities of the community nursing sister, there is now a clear recognition of the value of health visitors as members of the community health team and, in particular, of the important way in which their counsel and advice can complement that of the doctor. One demonstration of this partnership is that whilst health visitors formerly tended to concentrate their energies on the needs of mothers and young children they are increasingly concerned with the whole range of health problems — with the elderly, with the mentally ill and with patients who have a chronic disease or handicap.

As with the community nursing sister, the relationship between the doctor and the health visitor will be dependent on the doctor's understanding of the health visitor's skills and on the development of a mutual 'problem-solving' approach to patients and their difficulties. Because of her orientation towards preventive approaches, the health visitor will have a particular concern with certain groups of patients (such as young mothers) so that

*For a further discussion of these activities see Marsh, G.N. (1969) Visiting nurse — analysis of one year's work. *British Medical Journal* iv, 42 and Marsh G.N. & McNay, R.N. (1974) Team workload in an English General Practice. *British Medical Journal*, i, 315–321.

an important basis for collaboration will be in developing a joint programme of care for these groups. In the case of young children, this will include agreement about the advice and guidance that is given to mothers but it should also be extended to measures of the growth and development of infants and the identification of 'at risk' groups. The clinical practice of the doctor will often draw his attention to problems that are arising in families and early referral to the health visitor then becomes a means of introducing preventive action. Experience will suggest a variety of reasons for referral but it is worth recognising that they can range from easily identified difficulties such as the presence of physical or mental handicap to less definite impressions that all is not well — such as the mother who attends frequently with seemingly trivial complaints. In this latter instance, the health visitor may be able to take more time and may be able to develop a different rapport with the family with the result that the underlying problem is defined.

Clearly, the use of a joint 'team' record system will contribute greatly to the collaboration between members of the team and the use of problem-oriented records (or, at least, problem summary sheets) will help this process further. One group of patients to whom this argument applies particularly is the elderly where the difficulties of maintaining an independent life in the community often involve a combination of medical and social problems. With these and other groups (such as the mentally ill), regular review by the health visitor can provide the means of achieving a longer-term view of the patient's needs and for planning social as well as clinical goals for treatment and rehabilitation.

It will be evident that the health visitor can also contribute by providing advice and health education for patients such chronic diseases as diabetes or rheumatoid arthritis. In larger group practices or health centres where the numbers of patients with particular conditions is sufficiently large, there is a good case for encouraging the health visitor to develop group activities for these patients. These can be of special value in disabling conditions where they also permit patients to provide mutual support for each other and help to reduce the isolation that is sometimes their lot. One other kind of group activity (which can save the doctor frustration and disappointment) is the organisation of weight-reduction clinics which are run by the health visitor. Apart from providing an opportunity for dietary education, which can be sustained over a longer period than is usually available to the doctor, there is increasing evidence that the 'group therapy' aspect of such clinics is a significant component in their success.

The social worker
The health visitor and the community nurse share a common orientation towards the health of their patients

with the doctor; although the social worker also shares these goals she comes from a different background of training and experience and so often perceives a patient's problems in different terms and gives different priorities to the various aspects of the social problems she encounters. One consequence is that misunderstanding and confusion about the nature of social work is not uncommon amongst doctors and this, in turn, can lead to disappointment and irritation about their contribution to patient care. It is important to realise that social workers are not paramedical workers. Nor are general practitioners parasocial workers. Co-operation depends on mutual respect for one another's disciplines and being prepared to learn from one another (Daly & Faulkner 1973).

The simplest error in the doctor–social worker relationship is to see the social worker as a 'paramedical' who is a useful contact with various social and government agencies — as someone who knows about the right forms or the right telephone number. Since it is a part of the social worker's skills to deploy these various agencies on her client's behalf it is true that she may know more than the doctor about the operation of these aspects of the social service system but to see her role simply in these terms is to deny her basic skills in working with clients in order to identify and attempt to resolve their underlying social problems. To reduce the social worker to the status of a 'social agency clerkess' will cause resentment and dissatisfaction on both sides of the relationship.

The process of working with individuals or families in the attempt to correct social difficulties raises other aspects of potential misunderstanding. The social worker will tend to see ill-health in the context of the wider life-style of the patient and not necessarily as the central issue; in the terms of working towards an improved or more stable life-style, as she may consider that the resolution of an immediate problem is less important than some longer term goal. And, for her part, the social worker may have inappropriate expectations of the medical components of a problem situation so that she comes to feel that treatment is inadequate or misdirected.

These are all arguments for closer collaboration between the doctor and the social worker and, on the doctor's part at least, for a more sophisticated understanding of the potential of the social work contribution to the care of his patients. Referral to the social worker should be based on specific criteria in which the doctor is able to describe his perceptions of the problem and some appreciation of the contribution the social worker might make. In this sense, referral to a social worker is similar to referral to a hospital specialist.

One area of confusion relates to the respective roles of the social worker and the health visitor. Obviously, since the latter does have a concern with social problems, there is common ground between the two and some overlap in their functions. The difference, stated briefly, is that the health visitor is primarily concerned with the health problems of her patients and thus with the social circumstances that have a bearing on these problems. The social worker, on the other hand, takes the social circumstances of the client as the focus of her concern and involves herself with health problems in the context of their relevance to the client's social difficulties. This distinction may seem pedantic at first but it is important to make it in deciding on the appropriateness of a particular referral and the action that might be taken.

A number of studies have demonstrated the value of attaching a social worker to the primary care team but in Britain at the present time, both administrative arrangements and the general shortage of social workers mean that such a development is unlikely in the immediate future. Nonetheless, there are good arguments in favour of the doctor acquainting himself with the local administration of social work services and, where circumstances permit, getting to know individual social workers with whom he can discuss the patients he refers to them. Relationships between the two professions can be fostered further by inviting social workers to participate in case conferences when this would be appropriate and, in health centres or similar settings, by providing facilities which would allow social workers to work in closer proximity to the health care team.

'HE WILL KNOW HOW AND WHEN TO INTERVENE THROUGH TREATMENT, PREVENTION AND EDUCATION TO PROMOTE THE HEALTH OF HIS PATIENTS AND THEIR FAMILIES'

Key words — Treatment, prevention and education.

TREATMENT

In addition to a knowledge of drugs, their indications, actions and side-effects, the general practitioner should be aware of the possible consequences of inappropriate drug prescribing. These can include the creation of iatrogenic ill-health, the production of drug or doctor dependency and the strengthening of perhaps unrealistic and unwanted patient expectations. The prescription of a drug implies that a disease amendable to that treatment is present, reinforces the sick role and governs future patient behaviour. Marsh and his colleagues (1977) showed that formulating a practice policy on the avoidance of unnecessary prescribing for viral and other trivial self-limiting illnesses supported by a more comprehensive explanation of the illness to the patient ultimately resulted in a reduction in the prescribing habits of the practice and a fall in the number of patient consultations.

There are a number of non-drug management approaches that are more appropriate and more beneficial on their own in self-limiting illness and as an adjunct to drug treatment in many chronic or recurrent conditions. These range from simple explanation, discussion and advice, to a planned programme of supportive counselling. These are skills that have to be actively considered and constantly practised since they can easily be ignored in favour of the easier — and 'safer' — behaviour of prescribing.

PREVENTION

The increasing importance of such illnesses as hypertension, ischaemic heart diseases (IHD) and chronic respiratory problems in present day morbidity and mortality statistics gives support to the view that in general practice greater emphasis should be given to prevention. Prevention can be primary as in the correction of IHD risk factors, secondary as in the prevention, or minimisation by diabetic control, of target organ damage, and tertiary as in rehabilitation after a myocardial infarct. Prevention is discussed more fully in the following clinical chapters.

EDUCATION

Formal health education in general practice is of less value than the opportunity that every doctor/patient contact affords for education that is pertinent to the immediate medical problem. Advice to stop smoking, for example given to the patient with advanced chronic bronchitis at the time of an exacerbation, is likely to fall on more receptive ears than any amount of mass media opinion.

It could be argued that this is effectively shutting the stable door after the horse has bolted but most people require an immediate and direct incentive to break what may well have been a long-established habit.

Habits and ways of life are essentially established by parental and peer group example. Education therefore that is designed to correct the major self-inflicted illnesses related to alcohol, tobacco and drug abuse is likely to be more effective if directed to particularly receptive groups of people such as young adults, or at periods of life such as during a pregnancy when the patient is likely to be more motivated towards health. This kind of health education directed at current major health problems however is only part of the general practitioner's responsibilities in the field of education. The management of all diseases requires an educational input: to tell a young mother how to nurse her sick child, to make her aware of the kinds of problems that she can expect in child-rearing, to improve her mothering skills so that she can herself look after illness in the family, and to recognise the signs that tell her that professional help is required. The rehabilitation of the patient following some serious illness such as myocardial infarction cannot be assumed to be complete unless the patient is given some information so that he can help himself to full recovery and at the same time minimise the risks of a recurrence. In chronic illness the aim is that the patient should, to the best of his ability, manage his illness himself, even to the extent of altering any required drug treatment as is indicated by his changing symptoms or the development of an exacerbation. This, however, cannot be achieved unless the patient has a considerable knowledge of his condition, of what will improve or make it worse, of the warning signs of deterioration and of the indications for alterations in drug therapy and for seeking urgent medical help. In old age it is frequently the caring relatives who require the understanding and knowledge of how to care for an infirm and elderly patient.

The educational duties of the health visitor are more obvious and clearly understood. She has a major role to play in helping young families by ensuring that the health — physical and emotional — of young children is not impaired and is improved through correct attention to diet, exercise, clothing and play. She is the person primarily responsible for the childhood immunisation programme and through the well baby clinic can effectively deal with many problems while they are relatively trivial and before they become blown up out of all proportion. In recent years there has been a growing tendency for the health visitor to play an increasingly preventive educational role with the elderly and with the mentally ill in the community.

The district nurse has the education of a patient in self-care as one of her objectives and does not see her contribution simply as providing practical nursing procedures.

'HE WILL RECOGNISE THAT HE ALSO HAS A PROFESSIONAL RESPONSIBILITY TO THE COMMUNITY'

In addition to his duties to each and every individual patient the general practitioner has a responsibility to the community whether that is a geographically discrete area or is the population of patients registered with him or his practice. This added responsibility includes being aware of the social and environmental conditions within which his patients live and work, and an appreciation of special risk groups within his practice and their particular problems and needs. He has a duty to constantly strive to improve the quality of care offered to his patients through continuing education, audit and through research and to have the ability to develop new skills and to change methods and procedures in response to the changing needs of his practice and patients.

REFERENCES

Bain D J G 1981 Personal communication
Fry J 1979 Common diseases, 2nd edn. MTP Press, Lancaster
Howie J G R 1976 Clinical judgement and antibiotic use in general practice. British Medical Journal 2: 1061–1064
Kreig A F, Gambino R, Galen R S 1975 Journal of the American Medical Association 233: 76–78
Marsh G N 1977 'Curing' minor illness in general practice. British Medical Journal 2: 1267–1269
Robinson E T, Barber J H 1977 Early diagnosis of pregnancy in general practice. Journal of the Royal College of General Practitioners 27: 335–338

The organisation of general practice

In hospital practice, much of the organisation of the hospital and the facilities needed by doctors are provided as a part of the larger system of management. General practice is organised in a much simpler way but many of the organisational features of the hospital continue to be present — the need for records, for nursing services, for patient appointment systems and so on. These different activities are the direct concern of the general practitioner who must also organise them in such a way that they not only satisfy the needs of his own clinical practice but that they also contribute to the work of the other people — doctors, nurses and receptionists — with whom he is associated.

These needs fall into several categories. The level and the organisation of his own workload can be affected by the type of appointment system he employs. The effectiveness of patient care and the efficiency of both health visitors and nurses is influenced by the organisation and content of the record system and by the degree of emphasis that is placed on practice meetings and opportunities for case discussion. The continuity of care and the doctor's ability to develop a preventive or prophylactic approach to the management of chronic disease will depend on establishing 'at risk' and follow-up registers that will ensure that patients are not lost from view.

RECORD SYSTEMS

A discussion of records involves two main elements — the record itself and the system of which it forms a part. Records exist to maintain information which is thought to be of value in the future care of a patient and to make that information available to others who may need it. In thinking about both records and record systems it is possible to devise several criteria that they should meet:

RECORDS

Records:

— should present information in an easily accessible way

— should provide continuity of information
— should allow use by different people
— should be easy to use both in finding existing information and in adding new information
— should allow the extraction of information for numerical analysis e.g. morbidity data, information about workload

RECORD SYSTEMS

In a similar way, record systems:

— should allow economical and accurate handling (with a minimum of misfiling)
— should make it possible to identify different categories of patients (for example, old people or particular disease groups)
— should be easily operated by unskilled staff: that is individual records should be easily to identify
— should relate to other systems (for example, the appointment system)
— should allow numerical analysis

The last 5 years have seen an increasing adoption of the A4 folder as a standard general practice record. This folder allows more generous and efficient organisation of patient data and permits the inclusion of a number of special purpose enclosure sheets. Those that are normally available from Primary Care Divisions of Health Boards include a clinical notes sheet, immunisation and screening record, X-ray and laboratory report form mount, a childhood developmental screening record and a summary sheet for important illnesses or investigations. A strong case can be made for the inclusion of district nurse, practice nurse, health visitor and social work notes so that the record can be used by all members of a practice team and thus contain all information relevant to the patient. Many practices have gone yet further and have designed and included chronic disease review sheets, modelled on the ante-natal record where it is considered important that the patient is reviewed at regular intervals and that certain predetermined items of clinical and biochemical information be assessed at each review consultation.

There are still some practices however that for a number of reasons, principally amongst which is inadequate storage space for the A4 record, continue to use the now very old and dated medical record envelope and its insert card. By the criteria mentioned previously this record has many disadvantages but with careful use the same general principles can be achieved. One disadvantage is that the envelope easily becomes filled with redundant information so that it is important to avoid a 'squirrel complex' in retaining too many old letters or laboratory forms. The problem can be overcome by including a summary card in addition to the current 'clinical notes' card. The summary card is then used to enter significant items in the patient's history and complements the on-going clinical record. A good basis for planning such a card is on 'problem-oriented' lines; health visitors and nurses should also add information to the card. Information of continuing relevance is often lost in the continuous narrative of clinical notes. The inclusion of a summary card rescues the principle that significant information should be accessible.

One other principle, the identification of patients in particular categories, can also be difficult to satisfy with medical record envelopes. A traditional method involves the use of differently coloured tapes or other tags which identify individual records according to colour (so that red might signify 'drug sensitivity', brown — 'diabetes' ... and so on). This method has value in small practices but, on its own, creates difficulties in ensuring that *all* records are coded in this way and, in larger practices, in extracting them for analysis. A more satisfactory method is to establish separate index systems for these special categories which can combine identification data with arrangements for long-term follow-up appointments, or visits.

Another development in record keeping is the idea of the problem-oriented record. The argument for this particular form of record is that patients may have a number of clinical or social problems contributing to their need for medical care. The continuous narrative record often obscures relevant parts of the past history or focuses the doctor's attention on one aspect of the problem to the exclusion of other features. A problem-oriented form of record-keeping (or the inclusion of a 'problem sheet' as part of the record) allows the doctor to overcome this difficulty in two ways. Firstly, it provides an easily reviewed list of problems (whether 'active' or 'inactive') so that the patient's presenting problem is more easily seen in its proper context. Secondly, by establishing such a list, it is less easy to overlook problems that the patient does not present but which nonetheless may require action or influence treatment. The identification and recording of problems should not be restricted to strictly clinical conditions: the problems that are included may be either medical or social and health visitors, nurses and social workers should be encouraged to make use of such a record. This multiple use brings other advantages; it draws the doctor's attention to the patient's need for other services (such as social work) and provides his professional colleagues with an opportunity to record information which will come to the doctor's attention.

The actual filing and organisation of records in the system is dependent on both the type of record and the size of the system. In most group practices, the alphabetical filing of records provides a satisfactory system but their location in the practice premises and their accessibility to receptionists can influence the efficiency of the appointment system and are therefore worth careful consideration. In larger systems such as health centres there may be advantages to be gained from an integrated numerical system which is linked to practice registers. For obvious reasons, the maintenance of the system is important — the records of patients joining or leaving the practice should be entered or withdrawn without delay and amendments such as changes of name or address should be updated promptly. The efficiency of the record system influences the standard of patient care and should not be left to chance. Each aspect of the operation of the system should be carefully considered and formal procedures should be established for the guidance of all staff concerned with the system. This may sound pedantic but in a large group practice an inefficient record system is costly in staff time and results in a reduction in its value as a practice tool.

As well as providing a means of storing the records of individual patients, the record system also fulfills important functions in providing information about the work of the practice and about particular groups of patients. A number of additional registers or indices have been devised for these purposes. One of the most basic is the age/sex register which offers a means of identifying such groups as the elderly or pre-school children. Age/sex registers can be kept in many different forms; a common method is the use of 6 in × 3 in cards on which additional data can be handwritten. More sophisticated systems include the use of Copeland-Chatterson cards, which have the advantage that information concerning morbidity or social circumstances can be added in a coded form (by punching further holes in the card) and then sorted and analysed, the Jolly feature card system and of course computers which are increasingly being used to handle age/sex registers, morbidity and workload analyses and repeat prescription printing. The advances that are taking place in computer technology mean that a considerable variety of workload management, research and review procedures will be available to the general practitioner by means of small dedicated micro computers. Registers of this kind (which can also include disease-specific systems) are of value in analysing the workload of the practice but they have a more specific clinical use in enabling both doctors and health visitors to ensure that patients in need of periodic review do not become lost.

It is important to remember that the advantage of a computer is the speed with which it can handle data and its efficiency is wholly dependent on the quality of information entered. Before installing a computer it is essential that some decision is taken as to what functions it will be expected to perform, and there are a number of practices in the United Kingdom which are experimenting with the use of computers under a DHSS research scheme, from whom advice can be obtained.

Most practices will want to use a computer for management and patient care purposes rather than for research although this latter activity is an important potential benefit of the computer. Activities appropriate to a practice computer include the recall of patients for immunisation or other screening procedures such as cervical cytology or blood pressure checks, the printing and controlling of the repeat prescription system, providing problem and drug lists, notification of potential drug interactions, and special programmes of care for different population groups such as the very young and the elderly and for patients with chronic disease or disability. Practice management tasks such as payment to staff members, rota systems in large health centres and the control of medical and secretarial stocks are obviously also suited to computer use.

There are many arguments for undertaking the analysis of the work of general practice; perhaps the most succinct is that it is always advisable to know what one is doing! Workload patterns vary between practices and within a practice at different times of the year; their analysis provides a means of reviewing the organisation of the practice and of estimating the likely effect of changes — as with the idea of special clinics that are discussed below. An equally important reason is the need for 'self-audit'. In any medical activity it is difficult to know whether or not the goals that are set are really achieved and this is particularly difficult in general practice when continuity of care across a wide diagnostic range and responsibility for a defined 'population' of patients are added to the management of clinical episodes. In this context, the abstraction of information and its analysis provides the doctor with the means of assuring himself that his standards of practice are what he would wish them to be.

The argument for analysis of the work of a practice should also include a warning. Both the recording and abstraction of data can easily get out of hand and result in the accumulation of large quantities of information that are difficult to analyse and yet more difficult to interpret. This process of 'stamp collecting' is quickly discouraging and can result in the abandonment of the whole activity.

The alternative is simply stated but difficult in practice; it is that data should only be collected or abstracted if the question they are intended to answer has been clearly and precisely stated and the relevance of the data to the question well defined. The difficulty is in the formulation of the proper questions but the effort spent in doing so will be well repaid.

APPOINTMENT SYSTEMS

Appointment systems are now almost universally found in general practice and provide a method of regulating and organising the working day. In theory they allow the patient to be sure of seeing the doctor of his choice at a specified time yet appointment systems are one of the commonest causes for patient complaint. Many patients feel that such systems introduce a barrier between the patient and the doctor — a poorly designed system can increase the time taken to see the doctor from a 1 or 2 hours wait during a consulting session to a delay of 3 or 4 days before an appointment is available.

At its simplest, an appointment system is dependent on two assumptions: firstly, that the number of available appointments is approximately equal to the number of people seeking them, and secondlly, that the time allotted to each appointment is a rough average of the time that consultations actually take. In hospital practice, it is relatively easy to achieve these conditions but the variability of general practice is such that other factors must also be taken into account. It will be necessary to make allowances for seasonal variations in the rate of consultation and, in some cases, for variations in the day of the week. Figure 3.1 shows seasonal variations in an urban practice of 2500 patients and the number of hours needed each day for an *average* consultation rate of 7 minutes for each patient. It will be obvious that, in this practice, an arbitrary allowance of 2 hours each day will be appropriate for about 5 months of the year but that the system will break down and cause very significant delays (because of the cumulative effect of the 'excess' patients) in the other months. These figures do not take account of the other activities that also form part of a consulting session (such as telephone calls, letter writing or discussions with colleagues); the planning of the appointment system should also include an allowance of time for these. The ideal for an appointment system should be that it is sufficiently flexible to accommodate all 'new' patients seeking a consultation within 24 to 36 hours of their requesting it and that patients who feel that their problem is urgent should be seen on the day they request an appointment. It may not always be possible to achieve such a standard (and, of course, some patients may prefer a later appointment) but the measurement of actual practice against this goal will provide a guide to the effectiveness of the system.

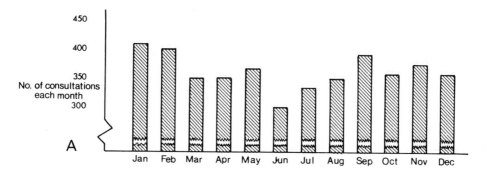

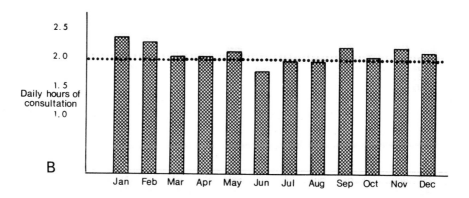

Fig. 3.1 A, Monthly consultations in a city practice of 2500 patients; B, Average number of hours needed each day for a consultation rate of 7 minutes for each patient.

The effectiveness of the system is not simply dependent on the provision of appointment times: different patients have different needs which will take more or less time so that, whilst the spacing of the appointments should be based on an *average* of these times, it is important to try to arrange the session to spread different demands evenly through it. To a large extent, success in this aspect of the system depends on giving careful guidance to the receptionist about the way she allocates appointments — clearly, first consultations take longer than return visits, the elderly take longer than the younger patients and consultations of a psychiatric or gynaecological nature take longer than simple organic illnesses. The proportion of consultations of these different types will vary from practice to practice but, in an 'average' consulting session of 25 patients about eight will be follow-up visits and three to four of an urgent or immediate character. A concentration of new patients at the beginning of a session, can mean that the doctor gets behind with the appointments and thus feels a need to hurry. The converse (which is more likely if the receptionist is not properly instructed) is a concentration of

return visits at the beginning of the session with the result that the doctor works ahead of his schedule, has a slack period in the middle of the session and still finishes late because of the new patients at the end of the appointment list.

There are several ways of overcoming these difficulties; the one that works best will depend on the individual's way of working and the time he takes to see different categories of patient. It is therefore important for the doctor to make simple work-study experiments of his own practice and to adapt the system in the light of these observations. One general approach is shown in Figure 3.2, which allocates three patients to each 15-minute time interval although the actual average consulting time is 6 minutes. By arranging that 'new' and return patients are seen in the ratio of 2:1 (a ratio based on practice experience) it becomes possible to divide the 15-minute period into different amounts of time for each patient and yet stay reasonably on schedule. The average consultation time is rather longer than the appointment intervals and, without correction, this would have the effect of making the system run about 25 minutes late by

New Patients	Return Patients	Time	No. of Pts seen	Duration of Session (mins)	Actual Cons. Time	Discrepancy (Minutes)
9.00 New 9.10 New	9.05 Return	9.00				
9.15 New 9.25 Urgent	9.20 Return	9.15	3	15	18	+3
9.30 New 9.40 New	9.35 Return	9.30	6	30	36	+6
9.45 New 9.55 New	9.50 Return	9.45	8	45	48	+3
10.00 10.10 New	10.05 Return	10.00	11	60	66	+6
10.15 New 10.25 New	10.20 Return	10.15	13	75	78	+3
10.30 10.40 New	10.35 Return	10.30	16	90	96	+6
10.45 New 10.55 New	10.50 Return	10.45	18	105	108	+3
11.00 11.10 New	11.05 Urgent	11.00	21	120	126	+6
11.15 New 11.25 —	11.20 Return Psych. Consultation	11.15	23	135	138	+3
11.30 Urgent 11.40 Urgent	11.35	11.30	25	150	156	+6
		11.45	27	165	168	+3

Fig. 3.2   Organisation of appointment system to avoid gross time delays

the end of the session. An approximate correction is achieved by including blank appointments at appropriate intervals during the session — these allow the schedule to be kept and also provide an opportunity for such other activities as telephone calls.

Two other aspects of the appointment lay-out in Figure 3.2 should be mentioned. The first is the division of new and return appointments into two separate columns. Provided that the approximate proportion of return visits is known, the lay-out has the effect of spreading them evenly over the week. It therefore avoids the risk of over-booking return visits on a particular day with the result that new patients have to wait longer for an appointment. In addition, it clearly separates the two types of visit and thus simplifies both the job of the receptionist and the task of analysing these records. Secondly, appointments are made from the beginning of the session (from 9 o'clock) and are not scattered throughout the whole period; combined with the '15-minute group' system this should mean that the doctor is

occupied throughout the period of the session that is booked and is not kept waiting as a result of gaps in the schedule; it also allows the spaces at the end of the session to be used to accommodate 'urgent' patients without disrupting the schedule in order to fit them in. These arrangements should permit an increase in the duration of the session during particularly busy periods. Doing so requires some advance planning on the part of the doctor or his receptionist: if, for example, it becomes evident on Tuesday that the appointment system is slipping behind (so that Thursday is already heavily booked) it will be desirable to extend the consulting sessions at the end of the week in order to prevent a further build-up over the weekend and on to the following Monday.

SPECIAL CLINICS IN GENERAL PRACTICE

In addition to the need to provide adequate provision for patients with acute disease, there is a need for a system of periodic review of patients in certain categories — those with chronic disease, the elderly and patients with psychiatric or socio-medical problems. Most doctors have appreciated the difficulty of seeing ante-natal patients in the midst of a general consulting session and have organised separate ante-natal clinics; this pattern of work can be extended to other conditions (such as diabetes, hypertension or chronic bronchitis) in addition to geriatric and paediatric screening programmes where a regular review of the patient is planned. This system has several advantages. It allows the doctor to see several patients with the same condition together and thus develop a more organised approach to their care, it enables the health visitor and the practice nurse to be present, it allows the nurse to organise and undertake preliminary investigations and it allows a different scheduling of appointments so that patients are seen at more appropriate time intervals and are not simply fitted into the more general schedule of Figure 3.2.

The organisation of review clinics is dependent on maintaining a register of patients for them and on making appointments up to about 4 weeks ahead but reviews at 3-, 6- or 12-monthly intervals require that appointments are sent to the patient about 2 weeks in advance. Whenever special clinics are organised it is vitally important that an efficient method is designed to note and arrange follow-up for those patients who do not attend for review on the expected date. In this the computer has a valuable role to play.

PRESCRIBING

The general principles of prescribing in general practice are, of course, much the same as those observed in hospital practice but the different setting of general practice (and the context in which the drugs are taken) introduces other factors that must be taken into account. In the hospital, the administration of drugs to in-patients is carefully controlled and the doctor can be reasonably sure that his instructions are followed; in general practice, the doctor relies on the patient to follow his instructions and has no way of knowing whether his advice is followed. In addition to the clinical indications for his prescription, he must also take account of the patient's ability to understand the instructions he has given. This does not present a problem in the majority of instances but complex multiple prescriptions can be confusing to the elderly and other factors, such as the nature of the patient's work, can interfere with the patient's capacity to comply with the management advice that he has been given. It is also necessary to take account of the possible effect of drugs on the patient's way of life. In most cases this will be of little consequence — on the other hand, the prescription of a drug with a sedative effect for a salesman or a long-distance truck driver who goes on working is clearly undesirable.

There are two ways in which prescribing in general practice must differ from prescribing in hospital practice. The first concerns the continuity of patient care and the doctor's need to view the drugs he prescribes in the context of the longer time-scale of patient care in the community. One obvious example is the prescription of psychotropic drugs which may often provide a simple solution to an immediate difficulty but which lead in time to the greater problem of a drug-dependent patient whose underlying complaint continues unresolved. A similar situation occurs in the case of patients with progressive chronic diseases (such as rheumatoid arthritis) where it is good policy to follow a progression of available drugs from the simple to the complex, only moving to the more powerful drug when the simpler remedy is no longer adequate. This practice allows drugs to be held in reserve and used in shorter, limited courses of treatment during acute episodes or exacerbations; since many of the more complex drugs carry the risk of undesirable and even dangerous side-effects, it also means that the patient's exposure to these risks is delayed for as long as possible.

The example of psychotropic drugs also illustrates the second way in which general practice prescribing differs from that of the hospital. Drugs and other medicines are commonly and widely taken by the population to the extent that they are the 'natural' response to the symptoms of day-to-day minor disorders that most people experience. In one survey (Dunnell & Cartwright 1972) 80% of the adults who were interviewed had taken some form of medicine in the previous 2 weeks even though two-thirds rated their health as 'good' or 'excellent'. About two-thirds of the medicines that were taken were self-prescribed; a tenth of those interviewed had taken sedatives in the past 2 weeks. The habit of medicine-taking has several implications for the doctor; the general acceptance of medicine as a way of relieving symptoms can mean that he is expected to prescribe and may find himself under pressure to do so in circumstances where it is against his clinical judgement. In a similar way he may find that some patients will regard him simply as someone who will facilitate their wish to obtain the drug they have decided they need. (This latter problem is complicated by the practice of patients experimenting with drugs prescribed for someone else.) It is important to recognise that patients have an increasing knowledge of drugs and that many will require a considered explanation of the doctor's reason for prescribing — or not prescribing — a particular medicine. Psychotropic drugs, in particular, are now so widely used that a wholly justified reluctance to prescribe them may be interpreted by the patient as a lack of sympathy or understanding. There are no easy answers to these difficulties; prescribing is so central to the doctor's clinical practice that his response to these aspects of it will be influenced to a large extent by his other approaches to his patients and his understanding of their needs. The concept of 'negotiation' between doctor and patient (and also the idea of the sick role) are important in this context because it is through insights of this kind that the doctor improves his awareness of the social features of medicine-taking and is thus able to exert some control over them.

One particular aspect of prescribing in general practice is the use of 'repeat prescription' procedures which allow patients on long-term therapy to obtain fresh supplies of drugs without consulting the doctor. The principle of repeat prescriptions is a good one although it is also a method that is open to considerable abuse if it is not carefully controlled. Obviously, it is important to give the receptionist clear instructions about repeat prescriptions and some method of maintaining a record of the prescriptions that are issued must be employed. The repeat prescription cards that are illustrated in Figures 3.3 and 3.4 provide an example of such a method. Two cards are illustrated — a coloured card is used only for antidepressants, hypnotics, tranquillisers and anticonvulsants, while a white card is used for other drugs. Both cards contain space for a list of current medications and spaces for recording the repeat prescriptions that are issued. The principle difference between the two cards is that items on the coloured card can only be repeated on three occasions without specific reference to the doctor. This procedure ensures that patients do not remain on potentially habit-forming drugs without review by the doctor and also provides a check on excessive consumption. In using both cards, the receptionist should be instructed to check that the frequency with which prescriptions are issued is reasonably in line with the dose that is prescribed and told that seeming deviations from the prescribed regime should be reported to the doctor. Again, as has been mentioned, this is a most appropriate role for a practice computer.

It goes without saying that the habit of signing blank prescription forms for repeat prescriptions is a bad one.

Current Medication					Date	Items	Receptionist's signature
DRUG	Strength	Quantity	Date	Date Discontd.	4.2.83	1 and 2	
1 VALIUM	5 mg	90	1/7 t.d.s.		4.3.83	1 and 2	
					1.4.83	1 and 2	
2 MOGADON	5 mg	30	1/7 nocte		Please see your Doctor on 29|4|83		
					Doctor's signature		
3							
4					Please see your Doctor on ☐☐☐		
					Doctor's signature		
5							
6							

Doctors note
This card is to cover only Antidepresants, Hypnotics, Sedatives, Tranquillisers and Anticonvulsants. Please use White Card for all other drugs.

Please see your Doctor on   ☐☐☐

Doctor's signature ....

Fig. 3.3   Repeat prescription card 1

Current Medication

DRUG	Strength	Quantity	Date	Date Discont.	Date	Items	Receptionist's signature
1 DIGOXIN	0.25 mg	60	$\frac{1}{1}$ b.d.		4.2.83	1,2,3	
					4.3.83	1,2,3	
2 LASIX	40 mg	30	$\frac{1}{1}$ name				
3 SLOW K	600 mg	120	$\frac{1}{11}$ b.d.				
4							
5							
6							

Doctors note
  This card must not be used for Antidepressants, hypnotics, Sedatives, Tranquillisers or Anticonvulsants.
  Please use Pink Card for such drugs.

Fig. 3.4   Repeat prescription card 2

Patients should be instructed to request the prescriptions they require at least 24 hours before their existing supply runs out and the receptionist should present the newly made-up prescriptions to the doctor for signature together with the patient's records. It is helpful to have a regular routine for this procedure — a common practice is to sign repeat prescriptions at the end of the morning consulting session.

The doctor in general practice is more heavily exposed to the blandishments of the drug industry than the doctor in hospital and it is easy to be beguiled by the plethora of different preparations that are presented. As a general rule, it is sensible to develop a range of drugs of first choice and to gain experience with their use; in addition, it will be helpful to have a range of alternatives (say two or three in each category) so that variations in therapy can be tried and individual patient idiosyncrasies accommodated. This policy provides a background of experience for assessing the new drugs or different preparations that become available. Although single drugs are to be preferred to mixed preparations as a general rule, the difficulty of relying on patients to follow different instructions for two or three drugs will make it preferable to prescribe combined preparations for some patients.

Some studies of general practice have suggested that patients often have difficulty in 'taking in' the details of the doctor's advice during a consultation; anxiety about their illness and concern with other aspects of it may reduce their ability to recall the treatment instructions they are given. Where it seems that the patient is likely to be confused or uncertain about the drugs that are to be taken (for example, some elderly people) it is often worth involving the nurse in a second explanation of the instructions. The nurse should also be encouraged to employ other devices that will help the patient — the preparation of a simple time-table sheet with the drugs identified (and the bottle marked) as '1', '2', etc. is one method.

CONCLUSION

Changes in the pattern of community morbidity and in the technology of medicine in the past two decades have emphasised specialist divisions in the medical profession. Much of this specialisation has occurred within the context of the hospital; more recently, it has become increasingly appropriate to regard the work of the general practitioner as 'specialist' and there has been a need to establish the principles on which the specialty is founded. As with other specialties, these comprise a set of particular skills but, in contrast to the trend in hospitals, such skills are not of a technical nature. The responsibilities of the general practitioner for the variety of people who make up his practice population, his concern for the whole range of diseases and the need to treat his patients in their social context over long periods of time all combine to define the skills he requires in different terms. Whilst maintaining his clinical standards. he must treat individuals rather than pathological states and must be prepared to adapt his therapies in ways that will best serve the patient's interest. Recognition of the needs of a population means that he must establish priorities in the use of his own resources (which include himself) and must develop an organisational basis for his practice which will allow him to achieve these objectives.

The variability of general practice is such that it is unlikely that there will ever be one 'best way' of organising or practising primary medical care in the community. As the literature on general practice grows, however, it becomes possible to look further than the variations that are reported and to identify those features of primary medical care that are common to different situations and which form the basis of the practice of the specialty. This chapter has attempted to review these more general aspects of practice; the following chapters apply them in the more specific context of particular illnesses or groups of patients.

REFERENCE

Dunnell K, Cartwright A 1972 Medicine takers, prescribers and hoarders. Routledge & Kegan Paul, London & Boston

Interviewing and counselling skills

INTRODUCTION

Interviewing and counselling are an integral part of a general practitioner's work. The former implies gathering information and the latter treatment, but the two activities merge in many if not most consultations. How we listen and talk to patients has a profound effect on our competence and their wellbeing. Until recently few medical students were taught about interviewing skills and there is still little training in counselling for family doctors.

It is said that 80% of diagnoses depend on the history, with physical examination and investigations accounting for the remainder. Good history-taking requires interviewing skills which affect the quality of information obtained, as well as the compliance and satisfaction of patients (Sanson-Fisher & Maguire 1980). These skills can be taught and are based on a knowledge of techniques which are common to all human communication.

About one-third of patients seen in general practice may have emotional problems (Goldberg & Blackwell 1970) many of which can be helped by counselling for which there are various approaches based on differing theoretical views of the nature of human behaviour. All these models, whether of behaviour therapy or psychoanalysis, depend on communiation. This chapter will therefore look first at basic human communication and the techniques which have evolved, and then at interviewing skills in a medical setting, before considering counselling for individuals, couples and families.

Doctors spend at least half their time with patients talking (Fletcher 1979). We should certainly listen more, but it is not for nothing that the word doctor used to mean a teacher, and that the snake-entwined caduceus of Aesculapius (the God of healing) which adorns the British Medical Journal was also the staff of Mercury — the messenger of the Gods and the divine patron of all communicators.

NON-VERBAL COMMUNICATION

INTRODUCTION

Human communication consists of messages which are encoded by a sender and decoded by a receiver. The behaviours involved have been studied by psychologists, sociologists and anthropologists, and their findings have implications far beyond the practice of medicine. The insights obtained form the basis of our understanding of the processes of interviewing and counselling. These processes may be conscious as in the case of verbal messages, or partly sub-conscious as in the case of many non-verbal messages which are an important part of communication. One investigator found that in normal two-person conversation, more than half the social meaning of the situation, or rapport, was linked to the non-verbal components (Birdwhistell 1952). Every doctor makes conscious or unconscious assumptions about patients from their appearance and dress, in the same way that a white coat signals a professional role with undertones of hygiene and technical competence. But there are other, perhaps less obvious factor which contribute towards non-verbal communication.

TYPES OF NON-VERBAL COMMUNICATION

Facial expressions

Facial expressions have evolved as a means of communication between animals, and are an important means of communicating emotional states in man (Ekman et al 1972). Basic emotions such as disgust, grief, and surprise seem to be expressed in a similar way throughout the world, but there are cultural display rules which modify personal control. It is not always easy to decode a smiling face, but equally a fleeting expression of anger or the corners of the mouth or eyebrows may tell us more than words about a person's feelings.

Gaze or eye contact

Gaze or eye contact when it is mutual, develops as a social signal very early in life and the mutual gaze of a baby with its mother first occurs at 4 weeks. When two people are in conversation each will look at the other for about half the time and there will be mutual eye contact for about 25% of the time, but the amount of gaze and eye contact depends on many factors (Argyle & Ingham

1972). A person will gaze at another twice as much when listening as when talking and gaze is connected to concentration in that people tend to look up at the end of speaking for feedback (Kendon 1967). As well as seeing non-verbal reactions, gaze helps to synchronise utterances, and also sends information in that it reinforces speaking and signals attention.

The amount of gaze increases when people like each other, and for those who are extroverted, friendly or self-confident. Women gaze more than men, as do those who are active and dominant, which can produce discomfort, as for instance a teacher's rebuke.

Avoidance of gaze is associated with negative emotions such as anxiety, shame or embarrassment as well as with depression and schizophrenia (Williams 1974). There tends to be more eye contact in 'contact cultures' such as the Middle East, Latin America, and Southern Europe, and less in 'non-contact cultures' such as Britain, Northern Europe and Asia, where too much gaze might be seen as threatening, disrespectful or insulting (Argyle & Cook 1976). Eye contact is a form of intimacy and has been found to be inversely proportional to distance. Emotional arousal affects the quality of gaze by increasing the amount of blinking and pupillary dilation, whereas receiving bad news is said to constrict the pupils. It is important for doctors to get into the habit of reading notes before a consultation, and of writing them up after the patient has left. Otherwise time for eye contact and interpersonal communication is lost and the quality of the consultation suffers accordingly.

Gestures

Gestures commonly accompanying human interaction, whether between individuals or in groups. There is a large range of hand and arm movements to which meanings are attached such as clapping, and thumbs pointing up or down. Some gestures are speech-linked and directed towards objects or events in such a way as to provide emphasis to what is being said, or to illustrate the verbal content of a message. In this way dialogue is supplemented and attention increased.

Gestures can also be largely unintentional and directed towards the self as a form of tension release, and therefore convey emotional states (Friedman & Hoffman 1967). The nervous wringing movements of hands or constantly moving fingers indicate anxiety as does the less obvious tapping of feet. Aggression and anger can be unconsciously conveyed in gestures such as a clenched fist, or elation by fast emphatic movements, in contrast to the slow hesitant movements of despair. In these contexts gestures could be seen as products of inhibited emotion and some observers have suggested more specific symbolism as for instance the constant playing with rings on a finger as an indication of marital conflict or frustrations at home (Mahl 1968).

Posture

Posture may reflect relative status, attitudes, emotions and personality. There are considerable cultural variations in the postures appropriate to status and attitudes, but in the Western world a more relaxed posture tends to be used by those of higher status (Goffman 1961) or those who are controlling an interview (Mehrabian 1969). Relaxation is characterised by leaning backwards or sideways with asymmetrical arm and leg positions. An attitude of empathy is indicated by leaning forwards which decreases social distance and suggests an attentive positive attitude towards the other person, as does an open position for the arms and legs. Whereas facial expression may convey more information about specific emotions, bodily posture shows the intensity of the emotion particularly in relation to tenseness or relaxation (Ekman & Friesen 1967). Depression may be indicated by a drooping listless posture, in contrast to the stiff intensity of anxiety. In the same way posture may reflect a type of personality or self-image. Psychoanalysts have attempted to interpret nuances of posture in various ways, such as people protecting various parts of their bodies.

Most prolonged communication between individuals takes place when both are either standing or sitting. If only one is doing so then the interaction is likely to be short and strained. Postures change during communication but not as fast as gestures. During psychotherapy patients appear to adopt three or four postures related to particular emotions or topics. These postures are specific for an individual and a definite pattern of movement can be seen between therapist and patient reflecting the empathy of an intimate interaction (Scheflin & Scheflin 1972). A patient may be helped to relax by the therapist deliberately copying his posture, and thus facilitating communication by his postural echo (Morris 1978).

Proximity

Proximity and relative position set the context for an interaction or interview, within which other forms of non-verbal communication such as posture and gesture can interplay. Individuals tend to maintain a personal space around them which has been classified into four zones (Hall 1959). For intimate relationships there is a zone of about 1½ feet (45 cm) where bodily contact is easy, and people can smell each other, feel body heat, and whisper but not see very well. Close personal relationships are conducted at a distance of 1½ to 4 feet (45–120 cm) where touch is possible and it is easier to see the other person. More impersonal relationships take place 9 to 12 feet (2.75–3.65 m) apart as for instance some professional consultations behind a desk. On public occasions speakers are usually placed at a distance of 12 feet (3.65 m) or more from their audience (Fig. 4.1). A closer proximity implies greater affiliation and intimacy. People tend to come nearer to women and to those they like. In

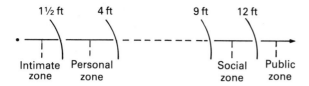

Fig. 4.1 Personal space

contrast dominant individuals, prisoners and those who are mentally disturbed or introverted (Mehrabian 1968), maintain a greater personal space around them. There are also cultural differences in that in Europe and North America more distance is usually maintained between people than in the Middle East or Latin America. If we are forced very close to each other as in lifts or trains, we tend to avoid their suggestions of intimacy such as conversation or direct gaze.

Territory is important for both man and animals. We have our personal territories of house and garden or surgery, and space can be manipulated to alter interaction or dominance. If chairs are placed in small groups instead of round the walls in an old people's home, communication increases. Similarly more height or distance between one person and a group will indicate dominance.

The relative position or orientation of two individuals at a table will affect the type of interaction. Competition is most marked when people sit opposite each other, whereas co-operation is most likely when individuals sit side by side. Conversation is easiest when two people sit at right angles, for instance round the corner of a desk, and this would seem to be the optimum position for a consultation if a desk is to be used (Sommer 1969, Cook 1970). However patients have been found to be more at ease if there is no desk at all between them and the consulting doctor (Pietroni 1976). Traditionally general practitioners have tended to adopt a dominant position for a consultation facing the patient across a desk, but this may not facilitate communication and empathy (Fig. 4.2).

Bodily contact and touch
Bodily contact and touch are the most basic forms of non-verbal communication and imply intimacy and often emotional arousal. The skin is the largest organ in the body and tactile stimuli are crucial for the healthy de-

velopment of babies and for an infant's perception of himself and others. As children grow up so they have less bodily contact with their parents and more with peers of the opposite sex (Jourard 1963).

In the Western world touch has been suppressed as a means of communication, so that for adults bodily contact is restricted to spouses, children up to adolescence, and to various forms of symbolic gestures such as handshakes. Between relative strangers and in public places touching is rare in a 'non-contact culture' such as Northern Europe, in contrast to Southern Europeans. In some African societies it is normal to hold hands or intertwine legs during conversation. Cultural norms of contact may change over time, as for instance the advent of ballroom dancing which permitted much closer bodily contact than previous dances or those in fashion since.

Touch is used to establish relationships and as a signal, for instance in greetings and farewells. There are also ceremonial aspects to bodily contact, such as the laying on of hands. All these factors may be present to some degree in a medical encounter, for which touch is often necessary. Part of a doctor's professional role is to give support and empathy through touching, and to receive clinical information, but not sexual gratification or emotional arousal. While we do not hesitate to touch a child, bodily contact with adults must be acceptable to both doctor and patient without the risk of misinterpretation.

There is a spectrum of feeling associated with touch ranging from avoidance, through affection, to sensuality and sexuality (Froelich & Bishop 1977). Where there is doubt or hesitation then it is better to clarify verbally or avoid bodily contact, but used with confidence the caring touch supports and reassures. This is particularly true for those who feel anxious, afraid, isolated or rejected. For them touching may bring great comfort and acceptance (Barnet 1972).

In a sense we should learn to touch more, and indeed there are groups in the community, such as the elderly on their own, who receive little bodily contact to cater for their emotional needs for which professional helpers could redress the balance. However it takes time for many doctors to feel confident about touching patients. The growth of encounter groups is an example of attempting to harness the therapeutic potential of bodily contact between human beings (Schutz 1967).

Paralanguage
Paralanguage is the term given to those aspects of vocalisation which are not verbal. These non-verbal signals may be linked to what is being said, or independent of it. The speed, loudness, pitch, and emphasis with which words are spoken convey information about emotions, attitudes and personality. A soft, slow, low-pitched hesitant voice with downward inflection, suggests depress-

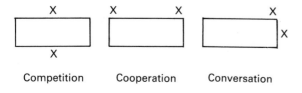

Competition   Cooperation   Conversation

Fig. 4.2 Orientation

ion, while a more rapid speech is associated with anger, excitement, enthusiasm, or joy (Davitz 1964).

Personal qualities and background may be inferred from the way in which people speak and from their accent, irrespective of the verbal content. Allowing silence in a consultation may be an important way of signalling acceptance to a patient, and pausing after asking questions may increase participation (Hargie 1980).

USE OF NON-VERBAL COMMUNICATION

Non-verbal messages are therefore an integral part of human communication, and it is important for doctors to be sensitive to such cues. Contraindications between verbal and non-verbal messages may be important clues as to a person's true feelings, which are more likely to be reflected by the non-verbal component (Shapiro 1968). Letting a patient know that you have picked up such messages may unlock the door to their real problem.

Non-verbal communication is used for a number of reasons. Firstly, there may not be appropriate words for such things as shape or personality, which are better conveyed by explicit gestures or implicit non-verbal messages. Secondly, emotional states are also communicated in non-verbal ways especially by facial expression and tone of voice. Although such messages may be culturally controlled, they are also less under personal control than words and therefore more likely to be genuine — for instance blushing. Non-verbal messages may contradict the content of speech, but may also be contradictory in themselves, as in a smile below angry or anxious eyes. A third reason for using non-verbal communication is that it provides a powerful reinforcer which emphasises the spoken word. Fourthly non-verbal messages are an important second channel of communication which regulates the flow of conversation by giving the speakers feedback about such things as stopping, starting and attention, like punctuation to the written word. Lastly non-verbal communication helps to define relationships such as intimacy, dominance, or liking, without making

them too explicit and therefore disturbing. Patients who are less socially skilled use fewer non-verbal messages than those who are more assured (Trower 1980).

VERBAL COMMUNICATION

INTRODUCTION

Language is an exceedingly complex attribute, but it is possible to categorise the types of response which can be made in an interview. A response is anything the interviewer says which is not verbally interrupted by the patient. Such categories are to a certain extent arbitrary and may not be mutually exclusive, in that one uninterrupted statement may contain more than one type of response. However there is evidence that more information is gathered more quickly and with greater rapport if doctors have some knowledge of these interviewing techniques (Marks et al 1975) as indicated by the following diagram (Fig. 4.3). One way of teaching these techniques is to use a check list of responses as defined below and then get interviewers to identify their own responses by playing back an audio- or video-cassette tape recording (Hannay 1980a). Such immediate feedback is the best way of illustrating vividly the importance of different types of questions and responses.

TYPES OF VERBAL RESPONSE

Open-ended questions are general questions with a broad scope which allow patients the maximum latitude in answering (e.g. How are you?).

Focused questions define the area of enquiry more precisely but allow some latitude in answering (e.g. What sort of chest pain is it?).

Closed questions are those which can be answered by 'Yes' or 'No', (e.g. Do you sleep well?) or by a particular number such as age, or the number of children.

Leading questions imply a specific answer, and should not be used as respondents will tend to agree passively with the interviewer (e.g. You don't sleep well do you?).

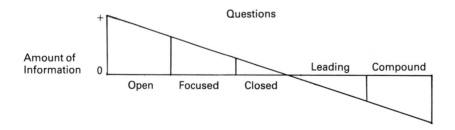

Fig. 4.3   Information gained by type of question

Compound or double questions ask more than one question at a time, with the result that a mixed message is sent and often the answer is incomplete or confused (e.g. Do you take sleeping pills and feel tired?). As with leading questions, compound or double questions should not be used.

Indirect questions are rhetorical statements which imply that a response is expected, without grammatically being an actual question (e.g. Some people find it difficult to get off to sleep).

Social exchanges are comments such as 'Good morning', 'Goodbye', 'It's a nice day'.

Facilitation is any response which encourages the patient to continue (e.g. 'Go on', 'Uh Uh').

Repetition or restatement means repeating all or part of what a patient has just said, either in their own words or restating in the interviewer's words (e.g. So you have difficulty getting off to sleep).

Confrontation is a response which confronts the patient with something incongruous in their appearance or answers (e.g. You said there was nothing worrying you, but you look miserable and now say you are depressed).

Clarification or interpretation means that the interviewer clarifies or interprets what the patient has been saying (e.g. It seems that your tiredness started after your sleep pattern was disturbed).

Reflected statements are responses which let the patient know that their feelings have been recognised and accepted (e.g. I can understand that this must be very worrying for you). This is not the same as reassurance or explanation, and is an important way of establishing rapport and letting patients know that their feelings have been understood.

Judgemental statements are responses which clearly state the value judgements of the doctor (e.g. Anyone who smokes cigarettes is foolish).

Instruction or advice, explanation and reassurance are all self-explanatory responses which are commonly used in interviews, particularly towards the end of a consultation.

USE OF VERBAL RESPONSES

If the same patient is interviewed by a number of doctors, each will show a different pattern of responses (Hannay 1980b). There is no right and wrong way of conducting a consultation but there are certainly better and worse ways. It is usually preferable to start with open questions before focusing down to closed questions. Leading or compound questions should be avoided as they invariably cause confusion. A knowledge of non-verbal and verbal techniques is an important basis for skill in interviewing, which implies using the appropriate techniques in the right way at the right time.

INTERVIEW SKILLS

INTRODUCTION

Skill in interviewing may develop from natural ability and experience, but there is no doubt that such skills are greatly improved by a knowledge of the non-verbal and verbal components of communication, as outlined above. These components need to be co-ordinated for communication to take place between two people, and this co-ordination is usually taken for granted. In most conversions there is enough talk to fill nearly all the time. If there was too much there would be interruptions or double-speaking, and if too little, long periods of silence. This synchronisation depends on verbal and non-verbal signals which also indicate the degree of dominance and intimacy involved, as well as emotional tone.

Any interaction takes place in a context, so that situations and roles are defined, and tasks or topics identified. Interaction sequences can be analysed in terms of categories of social acts (Bales 1950), which give rise to reactive sequences such as an open-ended question leading to a long answer. In a medical consultation the situation and respective roles are already defined to a considerable extent, although role distance may be altered by a doctor's style and self-image. The context of an interview is also important, and includes such things as the comfort of the waiting-room, the availability of reading material, and the type of receptionist.

There is now much evidence that the interviewing skills of medical students and doctors are deficient and can be improved by training (Maguire & Rutter 1976, Sanson-Fisher & Maguire 1980). This improvement leads to better rapport and diagnosis for the doctor, and for the patient results in improved compliance and recall of information, as well as increased satisfaction and ability to cope with pain or stress.

Audio- and video-tape recorders now make it possible to capture consultations for demonstration purposes or to provide feedback. Immediate individual feedback under supervision is an effective method of teaching, but it is time consuming and may be more efficient using small groups and simulated patients (Hannay 1980a, b). A number of scoring systems have been devised for analysing the structure and content of medical interviews which will be considered below, followed by a look at different types of interview and types of patient.

STRUCTURE AND CONTENT

The primary purpose of a medical interview is to establish rapport with a patient and to gather information. Interviews may also be supportive and involve therapeutic counselling, but initially medical students need a simple overall approach for the undifferentiated problems with which patients present in general practice (Hannay 1980a). Parts of the interview can be expanded where appropriate with detailed question about particular symptoms or a mental state examination, so that this approach does not conflict with hospital teaching but rather complements specialist knowledge and places it in context. By the end of an interview a student should have established a confident relationship with the patient, defined the exact nature of the presenting problems and gained a clear idea of the patient's background.

Clearly the structure and content will be different from an established doctor who knows the patient, compared to a medical student seeing someone for the first time. Good records should provide a data base for a doctor to relate what is happening to previous knowledge. There is also the ongoing nature of the consultation in general practice, although this can result in procrastination rather than development. However, the same principles apply to any medical interview for which a simple structure intended for medical students is shown in Figure 4.4.

It is not necessary to follow a predetermined sequence; indeed an important skill is to *follow associations* which means remembering when the patient mentions a relevant point and picking this up at the time or later in the interview. In this way the consultation proceeds more like a conversation, in which the doctor's control depends on having a mental framework which needs to be

Beginning (Establishing relationship)
Greet patient by name, and introduce self by name
Make patient feel at ease
— (e.g. offer to be seated)
Explain situation
— (e.g. medical student/trainee, taking history)

Middle (Gathering information)
Presenting symptoms or problems
— Clearly itemised
— Characteristics defined
— Duration established
Other medical history
— Past serious illnesses or operations
— Current chronic disease or disability
— Present medication
Family circumstances
— (e.g. Who else is at home?)
Social circumstances
— (e.g. How does the patient spend his or her day?)
Other symptoms or problems
— (elicited if relevant)

End (Closure)
Explanation and/or diagnosis
Advice and/or treatment

Fig. 4.4   Structure of interview

filled in, but allowing the patient to do this in his own time. This involves *actively listening* to what the patient is saying, which is much harder work than might appear. It is necessary to maintain an emotional neutrality so that one's mood is not affected too much by that of the patient, although obviously demeanour should respond appropriately to situations such as grief and humour. At the same time the doctor should be *aware of his or her own feelings* such as anxiety or uncertainty, and be prepared to discuss them with a colleague or even the patient. Feelings of confusion about a patient may be a pointer to early schizophrenia in the patient, and sexual attraction may warn of manipulation by an hysterical personality. There are three levels of *understanding another person*. We can understand *about* someone through the eyes of other people, or we can understand *with* someone through our own eyes (sympathy), or through their eyes (empathy).

It is particularly important to pick up *a patient's feelings* at the time they are offered, and to follow the magic carpet of what the patient says, rather than ignoring this and talking past the patient to one's own agenda. It is not that doctors are unaware of the patient's feelings, but rather they they do not know what to do about them. If a feeling such as worry or fear is presented, then the best response is often a reflected statement, followed if appropriate by an invitation to expand (e.g. I can understand that this is worrying for you. Would you like to tell me about it?). It will rapidly become apparent if the area is unimportant, but so often it is the key to the problem or even to the patient, which may have been missed for years.

Many people find *silence* during an interview difficult to tolerate, but it may be entirely appropriate. Being comfortable with a patient in silence may be a form of acceptance, depending on the situation. If the patient is silent because of confusion or embarrassment over something the doctor has said, then the matter should be clarified quickly. More usually a prolonged silence is due to the patient sorting out thoughts and feelings in which case he needs time, or because he is overwhelmed by emotion. If appropriate the patient should be allowed to release her emotions, for instance by crying which in itself is therapeutic, after which communication is usually easier, although crying can be used to avoid unpleasant issues. Reflected statements are often helpful in such situations, as they are when it seems that a patient is resisting questions.

It is useful to start an interview with open questions before narrowing down to closed questions which may need to be persistent in order to clarify a history, particularly with reference to time about which patients are often vague. As an interview proceeds there is usually a shift from focusing on the patient's frame of reference, to the doctor's frame of reference for explanation, reassurance, instruction and advice. When this happens it is important to be brief and simple, and not to use technical terms and language which the patient may not understand. It is also important to check that the patient understands, and to give him an opportunity to ask questions. Some interviews can be successfully conducted focusing completely on the patient's frame of reference leading to both patient satisfaction and compliance.

Teaching situations are often artificial; for instance, family doctors usually know the names of their patients and it is unnecessary for them to introduce themselves by name. They will also have notes available for details of medication and past medical history, but this may not always be so, and a basic framework ensures that important factors are not missed. If possible notes should be checked before a patient comes into the room, and written up after he has left. Good rapport and communication is disrupted by constant writing or reference to notes.

Many grading scales have been devised to rate the qualitative aspects of consultations such as the one shown

Please evaluate the consultation you have just seen by rating it on the following scales. Place a tick in such a position along each line to show how much you agree with each statement

1. Nature and history of problems adequately defined _____	Nature and history of problems defined inadequately
2. Aetiology of problems adequately defined _____	Aetiology defined inadequately
3. Patients's ideas, concerns and expectations explored adequately and appropriately _____	Ideas, concerns and expectations explored inadequately or inappropriately
4. Effects of problems explored adequately and appropriately _____	Effects of problems explored inadequately or inappropriately
5. Continuing problems considered _____	Continuing problems no considered
6. At-risk factors considered	At-risk factors not considered
7. Appropriate action chosen for each problem	Inappropriate actions chosen
8. Doctor's understanding of problems shared with patient adequately and appropriately _____	Sharing inadequate or inappropriate
9. Patient involved in management adequately and appropriately _____	Involvement in management inadequate or inappropriate
10. Appropriate use of time and resources in consultation _____	Inappropriate use of time and resources in long-term consultation
11. Use of time and resources in long-term management appropriate _____	Inappropriate use of time and resources in long-term management
12. Helpful relationship with patient established or maintained _____	Unhelpful or deteriorating relationship with patient

Fig. 4.5 Consultation tasks rating scale

in Figure 4.5 (Pendleton 1981). These scales are subjective assessments which are useful for learning and teaching, but are less precise than the quantitative presence or absence of certain aspects of an interview as indicated in the previous figure for the structure of an interview.

TYPES OF INTERVIEW

Three types of interview have been distinguished in general practice (Gill 1973). First is the *traditional medical interview* in which the diagnosis is illness-centred so that treatment and prognosis refer to the illness only, rather than the sick individual. This is the focus of traditional methods of history taking and examination, with an emphasis on increasing investigations and more refined diagnostic labels. Traditional medical interviews tend to be doctor-orientated in contrast to the second type of *detective personal interview* which is patient-orientated and tries to achieve an overall diagnosis of the patient as a person. This involves the doctor being aware of his own reactions to the patient whom he is observing as an object. The process may take some time and extend from general practice to lengthy psychotherapy, but the interviews and emotions concerned are largely controlled by the doctor.

A third type of interview has been called the *flash type* of interview, which is also patient-orientated but involves the doctor–patient relationship as well as the patient (Balint & Norell 1973). The barriers are lowered between the doctor and the patient, with a resulting flash of understanding which establishes a new relationship. The flash may happen in a long or short interview or during a general chat, and depends upon the doctor abandoning his own ideas of what is happening and turning in to the patient, rather than on asking more questions. The result is an interrelationship diagnosis which is often established by the patient and presented to the doctor, so that both work as partners in the new situation.

The concept of an intuitive flash of understanding based on the interrelationship of doctor and patient evolved from the work of Michael Balint. He brought his training in psychotherapy to bear on the problem of general practitioners and drew attention to the importance of doctors themselves as the main 'drug' used in medical practice. He emphasised the way in which patients offered or proposed various illnesses, and the crucial effects of the doctor's responses to the patient's offerings. Balint coined the phrase 'the apostolic function' to describe the individual ways in which general practitioners deal with their patients, so that doctors' personalities and beliefs are reflected and imposed, often with a lack of insight about themselves and their patients (Balint 1964).

A more quantitative approach to types of interviews in

general practice was developed by Byrne & Long (1976). They analysed almost 2500 audiotapes of consultations by some 60 general practitioners, and distinguished a gradation of interview-styles, ranging from those which were mainly *patient centred* to those which were largely *doctor centred*, depending on the incidence of particular behaviours, as indicated below. They concluded that consultations appeared to fall into four basic styles of diagnosis and seven basic styles of prescription, depending on whether the behaviour occurred before or after the point at which the doctor appeared to have made a decision about the condition of the patient. Byrne & Long (1976) further refined their rating system by giving weighted scores to various behaviours in the diagnostic and prescription phases, so that a numerical value for consultation style could be calculated. They found that about three-quarters of the consultations analysed were predominantly doctor centred, and only a quarter were patient centred. Those responses which were considered to be patient-centred are indicated in Table 4.1. Such responses lead to a more patient-orientated interview which produces more relevant information more quickly, by getting onto the magic carpet of what the patient says and following this rather than the doctor's preconceptions.

TYPES OF PATIENT

Anxious
Anxious patients need to be put at ease with more time for explanation and orientation. It is important to be sensitive to the non-verbal and verbal cues of anxiety, and helpful to reflect back to the patient that these have been picked up and accepted. Anxiety can lead to evasion, denial or the withholding of information, which may be due to the presence of others during the consultation. Some people are always anxious and lacking in confidence, whereas others may be anxious or embarrassed by a particular situation, in which case awareness of this with reflected statements and reassurance are important. A relaxed posture and attitude are infectious, and it may be helpful to state one's own experience and put situations in perspective. Some anxious patient have difficulty in talking, and can be encouraged by indirect and open question. It is important to check whether a non-talkative patient is depressed, by asking specifically about this.

Angry or hostile
Angry or hostile patients require calmness and an attempt to find out the reasons for their anger or hostility. The former implies an emotion and the latter a longer-term attitude, but both require clarification. If the anger is because of the doctor then this should be checked out, and if appropriate one's behaviour modified accordingly. It is important to see the other person's point of view and if necessary provide one's own interpretation and intent. This may require confrontation, but between two ways of looking at things, rather than between two people. Anger may be shown to reception-

Table 4.1   Types of behaviour in the consultation

Doctor centred behaviour	Patient centred behaviour	Negative behaviour
Offering self	Giving or seeking recognition	Rejecting patient offers
Relation to some previous experience	Offering observation	Reinforcing self position
Directing	Broad question or opening	(justifying self)
Direct question	Concealed question	Denying patient
Closed question	Encouraging	Refusing patient ideas
Self answering question (rhetorical)	Reflecting	Evading patient questions
Placing events in time or sequence of place	Exploring	Refusing to respond to feeling
Correlational question	Answering patient question	Not listening
Clarifying	Accepting patient ideas	Confused noise
Doubting	Using patient ideas	
Chastising	Offering of feeling	
Justifying other agencies	Accepting feeling	
Criticising other agencies	Using silence	
Challenging	Summarising to open up	
Summarising to close off	Seeking patient ideas	
Repeating what patient said for affirmation	Reassuring	
Giving information or opinion	Terminating (indirect)	
Advising	Indicating understanding	
Terminating (direct)	Pre-directional probing	
Suggesting		
Apologising		
Misc prof noises		
Suggesting or accepting collaboration		

ists for instance over appointments, and usually such difficulties are resolved if such patients are seen in a calm manner. Repeated hostility is often part of a more serious problem such as alcoholism.

The patient may already be angry with someone else, and again clarification is necessary, often helped by reflected statements so that the patient has the opportunity to express himself without the listener taking sides. It is important to remember that anger is often displaced from the real cause on to someone else such as the doctor, and patients may need time and empathy to become aware of this. Anger and aggression may be due to frustration perhaps because of an illness or life situation, and are a means of venting negative feelings of anxiety and helplessness. The patient may be overactive and try to control the situation, so that it may be necessary both to change the subject of conversation and also to bolster his self-esteem. There is also the hostility of the dependent patient who is always making demands, and the suspicion of the paranoid which should be recognised as such rather than disputed.

Depressed

Depressed patients are characteristically slow and pessimistic. The symptoms of endogenous depression, such as early wakening, should be looked for, and suicidal intent specifically asked about. Firm and kindly persistence is required, with appropriate treatment regimes and counselling strategies.

Over-talkative

Over-talkative patients may be aggressive or obsessional. In either case it is better not to facilitate but to guide courteously with more closed questions than usual. The same applies to the rambling elderly patient, who may need constant refocusing of attention and reassurance.

Seductive

The seductive patient may be an hysterical personality or psychotic playing out her fantasies. In either case it is important to recognise the situation, cope with one's own feelings, and respond in a firm professional manner.

Psychotic

Psychotic patients may be difficult to interview, being inarticulate, unresponsive and silently preoccupied with their fantasies or hallucinations. In some cases thinking and language may be obviously disorganised, but others with a functional psychosis may give a clear history and their condition may only become apparent on doing a mental state examination. Unlike those with organic brain disease, such patients are often orientated in time and place, with intact memory and recall, but they have difficulty in making personal contact and require pati-

ence and persuasion. However, those with paranoid delusions may find reassurance and support upsetting.

Patients with organic brain disease

Such patients may be delirious or demented, with defects of attention, memory, and abstract thinking. Those who are mentally defective will have limited abilities for comprehension and mental calculation, but it is important to remember that difficulties in communication may be due to deafness or dysphasia. In the latter case patients may be acutely aware of surrounding conversation, although with little ability to speak themselves.

Children

Children are a special case of interviewing because they are usually seen with others and have a short attention span, depending on age. It is helpful to have toys available to see how a child plays and to use open ended questions, if appropriate, with plenty of reassurance and support. Small children are very vague about localising symptoms and may project them on to toys such as a doll. Children should be treated seriously in their own right, and it is often helpful to see them alone, as otherwise they may try to please their parents. On the other hand, younger children often tell us a great deal by their behaviour in a family situation.

Mothers will usually provide the most information, but they have their own needs, and will try to present themselves as good mothers, trying to please the doctor and tending to normalise their children's behaviour. Fathers rarely have detailed knowledge about their children but they are important in ensuring compliance. Grandmothers should always be listened to, because they are usually right.

The information that needs to be known about child patients includes details of the pregnancy, and preschool illnesses, accidents and behaviour, together with developmental milestones and a systems review. Where appropriate enquiry should be made about behaviour at school, and relationships with parents, other adults, sibs and peers.

Adolescents

Adolescents may be suspicious of older people, resentful and hostile. It is important to try to get to know them and if necessary confront in a calm accepting way. Young people quickly see through phoney attitudes and need to know that the doctor is acting on their behalf and not in the interests of their parents. It is necessary to pick up cues and come to the point quickly, because adolescents tend to be intolerant of hesitation or silence.

Dying patients

Dying patients are not usually told by doctors that they

are dying, although the majority of those who are seriously ill will have considered the possibility of death. The failure of communication is largely a failure to listen and so enable patients to find their own way through the process of dying, just as we work through the process of living. Trust and faith in life and death are similar; both invoke mechanisms of defence which are normal providing they do not inhibit the constructive use of the personality. Denial is a common reaction to the possibility of bad news and protects people from anxiety until they are ready. Unless the denial is destructive, patients should be permitted the integrity of their own defences, while at the same time the doctor directs them towards reality.

Feelings of anger, resentment, fear, guilt, frustration and failure need to be unburdened and shared. Sometimes it is helpful to bring half-hidden worries and suspicions out into the light of consciousness where they lose their strength, but often it is empathetic listening which is therapeutic, although this can be disturbing for the listener. Some dying patients regress into infantile behaviour which is demanding and dependent. Others transfer the positive and negative emotions of their family life onto those who are caring for them, which is uncomfortable unless understood. The family of a dying person will also require support, and an opportunity to express their individual feelings such as guilt and resentment. The same applies to the grief reaction with its overlapping phases of shock, emotional release, covert hostility, depression, physical symptoms, guilt, overt hostility, inability to resume normal activities, waning of mourning and finally readjustment to reality. Such normal reactions may become morbid and prolonged.

Doctors also have feelings and internal conflicts. They are trained to cure and being aware that a patient is beyond curing may lead to guilt and resentment, and so to a turning away from the dying person. Some may be uncomfortable with the closeness of a dependent patient, while others may react against the negative feelings of those who are dying because of their own need to be loved. The dying require regular visiting, and the assurance that they are not being deserted. The patient should be helped not to put things off or to hold back from emotional contact. He needs to be able to express his independence and maintain his dignity, because dying is a unique experience for all of us. To do it well requires skill and compassion from those in attendance. It is important for doctors to be clear about their own feelings on such matters. If they believe that there is a meaning to life and death, even if they can not find it, then they are in a much better position to help (Lamerton 1972).

COUNSELLING INDIVIDUALS

INTRODUCTION

The aim of counselling is to enable people to cope more effectively and so adapt themselves better to situations and stresses in their lives. As such this is part of the essence of general practice, and could range from friendly informal advice to the formalities of traditional psychoanalysis. Even if desirable, the latter is not possible in general practice, but what is required is some professional approach to the many emotional problems with which patients present. The availability of modern psychotropic drugs may have increased the tendency to medicalise personal problems, but such medicines treat symptoms rather than causes, and provide busy doctors with both a label and a let out.

There is increasing evidence that counselling or short-term psychotherapy can be an effective help for many patients with neuroses and problems of an emotional or interpersonal nature. The field, however, is strewn with different methods and interest groups, many of them stemming from the work of Freud who by the 1920's had established the basic concepts of psychoanalysis. These include the nature of psychosexual development, defences and anxiety, the structure of the ego and superego, techniques of interpretation such as transference and dreams, and recall by free association. This last concept involves handing over the lead to the patient with a change in the doctor's role and has been called perhaps Freud's greatest discovery (Storr 1979).

Traditional psychoanalysis requires four to five sessions of 50 minutes a week for months or even years with the aim of symptom relief and personality change. This is achieved through the development of a regressive transference neurosis with a neutral analyst, who resolves the neurosis by interpretation, confrontation and clarification. Regressive transference is the process by which the patient displaces on to the analyst, feelings and ideas derived from his previous life experience. For those who are reasonably healthy and well motivated this approach appears to be useful, but there is little evidence that it is superior to simpler and more straightforward methods of psychotherapy based on more rational factors such as acceptance, advice and reassurance (Clare & Thompson 1981).

Early on the authoritarian nature of psychoanalysis produced break away groups. It has been suggested that Jung' emphasis on self-expression and fulfilment foreshadowed the present client-centred therapies based on a humanist-existential philosophy, whereas Adler's concern with the social dimension anticipated such developments as social skills training and family or group therapy (Crown 1979).

In the exuberant market place of North America counselling and psychotherapy have become part of the human potential movement, where specific treatments merge into cults for living (Clare & Thompson 1981). For many these have become a secular religion, by providing an explanation of human behaviour, a definition of values, a social and ritual focus, and for those tinged with Eastern philosophy an ultimate purpose in life.

In Britain there has been less interest in counselling and psychotherapy which have been more the preserve of the professions than private enterprise. Perhaps psychiatry and general practice have tended to rely more on physical or medical treatments because talking takes time and is difficult to justify in the context of a National Health Service. However, counselling strategies are being increasingly used, particularly under the stimulus of groups such as social workers and clinical psychologists. It is worth looking briefly at the broad types of psychotherapy which are available, before indicating that there are common elements to all and suggesting a specific approach for general practice.

TYPES OF PSYCHOTHERAPY

Psychodynamic therapies

Psychodynamic therapies have developed from traditional psychoanalysis and range from long-term psychotherapy to short-term interventions. There are a number of schools within the tradition which view conflicts as being the result of early experience and equilibrium as being maintained by effective personal defences. When these defences break down then symptoms emerge. Assessment is considered important and therapy may concentrate on helping the patient cope more effectively with problems, as in supportive psychotherapy for the chronically disabled (Bloch 1979), or aim to change personality style by uncovering the unconscious determinants of behaviour. This latter approach is closer to psychoanalysis as such, and although conducted face to face and for a shorter time, relies on transference, with an emphasis on interpreting the reactions of the patient to the interventions of the therapist (Storr 1979). Patients need to be well-motivated and appropriately selected.

For shorter-term therapies there is usually an agreed focus on symptoms, behavioural difficulties or conflicts, with a higher degree of therapist activity such as confrontation, clarification and interpretation. In longer treatments like psychoanalysis, the therapist would be less assertive and reluctant to take over from the patient and give advice. Sessions may be once or twice weekly, and range in number from three to six for crisis intervention, from six to 12 for supportive educational approaches, and from 12 to 20 for more extensive psychotherapy along dynamic lines (Wolberg 1980). One form of psychodynamic therapy involves a structural analysis of the games people play in social behaviour depending on whether they are using child, adult or parental roles (Berne 1966).

Client-centred therapies

Derived from the work of Carl Rogers such therapies are based on humanist theories of the trustworthiness of our own awareness as opposed to the unconscious motives of psychoanalysis. Instead of the negative aspects of human behaviour, the primary human drive towards personal growth and self-satisfaction are emphasised. Human dysfunction is seen as the result of incongruence between a person's own experience and their internalised views of themselves. Problems arise because an individual's need for acceptance is greater than his confidence in his image of himself so that he acts in incongruent ways. The discrepancy between the real and ideal self is reduced by unconditional positive regard. The most important factors in this non-directive client-centred counselling are the genuineness, caring warmth, and empathy of the therapists who use reflective responses rather than interpretations or directives. These principles are used to encounter groups where people are encouraged to remove their social facades and express their feelings openly. To be successful, encounter groups should strive to attain five objectives. Firstly, all participant concerns must become group concerns; secondly, participants must try out new ways of behaving in the group; thirdly, the group must establish a co-operative as opposed to a competitive goal structure; fourthly, the principal focus of the group must be the here and now; and lastly, immediacy is encouraged by using the word 'I' when speaking and being specific when talking about others (Clare & Thompson 1981).

Gestalt therapy founded by Fritz Perls also focuses on the here-and-now, with an emphasis on verbalising feelings and the immediacy of experience in a group setting. Neurosis is seen as a split between the mind and the body or the individual and his environment, so that anxiety develops in the struggle to unify parts of the whole (gestalt). Psychodrama and sensitivity training are methods of acting out, using techniques such as self disclosure, feedback from others, and here-and-now exercises, which are also found in gestalt and encounter groups, and increasingly in other forms of group therapy such as self-help groups. Psychodrama was developed by Jacbob Moreno who saw psychological problems as due to role conflicts, and these conflicts were re-enacted by group members. T-group or sensitivity training was devised on a similar basis for community leaders in America during the last war. At the same time the British army medical services were using analytical psychotherapy groups, with the work of Bion focusing on group dynamics as a reflection of the members' problems, while others such as Foulkes used the group to analyse individuals.

Behaviour therapy

Behaviour therapy consists of a number of training techniques based on learning theory. Dysfunction is due to faulty learning which is maintained by environmental and intrapersonal influences. These must be identified and the conditioned responses changed. The responses may be involuntary as in the classical conditioning of Pavlov, or voluntary as in the operant condition described by Skinner. A number of techniques such as desensitisation, aversion therapy and flooding are used to heal conditions like specific phobias. Anxiety management and assertiveness training are also forms of behaviour therapy, as is social skills training (Argyle 1981) and cognitive therapy which aims to restructure maladaptive thinking processes and has been used with some success in depression (Goldberg 1982). Although behavioural therapists have been primarily concerned with techniques, there is increasing interest in interpersonal skills and an awareness of the importance of the therapeutic relationship.

COUNSELLING AND PSYCHOTHERAPY IN GENERAL PRACTICE

General guidelines for counselling in general practice

These guidelines emerge from the different types of psychotherapy outlined above, which have a number of common factors. A characteristic of patients who seem to require more than a routine consultation and reassurance is that they are demoralised, with a loss of confidence in themselves and in their ability to master both external circumstances and their own thoughts and feelings. This results in a sense of failure, with feelings of guilt, isolation and resentment. The mood is one of anxiety and depression of varying severity. Most episodes are self-limiting, but prolonged states become self-perpetuating. It is the moderate forms of demoralisation with definable symptoms which are amenable to short-term psychotherapy, all types of which have common features which combat demoralisation and diminish symptoms (Frank 1981).

There are four factors common to all psychotherapies as follows:

1. An intense confiding relationship with a helping person, often within a group. The patient accepts the therapist's competence and goodwill, and becomes dependent by forming a therapeutic alliance, the quality of which is determined by the patient's confidence and the doctor's personal qualities.

2. A healing setting such as a general practitioner's surgery which reinforces the relationship by heightening the doctor's prestige.

3. A conceptual scheme which explains the cause of the patient's symptoms and prescribes a procedure for resolving them. The rationale must be acceptable and convincing to both patient and doctor, and to some extent is culturally determined by time and place.

4. A procedure which requires the active participation of both patient and doctor, and which both believe is the means for restoring health.

There are also five techniques which are common to all forms of treatment (Argyle 1978):

1. The doctor expresses a warm, accepting and uncritical attitude of interested concern in which both patient and doctor participate emotionally.

2. The patient is encouraged to talk about his anxieties, emotions and conflicts so that the sharing of feelings with someone who does not react critically acts as a catharsis and relief.

3. The doctor explores the patient's subjective world of feeling and thinking, and tries to understand the patient's point of view.

4. The doctor tries to give the patient insight into why he reacts as he does, by labelling his behaviour with a theoretical interpretation.

5. The doctor helps the patient make plans and positive efforts to try new ways of dealing with people and situations.

In many situations detailed techniques appear to be less important than the doctor's personality and the kind of relationship he can establish, particularly if this is warm, permissive, and empathetic. Nevertheless, psychotherapy is still a planned form of intervention. Despite marked differences in content, all types of psychotherapy share six therapeutic functions which are as follows (Frank 1981):

1. They strengthen the therapeutic relationship by giving contact, acceptance, and explanation within a shared belief system.

2. They inspire and maintain the patient's hope for help.

3. They provide the patient with learning opportunities, by offering both new information about his problems, and new experiences through the therapeutic relationship.

4. They provide the motive for change in attitudes and behaviour through emotional arousal.

5. They enhance the patient's sense of mastery, self-control, and competence, especially by labelling experiences as part of a therapeutic rationale, and by giving experience of success particularly in behaviour therapies.

6. They encourage the patient to work through and practice what he has learned in his daily living.

The above common factors, techniques, and functions all help to re-establish the morale of patients who are demoralised. In a sense it is not so much what the doctor does, but the way that he does it which matters. Brock (1980) has defined the principal aims of brief psychotherapy as firstly trying to understand the patient so that he has the experience of feeling understood, and secondly giving him the feeling that he can be 'held together'.

Some will employ additional methods such as relaxation or hypnosis, but most general practitioners will not have the time or training for the more specialised techniques of behaviour therapy and psychoanalysis, which may well be available for appropriate patients from clinical psychologists and psychiatrists. However, given the right attitudes of genuine concern there is a great deal which the general practitioner can do for patients with emotional problems, providing time is set aside for this. Short-term psychotherapy sessions usually last from 30 to 50 minutes and a variable number of sessions are involved, but much can be accomplished in three to six visits.

Short-term psychotherapy in general practice

A method for short-term psychotherapy in general practice has been developed by Lesser (1981). There are many different approaches, but this one is described specifically because it has been developed for family doctors, is taught to family medicine residents in Canada and has been successfully demonstrated to trainers in Scotland. The method has three main characteristics which are described below:

1. Behaviour-orientated.
2. Problem-orientated.
3. Paradigms or strategies are used as frameworks for treatment.

1. *A behavioural approach* does not require the use of psychodynamic concepts and fits best into the time constraints of general practice. The emphasis is on what the patient does in particular situations and three types of behaviours are examined. First are reported behaviours connected with events occurring in the daily life of patients which often serve to illustrate adaptive as well as maladaptive responses. Second are observed behaviours which are seen by the interviewer and are primarily non-verbal. Third are the self-reported behaviours of the interviewee such as 'why am I thinking or feeling this?'. An exploration of these might show the patient the problem he creates for others.

The main features of the behavioural method are:

a. A systematic description of the reported and observed problem behaviours.
b. A systematic description of the conditions and cues which precede, follow or reinforce the problem behaviour.
c. An attempt to change the conditions which seem causally related to the problem behaviour by getting the patient to replay the situation in a more adaptive manner in the consulting room.
d. Evaluating whether the patient has learned more effective problem solving. The behaviourally-orientated approach is a 'here-and-now' approach which does not force data into theoretical models.

2. *A problem-orientated approach* addresses itself directly to the problems which patients want clarified and solved. By examining the details of these problems, the doctor can assess their relative normality and the extent to which the behaviour is adaptive or maladaptive. If it is adaptive then the coping strategies will be geared to the realities of the present with open and appropriate affective expression. The main elements of the problem-orientated approach are as follows:

a. Obtain specific examples of the main conflictual problem (Describe an argument you have had).
b. Dissect out the problem so that the component parts can be visualised. (What and how were things done and said, and with what results?) Interviewers are encouraged to use a 'think, see, do, feel' approach in order to check out the cognitive, perceptual and volitional areas, so that feelings can be elicited more accurately.
   What did you think about it? How did you see it? What did you do (or say) about it? How do you feel about it?)
c. Allow the patient at every point to see the adaptive and maladaptive components.
d. Show the patient what he is doing and how he is doing it to himself and to others.
e. Encourage the accurate and honest labelling of the problem by the patient.
f. Replay in an adaptive fashion the behavioural transaction which was maladaptive so that the patient learns to deal with the situation more effectively.

3. *Paradigms or strategies are used as a framework* for treatment rather than psychiatric diagnoses, because patients come with problems which produce symptoms and limitations of function. They are not helped by sterile labels. For instance in marital problems, couples often present with a long-standing war and it is necessary to clarify what the couple wants. Do they want to go on as before, (in which case therapy is useless); or do they want to separate (in which case is it agreed and how to children fit in?); or do they want to work the problems out (in which case they must care, the war must stop, a new relationship must start, the past can be used to mature but not as a weapon against the other, problems must be resolved and tasks for growth defined). In dealing with marital disputes time is needed, and it is best not to become too friendly with the patients, or to see one alone too often. It may be necessary to take sides over issues, and extramarital affairs must be discontinued or discussed.

In teaching this approach to family medicine residents, audio-tape recordings of their own patient encounters are used with group discussion, so that feedback to individuals can be given and reactions shared. Video-tapes are used for interviewing families. Recurring themes which are stressed are: picking up affect-laden words and behaviours, clearly identifying problems, labelling maladaptive behaviours, and the need for rapid and efficient intervention. Certain patients are not suitable for this approach. These include patients whose present problems are based largely on past events, where knowledge of connections between the two does not result in change. Patients with multiple problems may need a disciplinary approach, and those who have not improved in six sessions need to be referred to a psychologist. At first a few trainees show anxiety at being recorded and exposed to peer criticism, and others have difficulty in confronting patients as well as each other. Some see counselling in a humanitarian sense, rather than as a 'therapeutic business venture'. It depends on a contracted agreement between patient and doctor for a particular purpose and time; if agreement breaks down then it is better to cut losses rather than waste time. Some trainees have difficulty in using simple descriptive language and others persist with formal diagnostic history taking rather than following the cues provided by the patient. In order to pursue a traditional diagnosis, they ignore 'the magic carpet' of what the patient says and the non-verbal communication. However, the great majority of family medicine trainees acquire the necessary skills of assessment and brief psychotherapy for patients in general practice (Lesser 1981).

COUNSELLING COUPLES

INTRODUCTION

There has been a steady rise in the number of divorces which have increased by seven-fold since the 1960's with a sudden jump in the early 1970's following introduction of the 1969 Divorce Reform Act. The fact that one in three marriages ends in divorce gives some indication of the extent of marital problems. This is partly due to changes in society such as greater equality between the sexes, and the liberation of women due to smaller families with modern contraceptive practice. In addition expectations are higher, both materially and emotionally. Private unhappinesses which were once endured have now become matters of general interest and concern. In the process, normality in marriage has been redefined and transferred from the area of morality to that of medicine.

Marriage guidance is now available from a number of agencies and professions. In general, marital counselling avoids working with unconscious mental processes and concentrates instead on a client-centred, non-directive approach. This has been the mainstream of marriage guidance in Britain, as opposed to the psychodynamic and behavioural approaches to marital therapy. The for-

mer aims to eradicate symptoms through the traditional psychodynamic methods of uncovering and 'working through' unconscious causes, whereas the latter is concerned with identifying specific problems which are amenable to behavioural modification. In practice, elements of the two approaches are often combined, depending on the personality and interest of the counsellor as well as the couple. Both methods will try to explore areas of disagreement and conflict, but psychodynamic approaches tend to be more reflective compared to the actively focused efforts of behavioural modification. Most marital therapy consists of weekly sessions in which the couple are seen together and rarely lasts longer than a few months. The main elements are clarifying the nature of the difficulties between the couple, linking aspects of the past with the present, confronting them with what is going on, interpreting motives, and generally encouraging the couple to take a cooler look at their relationship (Clare & Thompson 1981).

PSYCHODYNAMIC MARITAL THERAPY

There are certain aspects of personality development which may have an important bearing on marital problems. In early family life we learn to identify with parents and in marriage there is a tendency to relive these identifications. When the original ones have disturbed elements, then these disturbances may be repeated in marriage. People who marry may compensate for each other, or they may have the opposite effect. One scheme for marital therapy is to view marriage as a life cycle with several different types of relationship, any one of which can become disturbed, although some problems are more relevant to one phase of the life cycle than others. There are five main relationships between a couple (physical, emotional, social, intellectual and spiritual) all of which should be checked to see where the main problems occur. The nature of the problems will depend on the phase of the marriage life cycle. The first phase comprises the first few years of marriage; the second phase covers the period during which the children are growing up and ends when the youngest has left home; the last phase is when the couple are again alone together, until one of them dies (Dominian 1981).

In the first phase the physical relationship is usually uncomplicated, but there may be emotional problems depending on the readiness of the couple to form a stable relationship, and their ability to disengage themselves from their respective parents. One or both of the spouses may not be really ready to commit themselves to a permanent relationship, and there may be collusion due to the inability of parents to let go. At this stage the couple may discover that socially, intellectually or spiritually they are not compatible, and that the person they thought they were marrying is in fact rather different on prolonged intimate contact. In the second phase there may be a lack of interest in sex, associated with childbearing, and a growing independence of one or other of the partners who may move into a different social setting which causes conflict. During the third phase there is often a decline in sexual interest which may be one-sided and lead to extra-marital affairs. If the main emotional interest has been through their children, then a couple may feel empty when the children have left.

If possible the couple should be seen together, and be helped to perceive the way they see each other, the power structure of their relationship, how they communicate, and the areas in which they are not meeting each other's needs. Sometimes there is a dialogue of the deaf in that the couple are not listening to each other. By drawing attention to this the doctor can open up channels of communication so that each becomes aware of painful feelings in the other, and recognises the nature of the conflict between them. Genuine listening enhances acceptance and respect.

The transactional analysis devised by Berne (1966) is also used for marital therapy. Marital games or strategies are characterised by their ulterior motives and pay offs. The analysis depends on whether the spouses are using their child, adult, or parental ego states, and the nature of the transactions between them. There is also a be-havioural element to Berne's theories in that social inter-course depends on mutual 'stroking' which is con-ditioned by stimuli and learned.

BEHAVIOURAL MARITAL THERAPY

The basic principle of behavioural approaches is that a neurotic reaction is acquired through the simple process of conditioning. The answer to a problem is therefore not to search for underlying causes, but to decondition, by such techniques as aversion therapy and operant con-ditioning with rewards and punishments. Sexual prob-lems like impotence, premature ejaculation, vaginismus, and frigidity, have been particularly regarded as amen-able to behavioural techniques such as the systematic desensitisation of Masters and Johnson, who recognised that sexual problems exist in a relationship and insisted on treating couples as a unit. A behavioural therapist would pay particular attention to the presenting difficul-ties and try to assess areas of conflict and satisfaction in the marriage. Each partner would be encouraged to iden-tify their own needs or wants which can then be given and received by the other. The example given under a previous section for behavioural counselling for indi-viduals, illustrates such an approach which enables cou-ples to deal directly with their problems, and is simpler

and often less disturbing than seeking for underlying dynamic factor.

The distinction between counselling individuals, cou-ples and families is to a certain extent artificial, in that similar techniques and approaches apply. It may for inst-ance be appropriate to involve children in marital ther-apy, but in some ways the tradition of a one-to-one patient–doctor relationship inhibits general practitioners from seeing couples and families together although this is the context within which interpersonal problems take place. There are however special techniques and approaches for counselling families which will be consi-dered below.

COUNSELLING FAMILIES

INTRODUCTION

In recent years there has been a shift towards counselling families as well as individuals, particularly in North America. This stems partly from work with behavioural problems in child guidance clinics and partly from the growth of group therapy. The interactions and dynamics of the group were used by therapists to treat individual members. The success of this seemed to depend upon a number of factors, such as individuals learning to express their feelings, as well as receiving other people's impress-ions and so discovering previously unknown or unaccept-able parts of themselves. By seeing others reveal embar-rassing things and take risks, so individuals became more trustful of other people, and at the same time learnt to take ultimate responsibility for their own lives.

These considerations were reflected in a change in emphasis from the individual to the family and its in-teractions, as the unit of assessment and focus for treat-ment. This fitted in with general systems theory which states that a system is a whole and that its components and their characteristics can only be understood as func-tions of the total system. The whole constitutes more than simply the sum of its parts, and therefore the family with its interactinng members constitutes a whole system with definable boundaries.

Inevitably different approaches to family therapy have been developed as indicated below, but in general there is more emphasis on how the family operates in the present rather than looking for causes in the past of individuals. It is not so much that the past is unimportant, but rather that the present re-enacts the past in such a way that meaning can be sought within the boundaries of the present system. In order to assess what is going on within a family group and in order to intervene therapeutically, family therapists have developed various concepts and techniques which are outlined below. As yet there is little research on the outcome of family therapy in terms of effectiveness or efficiency, but common sense and experience would suggest that many problems which present to general practitioners have their origins in relationships within a family. This section therefore ends with a brief description of a method of family therapy specifically designed for family doctors.

APPROACHES TO FAMILY THERAPY

Psychodynamic

A psychodynamic approach to family therapy was developed by psychoanalysts who transferred their traditional concepts from individuals to the family group. The therapist is mainly an interpreter who makes family members aware how unconscious ideas and experiences affect present behaviour, so that insight leads to healthier functioning. Although such an approach does not grasp the reality of the family as a whole, some of the insights of psychoanalysis have been interpreted into the systems model, for instance the concepts of a family myth, family transference, and interlocking pathologies. A family myth is a pattern of mutually agreed but distorted roles which family members adopt as a defensive posture and which are not challenged from within the family. Family transference means the projection by family members on to each other, of child or parent positions which derive from their own past experience; these are a means of dealing with unacceptable, frightening or hostile feelings. Interlocking pathology implies that individuals in a close personal relationship within a family can affect each other by the exchange of symptoms, mutual secondary gains, and the unconscious transmission of feelings.

Communication

A communication approach to family therapy is based on the concept that family relationships depend on patterns of communication between membes, and when this is faulty then relationships become disturbed. The aim of therapy is therefore to promote a healthier pattern of communication. Some therapists like Minuchin (1974) are concerned with the structure of sub-systems within a family, such as parents or siblings. Family pathology occurs when sub-systems are either too enmeshed or disengaged, and this can be remedied by altering communication between members. Another example of focusing on communication is Parent Effectiveness Training (Gordon 1970), which seeks to prevent the emergence of behavioural problems and the deterioration of parent-child relationships. Parents are encouraged to listen actively to their children's feelings and to reflect these back in an accepting way. They are taught to communicate 'I' messages about their own feelings rather than blaming the child and to solve problems by mutual discussion.

Behavioural

A behavioural approach is based on the principles of learning theory as for counselling individuals or couples. Desired behavioural changes are specified and contracts between family members and with the therapist negotiated. Efforts are made to change the family's reciprocal reinforcing patterns, for other behaviours which are agreed to be more desirable.

SELECTION AND ASSESSMENT

The indications for family therapy depend upon whether a situation is perceived as being due to individual or family dysfunction. Children are the most dependent on their family and disturbances such as antisocial behaviour, conflicts with parents, sibling rivalry, school refusal, and anorexia nervosa may be treated with family therapy. Increasingly, problems of adults such as alcoholism are also being tackled by seeing the family as a whole. There may be circumstances in which the family group seeks help in crises such as divorce and bereavement. The situation may present in terms of family interactions, for instance scapegoating (when complaints about a child's behaviour camouflage marital difficulties), or inappropriate dependency, or the transfer of symptoms from one family member to another. Obviously key members of the family must agree to participate, and have the potential for achieving insight.

There are three main frameworks which can be used in assessing a family. The first concerns the family life cycle in terms of marriage, parenthood, the growing up of children, and then retirement and death. At each stage there are demands and challenges which have to be met and coped with. The second framework is the three-generation framework of family life, in which a knowledge of the families of origin of the parents may throw light on current problems. A parent's childhood experience may lead to a particular 'script' for child-rearing in the current family, or contribute to a family 'myth' which is handed down from one generation to another. The third framework concerns family functioning in the present. Successful functioning provides satisfactory models for socialisation and sexual identification, with appropriate boundaries. Family function can be considered under five headings:

1. *Communication* — both verbal and non-verbal. To what extent does communication occur, and how clear, open and direct is it?
2. *Feelings* — how are feelings expressed in a family and to what extent do they elicit a response?
3. *Atmosphere* — what is the predominant atmosphere in a family, for instance chaotic, aggressive, apathetic, humourous?

4. *Cohesiveness* — to what extent does the family have a sense of solidarity and belongingness?
5. *Boundaries* — are these sufficiently permeable between sub-systems to facilitate easy communication, and yet sufficiently intact to maintain the integrity of individuals?

These three frameworks provide a basis for assessing the presenting problem in terms of the main individuals concerned, and for understanding the origins of the problem and its maintenance in the family system. By encouraging the family to describe the presenting problems in detail, much information can be gained about family functioning, and how individual member interact with each other. A history of the family's past and development in terms of intergenerational issues may be helpful in understanding why the problem has occurred at this particular time.

TECHNIQUES OF FAMILY THERAPY

The word techniques implies a particular way of doing things, and as such certain techniques have been described by family therapists such as Minuchin (1974). In part these may be conscious ways of approaching situations, or an analysis of how some family therapists work subconsciously from experience. Families are transactional systems with a structure which is developing and adapting. Family therapy implies that a professional outsider joins this system temporarily in order to modify its functioning so that it can better perform its tasks. Families are structures with self-perpetuating properties and the aim of treatment is to initiate changes which will be maintained by the family through its own feedback mechanisms. However family members will only change if their present perceptions and behaviour are challenged in such a way that alternative transactional patterns can be initiated which make sense and produce new relationships which are self-reinforcing.

Every doctor or therapist has his own way of working, but certain *ground rules* have been developed by family therapists. Firstly, the family comes as a group, and all information is shared with the group so that there are no secrets with individuals. The emphasis is on openness so that feelings are expressed between members of the group including the therapist, who will also try to establish a meaningful relationship with each member. Secondly, after the initial assessment, it is usual to establish a contract with the family which defines the treatment goals for specific purposes. The goals may be modified but the responsibility is placed with the family group which must itself be defined. The contract would also specify where the group would meet, and the length and frequency of sessions. Before such a contract can be established, the therapist must create a therapeutic system by 'joining' the family so that restructuring can take place, and there are techniques for both these activities.

Coupling

Coupling techniques are those which enable the therapist to join and accommodate to the family so that a cohesive group is formed. *Joining* a family system implies accepting it as it is, and relating to the individual members. This may mean *accommodation* by the therapist, so that he adjusts himself in order to join the family. Minuchin (1974) has described a number of accommodation techniques for forming a therapeutic system. *Maintenance* means supporting the existing family structure, for instance by acknowledging the dominant decision maker. *Teaching* is a method of following the content of a family's communication by encouraging them to continue without confrontation, so that family structure can be explored. *Mimesis* is accommodation by the therapist to the family's style, mood and culture; this involves being sensitive to their feelings so that behaviour can be adapted accordingly and common experiences shared.

Restructuring

Restructuring techniques are those concerned with treatment after the therapist has joined the family, made an assessment, and established a therapeutic contract. The treatment techniques used depend on the situation, and the personality and training of the therapist, all of whom will develop their own style. Throughout family therapy, support, education and guidance is provided but the following techniques have been described by Minuchin (1974) and others. *Actualising transactional patterns* means getting the family to communicate with each other, rather than with the therapist. This can be done by encouraging them to re-enact particular situations, or to talk to other members rather than about them. *Marking boundaries* means emphasising the integrity of individuals or sub-systems, for instance by requiring that individuals should listen to each other, and that parent or children can talk to each other without interruption. *Escalating stress* may indicate dysfunctional coping behaviour, and can be produced by blocking transactional patterns, for instance by stopping a dominant member from speaking for another. Stress may be induced by emphasising differences and conflicts, or by joining one side or another in a conflict. *Assigning tasks* may be done within a session or at home and should have a defined purpose so that it can be performed and practised. The tasks may involve altering how a family communicates, and so illustrate the potential for change. *Utilising symptoms* can be a way of restructuring a family by getting members to focus on, or re-label individual symptoms so that relationships and insight are altered in the process. *Manipulating mood* by exaggerating and re-labelling predominant affects in a family may help to alter relationships. *Action methods* are used by some therapists so that family relationnships are recreated in space by what members do rather than what they say. This may involve the manipulation of seating arrangements or getting families to sculpt the emotional position of each member in a tableau vivant. In addition the techniques of encounter groups, gestalt psychologists, and psychodrama have been used to help families act out their conflicts or problems, and so gain insight. *Co-therapy* in which two therapists work together with a family is used in certain centres but requires experience and planning and is costly. Ideally the therapists are of opposite sex and so can provide role models for the family but there appears to be little evidence of the superiority of co-therapy.

Termination

Termination is explicit in the initial contract, but the aims may change as sessions continue. There may be problems of dependency developing, but this is more easily handled if the original goals are specific. There is no consensus about the time intervals and duration of treatment. Hourly sessions every 1 to 4 weeks are not unusual. Anything up to 6 months might be considered a brief intervention in America, but the situation there is different from the ongoing responsibilities of family doctors in the British National Health Service. Here the emphasis must be on shorter-term interventions for specific purposes when the whole family is seen together as a group. This in itself may be therapeutic at a common sense level, but it is necessary for the general practitioner to have a practical model with which to work, and realistic limits of time and goals. A method for short-term family therapy specifically designed for family doctors is indicated below. The justification for such an approach must be that it helps patients, although as yet there are few outcome studies. In the context of the National Health Service a reduction in morbidity should in the long-term save time and therefore resources, but it has yet to be demonstrated that family therapy is effective and efficient when used by general practitioners.

A METHOD FOR FAMILY THERAPY FOR GENERAL PRACTITIONERS

A method of family therapy has been developed at the McMaster medical school specifically for use by family doctors (Epstein & Bishop 1973, Comley 1973). The method is based on the McMaster model of family functioning and concentrates on present behaviour rather than past experience. In focusing on what happens in family transactions rather than why, families are taught to look after each other and to be their own problem solvers. The sessions usually last an hour each week, and about six sessions may be involved. The following is a brief description of the approach, which incorporates the McMaster model of family functioning in the assessment of the family.

1. Assessment (Determination of family's problems)

Orientation. Explain that the basis for family therapy is that individual problems may be a reflection of dysfunction within a family, and this is what is going to be assessed and treated with an agreed contract.

Data gathering. Collect information about family functioning both with regard to the presenting problem and in general, using the McMaster model of family functioning. This model views family functioning as consisting of three broad areas of tasks which involve six dimensions as indicated in Table 4.2.

Problem solving may be instrumental and concerned with practical matters such as finance and housing matters, or it may be affective and concerned with feelings. The reason for the family presenting for therapy may be only one instance of their inability to solve problems effectively. *Roles* are the repetitive patterns of behaviour by which individuals fulfil family functions, such as the provision of resources, mutual support and personal development. *Communication* may also be instrumental or affective, with some families being good at communicating practical matters but incapable of sharing feelings. In addition communication can be assessed along two other parameters, as to whether it is clear or masked, and direct or indirect. Masked communication does not state clearly what the person is thinking or feeling, and indirect communication is not addressed directly to those concerned. *Affective responsiveness* means the ability to respond with positive feelings such as love, tenderness, and joy, or negative feelings such as fear, anger and sadness. *Affective involvement* refers to the degree to which the family shows interest in, and values, the activities of family members. This may range from non-involvement,, through empathy to over-involvement. *Behaviour control* is the pattern the family adopts for handling behaviour in specific situations. The situations may involve normal functions such as sleeping, eating and aggression, or dangerous situations such as running on to the road and

Table 4.2   Model of family functioning

Dimensions	Task areas
Problem solving	
Roles	
Communication	Basic, Developmental,
Affective responsiveness	Hazardous
Affective involvement	
Behaviour Control	

reckless driving; or the behaviour control might be concerned with socialising both inside and outside the family. The style of behaviour control might be rigid, flexible, laissez-faire, or chaotic.

The family's functioning is assessed along the dimensions for the tasks which it has to carry out. The tasks may be *basic* for instrumental activities like the provision of food and shelter. Secondly the tasks may be developmental, either for individual members such as infancy, adolescence and old age, or for the family as a whole such as marriage and the birth of the first child. Finally the tasks may be *hazardous* and concerned with crises like illness, accidents, moves or unemployment.

Problem description and clarification. The family is asked to describe their presenting problems as they now see them, together with any other relevant problems which might be brought to mind. The doctor then describes the family problems as he or she sees them. If both the family and doctor agree about the nature of the problem then the next stage is negotiating a contract. However, there may be disagreement between family members, and this inability to agree could be part of the problem which needs labelling as such, or it may be necessary to return to gather more data. If the family disagree with the doctor the whole situation will need to be reviewed.

2. Contract (Establishment of goals and conditions of therapy)

Orientation. Establish agreement with the family that the assessment is done, and begin discussion of how the problems are to be handled.

Outline options. Indicate options open to the family at this point, e.g. continue as they are, seek other help, or work with the doctor. If the last is chosen, then the conditions of treatment are specified such as the number and length of sessions, and who is expected to be there.

Negotiate expectations. Determine through discussion what the family expects from therapy and convey to the family what is expected of them. It is mainly up to the family to indicate their expectations, and up to the doctor to clarify these in concrete terms.

Establish contract. Establish a written contract specifying the negotiated expectations and goals of therapy. The contract is often signed by both the family and the doctor, and includes details of the time commitment involved.

3. Treatment (Treatment of family's problems)

Orientation. Simply state to the family that treatment has begun.

Task setting. Establish priorities concerning the expectations of the family, and then define and assign tasks by negotiation. These tasks involve specific behaviours and represent a move towards meeting the family's expectations, and should follow certain principles. The tasks should be simple, assured of success, and reasonable in terms of the family's activities and the abilities of individuals. Usually there is a maximum of two tasks per session and they should be of obvious importance to the family. A task should be a positive act of commission, rather than stopping doing something, and should be clearly spelled out, particularly when involving the expression of emotions. Finally it is important that those involved in the tasks should be designated to report back at the next session.

Task evaluation. Check that the tasks have been achieved and move on to the next task if this is agreed. If the tasks have not been achieved, then it is necessary to discuss and clarify what went wrong, and negotiate new tasks. When all the tasks, and therefore expectations, have been met then it is time to move on to the final stage of closure.

4. Closure (Formal declaration that treatment is ending)

Orientation. Convey to the family that the agreed goals have been achieved and that the family is now functioning well.

Treatment summary. The family is asked to describe what they think has happened during treatment and what they have learnt. At the same time the doctor confirms or elaborates on the family's description.

Long-term goals. The family is asked to identify how they will be able to tell in the future if they are continuing to function well or not, and if not, what they would do about it. They are also asked if they wish to identify tasks or follow-up tasks to work on themselves.

The above description is a brief summary, but it does indicate the importance of family participation and the concentration on here-and-now behaviour. The emphasis on a negotiated contract may be more appropriate in a North American setting, but in any context of primary care it is necessary for doctors to be clear about what they are trying to do, and to set limits to what they hope to achieve. In short, some conceptual framework is required to enable general practitioners to start tackling the many problems which have their roots in family behaviour, and this is one example of a practical approach for use in primary care.

REFERENCES

Argyle M, Ingham R 1972 Gaze, mutual gaze and distance. Semiotica 6: 32–49
Argyle M, Cook M 1976 Gaze and mutual gaze. Cambridge University Press
Argyle M 1978 The psychology of interpersonal behaviour. Penguin Books, London
Argyle M 1981 Social skills and health. Methuen, London.

Bales R F 1950 Interaction process analysis. Addison-Wesley, Reading, Massarhusetts

Balint M 1964 The doctor, his patient and the illness. Pitman Medical, London

Balint E, Norell J S 1973 Six minutes for the patient. Tavistock Publications, London

Barnet K 1972 A theoretical construct of the concepts of touch as they relate to nursing. Nursing Research 21: 2

Berne E 1966 Games people play. Andre Deutsch, London

Birdwhistell 1952 Introduction to kinetics. University of Louiseville Press

Block S 1979 Supportive psychotherapy. In: Bloch S (ed) An introduction to the psychotherapies. Oxford University Press, London

Brock A 1980 Brief psychotherapy in clinical practice. Medicine 36: 1834–1836

Byrne P S, Long B E L 1976 Doctors talking to patients. HMSO, London

Clare A W, Thompson S 1981 Lets talk about me. British Broadcasting Corporation, London

Comley A 1973 Family therapy and the family physician. Canadian Family Practice, February 1975

Cook M 1970 Experiments on orientation and proxemics. Human Relations 23: 61–76

Crown S 1979 Individual long-term psychotherapy. In:: Bloch S (ed) An introduction to the psychotherapies. Oxford University Press, London

Davitz J R 1964 The communication of emotional meaning. McGraw-Hill, New York

Dominian J 1981 Marital therapy. In: Bloch S (ed) An introduction to the psychotherapies. Oxford University Press, London

Ekman P, Friesen W V 1967 Head and body cues in the judgement of emotion: a reformulation. Perceptual and Motor Skills 24: 711–724

Ekman P, Friesen W V, Ellsworth P 1972 Emotions in the human face. Pergamon, New York

Epstein N B, Bishop D S 1973 Family therapy: state of the art. Canadian Psychiatric Journal 18: 175–183

Fletcher C 1979 Towards better practice and teaching of communication between doctors and patients. In: McClachan G (ed) Mixed Communications, Oxford University Press, London

Friedman N, Hoffman S P 1967 Kinetic behaviour in altered clinical states. Perceptual and Motor Skills 24: 525–539

Frank J D 1981 What is psychotherapy? In: Bloch S (ed) An introduction to the psychotherapies, Oxford University Press, London

Froeloch R E, Bishop F M 1977 Clinical interviewing skills. C. V. Mosby Co., St. Louis

Gill C 1973 Types of interview in general practice: the flash. In: Balint E, Norell J S (eds) Six minutes for the patient. Tavistock Publications, London

Goffman E 1961 Asylums. Anchor Books, New York

Goldberg D P, Blackwell B 1970 Psychiatric illness in general practice. British Medical Journal May: 439

Goldberg D 1982 Cognitive therapy for depression. British Medical Journal 284: 143

Gordon T 1970 Parent effectiveness training. The New American Library, New York

Hall E T 1959 The silent language. Doubleday, New York.

Hannay D R 1980a Teaching interviewing with video-tape and peer assessment. Update June: 1439–1446

Hannay D R 1980b Teaching interviewing with simulated patients. Medical Education 14: 246–248

Hargie O D W 1980 An evaluation of a microteaching programme. Thesis, Ulster Polytechnic

Jourard S M 1963 An exploratory study of body-accessibility. British Journal of Social and Clinical Psychology 5: 221–231

Kendon A 1967 Some functions of gaze — direction in social interaction. Acta Psychologica 26: 22–47

Lesser A L 1981 The psychiatrist and family medicine: a different training approach. Medical Education 15: 398–406

Lamerton R 1973 Care of the dying. Priory Press Ltd., London

Maguire P, Rutter D 1976 Training medical students to communicate. In: Bennett A E (ed) Communication between doctors and patients.

Mahl G F 1968 Gestures and body movements in interviews. Research in Psychotherapy 3: 295–346

Marks J, Goldberg D, Hilber V 1979 Determinants of the ability of general practitioners to detect psychiatric illness. Psychological Medicine 9: 337–354

Mehrabian A 1968 Inference of attitudes from the posture, orientation, and distance of a communicator. Journal of Consulting and Clinical Psychology 32: 296–308

Mehrabian A 1969 Significance of posture and position in the communication of attitude and status and relationships. Psychological Bulletin 71: 363–367

Minuchin S 1974 Families and family therapy. Tavistock Publications, London

Morris D 1978 Man watching. Triad Granada, London

Pendleton D 1981 Learning communication skills. Update 22: 1708–1714

Pietroni P 1976 Non-verbal communication in the general practice surgery. In: Tanner B (ed) Language and communication in general practice. Hodder and Stoughton, London

Sanson-Fisher R, Maguire P 1980 Should skills in communicating with patients be taught in medical schools. Lancet Sept. 523–526

Scheflen A E, Scheflen A 1972 Body language and the social order. Prentice Hall, New York

Schutz W C 1967 Joy. Grove Press, New York

Shapiro J G 1968 Responsivity to facial and linguistic cues. Journal of Communication, 18:11–17

Sommer R 1969 Personal space. Prentice Hall, New Jersey

Storr A 1979 The art of psychotherapy. Secker and Warburg, London

Trower P 1980 Situational analysis of the components and processes of socially skilled and unskilled patients. Journal of Consulting and Clinical Psychology 32: 296–308

Walrond-Skinner 1976 Family therapy. Routledge and Kegan Paul, London

Williams E 1974 An analysis of gaze in schizophrenics. British Journal of Social and Clinical Psychology, 13: 1–8

Wolberg L R 1980 Short term psychotherapy. Thieme-Stratton, New York

FURTHER READING

Argyle M 1975 Bodily communication. Methuen & Co. Ltd, London

Argyle M 1978 The psychology of interpersonal behaviour. Penguin Books, London

Balint M 1964 The doctor, his patient and the illness. Pitman Medical, London

Balint E, Norell J S 1973 Six minutes for the patient. Tavistock Publications, London

Benjamin A 1974 The helping interview. Houghton Mifflin Co., Boston

Berne E 1966 Games people play. Andre Deutsch, London

Bloch S 1979 An introduction to the psychotherapies. Oxford University Press, Oxford

Clare A W, Thompson S 1981 Lets talk about me. British Broadcasting Corporation, London

Enelow A J, Swisher S N 1972 Interviewing and patient care. Oxford University Press, London

Gordon T 1970 Parent effectiveness training. The New American Library, New York

Lamerton R 1973 Care of the dying. Priory Press Ltd., London

Minuchin S 1974 Families and family therapy. Tavistock Publications, London

Storr A 1979 The art of psychotherapy. Secker & Warburg, London

Walrond-Skinner S 1976 Family therapy. Routledge and Kegan Paul, London

Wolberg L R 1980 Short-term psychotherapy. Thieme-Stratton, New York

Family planning

FAMILY PLANNING

Over the last 50 years or so, the importance of family planning and its implications for the physical, social and psychological well being of our patients has become self-evident. Childbirth in women over 40 years of age means a seven-fold increase in risks to their health compared with women under 20 years of age; an infant who is the fifth member of a family has twice the risk of dying at or around delivery compared with the first or second birth. Acknowledgement of an increased risk of non-accidental injury or emotional disturbance being greater in unwanted pregnancies means that the need for fertility control at both individual and community level has become increasingly obvious. The 'fifth freedom' advocated in 1965 was Sir Dugald Baird's answer to the tyranny of excessive fertility. Family spacing used to be facilitated by lengthy breast feeding, but its decline increased the hazards of inadequate family spacing.

Great improvements in family planning services have occurred since 1974 when Health Authority clinics began to provide free services. General practitioner family planning services became freely available to female patients in 1975. Both kinds of facilities have remained available and complementary, to all women, but evidence has recently suggested that many women prefer to use general practitioner facilities (Bone 1978) with the added incentive of combining the visit with a consultation about another member of the family.

Despite the increased availability of services and facilities, however, many unwanted pregnancies still occur possibly because present day 'acceptable' contraceptives may not be as satisfactory as is generally assumed. The popularity of different methods varies in different communities, different countries and different cultures: very different proportions of patients with intra-uterine devices or who are taking the pill are found, for example, in Finland, Holland and Scotland.

Adequate basic training is essential for providing the full range of services which patients can reasonably expect. All trainee practitioners are strongly recommended to undertake training to the standard of the Certificate issued by the Joint Committee on Contraception (RCGP 1981). The Joint Committee gives guidelines for and accreditation of appropriate courses of instruction for trainee practitioners, as well as refresher courses and seminars for instructing doctors who in turn give practical teaching sessions to trainees in a general practice setting.

Family planning is widely accepted as a multidisciplinary service and support and involvement of the practice nursing team (community nurses, health visitors, midwives and practice nurses) is essential to making the facilities of the practice known to the patients who need these services. Further reference to the contribution of the nurse in the family planning clinic is made on pages 50–51.

ORGANISATION OF CONTRACEPTIVE SERVICES IN THE PRACTICE

A structured family planning and well woman clinic is a great asset in a group practice. It should be an 'open' clinic — that is one to which patients can refer themselves either for a screening examination or for contraceptive advice, and to which any member of the practice team (whether receptionist, practice nurses, midwife, health visitor, community nurse, social worker or any of the doctors) can refer any patient in need of practical advice. Basic family planning training for all the nursing staff must be ensured and changes in organisation and clinical policy must be discussed and agreed by the complete clinic staff.

Records
A family planning record sheet is important. The one used in the author's clinic (Fig. 5.1) summarises each patient's history — medical, obstetric, gynaecological and contraceptive — and examination findings so that accurate counselling and advice may be given. The screening examination is similar to the post-natal examination, and the same proforma is used at these examinations as a basis for continued contraceptive super-

FORM
F.P.9

LOTHIAN HEALTH BOARD
FAMILY PLANNING SERVICES

Date of First Visit	Surname
Hospital Unit No.	Forenames
Name and address of doctor or partnership:	Address

| Date of Birth | Parity | 1-Mr   2-Mrs   3-Miss |

Contraceptive History

Social History: Including marital status and occupation

Family History – including cardiovascular disease; diabetes

Obstetric History

Previous Medical History – including: cardiovascular, liver and breast disease; headaches; endocrine disorders; psychiatric history; relevant operations; current drug therapy; contact lenses; smoking habits.

Gynaecological History

Menstrual Cycle:
(pre O.C., pre I.U.D.)   Amenorrhoea

Blood loss.............................. ......

Dysmenorrhoea: Discharge:

Pre-Menstrual Symptoms: Dyspareunia:

Gynae. Operations: Pelvic Inflam.
                                        Disease:

| Outcome of last pregnancy | Baby's Health | Breast Fed YES/NO | Mother's Health |

First Examination

General:

Breasts:

Abdomen:

Pelvis:

vulva:

vagina:

cervix:

uterus:

appendages:

C.S.   YES/NO

Date..

Weight...........KG B.P......../.......

Date of Last:
Menstrual Period ....

Cervical Smear...........................

Haemoglobin	
Urinalysis	
Pregnancy Test	

OTHER INVESTIGATIONS:

COMMENTS – Method agreed today: Follow up (where and when) etc.

Fig. 5.1 Family planning sheet

CRAIGSHILL HEALTH CENTRE   **FAMILY PLANNING FLOW SHEET**

Surname				Initials	Marital Status		Computer No.		Practice Number	

RECORD OF VISITS (Continued)

Date	L.M.P.	Weight	Present Contraception			B.P.	COMMENT (including current relationship. change in parity: cervical smear)	Smear		Review Appt	M.O. Initials
			O.C.	CAP.	I.U.D.			Date	Result (Grade)		

Fig. 5.2   Family planning flow sheet

vision. A flow sheet is filed in the practice record (Fig. 5.2) as a way of recording observations at successive review assessments so that continuing changes are readily noted, and more importantly so that the patient's own practitioner can see at a glance during a subsequent consultation what the contraceptive status of the patient is at that particular time. Similarly, since the practice records are available for all clinic visits, the doctor (or nurse) in the clinic is aware of any illnesses since the patient's last assessment.

Nursing assistance
The nurse can make valuable contributions to the clinic in a number of ways:

1. She has a role in educating the younger patient, in emphasising the importance of contraception, in proper family spacing, and in informing patients, either at home, in the clinic or treatment room, of the services and facilities available at the practice surgery.

2. In the clinic, the nurse can take a history from a new patient and assist the doctor with different aspects of patient assessment, for example weight, blood pressure and blood tests such as Rubella antibody titre or haemoglobin.

3. With appropriate training, the clinic nurse can take high vaginal swabs and cervical smears, and with further medical supervision in both theory and practical techniques, she can review patients who are an oral contraception, or are using a diaphragm, and can check intra-uterine devices. She can also teach patients about the self-examination of breasts.

4. She assists the doctor in inserting intra-uterine devices:

a. For pre-packing the equipment required (either sterilised on the premises, or autoclaved by arrangement with the local district hospital). Several sets of instruments are required to mantain a readily available pack, since occasionally an 'urgent' insertion arises where mitigating social circumstances exist, or where the post-coital insertion of a device is deemed necessary.

b. Good rapport of nurse and patient is a great asset during a series of insertions of intra-uterine devices, when 'verbal anaesthesia' from an experienced nurse can assuage much of the patient's anxiety.

5. She can give patients initial counselling in the various methods of contraception, including sterilisation, and supply appropriate leaflets and information. Nurses respond well to this changing clinical role and team in-

volvement in an important area of preventive medicine and patients appreciate the familiar face of the practice nurse in this aspect of family health care. Tasks undertaken in the family planning clinic within the practice are allocated at the discretion of the responsible doctor, provided that he (or she) is satisfied with the nurse's level of experience and practical competence. The doctor in charge must accept legal responsibility for the nurse's functions within the clinic and should be available to discuss any questions the nurse may have, and to assess appropriate patients as necessary. It is also the doctor's responsibility to ensure that members of the clinic are kept up to date in trends of family planning and contraceptive techniques.

Requests may be received for having students from many disciplines as observers. Prior notice should always be obtained and careful schedules arranged since no more than one observer should be accepted in any clinic room. Family planning questions and contraceptive problems are usually very sensitive areas, and by and large, patients have plucked up considerable courage, or have been assiduously persuaded by a colleague, to attend the clinic. It should only be with the patient's permission that any observer, other than the actual clinic staff, is allowed within the consulting room.

THE CONTENT OF NEW AND FOLLOW-UP CONSULTATIONS

The new consultation

The initial assessment of a patient attending the clinic for the first time includes a complete health profile of the patient. Precise details of age, parity, medical, obstetric, gynaecological and contraceptive histories form an important data base for future reference. Although a physical examination, and an examination of the breasts, may be carried out a pelvic examination (including taking a cervical smear) is usually postponed until a subsequent visit — particularly in the case of the young single girl or the patient who has not previously had intercourse. Some authorities consider that a pelvic examination is not necessary for effective contraceptive advice since about 75% of patients will anticipate using the oral contraceptive by choice. Pelvic findings rarely influence the choice of pill, but, on the other hand, a number of young patients are relieved when reassured that they are anatomically normal. Pelvic examination affords the opportunity to take a cervical smear, and to detect any uterine or ovarian swellings. It may be argued that screening is not the function of a contraceptive clinic, but the general practitioner has a responsibility for the patient's overall health and a family planning clinic provides an extremely useful setting both for screening tests and for health education. Weight and blood pressure estimation, and

urine culture in patients with a past history of urinary tract infection should be carried out. A Rubella antibody titre check should be offered to all new patients. Time must be available in the clinic for answering patients' questions and for discussing problems; counselling and the provision of professional advice and information are important functions of the clinic.

It is important to be aware however that complete care of all the patients in a practice who need these services cannot be expected in a weekly clinic of this kind. A number of patients are genuinely unable to attend because of priorities at work even though more managers and personnel officers do nowadays give patients short leave of absence to attend a medical appointment. Other problem patients and well known 'poor attenders' remain immune to any persuasion or invitation to attend. This group of patients should be well known to the practice team, and the doctor should make appropriate enquiries and examination of such patients when the opportunity presents by the patient consulting for any reason. It may be difficult for the patient to relate a complaint of hoarseness due to heavy smoking with having a cervical smear and IUCD check carried out but the reasons for the doctor's apparently illogical actions should be explained.

The follow-up consultation

This is a much more brief meeting primarily to afford the patient an opportunity to raise questions which may have arisen since she began using contraception. The significance of any deviation from normal patterns of the menstrual cycle should be assessed, and appropriate reassurance given. Examination should be confined to weight and blood pressure checks where these are indicated. Where a pelvic examination was not done at the first visit, this should be considered at either the first or second review visit and should include a cervical smear. If problems have arisen following insertion of an IUCD, for example, then speculum examination with bimanual examination would be obligatory.

The flow sheet (Fig. 5.2) has proved extremely useful as part of the practice case record, and changing trends in observations — together with the results of investigations — are obvious at subsequent follow-up visits to the clinic, as well as to the patient's own doctor who may be managing some intercurrent illness. The value of nursing assistance in the follow-up clinic has been stressed already. Many patients have an easy rapport with the practice nursing staff, and find discussion of 'minor' problems easier with them. The fear of 'wasting' the doctor's time may inhibit patients from airing their anxieties regarding contraceptive problems or indeed their associated domestic or marital worries. The nurse's role in the follow-up clinic may well contribute significantly to the continuation rate of a particular contraceptive with a good number of patients. Continuing education is necessary in the follow-up clinic, because patients do talk amongst themselves and may come with growing fears of problems whiich almost invariably prove unfounded. These can however provoke such anxiety that, despite continuing counselling, a change in the method of contraception is indicated.

It is widely accepted that the form of contraception which is uppermost in the patient's mind or which she has firmly decided upon, is the form she is most likely to continue over the longest time. The role of the doctor or nurse in the family planning clinic should be primarily that of a counsellor seeking to exclude any contraindication to the patient's preferred method of contraception. If a contraindication is found suitable alternative forms should be discussed in detail and without haste; preferably the patient should be given written information in leaflet or brochure form so that she can discuss the method with her consort before a final decision is made.

An illustration of the importance of assessment and counselling of patients came to light in a review of the first 50 multiload Cu 250 intra-uterine devices inserted in the author's clinic after a period of 12 months. This particular device has been claimed as a major advance in IUCD technology, and its early evaluation claimed improvements over existing IUCD therapy in terms of ease of fitting, the incidence of pregnancy, expulsion and removal for bleeding or pain.

A review of the Health Centre clinic showed that of the 50 insertions (none of which were in nullparous patients) four were removed within 6 months and a further two within 12 months to allow for a planned pregnancy — that is 12% had changed their minds, although an explanation of the 3-year life span of the device had been given to each patient. 10% of the devices were removed because of side effects or 'complications' within the first 6 months, and a further 14% in the second 6 months. From this small internal 'audit' within one practice several questions were posed:

1. Was our attitude or approach to the introduction of the IUCD correct?
2. Was the selection of patients sufficiently thorough and deliberate?
3. Was the initial patient counselling adequate in detail?
4. Could patient management have been improved?

Technical details apart, a major result of this small audit was to emphasise the importance of adequate counselling of the patient, including the giving of information about the IUCD (with its advantages and disadvantages) and a full discussion of the patient's own needs and intentions. Although 38% of removals occurred within 12 months of insertion, the majority of problems were relatively minor, and only two had proven acute pelvic inflammatory disease (one was confirmed at laparoscopy,

and the other was found to have a tubo-ovarian abscess at laparotomy).

One further problem in follow-up is the movement of the patient to another area or practice. Provided the patient informs the clinic of the intended move, the month of her next review can be written on her appointment card and she can be advised to attend her new general practitioner for continued follow-up.

FORMS OF CONTRACEPTION AND CRITERIA OF SELECTION

There is a risk in the field of family planning of becoming obsessed with one method, one approach, one sex, and one answer. The pill was hailed as the solution to unwanted pregnancies; next it was the intra-uterine device with a variable demand for occlusive methods depending on the latest press 'scare' over the pill. However, experience over the last decade makes it quite clear that there is no single solution to the complex and personal problem of excessive human fertility. What is appropriate or acceptable to one couple or one social level may not be suitable for another. Of all the health services, family planning must be one of the most patient orientated areas in medicine, with a multi-contraceptive, multi-disciplinary approach, rather than a doctor-orientated organisation.

The general practitioner requires a sound practical knowledge of the known forms of contraception, so that he can offer informed advice on any method, discuss its advantages and disadvantages and thus dissuade patients from any contraceptive technique which he feels is contraindicated for any reason. There is still a considerable lack of knowledge among patients in general about the various acceptable forms of contraception. The general practitioner is by far the best placed to enquire about a patient's contraceptive practice in a variety of situations — for example during pregnancy and in the puerperium, at the time of an abortion whether spontaneous or therapeutic, when the patient presents with a 'scare' of pregnancy, or when the complaint involves gynaecological symptoms or a sexual problem. The doctor should introduce the question of contraception since in such situations patients seldom raise the subject themselves.

Coitus interruptus
As the name implies, this method involves the interruption of sexual intercourse by withdrawing the penis from the vagina shortly before ejaculation. Due to its apparent simplicity, it is one of the earliest methods known, being widely used before the introduction of more sophisticated techniques of contraception. Various studies (Cartwright 1970, Peel 1972) have shown that about half of

respondents had used withdrawal at some time. Many who use this method do so by choice rather than through ignorance of other alternatives. Failure of this method seems to result in unplanned rather than unwanted pregnancies; the intention is to delay a pregnancy rather than to avoid a pregnancy altogether.

Apart from the unacceptable failure rate of coitus interruptus there can be considerable anxiety for both partners lest it fails. Although it is alleged to contribute to loss of libido, to psychosexual problems or to a depression, coitus interruptus can be highly satisfactory for some couples where the technique has been perfected (e.g. maintaining erection and delaying orgasm until after his partner's). So long as such couples accept that an unplanned pregnancy is possible while at the same time obtaining mutual sexual satisfaction in its use, the doctor should not discourage them. In a study in Finland (Leppo 1978) 'withdrawal' was, along with the condom and the pill, the most commonly used method of contraception. Older patients were thought to have used withdrawal throughout their lives, with satisfactory results. Perhaps the old adage 'some methods are better than others, but any method is better than none' should still be acknowledged.

Natural methods of family planning (NFP)

Natural methods depend on the biological fact that ovulation normally occurs 14 days before the next period. Given a regular (28 day) menstrual cycle, abstinence around the time of ovulation should therefore prevent conception occurring. However, when menstruation is irregular there are obvious difficulties in pre-empting ovulation. A number of methods have been devised to define the beginning and the end of the fertile time in a given cycle.

The calculation method

This was based on a formula produced on the basis of allowing 72 hours for sperm survival, and up to 24 hours for ovum survival. A fertile time of 7 days can be shown to occur with a normal menstrual cycle. However, many women have irregular cycles so that the prediction of ovulation becomes difficult, and the method is fraught with the risk of failure. It can, however, be combined with other methods.

Temperature method

The date of ovulation can be observed with greater accuracy by recording the patient's basal body temperature, which shows a sustained rise at or just after the time of ovulation. Patients require careful teaching of temperature recording, and the nurse in the clinic is the ideal person to do this. It is worth pointing out to the patient that the thermometer can be left by the bedside after taking her temperature, and both reading and recording can be done later in the day when more time may be available. A suitable chart is provided by the National Health Service (see Fig. 15.11, p. 187). As an aside, it should not be forgotten that a continuing raised temperature recorded after ovulation can also detect early conception (Fig. 5.3). This is of value both to the infertile patient, and as evidence of failure of the 'rhythm'

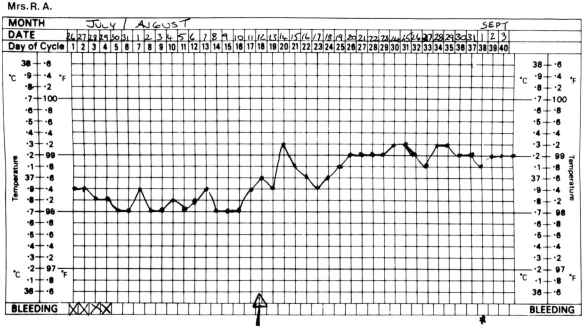

Fig. 5.3 Basal temperature chart showing early conception. (This pregnancy continued uneventfully)

method. To avoid a pregnancy with this method alone, intercourse would have to be restricted to the post-ovulatory infertile phase. Thus this method also should be combined with other signs and symptoms of ovulation.

Ovulation method

Definite cyclical changes occur in the cervical mucus in the course of a menstrual cycle. This is the basis of the 'Billings method' of natural family planning. The changes in cervical mucus are gradual, and have been divided into four phases:

1. 'Dry days' — immediately post-menstruation (associated with low oestrogen levels).
2. Cervical secretion becomes cloudy and sticky (oestrogen levels are rising).
3. 'Wet days' — the cervical mucus increases in volume and becomes clear fluid, the 'ovulation cascade' — marking the peak of fertility (oestrogen levels are at their highest).
4. The cervical mucus decreases sharply, becoming sticky and cloudy (the progesterone levels are increased).

Some women can learn to recognise the changes in the characteristics of their cervical mucus and in particular can assess a reduction in the viscosity of cervical (and vaginal) secretions at the time of ovulation. The fertile period extends from the start of the post-menstrual 'wet' sensation until the fourth day post-peak, averaging 7 to 9 days.

Individual patients can be encouraged to observe several clinical indices of the physiological processes taking place during each cycle. Temperature charting can be combined with observations of cervical mucus changes, mid-cycle pain (Mittelschmerz) and breast sensitivity.

More interest is being shown in NFP, due perhaps to its simplicity, to patients' disenchantment with other methods of contraception and with motivation on religious grounds. With adequate and accurate teaching, the acceptability and effectiveness of NFP has been demonstrated (Flynn 1980). It is estimated that NFP is used by 10–15 million couples world-wide, compared to 50–80 million on the pill and 100 million relying on male or female sterilisation.

Occlusive methods

The female

The use of a vaginal diaphragm or cervical cap means that contraceptive responsibility is very much that of the female. Much debate has taken place as to whether it is the effect of mechanical occlusion or merely the action of the spermicidal jelly or cream which acts as the contraceptive. Modern vaginal occlusive appliances are looked upon as carriers for the spermicidal cream or jellies, with pessaries as further 'back-up'. Types of occlusive devices are:

The vaginal diaphragm. The most popular type of device, consisting of a circular dome of thin rubber with a flat watch spring or coil spring enclosed at the base. Sizes range from 50 mm to 100 mm. In position, the posterior part of the device rests in the posterior fornix, while the anterior rim should tuck comfortably behind the pubic symphysis. The action of the watch spring in the rim is to maintain the rim of the appliance against the vaginal wall, while the pelvic floor muscle tone (albeit resting) pushes inwards, maintaining an occlusive barrier against ascending spermatozoa. Where significant laxity of the vagina, poor pelvic floor musculature, or genital prolapse exist, the vaginal diaphragm is unsuitable (Fig. 5.4).

The cervical cap. A much smaller cup shaped structure which fits directly over the cervix. The rim of the cap

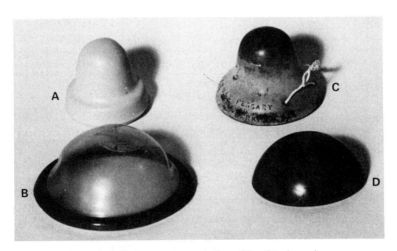

Fig. 5.4 a. Cervical occlusion cap; b. vaginal diaphragm; c. cervical cap (Vimule); d. vault cap

(properly fitted) should fit snugly into the vaginal fornices. Cervical caps are available in four sizes — small, medium, large and extra large. A test of proper fitting is that it should remain in position on straining, and that two examining fingers should not reach the cervix or dislodge the cap. The cervical cap is unsuitable where cervical erosion or chronic cervicitis exists or where the cervix has previously been lacerated.

The vault cap. Fits in the vaginal vault and depends on suction to keep it in place. Unlike the vaginal diaphragm, it has not a watch spring in its base (Fig. 5.4). It is useful where there is marked laxity of the vaginal walls, including genital prolapse, and in cases where the cervix is very short.

Assessment of patients for a diaphragm

The patient who is most interested in the diaphragm method is likely to be intelligent and widely read, aware of the side effects of other forms of contraception, and probably in a higher socio-economic group. A recent survey in England (Allen 1981) showed that the diaphragm was the contraceptive choice of between 1 and 2% of the population and that these women were of an older age and in the higher socio-economic levels. The survey showed the diaphragm to be decreasing in popularity but the impression in family planning circles is of increasing use, particularly following the published evidence of the Royal College of General Practitioners (Beral & Kay 1977).

Continuation rates depend so much on patient motivation, as with most other forms of contraception. Detailed assessment of a patient must include a bimanual pelvic examination at which a cervical smear can also be taken. The distance from the tip of the examining finger deep in the posterior fornix to the inner margin of the pubic symphysis indicates the size of the diaphragm required. The appropriate diaphragm is then squeezed flat and inserted horizontally (in keeping with the cross section of the vagina) taking care to dip the leading part below the cervix, to reach the posterior fornix. The anterior rim of the diaphragm can then be tucked neatly behind the pubic symphysis. Allowing for the tenseness of the patient during examination and fitting, the anterior rim should not protrude from the posterior margin of the symphysis. Nevertheless, the largest size of diaphragm which is comfortable to the patient and which is not protruded on straining, should be used, since considerable relaxation of the vagina can be expected in association with sexual intercourse. Mechanical introducers of the diaphragm are available for patients who have difficulty in inserting it digitally.

The patient herself should be asked to feel the position of the cap following its initial insertion, and to feel the cervix through the diaphragm. Thereafter she should remove it herself, under supervision, by dislodging the rim of the diaphragm from behind the symphysis pubis with a finger, and pulling it out. The patient is then encouraged to practise insertion, either standing with one foot on a chair, or lying in the dorsal position with her knees flexed. The clinic nurse can supervise this practice, and instruct the patient regarding the use of spermicidal jelly, or cream. The patient should be asked to return in a week, with the diaphragm in position, so that its size and current fitting can be checked. When this has been confirmed to the doctor's satisfaction, a new diaphragm is then supplied, or prescribed, together with a further supply of cream, and reviews are usually at 6-monthly intervals. Each new cap is guaranteed only for 12 months and this factor should be explained to the patient, to emphasise the importance of regular reviews. It is important to remember that the size of diaphragm may require to the changed following a confinement, after significant changes in weight, after a vaginal operation, or during the menopause.

A fitting ring set is available containing samples of diaphragms extending through the whole range of sizes, so that an assessment can be made of the optimal size of diaphragm for each patient.

Similar principles apply to the Vault (Dumas) Cap and the vimule (Fig. 5.4) cap with their position over the cervix being maintained by suction. Correct positioning is confirmed by feeling the cervix through the dome of the vault cap. The vault cap or vimule cap is suitable for the woman with a cystocoele or a prolapse, or with a markedly retroverted uterus, when it is unlikely that a diaphragm would be retained.

The male

Sheaths are made of very fine rubber, and are also known as a 'prophylactic', 'protective' 'French letter' or by specific brand names. They are tailored to fit the 'erect penis' closely with the closed end either plain or teatended. Unless spermicidal sheaths are used, it is recommended that the woman uses a contraceptive cream, jelly, foam or pessary since the main cause of method failure is condom breakage discharging semen into the vagina. Care with lubrication (with a spermicide), fitting the sheath well before ejaculation, and care in withdrawal of the penis soon after intercourse while the sheath is closely applied will all help to increase its contraceptive effectiveness. There are a number of situations where the sheath is particularly useful, such as in the early postpartum period, while the woman is waiting to start an oral contraceptive, during the period of instruction with the diaphragm, or during the interval before fitting an intra-uterine device.

The effectiveness of the sheath properly used should not be understated, and Peel (1969) demonstrated a pregnancy rate of 3.1 per 100 woman years — a level which is comparable with the intra-uterine device or the progestogen only pill. In some parts of the world it is the most widely used form of contraceptive. Most failures occur because the sheath is not used regularly. Current use of the sheath varies from country to country, for example in Finland (Leppo 1978) it has the greatest frequency (71%) of all accepted methods, while the figure in two Area Health Authorities in England was of the order of 15% (Allen 1981).

Chemical contraceptives (spermicides)
Spermicides (chemical agents capable of killing spermatozoa) are widely available commercially, in various forms — tubed products (creams and jellies), aerosols (foams), suppositories (soluble pessaries), foaming tablets, or C-film (a water soluble polyvinyl alcohol film). They are intended to be inserted high into the vaginal vault, around the cervix, shortly before intercourse. With the diaphragm, for example, a spermicidal cream *and* pessary are recommended by some authorities, but it is generally accepted that the use of spermicidal cream or jelly is sufficient, although for a second intercourse, the combination is advisable. Spermicides recommended by the Family Planning Association have to pass a series of stringent tests, but it is noteworthy that none of these tests have any legal standing.

The intra-uterine device
The principle of intra-uterine contraception dates back many centuries when small stones were put into the uteri of camels prior to long treks across the desert. During the last century 'wish-bone' and collar-stud pessaries were used. Grafenberg rings (made of coiled silver wire) were not accepted by the medical profession in this country, and the principle of inserting a foreign body into the uterus was condemned, since it was thought that any contraceptive effect would be due to the infection thus produced. However, in the last four decades, there has been a swing in medical opinion towards widespread (but not complete) acceptance of the intra-uterine device (IUD). The number of IUD users throughout the world is steadily increasing, due in part perhaps to anxieties about or disadvantages of alternative methods of contraception, and to the increasing number of personnel now trained to insert intra-uterine devices.

The shape, size, composition and configuration of the devices have changed rapidly in the past 25 years. The earlier models did not contain any active metals or chemicals for slow release within the uterus, and were known as 'first-generation' devices — for example the Birnberg bow, Lippes loop, Margulies spiral, or the Saf-T-Coil. Second-generation or bioactive devices contain copper in the form of wire or bands, releasing copper ions, and others contain hormones, such as progesterone in small regular amounts. A number of devices which either have been in common use, are presently widely used, or coming into vogue are shown in Figure 5.5.

In practice, the types of device now in general use are second generation in type, containing copper — the Copper 7 (Gravigard), the Copper T, the Multiload, and most recently, the Novagard — a modification of the Copper T — which has undergone encouraging trials in Scandinavia (Nygren & Nielson 1981) and which has very recently been marketed in the United Kingdom. Presumptions cannot be made about the reliability or acceptability of a particular device in different parts of the world. The actual device used may be exactly of a defined standard, but difficulties in comparison of results arise due to differences in the level of acceptability of a device — such as the incidence of bleeding or pain for which removal of the device is required. Experience shows that in the analysis of multicentre trials, for example, the variation in recorded events such as bleeding and pain is marked. Such multicentre data illustrate that successful IUCD use depends as much on environmental factors such as who is responsible for the fitting, and the rapport between the person fitting the IUD and the patient, as upon the IUD model itself (Snowden 1982). Time spent in counselling the patient beforehand, in answering any queries and dispelling any doubts, is time well spent. Nursing assistance during insertion is also

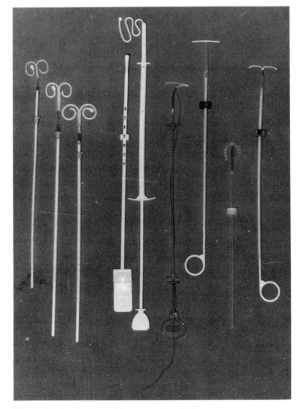

Fig. 5.5 A selection of intra-uterine devices

extrmely important in improving and maintaining the state of relaxation of the patient during the procedure. Skill in terms of manual dexterity with a 'light touch' is important in carrying out the procedure with the minimum of discomfort to the patient. The results (in terms of continuation rate) are enhanced by the psychological effects of the rapport between patient and operator at the time of fitting the device, together with regular reviews and reassurances.

Mode of action of the intra-uterine device

To date, the precise mechanism of action of the IUD remains unclear. The contraceptive effect is thought to involve more than one mechanism — interfering with the chain of events involved in the blastocyst attaching to the uterine well, or by direct action on the blastocyst, or the sperm, or perhaps by a combination of both. Since the effect of the IUD is immediate on fitting, or on removal — or even displaced into the cervical canal — the action of the device must be mainly in the uterus, with its greatest effect around the time of nidation. The action of the bioactive devices is probably more complex than the inert (first generation) devices.

Insertion of an intra-uterine device

Adequate counselling of the patient, including time to talk it over with her consort with all available information, is essential. The warning of possible effects on menstruation must be given, and an initial detailed history will suffice to advise a patient with heavy or irregular periods against an intra-uterine device. The expectations of the method must be discussed with the patient so that she can balance the advantages and disadvantages against, for example, potential problems with oral contraception. An IUD can be fitted any time during the menstrual cycle, but it is usually advised towards the end of, or just after menstruation. There is least risk of pregnancy having occurred, and any slight blood loss due to the fitting will be least noticeable. Adequate alternative contraceptive cover should be ensured if the patient is asked to wait until after her next period.

The post-natal examination at 6 weeks is a suitable and convenient time to insert an IUD provided the patient has been carefully counselled. The device can also be easily fitted immediately after a therapeutic abortion, or at the follow-up examination 2 weeks later. Likewise following evacuation of the uterus for incomplete abortion a device can be fitted at the time, particularly for 'at risk' patients and for those who may be, by habit, poor attenders. Devices inserted within a few days of confinement are more liable to be translocated, or expelled.

Contraindications to insertion of an intra-uterine device

An accurate history is essential as part of initial patient assessment to exclude amenorrhoea due to early pregnancy, and conditions such as recent pelvic inflammation, severe dysmenorrhoea (sometimes exaggerated after insertion of an IUD), known allergy to copper, and valvular heart disease (with the possibility of sub-acute bacterial endocarditis). Menorrhagia (severe enough to cause anaemia), intermenstrual bleeding, or vaginal discharge require investigation, and the treatment of these conditions can eliminate the contraindication.

Pelvic examination is obligatory to confirm the direction and position of the uterus, and a cervical smear can be taken at the same time as well as swabs for culture if indicated. At examination, the following contraindications can be excluded:

1. Established pregnancy.
2. Uterine fibroids — especially if distorting the uterine cavity.
3. Some forms of congenital uterine abnormalities.
4. Acute or subacute pelvic inflammation.
5. Active vaginal infection. A past history of infection need not contraindicate insertiion, but *recurrent* infection in the past should lead one to consider other methods.
6. Genital neoplasms (excluding carcinoma-in-situ of cervix)
7. Uterine scars. Caesarean section scars — especially hysterotomy or myomectomy scars, merit careful consideration before selection of this method.

Nulliparous patients frequently find insertion of a device painful without dilatation of the cervix. Smaller devices have the risk of higher pregnancy rates. The possibility of infection is of greater significance in the nulliparous patient, with its risk of tubal damage, and possible sterility. It has been found in this context that the risk of infection and its complications in nulliparous patients is greatest in women below the age of 25 years (Luukkainen et al 1979).

Most IUD's are now available with their introducers, already sterilised, in pre-packed containers. The necessary equipment for insertion of a device should ideally be pre-packed and autoclaved (many larger health centres are now equipped with small autoclaves). Alternatively, presuming good relations with the local district hospital. IUD packs can be accepted, by arrangement, for dry heat sterilisation. Removal hooks can be boiled or autoclaved.

Equipment for insertion of an IUD

Sterile dressing packs with, preferably, leg drapes
Face mask
Dressing towel
Sterile gloves
Cusco's vaginal speculum
Bowls for antiseptic solution and cream
Teneculum forceps
Sponge-holding forceps with swabs

Uterine sound
Intra-uterine device and introducer
Scissors (preferably 15 cm (6 in) long)
Vulval pad

Technique of insertion

With a pre-prepared autoclaved pack, the instruments are laid up (Fig. 5.6) whilst the patient having previously emptied her bladder is settled on the examination couch. If a cervical smear has not been carried out at a recent assessment, a speculum is passed, and a cervical smear taken, before swabbing down with a solution of cetavlon (2%) or povidone-iodine. Any significant vaginal infection noted at this time would, of course, necessitate swabs being sent for culture, and insertion of the device postponed until after treatment had been successful. A bimanual examination is carried out to confirm the position of the uterus. It is best if the patient is in the lithotomy position since better visualisation of the genital tract is obtained while the operator is 'sitting comfortably' with good lighting over either shoulder.

A Cusco's bivalve speculum (see Fig. 15.2, p, 172) is then inserted, and clamped in position to allow visualisation of the cervix throughout the procedure, while leaving the operator's two hands free. The cervix is gently grasped with the tenaculum forceps, and steadied while the uterine sound is passed along the axis of the uterus to assess the length of the uterine cavity and cervical canal. The flange on the axis of the IUD can then be adjusted to this length so that on inserting the device (while steadying the cervix with the tenaculum forceps) it is known when the end of the device reaches the uterine fundus. It should be remembered that linear plastic de-

vices lose their 'memory' quite readily so that the introducer should not be loaded for more than 2 minutes before insertion. Loading of some devices has the advantage of requiring no such manoeuvre, while at the same time carrying minimal risk of perforating the uterine fundus. Detailed instructions for insertion are supplied with each device and should be carefully followed. About 3–4 cms of thread should be left at the external cervical os, after careful removal of the introducer, since with some devices (e.g. the multiload) the threads run through the cylinder of the introducer.

On completion of the insertion, it is prudent, after swabbing the vagina, to examine bianually to ensure that there is no pelvic tenderness. It should then be explained to the patient that it is quite feasible for her to examine herself vaginally, to feel the threads of the device. It is useful to have a device for demonstration purposes, to allow the patient to feel both the threads of the particular device, as well as the lower end of the axis of the device. Since the threads are stiff initially it is best for the patient to use a pad for the first two or three periods, after which the threads soften and become quite closely apposed to the cervix.

The possibility of expulsion, albeit remote, should be explained to the patient, and that this is more likely to occur during or just after menstruation. It is wise to suggest to patients with an IUD that they examine themselves vaginally from time to time to feel for the tails of the device. This manoeuvre reassures the patient that the device is in its normal position; if partial or total expulsion of the device has occurred, then self-examination is likely to discover this problem.

The first review appointment for the patient is recom-

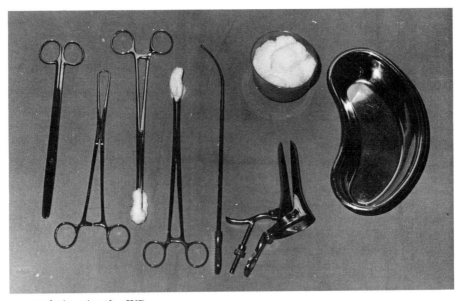

Fig. 5.6 Instruments for insertion of an IUD

mended at 6 weeks, so that she has had a chance to assess her menstrual loss and to report it accordingly. It is always advisable to warn patients of possible side-effects such as bleeding or pain after insertion, but to make it clear that such problems are usually of short duration. It is worthy of note that the patient who experiences considerable discomfort at the time of insertion is invariably the one who will have the shortest continuation rate with any device.

Problems of insertion of an IUD

Most insertions of an IUD are easy, but one in 10 can be expected to be a little difficult, with an occasional one impossible to fit. The routine of bimnual examination prior to insertion of a device is essential since passage of a uterine sound anteriorly when the uterus is retroverted can readily perforate the uterus. Similarly, the uterus is also easily perforated early in the puerperium, and insertion should be avoided at this time, save in exceptional circumstances (such as with a particularly 'at risk' patient). Occasinally, either due to spasm at the internal cervical os, or to an ill-defined cervical canal, it may be impossible to pass an introducer or the device itself. A gynaecological colleague with full theatre lighting and anaesthetic assistance can safely overcome such hurdles without losing the confidence of the patient.

Despite every precaution some patients will experience severe pain during insertion, similar to dysmenorrhoea, though commonly this is transitory. A hot water bottle applied to the abdomen generally relieves the pain, but if it persists, analgesics such as paracetamol may be required. Rarely the pain may persist and be so severe that the device has to be removed, although removal is rarely necessary to aid recovery.

Bleeding at the time of fitting is usually slight, and the most common cause is due to damage to the cervix by the tenaculum forceps — particularly if insertion is being carried out in the post-partum period. Considerable bleeding could result if a device was fitted into a pregnant uterus, but careful initial assessment of the patient by both history and examination should exclude pregnancy if, by habit, devices are inserted in the early post-menstrual phase.

A syncopal attack happens rarely during or just after fitting a device. Treatment consists of slackening any tight clothing, lowering the patient's head, and raising the legs, while at the same time maintaining a good airway. Atropine 0.6 mg should be given intravenously if brachycardia of 50 beats per minute persists. A Brook's airway is also an essential requirement for the resuscitation tray.

Side-effects after insertion of an IUD

Bleeding. A little bleeding after insertion of a device is to be expected and patients should be advised that this is a normal occurrence. The first two or three periods afterwards may well be heavier than before and patients should be warned to expect this. Intermenstrual bleeding (usually 'spotting') is also quite common and should settle within 2 or 3 months. Sometimes, however, heavy periods can persist, giving rise to anaemia, and in some cases, the only solution is to remove the device. In a survey of patients in the author's Well Woman/Family Planning clinic, the six patients with a demonstrable anaemia (except one with a folate deficiency) each had an IUD. A haemoglobin estimation is recommended annually as part of the follow-up for patients with an IUD. The doctor is entirely dependent on the patient's interpretation of heavy bleeding or heavy periods; where the patient seeks the removal of the device in view of continued unacceptable menstrual loss, then her wishes should be acknowledged and the device removed. Prolonged periods, even if not heavy, may lead to an avoidance of intercourse and eventually, on those grounds, cause the patient to seek removal of the device.

Pain. Cramp-like pain can occur in the lower abdomen, similar to dysmenorrhoea. This usually passes off in a day or two, but patients, while reassured, should also be warned that intermittent pain or low backache can continue over the first few weeks. Analgesics can be suggested for recurrence of pain after the diagnosis has been established. In some cases, pain soon after insertion can be due to incorrect fitting of the device — where it is not lying 'flat' in the transverse plane of the uterus; removal of a distorted device can confirm the suspicion of incorrect insertion.

A careful abdominal and bimanual examination is required where pain has occurred following insertion of a device. Negative findings should be used as first hand reassurance to the patient. Absent tenderness should reassure the operator that perforation of the uterus has not occurred but it is possible for a 'silent' perforation to occur. Continuing severe pain makes removal of the device obligatory; where distortion of the device appears to have been the problem another device can be inserted, provided that the patient is agreeable.

Expulsion. Any intra-uterine device can be expelled spontaneously from the uterus. Expulsion is most common during the first 3 months following insertion, and only rarely after the first year. In the review of 50 multi-load devices inserted in the author's clinic, referred to previously, two were expelled — one after 2 months, and the other after 7 months. One of these was the second (different) device to be expelled from one patient who interestingly, although only 23 years of age, had had a very stormy obstetric history — two miscarriages, spontaneous rupture of membranes in two other pregnancies, with premature labour ensuing in one. It is generally accepted that explusion of a device occurs more frequently in younger women of low parity than in older women of high parity. Despite using a device with a known lower expulsion rate, as many as one-third of all reinsertions end in expulsion of the device. It has recently been shown (Emens & Shah 1982) that the expulsion rate of an IUD is unacceptably high (in the region of 25%) if fitted less than 1 week after delivery.

Expulsion may be complete, with the device lying in the vagina, or attached to a large clot on a pad, or it may be lost altogether. Occasionally a woman can be unaware that expulsion has occurred, and often unplanned conception can ensue. Ultrasound examination will locate the device whether within or outwith the uterus, but if scanning facilities are not available, an abdominal X-ray should be carried out (since all devices now used are radio-opaque), provided that an early pregnancy has been excluded.

Extrusion. Apart from perforation of the uterus occurring at the time of insertion, IUDs can occasionally invaginate themselves through the uterine wall, to escape into the peritoneal cavity (particularly to the Pouch of Douglas) or to be trapped between the leaves of the broad ligament. This is termed extrusion, or translocation, as distinct from traumatic perforation at the time of insertion. Surprisingly, perhaps, extrusion may not cause any pain, bleeding or shock, and may not be suspected until, at the patient's next follow-up, the threads of the device are not visible at the external os, the threads however may not have disappeared from view. It is important to check quickly whether the device has been expelled or translocated, since copper devices in the abdomen rapidly form adhesions, and may damage the bowel. First choice method of removal is by laparoscopy, but should this fail, mini-laparostomy is indicated under general anaesthesia.

Where the tails of the device have disappeared, and the device has been shown to be within the uterus, there are a number of methods which can be attempted to rescue the tails. Sometimes they can be caught by Spencer Walls forceps, in the cervical canal, and pulled down to the usual 3 cm length. Suction through a narrow canula can help to retrieve threads which are not visible at the cervix. Alternatively one of a choice of hooks can be used to retrieve the tails, or even the device itself. Rarely, when a device has lost its threads, a hook is necessary to displace the device outwards: the device should always be grasped near the cervical end, to facilitate its uncoiling during removal.

Pregnancy. The failure rate of the traditional inert devices is in the order of 2 to 4 per 100 woman-years (IPPF 1980). Pregnancy is more likely to occur within the first few months of insertion than later; certainly pregnancy rates in the first year are greater than in later years. Incorrect positioning of the device will inevitably be reflected in an increased pregnancy rate.

Two out of three pregnancies occur with the device in situ, while the remainder are associated with unrecognised expulsion, or with translocation. Pregnancy with a device left in situ incurs a greater risk of spontaneous abortion that if it is removed. One Edinburgh study (Steven & Fraser 1974) showed only 14 spontaneous vaginal deliveries occured out of 82 pregnancies with a device in situ. In a number of cases the tails of the device retract within the enlarging uterus. There is no place for attempted removal in those instances, but if the tail remains accessible, the device should be removed. The Central Medical Committee of the International Planned Parenthood Federation agreed in 1975 that 'termination of pregnancy and removal of IUD should be offered to a woman with an unwanted pregnancy where national laws permit this'.

The device can usually be removed in early pregnancy by gentle traction. If this opportunity is refused by the patient, thereby electing to continue with the pregnancy, careful observation is necessary. Advantage can be taken of ultrasonic scanning in early pregnancy, to confirm that the device has not been expelled previously. At confinement, careful inspection of the membranes must be made. If it cannot be found, then the uterus must be explored to remove it, and to confirm that perforation has not occurred. The risk of infection at this stage must be borne in mind.

Ectopic pregnancy. Of pregnancies occurring with an IUD in situ, approximately 5% will be ectopic, compared with about 0.3% of all pregnancies, although this varies in different parts of the world. This increased likelihood of ectopic pregnancy in IUD users emphasises the need for continued alertness in this respect. Any pelvic inflamation or infection associated with an IUD would in the course of tubal involvement interfere with tubal mobility making ectopic pregnancy more likely. It must be remembered however that since there is considerable evidence of significant increase in the incidence of pelvic inflammatory disease (the rate has doubled in the United States, although less than 10% of American women of reproductive age use the IUD) other important factors must be implicated in the rising incidence of ectopic pregnancy (Sivin 1979).

Infection. Controversy over the association of inflammation in the pelvis with the use of IUD's has been long-standing. A major difficulty in quantifying any such association has been in defining the term 'pelvic inflammatory disease'. However, the increased use of laparoscopy in both developed and developing countries has provided opportunities to observe the pelvic organs and the tubes, for assessing and comparing more reasonably, the frequency of pelvic infection. The risk of infection has been shown to be seven times more likely in nulliparous than in parous patients (Lestrom 1979) It is suggested that decreased host resistance to bacterial infection is the explanation for IUD-related inflammatory morbidity. It could also be speculated that organisms gaining entry to the genital tract at the time of menstruation are dealt with less well by the chronically inflamed endometrium and oviduct. Measures to prevent or minimise the risk IUD-related pelvic infections have largely centred on the insertion of the device and the use of sterile equipment at the time of insertion is essential.

Women with evidence of pelvic infection should not be fitted with an IUD until the infection has been cleared. Current opinions recommend immediate treatment with an antibiotic, with removal of the device only if the patient does not respond to treatment within 48 hours. Some protection from bacteraemia should be afforded if the decision is made to remove the device.

Long-term side-effects.

1. There is no evidence that the use of an IUD predisposes to either cervical or endometrial cancer.

2. Given the association between IUD use and pelvic inflammatory disease, with its risk of tubal damage, there has been no confirmation of significantly reduced fertility in the longer term. Vessey et al (1978) in a British study of subsequent fertility of IUD users compared with similar cohorts of women abandoning diaphragms or other traditional contraceptive methods, showed a marked reduction in fertility in IUD users in the first year, but by three and a half years there was no difference between the two groups. This would suggest that some IUD users were slow to recover their fertility, but almost all did so eventually.

Follow-up of patients with IUD

The routine review of a patient fitted with an IUD should be about 6 weeks after fitting, at 6 months, and again at 12 months. If all is well at that time, annual review thereafter is adequate. Practitioners should of course be prepared to see their patients at short notice, should some unforeseen problem appear. They should not be disconcerted if a patient who has had a device inserted in a Health Board Family Planning Clinic consults them as a matter of some urgency with a complication, particularly outwith clinic hours. There should be adequate communication from the clinic with information being given to the general practitioner on the type of device fitted, the findings at examination, and the length of tails left in the vagina. A patient, for example, may attend with considerable anxiety having discovered that she cannot feel the tails of the device. The clinic that inserted the IUD should be informed accordingly.

The oral contraceptive

Combined oral contraceptives

Combined oral contraception first went on trial in 1956, and has been available in the United Kingdom since 1961. The composition of the pill has been modified over the years, with a reduction in the dose of the constituent hormones (oestrogen and progestogen) to the smallest amount that will protect against pregnancy, and yet control the mestrual cycle. The possibility of a steroidal contraceptive for males continues to be explored but remains elusive. The question of acceptability by the male population remains unanswered, although, as evidenced by the increasing demand for vasectomy, an increasing number of men appear to be undertaking responsibility for contraceptive practice.

The most widely used regime is a 21-day course of an oral preparation of oestrogen and progestogen, followed by an interval of 7 days without steroids, during which a 'period' (withdrawal bleeding) will occur. A number of 'combined' pills are marketed to be taken continuously, with inert pills being taken on the days when no hormones are required. This regime was designed to make it easier for women to take a pill *every* day without stopping, but in practice, women who remember tablets at all remember either method equally well.

With the more recent formulae and 'low-dose' permutations, relatively few varieties of preparation are required for the great majority of oral contraceptive users. A number of formulae are manufactured in precisely the same form by different companies, but under different names: this reduces further the number of types to remember. Reference to the British National Formulary, Chapter 7 (Obstetrics and Gynaecology) will confirm the 'pairing' of a number of preparations.

A recent addition to the selection of combined pills has been the 'triphasic' pill — containing three different ratios of combined hormones, and a biphasal variety containing only two ratios. In the triphasic type, the proportion of ethynyloestradiol is increased from 30 μg to 40 μg for 5 days over mid-cycle, while the levonorgestrel is gradually increased from 50 μg to 75 μg and for the last 10 days to 125 μg. The rationale of this variation is to achieve a more accurate physiological imitation of the normal menstrual cycle. Improved cycle control can be expected with this triphasic pill. The biphasic type contains 35 μg ethinyl oestradiol throughout the 21-pill pack, while the progesterone is norethisterone 0.5 mg in the first seven pills, and 1 mg in the remaining 14. These types are claimed to have less effect on blood pressure, and minor side effects such as headache or depression are negligible. They might be expected to improve acne, and to be of some value for patients with greasy hair, a dry vagina, or mild hirsutism. Despite these advantages, it should be remembered that if one pill is forgotten, the margin of error is probably less than with the 'higher dose' standard pill. Nevertheless, the triphasic pill has a useful place, for example, in patients with cardiovascular risk factors who are not happy on the progestogen only pill, or in patients who have recurring breakthrough bleeding on the traditional type of pill.

Continuous oral progestogens

An alternative to combined oral contraception is the progestogen only pill, or 'mini-pill' which consists of a synthetic progestogen. This pill is taken continuously from the first day of menstruation, or after childbirth, and should always be taken at the same time of day. It is particularly useful during lactation and does not affect the milk supply. Neither does it inhibit ovulation in every cycle, nor control menstruation as does the combined pill. The menstrual cycle may, in fact, be somewhat irregular. However, it is very useful for women in the perimenopausal era, for whom combined oral contraception may not be recommended. Side effects of 'combined' hormone preparation, such as weight gain, headaches or cholasma, are usually reduced with a progestogen only preparation. Patients with a history of venous thrombosis with or without pulmonary embolism can be prescribed a progestogen only pill. Recent evidence does suggest some progestogens can also be associated with hypertension, but to a lesser degree than is the case with the combined pill.

The 'morning after' pill

As an 'emergency' means of contraception post-coital contraception is available by prescribing two tablets of a 50 μg oestrogen-containing preparation such as Eugynon 50 repeated 12 hours later, provided that this can be implemented within 72 hours of unprotected intercourse. Experimental work suggests that the oestrogen stimulates ciliary tubal activity and hastens the passage of the ovum into the uterus. Implantation is generally regarded as the beginning of independent life for the developing embryo, and this is thought not to occur for at least 5 days after fertilisation. Earlier work had been done with stilboestrol and ethinyl oestradiol in high doses for 5 days but gastro-intestinal intolerance prevented that regime from gaining in popularity unless an anti-emetic was also administered (Haspels 1976).

Mode of action of the oral contraceptive

The combined oral contraceptive has a number of sites of action which are dependent on a negative neuro-endocrinological feedback within the hypothalamic-pituitary-ovarian axis.

1. First the oestrogen in the pill suppressed the production of follicle stimulating hormone (FSH) resulting in the prevention of ripening of the follicles and of maturation of the ovum. Occasionally, however, ovulation does occur.

2. The lutenising hormone (LH) 'surge' is prevented so that the follicle does not rupture.

3. The production of normal ovulatory mucus by the cervix is prevented; ferning cannot be demonstrated.

4. Cyclical endometrial reaction becomes suppressed thereby reducing the chances of nidation even though ovulation has taken place.

These multiple modes of action of the pill collectively contribute in the high level of effectiveness of the combined oral contraceptive. Even if evaluation were to occur, such is the influence of the pill on the endometrium, the cervical mucus and possibly also on tubal activity, that implantation and therefore pregnancy is extremely rate (about 0.1 per 100 woman years).

The progestogen only pill

This produces a viscous cervical mucus, tends to cause a relative atrophy of the endometrial glands, and is thought to reduce tubal activity. The main site of action is the cervix where the thickened mucus makes it virtually impenetrable to sperms. Ovulation is not prevented in more than 40% of cycles but if fertilisation should occur, the suppressed endometrium makes nidation very unlikely (1–4 per 100 woman years). It is probably the only acceptable oral contraceptive for women over 45 years old, or over 35 years if they smoke cigarettes. The main problem for the patient taking the progestogen only pill is the variability of menstruation. It is wise to forewarn these patients who will then accept the changes more readily and without undue alarm.

Effects of the oral contraceptives

General aspects. Of any cohort of women taking combined pills, 70–80% will have no problems with any formulation. The remainder have side effects to some extent; some of these may be improved by a change of formula, either by a change in proportion of the same constituents or by changing either the proogestogen or the oestrogen components. It must not be forgotten that psychological factors may play a considerable part in the sphere of contraception. It may be that the most potent cause of side effects from the pill may be the attitude of the physician, and the influence of his approach to the patient on this subject is very important. Varying the dose and effectiveness of the progestogens is facilitated by the fact that a number of companies market pills with different doses of the same compounds, combined with an identical amount of oestrogen. If a woman normally has menorrhagia or dysmenorrhoea, then a preparation with a higher amount of progestogen is indicated. When a satisfactory response has been obtained the proportion of progestogen can be reduced after, say, 6 months, to reduce the total steroid load. On the other hand, where a patient's main anxiety is with acne, or hirsutism, then a low dose of progestogen would be indicated. Either way, the lowest dose pill will have the least effect in enhancing the appetite thereby decreasing any risk of weight gain.

It should always be remembered that women who choose to use oral contraceptives tend to differ from those who choose the IUD or barrier methods in factors such as their past fertility, coital frequency, standard of sexual hygiene, smoking, and age. Comparisons between patients using oral contraceptives and those with IUD's or barrier methods are rarely valid; some other significant factors may be present in the oral contraceptive users.

Endocrine effects. The pill causes marked suppression of the release of gonadotrophins, and the oestrogen component of the combined pill increases the total plasma cortisol levels. The 'progestogen only' preparations do not have this effect on plasma cortisol levels.

Thromboembolism and cardiovascular disorders. The link between venous thromboembolism and the combined oral contraceptive was the major stimulus to the development of the low oestrogen type and progestogen only pills. Oestrogen was recognised as the major cause of the changes in blood coagulation factors, so that most combined preparations have 30 μg or 35 μg of oestrogen. The progestrogen-induced fall in high density lipoprotein cholesterol was a later discovery, as was the tendency to hyperinsulinism associated with the androgen-related progestogens such as levonorgestrel and norethisterone. These changes are thought to be relevant to the causation of arterial disease, principally to myocardial infarction and strokes. The incidence of myocardial infarction and cerebrovascular accidents is fortunately rare, particularly in non-smokers, and the latest RCGP Report (March 1981) shows no effect of duration of use. In fact, a review of death registrations in a number of developed countries with a high use of oral contraceptives shows a decline over time in the mortality from cardiovascular disease (International Planned Parenthood Federation 1981).

Oral contraceptive users have a slightly higher morbidity than non-users from venous thromboembolism. Since the oestrogen component is the implicated factor, the lowest effective dose of oestrogen should be used. When major surgery is contemplated, oral contraception should be stopped at 6 weeks before operation, alternative effective contraception should be advised, and the pill can be restarted 4 weeks after surgery. For emergency procedures, the surgeon may consider the use of prophylactic anticoagulant measures.

The potential risks of the oral contraceptive should be adequately explained to patients and possible alternative contraceptive methods discussed, especially for some 'at risk' groups of women such as those aged over 40, those who smoke and are over 35 years old, those with proven hypertension, or epilepsy, nulliparous women with a history of dysmenorrhoea or amenorrhoea.

Since in general practice the doctor has a responsibility to only a small population of women of childbearing age, each patient merits individual consideration in terms of her priorities, presence of risk factors, together with the risks of possible pregnancy in her particular case. The older woman who smokes, for example, should either give up smoking, or be counselled in other methods of contraception. The compounding risk factors such as smoking, obesity, age and mild hypertension should be made quite clear to patients in discussions on oral contraception. Where alternative methods of contraception are available for substitution, it would be prudent to be cautious where relative contraindications exist.

Hypertension. The blood pressure should be measured as a baseline at the initial assessment of a patient, prior to the use of an oral contraceptive. Although a number of patients develop minor increases in blood pressure while using oral contraceptives, about 5% become frankly hypertensive after years of use. If a patient's blood pressure rises to levels of 160 mmHg (systolic) and 100–105 mmHg (diastolic) on an oral contraceptive, having been normotensive originally, the pill should be discontinued, and an alternative form of contraception agreed upon. Patients showing minor increases in blood pressure readings at successive visits should be reviewed at more frequent intervals, such as 3-monthly, so that any further increases can be identified. Where risk factors such as previous hypertension exist careful monitoring must be maintained if such a patient is to be prescribed an oral contraceptive.

Depression. Although there is reasonable evidence that the oral contraceptive relieves the premenstrual syndrome in many women, occasionally it can be associated with episodes of depression. If symptoms are significantly affecting the patient's life the pill should be discontinued, but it must be remembered that the patient with a psychiatric disorder may not take kindly to alternative forms of contraception, nor to the stress of an unwanted pregnancy. Pyridoxine (Vitamin B6) may be tried on an empirical basis in such cases — sometimes with good effect — obviating any change in type of pill, or of method.

Drug interaction. Drugs may interact with oral contraceptives in several ways. Firstly, they influence the absorption of the oral contraceptive by decreasing its solubility in water, by altering the gastro-intestinal pH, or by causing gastro-intestinal hurry or slowing. Secondly, drugs can activate or inhibit the metabolism of the oral contraceptive. Thirdly, there can be competition for a common receptor, for example the administration of a contraceptive steroid at the same time as a corticosteroid may produce a synergistic effect on the corticosteroid action thus necessitating a reduction in the dosage of the steroid.

'Breakthrough' ovulation may occur when an oral contraceptive user is treated with an antibiotic such as rifampicin, ampicillin, amoxycillin, and tetracycline or with an anticonvulsant such as phenytoin and phenobarbitone.

During short-term chemotherapy, another form of contraception should be considered as an adjuvant; with long-term therapy such as with an anticonvulsant, either a 'higher dose' preparation (with 50 μg ethinyl oestradiol in combination) should be used, or a long-term contraceptive alternative chosen. Conversely, oral contraceptives can alter the effect of some drugs such as Marevan or the tricyclic drugs, and again when such therapy is given, it is preferable to advise an alternative form of contraception. It should be noted that the number of reported drug interactions is still low but the risks of interaction must be somewhat greater with the present day low dose combined contraceptive steroids.

Lactation. Breast feeding has increased in popularity in recent years, without as yet reaching the level attained in developing countries. There is increasing evidence that oral contraceptive preparations have an adverse effect on the quantity and possibly the quality of milk, and on the duration of lactation. To encourage the maintenance of adequate breast milk supplies, the progestogen only pill should be recommended until the infant is weaned.

Subsequent fertility. Since a small number of women can be expected to have a short episode of amenorrhoea on discontinuing the oral contraceptive it could be deduced that there may be relative infertility during this time. Any such reduction has been shown to be nullified within 2 years and a period of amenorrhoea for up to 6 months does not itself merit special referral or investigation. Women whose ovulation is significantly suppressed usually respond to 'fertility' drugs such as bromocriptine, or clomiphene citrate.

Attempts should be made to find the cause if amenorrhoea persists for more than 6 months. Specialist referral is wisest, so that aetiological factors such as pituitary or adrenal tumours can be excluded. Occasionally, post-pill amenorrhoea can be associated with hyperprolactinaemia, so that a pituitary tumour has to be excluded. Following exclusion of a pituitary lesion, bromocriptine will successfully reduce the elevated prolactin levels. There is no evidence that the oral contraceptive can induce a pituitary adenoma; nor does post-pill amenorrhoea appear to be related to duration of therapy. For patients with a past history of amenorrhoea when periods have spontaneously returned to normal, the combined pill does not appear to be contraindicated. However, in cases of amenorrhoea which require specific therapy to induce ovulation, further use of the pill is probably inadvisable.

Jaundice. Reports of jaundice in patients on oral contraception have appeared in the UK and in Scandinavia. Patients who have a history of recurring idiopathic jaundice of pregnancy should avoid oral contraception. Likewise the patient with a past history of infective (viral) hepatitis should be advised against oral contraception until the liver function tests have returned to normal for 12 months. Where gall stones are known to exist an alternative to oral contraception should be advised, since the pill could possibly increase the production of further gall stones.

Injectable steroids

Injectable contraceptives, although suitable for a small group of particularly vulnerable, 'at risk' patients nevertheless do have a number of advantages which mean that this method should be available in any family planning programme. Much scientific evaluation on this group of contraceptives has been done; for example, depomedroxyprogesterone acetate has been subjected to more scientific study throughout the world than any other single hormonal contraceptive preparation (IPPF 1981).

The steroid is given by intramuscular injection (150 mg every 3 months) and this is an acceptable method of contraception in countries where injections are a familiar part of preventive or therapeutic health care. The steroid can be administered in privacy, and because of the medical supervision required is well suited to the forgetful patient, or to the patient of lower intelligence, who has not understood or is not capable of the responsibilities of the traditional methods of contraception.

Although the World Health Organization stated in 1979 that there were no toxicological reasons for discontinuing the use of medroxyprogesterone acetate in family planning programmes, the Committee on Safety of Medicines recommends its use only in two short-term situations:

1. For wives of men undergoing vasectomy for contraception until the vasectomy becomes effective.
2. In women being immunised against rubella, to prevent pregnancy during the period of activity of the virus.

Fears of possible long-term effects of the drug have to be balanced against the immediate effects of a rest from repeated childbearing which is so vital for the health of the most deprived patients. In such circumstances, practitioners who select the injectable method for particular patients must keep careful and accurate records, with a detailed summary of the rationale and indications for this method. Menstrual irregularity may be quite marked with medroxyprogesterone acetate — varying from periods of amenorrhoea for the full 3 months, to an increased or prolonged loss, or a decreased flow. The most unpredictable effects on the menstrual pattern occur during the first few months of use, and the normal schedule may be replaced by intermittent slight bleeding, or staining of unpredictable duration, interval, and rate of flow. A number of women will demonstrate amenorrhoea immediately, and by the end of 2 years, about 40% of patients on the injectable method tend to be amenorrhoeic. It is therefore of paramount importance that these patients be counselled fully beforehand about the possible disturbances of the menstrual pattern and the risk of ensuing amenorrhoea. Such an occurrence would then be rightly regarded as minor inconvenience, and anxiety allayed. There is a tendency to weight gain with depo-provera but this levels off after about a year. Dietary advice however should be offered at the start of therapy, since most women experience an increased appetite.

With some high risk groups of patients the injectable contraceptive has had a high continuation rate. This method avoids the side-effects of oral contraceptives and intra-uterine devices. It is useful for the lactating woman, and provides an alternative method for women who cannot tolerate the oestrogen-related side-effects of the pill, or the pain and bleeding of intra-uterine devices. There are no demonstrable adverse metabolic effects, and although the return to fertility may be delayed for up to 12 months, there is no known long-term impairment of fertility.

Despite the acceptance of depomedroxyprogesterone acetate (Depo-Provera) by the Committee on Safety of Medicines as a long-term contraceptive, the Minister of Health, in September, 1982, upheld the licensing authority's view that the risk of using Depo-Provera outweighs the benefit from such use. The World Health Organization, however, has already published a memorandum in which its use is endorsed (WHO 1982).

ABORTION

COUNSELLING

The realisation of an unplanned pregnancy is invariably an emotional shock for a woman. In the UK it is customary for such a patient to approach her general practitioner, or to attend a family planning clinic for advice. The doctor has firstly to come to terms with his own immediate responses to such a situation. Abortion counselling — and that is precisely what such a consultation constitutes — must avoid any 'directive' tendency, and the doctor as counsellor must remain 'detached' from the problem. Counselling is time consuming, but every general practitioner who provides contraceptive services should also be prepared to provide abortion counselling whenever necessary.

The patient requires guidance and help in coming to a decision on whether or not to seek an abortion. The alternatives to abortion must be explained to her as well as its implications and problems. At the same time future contraceptive measures should be discussed, information supplied, and, if possible, provisional plans can be made even at this stage. All reasonable help should be afforded the patient in preventing a recurrence of an unwanted pregnancy. Frequently the patient needs a little more

time to think over her situation in the light of what she has been told. Girls under 16 years of age should be encouraged to discuss their problem with their parents. Most mothers, at least, come round to a sympathetic understanding of their daughter's plight, and take some of the burden from the girl's shoulders after she has perhaps suffered some weeks of fear and guilt without confiding in anyone.

Only a matter of days should be allowed for further thoughts and deliberation on the patient's part, since, if abortion is decided upon, the earlier it is done, the greater the safety of the procedure and the less the risk of complications. In the meantime, a pregnancy test should be done to confirm suspicions of an early pregnancy.

In considering abortion for any patient, all relevant personal, economic and medical details should be obtained, as well as a gynaecological history. The present relationship of the patient with the putative father should be established: if married, are divorce proceedings being instigated?, does the husband know of the pregnancy?, is it his child? If the patient is single or divorced, is the relationship stable, or was it merely a casual encounter?, is marriage (or remarriage) planned? There may be extenuating circumstances, such as other young siblings in the same household, or the patient may be a single parent with one or more children already in the family.

In these varying situations, the plight of the individual patient, together with the plight of existing child or children within a home which is already broken, merit detailed consideration in relation to the various clauses of the Abortion Act. The involvement of a social worker is of considerable assistance. A detailed background knowledge of the family, the care of other children, the support available from relatives, as well as conditions of living accommodation (whether rented (and paid up) or unofficially sub-let, or due for demolition) and an appraisal of her financial circumstnaces all provide a valuable backcloth to further counselling and to a decision regarding abortion. The World Health Organization (1971), in its analysis of abortion laws in different countries, accepted that a complete spectrum existed — from the extremes of abortion not being permitted under any circumstances, to abortion being permitted at the request of the pregnant woman.

The clauses of the Abortion Act (1967) of the United Kingdom include specific well-defined criteria — more than one of which may refer to a particular case:

1. The continuance of the pregnancy would involve risks to the life of the pregnant woman greater than if the pregnancy were terminated.

2. The continuance of the pregnancy would involve risk of injury to the physical or mental health of the pregnant woman greater than if the pregnancy were terminated.

3. The continuance of the pregnancy would involve

risk of injury to the physical or mental health of the existing child(ren) of the family of the pregnant woman greater than if the pregnancy were terminated.

4. There is a substantial risk that if the child were born, it would suffer from such physical or mental abnormalities as to be seriously handicapped.

Certificate 'A' (Fig. 5.7) must be completed, signed, and dated, by two registered medical practitioners prior to the termination of the pregnancy (whether in Scotland or England). The usual procedure is that on referral of the patient to a gynaecologist the general practitioner signs the form, having ringed the appropriate number(s) of clause(s), and forwards it with a detailed covering letter. With the relevant information and background available, following assessment and examination, the gynaecologist is then in a position to confirm the indications for abortion. General practitioners should remember, however, that should they not be in agreement with the patient's wishes regarding termination of pregnancy, they are duty bound to refer her forthwith for another opinion, or to ask the patient to consult another doctor, or to attend the nearest Family Planning Clinic. Delay should be avoided at this stage of the proceedings, and a judicious phone call to the appropriate gynaecological clinic secretary usually obviates this risk.

Written consent of the patient is always obtained before operation. A patient aged 16 years or over may give consent, but for those under 16, the consent of a patient must be obtained. With a married woman, however, the husband's consent is not necessary — a fact of considerable help where the husband is not the putative father.

In an emergency, to save a patient's life, or to avoid serious permanent physical or mental injury, a registered medical practitioner may perform an abortion without delay. Certificate 'B' (Fig. 5.8) requires to be signed by the practitioner either before performing the abortion, or within 24 hours after it. A second signatory is not necessary.

Follow-up and future contraceptive practice
It is extremely difficult to estimate accurately the use of accepted forms of contraception in patients attending for abortion counselling. The stressful situation is self-evident and in these circumstances correct answers may not be given as to whether contraception was used (and failed) or not. Studies have shown that as many as 80% of girls who were pregnant for the first time had used no form of birth control. With the traditional methods of contraception, it is accepted that there is a failure rate, and abortion becomes a back-up for the estimated 5% who do fail. The resultant thousands of unplanned and probably unwanted pregnancies reflect the present era of society and social conditions. The trend towards women having educational or employment careers has undoubtedly had a significant influence on the opinions of

women over 30 years with regard to abortion, and indeed to sterilisation also.

Follow-up of an abortion patient is important since for many young girls who have just had their first pregnancy terminated, this is their first experience of proper contraception. Many may not have known how to seek advice, or where to get supplies, but having matured throughout the experience of a therapeutic abortion, most girls and young women begin to understand the raison d'être of adequate contraceptive practice.

Early follow-up of abortion patients (after 2 weeks or so) is thought to be the best, since later arrangements appear to produce a larger number of defaulters. Many, if unsupervised at this stage, would be at precisely the same risk as before, without proper contraception. A patient going on the pill after a therapeutic abortion is advised to start on the night of her operation to afford immediate cover. Likewise, the patient who wishes to have an intra-uterine device fitted can have it inserted at the time of operation, or certainly within 2 weeks of operation, assuming that there are no contraindications. It has been shown that the insertion of an IUD immediately after a suction evacuation of the uterus gives rise to no greater risk of infection than does insertion at a later date. Continuation rates correspond to those fitted inter-menstrually. After a pregnancy is terminated all patients should be offered a choice of follow-up via the hospital, a local clinic or her family doctor. Many such patients may not have family doctors in the neighbourhood, and ideally, each Area Health Board should have an arrangement for follow-up of non-attenders.

Neither ignorance nor naivety can explain the high incidence of unwanted pregnancies. Illegitimate pregnancies continue to increase in Scotland and the abortion rate for teenage pregnancies continues to rise (Scottish Health Statistics — Scottish Health Service). Following termination of a pregnancy explanation and encouragement are required to maintain contact with the patient and to extend the continuation rate of the chosen method of contraception, since it is possible for the use of contraception itself to induce feelings of guilt and conflict.

Sequelae of abortion
The length of hospital stay for patients undergoing termination of pregnancy is usually short; some units having a 'day-case' policy for selected patients at a very early stage of pregnancy. Follow-up is invariably scanty unless it is positively organised by the family doctor and patient compliance can leave much to be desired.

Morbidity and complications increase with increased duration of pregnancy, and not unexpectedly, some variation occurs dependent upon the method of termination used. With a short stay in hospital, more patients

> **IN CONFIDENCE**

Certificate A
(Schedule 1)

Not to be destroyed within three years of the date of the operation

ABORTION ACT 1967
Certificate to be completed in relation to abortion under Section 1(1) of the Act

I,...
(Name and qualifications of practitioner in block capitals)

of...

....
(Full address of practitioner)

Have/have not* seen/examined* the pregnant woman to whom this certificate

relates at ....
(Full address of place at which patient was seen or examined)

....

on ....

and I,...
(Name and qualifications of practitioner in block capitals)

of...
(Full address of practitioner)

....

Have/have not* seen/and examined* the pregnant woman to whom this certificate

relates at ....
(Full address of place at which patient was seen or examined)

....

on ....
*Delete as appropriate

We hereby certify that we are of the opinion, formed in good faith, that in the

case of...
(Full name of pregnant woman in block capitals)

of...

....
(Usual place of residence of pregnant woman in block capitals)

1. the continuance of the pregnancy would involve risk to the life of the pregnant woman greater than if the pregnancy were terminated;
2. the continuance of the pregnancy would involve risk of injury to the physical or mental health of the pregnant woman greater than if the pregnancy were terminated;
3. the continuance of the pregnancy would involve risk of injury to the physical or mental health of the existing child(ren) of the family of the pregnant woman greater than if the pregnancy were terminated;
4. there is a substantial risk that if the child were born it would suffer from such physical or mental abnormalities as to be seriously handicapped.

Ring appropriate number(s)

This certificate of opinion is given before the commencement of the treatment for the termination of pregnancy to which it refers.

Signed ....

Date...

Signed ....

Date...

(OVERLEAF: CERTIFICATE B—FOR USE IN CASES OF EMERGENCY)

Fig. 5.7   Certificate A (Abortion Act)

```
┌─────────────────────┐
│   IN CONFIDENCE     │
└─────────────────────┘
```

**Certificate B
(Schedule 1)**

**Not to be destroyed within three
years of the date of the operation**

ABORTION ACT 1967
**Certificate to be completed in relation to abortion performed
in emergency under section 1(4) of the Act**

I...
(Name and qualifications of practitioner in block capitals)

of..

....
(Full address of practitioner)

hereby certify that I *am/was of the opinion, formed in good faith, that it *is/was necessary
immediately to terminate the pregnancy of

....
(Full name of pregnant woman in block capitals)

of..

....
(Usual place of residence of pregnant woman in block capitals)

(Ring
appropriate
number)

in order 1. to save the life of the pregnant woman; or

          2. to prevent grave permanent injury to the physical or mental health of the
             pregnant woman.

This certificate of opinion is given—

(Ring
appropriate
letter)

    A. before the commencement of the treatment for the termination of the pregnancy to
       which it relates; or, if that is not reasonably practicable, then

    B. not later than 24 hours after such termination.

Signed ....

Date..

*Delete as appropriate

(OVERLEAF: CERTIFICATE A)

Fig. 5.8   Certificate B (Abortion Act)

come immediately under the responsibility of their general practitioner, who is under no obligation to report any complications he may meet. Management may involve admission of the patient to the unit where the termination was carried out, or to a hospital in a different part of the country. Alternatively, the patient may be managed at home. The immediate risks of abortion are:

1. Perforation of the uterus.
2. Laceration of the cervix.
3. Haemorrhage.

Short-term risks (within a week or so of operation) are infection and secondary haemorrhage. Longer-term sequelae and future obstetric performance are presently being studied on a combined basis by the Royal College of General Practitioners and the Royal College of Obstetricians and Gynaecologists ('Attitude to Pregnancy' Study).

The 'immediate' risks are minimised by early termination of pregnancy; the earlier this is done the less are the complications — both immediate and longer term. There is convincing evidence in Scandinavia of reduced morbidity in patients who are aborted early, and in patients who are counselled, assessed and operated on by an experienced doctor, and as far as possible by the same doctor.

The method of termination of pregnancy also influences sequelae. Vacuum extraction (used for suction evacuation of the uterus up to 12 weeks gestation) appears to have no obvious effect on the next pregnancy. Comparison of subsequent pregnancies to either spontaneous or induced abortion showed no differing effects relating to short gestation or low birth weight. Dilatation and curettage, on the other hand, especially in less experienced hands, or with inappropriate anaesthesia, can cause trauma to the cervix, with resultant incompetence precipitating premature labour or second-trimester spontaneous abortion in future pregnancies.

The psychological effects of abortion are very variable. Women who are in good physical and mental health are unlikely to suffer psychological trauma from abortion — provided they wanted it, and did not have it forced on them by others. Women with a pre-existing psychiatric illness, however, may well find that termination has precipitated an exacerbation of their condition. Alternatively, they may suffer greater psychological morbidity if they were refused abortion, and forced to go through with the pregnancy and to look after an unwanted baby later. Such women need a particularly sympathetic approach throughout counselling and continued support afterwards. Patients undergoing second trimester abortions are more likely to be immature, may be more ambivalent towards abortion in the first place, and may have long-standing poor relationships within the family. These patients can be expected to need more support

after termination of pregnancy than those who sought and obtained early abortion. It is hoped that further light will be shed on psychological sequelae or behavioural changes following abortion by the 'Attitude to Pregnancy' Study.

Quite apart from the possible sequelae for the mother, if abortion were refused, the question of the potential environment of the unborn child must also be considered. Factors such as the maturity or immaturity of the mother, domestic or financial insecurity (particularly where parental rejection has resulted), mental or physical cruelty by the putative father, or the likelihood of subsequent psychiatric crisis, must be weighed against possible neglect of the baby, or non-accidental injury precipitated by the adverse emotional effects of an unwanted pregnancy.

STERILISATION — MALE AND FEMALE

Sterilisation has in recent years become an increasingly popular alternative method of fertility regulation by which individuals have the right of control over their own fertility. The indications for sterilisation have widened from eugenic reasons and genuine medical indications as a way of preservation of health, to the decision of an individual couple that their family is complete. Family sizes are, on average, now considerably less than they were two or even one decade ago. The older patient with her completed family is aware that no one of the accepted reversible methods of family planning is without failure; she also recognises the increased risks for the older patient of pregnancy and childbirth.

With the development of modern techniques of sterilisation (by laparoscopy) and the use of silicone rings or metallic clips to occlude the fallopian tubes, there is no reason for restricting sterilisation to patients above a particular age or parity. Sterilisation counselling is of the utmost importance since the procedure, in contrast to other, reversible, forms of fertility control, is likely to be permanent. Provided the operation and its implications are discussed thoroughly and the couple is given some time to come to their own conclusions with the help of appropriate information, there is no reason why sterilisation should be withheld once it is decided that it is, for them, the most acceptable and efficient method of birth control.

The risks of the operation, or of the long-term use of oral contraceptives with increasing age, have to be weighed against the risks of an unplanned pregnancy, towards the end of the woman's reproductive life. Apart from recommending sterilisation on medical grounds, the onus is on the doctor to look for any contraindications to such a decision when it is opted for by the patient on socio-economic grounds. It is the doctor's responsibility to review the psychological and sociological state of the man or woman requesting sterilisation, and to assess the stability of the marriage. A high age differential between husband and wife immediately introduces a note of caution regarding possible sterilisation of the younger partner, particularly if the woman is by far the younger.

MALE OR FEMALE STERILISATION?

Health reasons can constitute one reason why one partner rather than the other should be sterilised. Psychological and social actors may themselves lead to the couple's own rational decision as to which partner should be sterilised. Male sterilisation (vasectomy) is largely done on an outpatient basis, under local anaesthesia, thus causing little interruption to home life, and to bread-winning. Sterilisation of the female, however, commonly involves hospitalisation for at least one or more (usually two) nights so that home and family life is disrupted for a matter of days until normal activities of motherhood can be resumed. Vasectomy is not necessarily a quicker procedure than laparoscopic (female) sterilisation, nor is waiting time for vasectomy shorter despite a number of options for operation — by a urologist, general surgeon, family planning clinic, or general practitioner. In this country laparoscopic sterilisation is very much the province of the gynaecologist and has to take its place with a variety of other procedures in gynaecological surgery — including termination of pregnancy — so that waiting lists develop readily. Also, laparoscopy itself is not without hazard, such as puncture of the bowel or of a major blood vessel, and technical difficulties such as obesity or adhesions from previous abdominal surgery may necessitate formal laparotomy. A confidential enquiry into Gynaecological Laparoscopy by the Royal College of Obstetricians and Gynaecologists (1977) showed that 41 of every 1000 laparoscopic sterilisations had immediate complications.

Neither male nor female sterilisation is 100% effective. Waiting time for vasectomy may be shorter, but its disadvantages include a period of 4 months postoperatively when sterilisation is not complete, and spontaneous re-canalisation is relatively common following vasectomy.

Female sterilisation

No counselling should omit details of the procedure, nor should any queries of the patient be avoided. Common worries include the after-effects of the operation, its effect on sexual intercourse or on menstruation. The patient should be warned that no method is perfect, and that it is possible for a pregnancy to occur (1 in 100 after 7 years) after sterilisation. Occasionally questions will be asked about the feasibility of reversal of the operation, but it is important to emphasise that, if there are genuine

indications for the operation, it should be accepted as permanent. Reversal of sterilisation can be carried out but the patient should be warned that the success rate is in the region of 50%, and that the risk of ectopic pregnancy is increased.

An outline of the usual procedure with sterilisation should always be included in the counselling, mentioning briefly the type of operation (tiny incision, two clips), the type of anaesthesia, and that discharge from hospital is usually 24 hours after the procedure. Some gynaecologists allow the patient home later the same day, but with the ring technique some post-operative pain is not uncommon (Lawson et al 1976). Clips of plastic or metal are easy and safe to apply, and damage only a small piece of tube. Reversal of sterilisation is easier with the use of clips since only a small piece of tube has been damaged, and the lumen of each part to be anastomosed is of equal diameter. The surgical techniques of sterilisation will differ, depending on whether the woman is obese, has concomitant pelvic or systemic disease, or whether the operation is post-partum, post-abortion or as an interval procedure. Elective sterilisation is to be preferred since the risks of regret, of failure and of surgical complications are least. Even in the presence of symptoms attributable to pelvic disease few women are likely to prefer the major operation of hsyterectomy to the relatively minor procedure of laparoscopy.

Complications
1. At *operation* (laparoscopy):
a. Perforation of a blood vessel, either by the needle used to introduce the pneumoperitoneum, or by the trocar for the laparoscope.
b. Direct trauma to the bowel by the trocar.
2. *Later:*
a. Bleeding can occur from the abdominal wall, or from the mesosalpinx. Evidence of intraperitoneal bleeding or haematoma formation necessitates laparotomy to examine the extent of any damage, and to effect haemostasis. Small haematomas of the abdominal wall can be treated conservatively.
b. Peritonitis following inadvertent burns of the bowel used to be a problem when diathermy of the fallopian tube was the technique used. At the time, no obvious damage such as perforation would necessarily have occurred, but ischaemic necrosis gradually develops over a few days, resulting in sloughing in the central part of the burn, with the escape of bowel contents into the peritoneal cavity. The sloughed area requires to be removed, with appropriate end-to-end anastomosis thereafter.
c. A ureteric fistula can occur, where diathermy of the mesosalpinx has similarly produced ischaemic necrosis to the base of the broad ligament, damaging the blood supply of the ureter, with consequent escape of urine into

the peritoneal cavity instead of into the bladder.

3. *Longer-term sequelae:*

a. *Ectopic pregnancy.* Rarely a fistula can arise at the uterine end of the tube, and by this means (via the peritoneal cavity) sperms can reach the fimbrial end of the tube, and fertilise the ovum, which becomes 'impacted' in the occluded portion of the tube. The clinical picture is as for the classical ectopic pregnancy but the doctor can be misled by assuming that following sterilisation, no pregnancy is possible.

b. *Intra-uterine pregnancy.* The failure rate of abdominal sterilisation varies from 0.3% to 1% depending on the type of procedure used and the experience of the operator. In these circumstances the patient's request for termination of the pregnancy should be met.

c. It is possible for torsion of the distal segment of the tube to occur after tubal ligation. Symptoms resemble those of torsion of an ovarian cyst without a palpable significant mass.

Male sterilisation

Vasectomy has increased in popularity over the last 15 years. As with female sterilisation, similar thorough initial counselling is of great importance. The male must be reassured that his sexual performance will in no way be affected, and a clear explanation of the mechanism of continuing ejaculate, without alteration in its volume, must be made to the patient. The best recommendation for this method of contraception usually comes from a friend who has had the operation, and who can reassure the patient that his future sexual performance will not be inhibited in any way.

As for female sterilisation, it should be explained to the couple that the operation is intended to be permanent, but very rarely, a pregnancy can occur. Sterilisation does not, of course, result immediately after the operation. Two specimens of ejaculate are tested at intervals of 3 and 4 months after the operation. When two successive samples of semen have been confirmed a sperm-free, the patient is acknowledged as being sterile.

The history-taker should exclude any previous scrotal swelling or operation, such as herniorrhaphy or excision of varicocele, and orchitis following mumps. The presence of diabetes or of significant anaemia can influence the incidence of post-operative infection. Any allergy or previous reaction to local anaesthesia should also be excluded.

The surgical approach is via the skin at the neck of the scrotum, where the spermatic cord can be located, and a small incision is made over it. Up to 4 cm of cord is removed: it is argued that removal of a small portion facilitates possible reconstruction in the future, while re-canalisation of the vas is less likely if a longer portion of cord is removed. The excised portions of vas should be sent for histological examination — for confirmation of the procedure in case any question of litigation should arise at a later date. Most surgeons make a separate approach to each vas but a few use a single midline incision in the scrotum, and expose each vas in turn prior to double ligation and removal of a segment. Skin sutures are usually subcuticular, and of absorbable material, thus obviating any need for removal of sutures. Superficial bruising and haematoma formation is usually avoided by strict haemostasis at operation. After a day's rest the patient should be encouraged to return to work unless it involves heavy manual work. Firm underwear or swimming trunks should be worn for 2 weeks after operation, to avoid the dragging pain from the distended testicles.

Complications

1. *Bruising* of the skin or haematoma (small ones are not uncommon). Larger haematomas are invariably painful and require evacuation since they can be a nidus for infection. Up to 5% of patients may have some degree of haemorrhagic sequelae — usually mild in degree, but occasionally a haematoma may reach the size of an orange.

2. *Pain* may be expected when the effect of the local anaesthetic wears off, and the patient should be warned of this possibility. Severe pain may suggest significant haematoma formation; rest coupled with a prophylactic antibiotic will minimise the risk of infection: rarely surgical drainage will be necessary.

3. *Infection* can also occur, but is less common than haematoma. An antibiotic will be required, and if clinical impressions suggest the formation of pus, it should be drained — via the incision if possible. Rarely an abscess may form, necessitating drainage.

Mention should also be made of a few remote complications, such as epididymitis, orchitis, sinus formation, spermatic granuloma, or spontaneous re-anastomosis.

Until such time as the vasectomy can be confirmed as successful, effective contraception must be continued. One of the indications for the injectable form of contraception is to cover the waiting period after vasectomy. Alternatively, the oral contraceptive should be continued until proof of sterility is obtained, and the patient with an IUD in situ should not have it removed until success of the vasectomy has been confirmed. Seminal analysis should be carried out should a pregnancy occur subsequent to vasectomy, since, if spermatozoa are demonstrated, the vasa must be explored under general anaesthesia, re-ligated and divided.

Reversal of vasectomy, when attempted, is undertaken by microsurgery, but the success rate in terms of pregnancy following the reversal operation is little more than 25%. Auto-immunity to spermatozoa can occur; in such cases the semen may appear quite normal in every respect, but the sperms are unable to cause fertilisation. Few centres have urological surgeons with sufficient time and experience in microsurgery to justify reversal of male sterilisation, save in exceptional circumstances.

Why not a pill for men?

Spermatogenesis can be suppressed successfully by the antigonadotrophic action of progestogens, or oestrogens used alone, or in combination. The major problem hinges on the adjustment of doses to provide adequate spermatogenic suppression without loss of libido. The majority of substances that act directly on the testes appear to be toxic or to suppress spermatogenesis reversibly. Interference with sperm maturation is possible for example, with $\propto$-chloroydrin, but toxic effects have precluded the use of this compound. Analogues with similar actions have been isolated, and investigations on their toxicity continue.

It is uncertain whether such a preparation or method of contraception would be acceptable to the male population. In the light of an increasing number of men undertaking responsibility for contraception, as evidenced by the increasing demand for vasectomy, the acceptability of such preparations may be much greater than is at first thought.

The most recent possibility in the field of oral male contraception is gossypol — a yellow pigment found in the cotton plant and its seeds. Apart from its known nutritional value, its toxic effect on the testes was later recognised and, in 1978, glossypol was used in contraceptive trials in men in China. An initial daily dose of 20 mg gossypol acetic acid was given, followed by a maintainance dosage of 50 mg weekly; a success rate in terms of necrospermic or agoospermic ejaculates of 99% was achieved. Recovery of testiculo function appeared to be delayed for one to four and a half years. The potential for male contraception with a non-steroidal chemical is thus feasible, but its range of action and toxicity requires more limited definition.

Advances in female contraception

1. Trials of various vaginal sponges ('collatex' and 'collgen') are presently being conducted on a multicentre basis to assess both efficiency and patient acceptability.

2. Vaginal rings impregnated with a progestogen on a 'slow-release' basis have been assessed, but menstrual losses have been variable and irregular, making such devices unacceptable for widespread use.

3. Analogues of LHRH (luteinising hormone releasing hormone) have some theoretical advantage in that ovulation can be prevented by daily administration of an LHRH agonist. Alternatively a large dose of LHRH given just before ovulation results in an inadequate luteal phase and if this dose is given late in the luteal phase of the cycle, lysis of the corpus luteum will be induced.

This alternative method of contraception would be useful in the older patient (over 35 years of age) or in those with other risk factors present, since no exogenous oestrogens are taken. It would be preferable to the combined pill in lactating women, and patients with menorrhagia or persistent pre-menstrual symptoms would also benefit.

4. The use of prostaglandins in the form of vaginal pessaries for the interruption of a very early pregnancy is presently being assessed. Recent trials with new PGE analogues for very early (post-conceptional) termination have demonstrated a success rate of over 90%. The possibility exists of such a 'medicinal' method being used on an outpatient basis, under medical supervision, given careful patient selection, appropriate counselling and the availability of in-patient gynaecological facilities.

5. About 5% of infertile women have, as a cause of their infertility, circulating antizonal antibodies — antibodies which disrupt the interaction between spermatozoa, and the zona pellucida of the ovum. The inhibition of sperm binding depends on the production of an immuno-precipitate on the outer zone surfaces; this 'shell' of carbohydrate rich glycoprotein (on the outer zone surface) is the target for antizonal antibodies. The contraceptive properties of these glycoproteins depend on two factors — their specificity (no cross reacting antigens have been found elsewhere in the body) and their immunogenicity (infertility has been induced in primates using weak adjuvants such as alum). Since the zona pellucida is a 'solid' structure situated within the ovary, the potential advantage of this method of contraception is that the risk of complications due to immune-complex formations should be slight. The action, basically, therefore, is one of disruption of fertilisation.

THE WELL WOMAN CLINIC

There is little doubt that a structured clinic offering 'well woman' screening and family planning services is a great asset within a modern group practice.

There are a number of reasons for this:

1. The general practitioner is best places to provide facilities and expertise for well-woman screening and for contraceptive services.

2. The nursing team (midwife, health visitor and community nurse) can with approppriate training be a valuable asset in such a clinic. In the course of their professional contact with patients — particularly the 'at risk' socially underprivileged mothers.

3. Senior nurses in the practice team, following an approved course of family planning training, and with some supervised practical sessions, can see patients for review in the same clinic, while the doctor is involved in the examination of new patients, or in the assessment of problems. The trained nurse can, in the course of her

review of patients, answer any queries while assessing the patient's contraceptive status, and record data regarding menstruation, weight and blood pressure. Where the nurse has undertaken further supervised practical experience, she can be responsible for taking cervical smears and vaginal swabs and can check on the position of intra-uterine devices. Such extension of the nurse's role is possible as long as she is acting under the doctor's supervision. The doctor accepts legal responsibility for the actions of those to whom he delegates and he must thereafter satisfy himself that her training, experience and abilities are appropriate.

4. The clinic should be an 'open' clinic, that is patients can make their own appointments, in familiar practice premises and with familiar doctors and nurses.

5. Any of the doctors, nurses and receptionists in the practice should be able to refer patients to the clinic which in turn should be able to cope with counselling and with queries on any accepted method of contraception. Should any untoward abnormality be demonstrated appropriate arrangements should be made to refer the patient to her own doctor.

6. Facilities for insertion of intra-uterine devices should be available, and, in the clinic setting, a nurse will be present — a valuable asset for this procedure.

7. Secretarial assistance can help to ensure that there is accurate completion of the various case sheets, and claim forms; good records (including a flow sheet) are of great assistance to the patient's own doctor should any intercurrent illness arise.

8. The non-attenders at the clinic, some of whom may be known to the nursing team, can be checked from the appointment list, and known 'at risk' patients can be visited, and offered an alternative appointment.

9. Follow-up appointments should be made as required or at the end of the patient's consultation so that the practice notes of all expected patients can be made available for each clinic.

A detailed survey of the author's Well Woman Clinic at Craigshill Health Centre, Livingston (practice population 9600 patients) revealed some interesting information.

ATTENDANCE

Table 5.1 shows the age group of patients attending in the first 18 months of the clinic. Patients in the over 50 group were selected from the practice age/sex register. Each was sent a letter intimating the introduction of the clinic and inviting their participation. The numbers of such patients in Craigshill suggested that a clinic on alternate weeks could provide a screening examination for each patient every 5 years — a frequency advised by Baird (1968). The present policy, now adopted by

Table 5.1 Age group of patients attending in first 18 months of Well Woman Clinic

Age distribution	Numbers
Under 20	18
20–24	113
25–29	148
30–34	92
35–39	48
40–49	50
Over 50	89

Lothian Area Health Board, is that provided two negative smears have been obtained within 12 months, a repeat every 5 years will suffice. Patients attending the health centre for contraceptive advice during normal consulting sessions were invited instead to attend the new Well Woman clinic. More importantly, less motivated patients (some of the 'high risk' mothers) were informed of the clinic by any member of the primary care team, and urgent referral, if this was thought necessary, made at the time of contact. It is interesting to note that 17% of the patients were seen in the vulnerable groups of social class IV and V, while only 9.4% of householders in Livingston were recorded in those categories. Also of interest is that the attendance rate improved noticeably following a press release made in co-operation with the Health Board public relations officer; at the same time, two senior members of the nursing team gave talks to all the local women's groups on an informal basis, with generous question and answer sessions. Increasingly, referrals of high risk patients have been from the nursing team, emphasising one of the advantages that district nurses and health visitors have in their direct contact with such patients.

RESULTS

General

The 'general' abnormal findings in the early survey are shown in Table 5.2. An area of concern is the surprising level of 'positive' findings in the younger age group — for example, obesity, hypertension, anaemia, and breast lesions.

With the exception of one, patients with demonstrable anaemia had intra-uterine devices; and an iron deficient picture was the rule. The exception was a 40-year-old patient whose folate deficiency could reasonably have been attributed to the contraceptive pill, or to her recurrent urinary tract infection. Further investigation, however, including a jejunal biopsy, demonstrated mild coeliac disease. The effective absorption of the oral contraceptive in this patient was therefore in question, and after appropriate counselling, sterilisation was accepted.

Table 5.2   Abnormal findings (general)

	Child bearing age group (16–49 years)	Post child bearing group (over 50 years)
New glycosuria	Nil	1 (1.1%)
Obesity (75 kg)	42 (11%)	15 (17%)
Hypertension (Diastolic 100 mmHg)	22 (4.7%)	19 (21%)
Anaemia (Hb 10.4 g)	7 (1.5%)	Nil
Breast lesion — Benign	2 (0.4%)	Nil
Malignant	Nil	Nil

Gynaecological findings

The gynaecological abnormalities detected at the screening clinic are shown in Table 5.3. None of the patients with demonstrable genital prolapse was felt to require operative treatment and no true association with urinary tract infection was noted. Vaginal infections, more common in the sexually active age groups, appeared most prevalent in the 40–49 year group, with confirmatory evidence by swab culture. Cervical erosions, as one might expect, were more frequent in the younger age groups: 82% of the patients with cervical erosions were taking an oral contraceptive. Only 2.8% of the erosions required cautery to the cervix (four patients, one of which was done at the time of sterilisation). Two of the patients with ovarian cysts had plans for future pregnancies. Figure 5.9 and Figure 15.13 (see p. 195) show the cysts after removal. In both patients contraceptive supervision continues in the Well Woman Clinic following successful pregnancies. Of the six patients with fibroids, three required active treatment:

1. Myomectomy: oral contraceptive taken for 8 years previously was continued for 12 months after question, before conception was planned.

2. In one patient a hysterectomy was recommended instead of continuing oral contraceptive.

3. The third patient was found to have seedling fibroids at examination under anaesthesia and normal endometrium was demonstrated on histology. Her follow-up continues in the Well Woman Clinic.

Table 5.3   Abnormal findings (gynaecological)

Positive findings	Child bearing age group	Over 50 age group	Practice total
Prolapse	1	4	5
Infection	24	4	28
Cervical erosion	92	3	95
Cervical polypi	Nil	4	4
	3	3	6
Fibroids	3	Nil	3
Ovarian cyst			

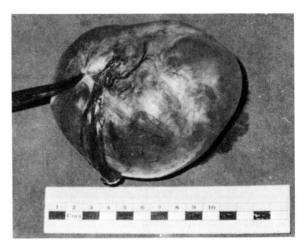

Fig. 5.9   Serous cystadenoma of ovary (benign); discovered in the Well Woman/Family Planning clinic. Further pregnancy planned.

COMPLICATIONS OF CONTRACEPTION

As might be expected, elevation of blood pressure was confined to patients on oral contraception. Anaemia in those patients with an IUD was in keeping with the high incidence of irregular bleeding with this device. Some of the complications of contraception are shown in Table 5.4.

In an audit of 50 consecutive insertions of intra-uterine devices, the author found that patients, once they had decided the device was not for them, tended to over-emphasise symptoms such as pain or intolerable bleeding, until removal of the device became obligatory.

The incidence of abnormal cervical smears in this clinic and in West Lothian as a whole is discussed later (ch 15, p. 192). Suffice it to say here that the continued motivation of all the primary care team is essential in the long term to effectively screen a practice population, since an inevitable group of high risk patients will not attend a special clinic by invitation. If the evidence of Baird (1968), and Spriggs (1977) is to be believed, screening should continue on to old age — at least once every 5 years, or at 3-yearly intervals should resources permit if the greatest benefit in terms of early detection of cervical cancer is to be achieved.

With regard to contraception, it must be accepted that

Table 5.4   Some complications of contraception

Problem	IUCD	Oral contraception
Irregular bleeding	15%	2.2%
Hypertension (diastolic 100 mmHg)	—	1.9%
Anaemia (Hb < 10.4 g)	1.5%	—

no method is perfect. Counselling must be more than adequate: it must be simple and precise, giving a clear idea to the patient of the advantages and disadvantages of each potential method so that a mature decision can be made. The better the counselling, the more informed is the patient's decision: thereupon the better will be the continuation rate of the contraceptive method used and the less the chance of unwanted or dangerous pregnancies.

REFERENCES

Allen I 1981 Family planning, sterilisation, and abortion services. Policy Studies Institute 595: 27

Baird Sir Dugald 1968 Office of Health Economics: The early diagnosis of carcinoma of the cervix

Beral V, Kay C R 1977 Mortality amongst oral contraceptive users, Royal College of General Practitioners Study. Lancet 2: 727

Bone M 1978a The family planning services: changes and effects. Office of Population Censuses and Surveys, Social Services Division. HMSO, London

Cartwright Ann 1970a The medical care research unit national survey. Routledge and Kegan Paul, London

Emens J M, Shah S R 1982 Early post-partum insertion of the multiload Cu 250 intra-uterine device. British Journal of Obstetrics and Gynaecology, Supplement No. 4: 43

Family Planning 1981 An exercise in preventive medicine. Royal College of General Practitioners, p 6

Flynn A 1980 Natural methods of family planning. British Journal of Family Planning 6: 9–14

Haspels A A 1976 Interception: post-coital oestrogens in 3016 women. Contraception 14: 375–381

International Planned Parenthood Federation May and October 1981 Medical Advisory Panel Meetings: Policy Statement

International Planned Parenthood Federation, Family planning handbook for doctors 1980. Evaluation of intra-uterine device. IPPF Medical Publications, p 77

Lawsons, Cole R A, Templeton A A 1976 The effect of laparoscopic sterilisation by diathermy or silastic bands on post-operative pain, menstrual symptoms and sexuality. British Journal of Obstetrics and Gynaecology 86: 659–663

Leppo K 1978 Contraception in Finland in a public health perspective. ch 3, p 48

Lestrom L, Bengtsson L P et al 1979 The risk of pelvic inflammatory disease in women using intra-uterine contraceptive devices as compared to non-users. Lancet 2: 221–224

Lukkainen T, Nielsen N C, Nygrenk G, Pyorala T 1979 Nulliparous women, IUD and pelvic infection. Annals of Clinical Research II: 121–124

Newton J R (In press) Evaluation of multiload Cu 250. Institute of Population Studies, University of Exeter

Nygren K G, Nielsen N C 1981 Contraception 24: 529

Peel J 1972 The Hull Family Survey II. Journal of Biosocial Science IV: 333

Peel J 1969 Male-oriented Fertility Control. Practitioner 677: 202

Report of Working Party of the Confidential Enquiry into Gynaecological Laparooscopy of Royal College of Obstetricians and Gynaecologists 0000

Sivin I 1979 Copper-T IUD use and ectopic pregnancy rates in USA. Contraception 19: 151–173

Snowden R 1982 Why an international IUD standard is not possible. In: International Planned Parenthood Federation (IPPF). Medical Bulletin 16: 2

Spriggs A I, Hussain O A N 1977. British Medical Journal I: 1516–1518

Steven J D, Fraser I S 1974 Pregnancy after IUD failure. Journal of Obstetrics and Gynaecology of the British Commonwealth 81: 282

US Department of Health, Education and Welfare 1978 Food and Drug Administration, Advisory Committee on Obstetrics and Gynaecology. Second report on intra-uterine contraceptive devices. US Government Printing Office, Washington D C, p 102

Vessey M P, Wright N H, McPherson K, Wiggins P 1978 Fertility after stopping different methods of contraception. British Medical Journal I: 265–267

World Health Organization (WHO) 1971 Abortion Laws, Geneva

World Health Organization (WHO) 1982 Bulletin of World Health Organization 60: 119–210

SUGGESTED READING

Oldershaw L Contraception, abortion and sterilisation in general practice

International Planned Parenthood Federation 1980 Family planning handbook for doctors

The management of pregnancy

INTRODUCTION

The care of a woman during and immediately following her pregnancy is one of the most satisfying duties that befalls a general practitioner. Maternity work is an area of practice which he can develop and use his skills in preventive medicine and unlike many other aspects of medical care he is able to measure the outcome of his work. Good personal care during this period can establish a relationship between doctor and patient which is of great value in the later care of the family.

The quality of care that can be given in practice is often greater than can be offered by the hospital ante-natal clinic, partly because of the continuing personal care which the family doctor can give as he is more able to take account of all the patient's problems. The optimum management of the patient can only be achieved if both community and hospital staff work closely together. This need has been widely recognised and systems of shared care are now common and frequently involve a unified general practice/hospital record system. A recent report by Hull and her colleagues in 1980 casts doubt over the value of the number and timing of ante-natal attendances as a means of identifying hazards to mother and child. The report concluded that it was likely that too much routine, and relatively ineffectual, ante-natal care is given to too many mothers. A work party of the Scottish National Consultative Committee (Obstetrics) (1982) has recommended a reduced number of ante-natal attendances for those mothers for whom the pregnancy is expected to be normal, based on previous menstrual, physical, obstetric and gynaecological history.

The programme recommended by the Committee included the following timing and content of ante-natal examination:

Gestation	Visit to	Principal content of consultation and examination
Less than 8 weeks	G.P.	Diagnosis of pregnancy. General discussion of and advice about pregnancy.
12 weeks	G.P.	1. Confirm pregnancy diagnosis. 2. Confirm stage of gestation by ultrasound. 3. First obstetric examination: a. Full history and examination. b. Blood tests: i. FBC ii. Blood and rhesus grouping iii. Rubella titre iv. VDRL 4. Cervical smear if high risk patient. 5. Refer to hospital clinic.
16 weeks	Consultant	1. Plans made for ante-natal care and confinement. 2. MSAFP Screening and appropriate follow-up. 3. At this and subsequent visits: a. Weight. b. Blood pressure. c. Urinanalysis. d. Fundal height in centimetres above symphysis pubis. e. Information and advice to mother.
20 weeks 24 weeks 28 weeks	G.P.	+ Rh antibodies if Rh −ve. Hb.
32 weeks		+ Foetal lie and presentation.
36 weeks	Consultant	Hb.
38 weeks 39 weeks	G.P.	
40 weeks and 40+	Consultant or G.P.	

More than 95% of all births now occur in hospital, either in specialist units or in general practitioner maternity units (Social Trends 1981). General practitioner obstetrics is thus for most doctors restricted to pre- and post-natal care. There is however a small but growing patient movement in parts of the United Kingdom for a return to domiciliary confinements for selected mothers. It is probable that this trend will continue and all general practitioners offering full maternity services should therefore be prepared to face the possibility of being responsible for intra-partum care either as a result of agreement between patient and doctor or in an emergency.

ACCOMMODATION

Access to suitable accommodation can be a major problem for many general practitioners. The essential needs of an ante-natal clinic include an adequate reception and waiting area for patients, and a good appointment system. The combined consulting and examination room should have an area of at least 180 square feet (17 m^2) and there should be access to a changing cubicle — this may simply be a screened-off area within the consulting room. A separate interviewing room of about 120 square feet (11 m^2) is of value, especially when a nurse assists at the clinic.

EQUIPMENT

Little additional equipment is required over and above that which is usually found in the normal consulting room. The weighing machine should be sturdy and accurate and should be checked periodically by the local Weights and Measures Department. A good light source is important, preferably from a mobile anglepoise lamp. Both a binaural and foetal stethoscope are required, as is an accurate sphygmomanometer. Syringes (2 ml, 5 ml, 10 ml and 20 ml), hypodermic needles and various sample collection tubes should be set out on a 'tray' or 'trolley'. Sequestrene tubes are required for blood counts, clean tubes for the collection of clotted blood for blood grouping rhesus and rubella antibody checks, VDRL tests, and a few fluoride oxalate tubes should be available for blood sugar estimation. Universal containers, both plain and containing boric acid preservative, are required for early morning and midstream specimens of urine. Uristix strips and Clinitest tablets should be available for testing for glycosuria and proteinuria. A pregnancy test outfit is useful and the Organon Pregnancy Test is particularly suitable for general practitioner use as the reagents are incorporated in a dried form on the surface of a cardboard slide — no refrigeration is therefore necessary. Glass slides, Ayre's spatulas and a fixative are required for taking cervical smears, and charcoal swabs with the appropriate transport medium (Stuart's medium) should be available for cervical and vaginal swabs. Sterile and non-sterile polythene gloves and disposable speculae are adequate for most vaginal examinations and a supply of 1:5000 hibitane solution should be available. Hibitane or Dettol cream, and K.Y. jelly are also necessary.

PERSONNEL

Ante-natal care is best undertaken by a team, each member of which has differing skills and a different but important role to play in the overall care of the patient. The basic team consists of the general practitioner, a midwife, health visitor and a receptionist. Help will be required on occasions and for particular problems from others, and the specialist obstetrician, the physician, the social worker and the dentist may all be involved. The importance of defining a basic team which is augmented, when necessary, by other disciplines emphasises the need to identify maternity care as an essential component of family practice.

A further and important responsibility for the general practitioner is the need to identify women at risk. This group includes the unmarried, the very young, those of high parity, and the emotionally and socially deprived. It is largely from this group that mothers who book late and who are poor attenders at ante-natal clinics are derived. It is thus a group of mothers who are particularly at risk of perinatal, neonatal and maternal morbidity and mortality.

APPOINTMENT SYSTEM

An efficient appointment system minimises the time that the patient spends waiting before being seen and helps to avoid the irritating effect that erratic bursts of pressure can have on the staff. The appointment system should not be too rigidly applied as the waiting period is often the only opportunity that patients have for mutual discussion, and this can often be of considerable benefit.

The first visit of the patient to the ante-natal clinic should be relaxed and unhurried and not less than 15 minutes should be allowed on the appointment sheet. Return visits require rather less time (8 to 10 minutes) and if the doctor and the midwife are working simultaneously, patients can be booked at twice this rate. In an urban practice there are approximately 12 births per 1000 population each year and it is generally accepted that, unless complications arise during the pregnancy, the patient should be seen every month until the 28th week, every fortnight until the 36th week and then weekly until delivery. Each patient will therefore require not less than 14 visits during her pregnancy and at least one post-natal consultation (but see above, p. 76). The organisation of the ante-natal clinic must allow for those patients who arrive without an appointment but the additional patient is usually balanced by the occasional defaulter. As with normal surgeries the workload may vary during the year and the time required for the ante-natal clinic should be adjusted accordingly. At the end of each clinic the records of those patients who fail to attend should be reviewed and further appointments or domiciliary visits arranged as indicated.

RECORDING AND COMMUNICATION OF INFORMATION

If the patient is to receive good ante-natal care it is important that accurate and complete records are kept and that the information is available to every member of the team involved with the patient. Communication by letter may be unavoidable but every opportunity should be taken for those caring for the patient to meet together and discuss problems. This is as true of the need for the general practitioner and the hospital specialist to meet as it is of the easier communication that can occur between doctor and midwife.

One method of recording information and of making it available, both to those caring for the patient in the community and to the hospital staff, is a no-carbon-required (NCR) duplicated A4 size ante-natal record sheet. The patient takes one part of this record to the specialist when she attends the 'booking clinic' at the hospital and it is retained by her from about the 32nd week of her pregnancy until delivery. The other part of the NCR sheet is left in the patient's general practice record. On admission to hospital, the patient's copy becomes part of the hospital casenotes.

Whatever the format of the ante-natal record it should be designed in such a way as to make it obvious when any specific item of information is not recorded or when the patient's progress becomes abnormal. This can best be achieved by recording the information in columns, or in a graph form similar to the percentile charts used in child-growth assessments. The record should indicate what information should be collected at each consultation and also show the range which would be accepted as normal. This allows each member of the team to be aware of any deviation from normal which might influence their decisions regarding their part in the total care.

EARLY PRESENTATION AND DIAGNOSIS OF PREGNANCY

The expected history is of simple amenorrhoea and morning sickness but in practice the presentation of a pregnancy can take many forms. Some multiparous patients can tell when they are pregnant at an early stage and occasionally may be able to do so despite an apparently normal previous period. On the other hand it is not uncommon for the patient who is pregnant for the first time, and especially when she has been married for some years, to present with a complaint of nausea or vomiting, frequency of micturition and unusual tiredness, completely unaware of the possibility of a pregnancy. The presentation can also be of vaginal bleeding associated with lower abdominal cramp-like pain — a threatened or inevitable abortion. In the unmarried girl any abdominal symptoms which appear to have no organic basis should arouse the suspicion of a pregnancy or a fear of pregnancy. The abrupt question — 'Do you think you might be pregnant?' — is likely to produce a negative reply and a gentle, but obvious, approach is best. Many girls are not as innocent as they appear, conversely there are still many adolescents who are ignorant about procreation and contraception.

Simple amenorrhoea occurring while the patient is using apparently adequate contraception (particularly the pill) can give rise to the request to exclude pregnancy as a cause. Amenorrhoea occurring at the menopause or prolonged amenorrhoea following a confinement can arouse anxiety and the fear of a further pregnancy.

Patients frequently ask for a pregnancy to be confirmed or excluded as early as 7 to 10 days after the first missed period. At this early stage it is difficult to make an accurate diagnosis and the patient should be asked to wait until at least 2 weeks after the missed period when the immunological tests become reliable. However, a diagnosis should not be delayed unnecessarily. The patient's normal menstrual cycle and the date and character of the last menstrual period should be determined as they will usually indicate whether the period of amenorrhoea is abnormal for the patient. The history of the frequency and timing of coitus is also helpful. The presence of 'secondary signs' of pregnancy should be sought. Morning sickness is well recognised, but not invariable, and frequency of micturition, tiredness and the presence of tingling, tenderness or fullness in the breasts, with dilated superficial breast veins, will all contribute to the overall clinical impression. The abdomen should always be examined for a fundus regardless of the date of the last normal period. This is particularly important in the young unmarried girl who may state that she has missed one period and be found on examination to have a palpable fundus.

Vaginal examination is unlikely to be helpful in the diagnosis of pregnancy before the eighth week, particularly in the obese or tense and anxious patient. After this time an accurate diagnosis of pregnancy can be made by vaginal examination if this is thought necessary. Pulsation of the uterine arteries is readily felt in the lateral fornices and the enlarged uterus can be recognised by bimanual manipulation.

IMMUNOLOGICAL TESTS

Immunological pregnancy tests are included in most hospital laboratory services offered to the family doctor, but frequently the laboratory is unable to handle large numbers of such requests, and may impose limitations related to specific medical indications for the test. Even when pregnancy tests are available, there may be difficulties in transporting the urine specimens to the laboratory and there can be a delay of several days before the doctor receives the test result. This delay can at the least cause the patient several days anxious waiting, and in some cases, such as when the patient is thought to have rubella, any delay in establishing a diagnosis of pregnancy can be more serious. A case can therefore be made for having an immunological test set in the surgery. The speed with which the result is obtained amply justifies its use, and there is evidence that the results obtained in the surgery are as accurate as those in the laboratory (Robinson & Barber 1977). There is an obvious benefit to the patient in being given a definite diagnosis of pregnancy at her first consultation, particularly when a patient with simple amenorrhoea is anxious for an immediate diagnosis. It is also important to be able to make an immediate and definitive diagnosis of pregnancy when the patient has an important co-existing medical condition or where termination of the pregnancy might be considered necessary.

A suspected ectopic pregnancy or an abortion, particularly if 'threatened' or 'missed', are other situations where the use of an immediate pregnancy test will give valuable information.

Pregnancy tests should preferably be performed on an early morning specimen of urine and a reliable result can usually be obtained as early as 10 days after the first missed period. The urine should be filtered if it is cloudy or contains sediment to ensure that there is no protein present which may give a false positive result. The presence of gelatine in the capsule of boric acid which is often used as a preservative in MSU collecting bottles also gives a false positive result. Care should be taken in women over 40 years of age as the raised levels of pituitary hormone associated with the menopause can give a false positive result. This error can be avoided if menopausal urine is diluted with an equal quantity of water.

ULTRASONOGRAPHY

This examination is likely to be of great benefit to the general practitioner and his patient when 'open access' to it becomes more readily available, as a diagnosis of pregnancy can be made as early as the sixth week after the last menstrual period.

THE FIRST VISIT TO THE ANTE-NATAL CLINIC

HISTORY

There is less need in practice than in hospital to take a full and exhaustive history at the first visit, as much of the essential information is already recorded in the patient's medical record. It is preferable, however, to record a summary of the relevant information on the ante-natal sheet rather than to rely simply on a knowledge of the patient, and this has the added advantage of making the information readily available to other members of the team. In many instances much of this information can be entered in the ante-natal record by the midwife, the doctor, or the receptionist, in advance of the patient's consultation. This is particularly so when the case notes contain a summary sheet or a summary of the patient's past medical and obstetric history or a previous ante-natal record.

The patient's first ante-natal consultation is then only concerned with updating this information and can be more relaxed and unhurried. The ante-natal record sheet should have a printed list of the information which should be collected. In the past history, the important medical conditions are rheumatic fever, chorea, epilepsy, diabetes, hypertension, chest diseases (such as bronchitis and asthma), tuberculosis, urinary tract infection, and psychological illness. All previous surgical operations should be recorded, as should any current symptoms, problems or medication. The 'family history' should include hypertension and diabetes. The 'marital history' should contain details of the date of the patient's marriage, whether there seems to have been difficulty in conceiving and whether there are any adopted children. It is essential to record the date of the last menstrual period and to ask the patient if she is sure of her dates. Some women will not recall the date easily and should not be pressured into agreeing to a date. The parity, the patient's normal menstrual cycle and any irregularities in menstruation should also be recorded. The 'obstetric history' should include details of previous confinements; the date and place of each, the maturity (in weeks) of the infant, whether labour was spontaneous or operative, and whether there were any complications during any stage of labour. Certain details about each infant should also be recorded; whether it was born alive, stillborn, or was aborted, and its sex and birth weight. Perinatal death should be noted with the cause of death.

EXAMINATION

Much of the initial examination at the 12-week visit can be completed by the midwife or the practice nurse. The patient's height, weight and sitting blood pressure are taken and are recorded in tabular form in the ante-natal record. During the later weeks of pregnancy the blood pressure may be abnormally low if it is taken when the patient is lying flat, due to the pressure of the enlarged uterus on the inferior vena cava. While the sphygmomanometer cuff is round the arm, 15 ml of blood should be taken for a full blood count, blood grouping, rhesus and rubella antibody titres, and for VDRL tests. The urine should be checked for glucose and protein and, if vomiting is troublesome, for acetone. Screening for bacilluria is of value if facilities are available, but dip-slides or 'uriglox' are necessary. The patient should be specifically asked about urinary tract symptoms and an MSU should be sent for culture and antibiotic sensitivity if there is any evidence of infection. A vaginal discharge which is unusual or troublesome should be swabbed and sent for microscopy and culture. The value of a cervical smear taken at this time is doubtful.

At this first visit a full physical examination should be made with special attention being paid to the condition of the teeth, breasts, legs, chest and heart. The presence or absence of a palpable fundus should be noted on abdominal examination.

It is important to ask the patient if she has any problems which have not been discussed and if a problem does exist, an explanation should be given in simple terms. The patient should be asked to note when she first feels the baby moving, and it should be explained to her that this can be expected at between 18 and 20 weeks in a first pregnancy, and between 16 and 18 weeks in a second or subsequent pregnancy. At the end of the consultation it is important to make a point of telling the patient if all is well and the pregnancy is progressing normally.

At subsequent visits to the ante-natal clinic, the patient should be asked about any symptoms she may have, particularly those of urinary tract infection, troublesome vaginal discharge, heartburn or insomnia. The presence of ankle oedema or varicose veins should be noted and the blood pressure taken at each visit with the patient relaxed and sitting. The patient's weight should be accurately measured and the gain in weight should not normally be more than 2 kg in any month or 1 kg in any week. The total weight gain to be expected during the pregnancy is 9.5 kg, a 3 kg increase over the first 20 weeks, 3 kg between the 20th and 30th week and 3–3.5 kg from the 30th to 40th week. The urine should be checked for sugar and protein.

Anaemia is one of the most important abnormalities to be detected in pregnancy and the patient's haemoglobin should be checked at the 12-week visit, at the 28th and the 36th week. A repeat check for rhesus antibodies should be made at 28 weeks.

The important features of the abdominal examination are the height of the fundus, the lie of the fetus, the presenting part and its position, and whether it is engaged or free. A note should be made of whether fetal movements have been felt and whether the fetal heart is heard. The traditional fetal stethoscope is still commonly used but fetal heart detectors are now available at a cost which is acceptable to a group practice. Before she leaves the clinic, the patient should again be asked if she has any problems and time should be spent in explanation and reassurance no matter how minor they appear to be. If the pregnancy is progressing normally, again the patient should be specifically told of this.

SELECTION OF CASES FOR CONFINEMENT IN A SPECIALIST OBSTETRIC UNIT

Confinement in a specialist unit should be arranged for any patient whose previous history includes any of the following conditions:

A. Previous medical history

1. Cardiac disease
2. Hepatitis
3. Chronic nephritis and recurrent urinary tract infections
4. Chronic bronchitis and bronchiectasis
5. Hypertension
6. Thyroid disease
7. Diabetes
8. Tuberculosis
9. Epilepsy and other CNS diseases
10. Chronic debilitating diseases
11. Prolonged steroid therapy
12. Haematological disorders
13. Mental illness

B. Previous surgical history

1. Conditions affecting pelvic capacity, e.g. congenital dislocation of hip, fracture of the pelvis, neoplastic bone conditions, infective conditions affecting the pelvis, e.g. TB, poliomyelitis
2. Crohn's disease
3. Ulcerative colitis
4. Megacolon
5. Previous deep vein thrombosis, pulmonary embolism or history of severe phlebitis
6. Operations on the thorax

C. Previous gynaecological history
1. Uterine scars, e.g. myomectomy, hysterotomy
2. Previous pelvic floor repair
3. Previous cone biopsy of cervix
4. Genital anomaly, e.g. double uterus, septate vagina

D. Previous obstetric history
1. Recurrent abortions — two or more
2. Previous prematurity
3. Previous Caesarean section
4. Previous difficult forceps delivery
5. Previous Rh or other antibodies
6. Previous eclampsia or severe pre-eclamptic toxaemia
7. Grande multiparity — five or more
8. Previous stillbirth or neonatal death
9. Previous post-partum haemorrhage or placental retention
10. Previous 3rd degree tears
11. Previous puerperal mental illness
12. History of amniotic embolism
13. Previous gross fetal abnormality
14. Cervical incompetence

ANAEMIA

Anaemia in pregnancy may first be suspected clinically and then proved by finding a low haemoglobin, or its presence may be detected by one of the routine haemoglobin tests. The normal haemoglobin differs from that of the non-pregnant woman and varies with the stage of the pregnancy. The blood volume increases by about 30% and as the increase in plasma is greater than that of the red cell mass a haemodilution results. The PCV is at its lowest level at about 32 weeks and the haemoglobin may drop to 10 g/100 ml at about this stage.

The incidence of anaemia in pregnancy varies with the social class of the patient and may be as high as 50% in social classes 4 and 5. 95% of anaemias are of an iron deficiency type and incipient iron deficiency anaemia occurs when the saturation of the total iron binding capacity is less than 16% with a haemoglobin greater than 12 g/100 ml. In a true iron deficiency anaemia, the haemoglobin is less than 12 g/100 ml, the PCV is less than 35%, the serum iron is low but the total iron binding *capacity* is raised with a saturation of 10% or less. Women who go into labour with a co-existing severe anaemia are at risk and the effect of hypoxia on the myocardium may cause concern. Complications in the post-partum period are also more common and the anaemic patient is especially prone to infections. There is evidence to suggest that perinatal mortality and morbidity are also increased by maternal anaemia.

The prevention of iron deficiency anaemia is important and the pregnant woman should be given iron and vitamin supplements throughout her pregnancy. Many pregnant women, especially those in the lower social classes (4 and 5) have an inadequate dietary intake of folic acid and a preparation which contains iron and folic acid should be prescribed (Pregaday — 100 mg elemental iron, 350 μg folic acid — 1 tablet daily). If a dosage of three tablets each day is preferred, a preparation such as Pregamal is indicated (65 mg elemental iron and 100 μg folic acid). The patient who is found to be anaemic at the first visit or who develops anaemia later in pregnancy, due either to her failure to take the iron and folic acid prescribed or to insufficient absorption of the preparation given, requires close supervision and treatment. If there is doubt as to whether the patient is taking her iron tablets, a specimen of faeces should be obtained by a rectal examination and tested for iron.

If the patient can be relied upon to take oral iron ferrous sulphate (200 mg three times daily after food) should be prescribed. Response to treatment can usually be detected after 10 days by an increase in the reticulocyte count. If oral iron is ineffective, either due to the patient's intolerance of the preparation, refusal to take the iron regularly, or to poor absorption a course of parenteral iron (Jectofer) should be given. It should be remembered that inter-current infections, particularly of the urinary tract, adversely affect the response to iron therapy. Treatment with parenteral iron may also be required if the patient is less than 8 weeks from term and there is thus insufficient time in which to correct the anaemia with oral iron. Jectofer is given intramuscularly daily or on alternative days, in a dosage of 1.5 mg/kg body weight, and 200 mg is required to raise the haemoglobin by 1 g%. The course of injections should be continued until the serum iron level is within normal limits. Patients with a haemoglobin of less than 8 g/100 ml in the last 4 weeks of pregnancy should be admitted to hospital as a transfusion with packed cells may be necessary to correct the anaemia.

MEGALOBLASTIC ANAEMIA

Megaloblastic anaemia in pregnancy is almost always due to a folic acid deficiency. The argument that the routine use of folic acid may mask a pernicious anaemia is not valid as patients with a low serum B_{12} seldom conceive. Co-existing iron deficiency anaemia, however may complicate the blood picture. The incidence of megaloblastic anaemia in pregnancy is of the order of 2 to 4% and is more common in multiparous patients over 30 years of age and in multiple pregnancies. Poor dietary intake of folic acid due to bad nutrition, persistent vomiting, or alcoholism is the usual predisposing factor. The anaemia normally first presents between the 7th and the 8th month of pregnancy; the haemoglobin is less than 10 g, the erythrocyte count is usually less than 2 000 000/ml^3, and the red cells show a megaloblastic picture. A marrow biopsy is not indicated. Folic acid supplements of about 300 μg per day will prevent megaloblastic anaemia and the established condition can be treated by giving folic acid (5 mg t.d.s.) in addition to iron supplements and a high protein diet. The prognosis is good if the treatment is started at least 4 weeks before term, but admission to a specialist unit is required if the diagnosis is not made until after this stage of pregnancy. It should not be forgotten that anaemia due to blood loss can also occur in pregnancy.

HYPERTENSION

The majority of pregnant patients consult the family doctor during the first trimester when a base line blood pressure is recorded and can be compared with previous pregnancy or non-pregnancy readings in the patient's medical record. As with hypertension in the non-pregnant patient there is no universally accepted level above which a diagnosis of hypertension can be made. Diastolic pressures of 110 mmHg or above are clearly abnormal but the same cannot be so confidently said of diastolic pressures in the 90's.

As there is a considerable fluctuation in the blood pressure in any 24 hours in both the hypertensive and non-hypertensive person, it is probable that similar variations occur in pregnancy. A single BP reading is, therefore, of little value unless it is grossly elevated. To avoid spuriously high readings, which can cause the patient to be unjustly labelled as hypertensive, the pressure should be recorded with the patient in the sitting position and when she is both physically and emotionally relaxed. This is usually easier to achieve in the familiar surroundings of the surgery than in the hospital out-patient department. Unless the reading is very high, a diagnosis of hypertension should not be made until similar readings are found on at least three occasions (Hartley et al 1983)). The first indication of the possible development of hypertension is a rise in blood pressure from previously recorded normal levels. If the blood pressure is normally taken by the midwife or the practice nurse, the need for accuracy and good technique should be explained and stressed. Developing hypertension can also be suspected if there is an excessive gain in weight or if oedema or albuminuria is found. The sudden onset of headaches, particularly if they occur in the morning, is also a suspicious symptom. Although hypertension in a pregnant woman may present in a variety of ways, the problem is usually one of a pregnancy occurring in a patient with known hypertension or when an elevated pressure is recorded at a routine ante-natal check. The care of the ante-natal patient with established hypertension or pre-eclamptic toxaemia must always be the joint responsibility of the family doctor and the appropriate hospital specialist, as the patient may require in-patient care in a specialist unit.

URINARY TRACT INFECTION

Patients who are found to have an infection of the urinary tract during pregnancy can be divided into three main groups. The first, (about 8% of patients) are those with asymptomatic bacteriuria — apparently healthy women who are found to have more than 100 000 pathogenic organisms per ml of urine. The second group contains those who present at some time during pregnancy with an acute illness characterised by loin pain and tenderness, which may be severe, accompanied by dysuria, nausea, vomiting and pyrexia — acute pyelonephritis. The third group have milder symptoms of frequency, nocturia, and dysuria without systemic upset — a 'cystitis'. In pregnancy, frequency of micturition and nausea are of course unreliable symptoms of urinary infection: however in patients who have a proven infection, frequency will be present in about 77% of cases, nocturia in 58%, dysuria in 57%, and loin pain in 42%. The incidence of urinary tract infections in pregnancy is higher in the primigravid than in the multiparous patient.

There is a close relationship between asymptomatic bacteriuria and acute pyelonephritis. 30% of patients with the former will later develop an episode of acute infection, and 20% of those with acute pyelonephritis will be found after treatment, to have asymptomatic bacteriuria. The importance of this association is that 75% of patients with an acute pyelonephritis and 40% of those with asymptomatic bacteriuria are later found to have an abnormality in their intravenous pyelogram. Cystitis, on the other hand, does not have the same serious prognosis although a small number of patients will at some time develop either pyelonephritis or asymptomatic bacteriuria.

Only about 50% of patients with 'cystitis' are found to have a significant bacteriuria. The precise aetiology of the remainder is uncertain — some may be due to viral infections and in others the symptoms may be related to a co-existing vulvo vaginitis. In general practice, *Escherichia coli* is the commonest pathogen (about 70% of cases) and it is usual for it to be sensitive to the commoner anti-bacterial agents such as amoxicillin or ampicillin. Midstream urine samples should be collected in a sterile disposable foil gallipot or directly into a sterile universal container. 0.5 g of boric acid may be used as a preservative in a universal container. The MSU sample should be refrigerated (at 4°C) until it is transported to the laboratory for bacterial count, culture and sensitivity. If hospital laboratory facilities are not available approximate results can be obtained from dip slides (such as Uricult) innoculated in the surgery and incubated for 24 hours at 37°C. It is valuable to include urine culture as a routine part of ante-natal care and MSU samples should be taken at the patient's first visit to the clinic and again at 32 weeks.

Acute pyelonephritis can usually be confidently diagnosed on clinical grounds and confirmed later by the results of urine culture. The patient is usually first seen at home confined to bed by an illness which is severe and distressing. The symptoms tend to be more marked in the first episode and to be come less severe with each successive attack. Bacterial cystitis, on the other hand, is characterised principally by dysuria and frequency and, although the symtpoms can be disturbing, the patient may not feel unduly ill.

A high fever during pregnancy is a threat to the fetus and the treatment of acute pyelonephritis must therefore be energetic. Tepid sponging may be necessary to lower the temperature during the first 24 hours of the illness, until the antibiotic becomes effective. Initially the only diet likely to be tolerated is one which contains fruit juices and food high in carbohydrates. The fluid intake should be sufficient to produce a urinary output of abut 1500 ml daily and frequent and complete emptying of the bladder should be encouraged. Double or triple voiding of urine is helpful in reducing urinary stasis. An approximate measure of the urinary output can be achieved at home using a Winchester bottle and an appropriate filter funnel.

All pregnant patients with a proven bacterial urinary infection should be treated with an adequate course of an antibiotic. The principle of this therapy is to give a 1 week course of antibiotic and to culture a midstream urine 4 days after the end of the course. This regime is repeated until the post-infective sample is found to be sterile.

The patient with an acute pyelonephritis should be given an antibiotic (such as ampicillin — 500 mg 6-hourly) when first seen and before the result of the MSU is received. Only rarely will it be necessary to change the therapy in the light of the sensitivity report. Active treatment should be continued until an MSU sample is reported as sterile. Further MSU's should be examined at each successive ante-natal visit as 30% of patients will have a recurrence of acute pyelonephritis, and 20% will later be found to have asymptomatic bacteriuria. A final MSU should be examined at the post-natal visit when a decision can be made on the need for further investigation of the urinary tract. Due to the frequency with which acute infections recur, and the increased possibility of there being an underlying abnormality of the renal tract, there is a case for the prophylactic use of amoxicillin 250 mg t.i.d. for the remainder of a pregnancy following the treatment of an acute pyelonephritis.

MINOR PROBLEMS OF PREGNANCY

An unexpected increase in weight which is not associated with hypertension or albuminuria, merits more frequent ante-natal checks. The increase in weight may be due to occult oedema but is more likely to be due to a high calorie or excessive food intake. Advice on diet is an essential part of the health education given in pregnancy and is usually undertaken by the health visitor.

Albuminuria occurring without hypertension or oedema is usually associated with a urinary tract infection or a vaginal discharge which has contaminated the specimen. *Glycosuria* in pregnancy is not uncommon and is usually only discovered during the routine examination of the urine. A further specimen should be checked quantitatively and if a significant amount of glucose is present (0.5%) a modified glucose tolerance test will distinguish the commoner low renal threshold glycosuria from diabetes mellitus. The patient who has glycosuria due to a low renal threshold simply requires reassurance that all is well — the patient with diabetes mellitus must be referred to a specialist for the initial management and stabilisation of the diabetes. Thereafter, the ante-natal care will involve the hospital physician and obstetrician as well as the family doctor. *Heartburn* is a common problem in pregnancy but because of its relatively harmless nature the patient may not receive much sympathy. It is, however, distressing to the patient, particularly in later pregnancy when it can be particularly severe at night, often disturbing the sleep. The patient may consider that heartburn is a normal feature of pregnancy and may not mention the problem unless she is specifically asked about it at the ante-natal clinic. The attitude that if a problem is not mentioned it is not severe enough to warrant treatment, is not worthy of the good physician. Heartburn can be successfully managed by advising the patient to take small and frequent meals, to avoid stooping and to raise the top of the bed by 6 in (15 cm). Antacids may be necessary if these simple measures are ineffective, and Mucaine, which contains an antacid and a local anaesthetic, is particularly effective if taken after meals at night. The patient should be warned against drinking anything after taking this antacid, as this will diminish the effect of the local anaesthetic.

Varicose veins may be troublesome, particularly in the multiparous patient. Not only are they unsightly and embarrassing but they often cause tiredness and discomfort in the legs, particularly in the evening. Vulval varicosities cause some discomfort but may be very alarming to the patient who may be afraid that these veins may burst during delivery. The ache from varicosities of the legs and the vulva can be eased by the use of support tights. Elastic stockings are useless in pregnancy because of the difficulty of holding them up with a suspender belt. *Haemorrhoids*, particularly in the later stages of pregnancy, often receive unsympathetic management and like heartburn, can cause considerable anxiety and distress. The pain can be so severe that the patient finds it difficult to move about to do her housework and sitting down becomes almost impossible. Acutely painful or thrombosed haemorrhoids may be eased by the application of packs soaked in warm saline or eusol solution. Haemorrhoidal ointments containing a local anaesthetic are helpful in milder cases. The condition is often exacerbated by constipation and the use of a faecal softener (such as Dorbanex or liquid paraffin) with a laxative (Senokot) may do much to ease the pain during defaecation. Surgery should always be considered if the patient is incapacitated by severe prolapsing haemorrhoids but this rather drastic measure is seldom necessary. Sclerosant treatment should not, of course, be used during pregnancy.

The problem of the patient with *sickness* is also affected by the attitude of the patient and her doctor. Most patients accept morning sickness as an integral part of being pregnant but it is wiser to list vomiting in pregnancy as a problem no matter how mild it seems to be. Nausea and vomiting in pregnancy appear to have a multifactorial cause. Certainly, the condition is adversely affected by emotional upsets or tension and it can be particularly troublesome in the primigravid patient who has an over-anxious or protective mother. Mild nausea and vomiting can be controlled by dietary advice. A carbohydrate diet with fruit juices is usually well tolerated whereas even the smell of fried food can cause nausea. When it is more persistent the addition of doxylamine succinate (Debendox) — 2 tablets at night and then one in the morning and one mid-afternoon if necessary — can often give relief. When vomiting is severe or persistent the electrolytes should be checked and the patient admitted to hospital if the electrolytes are abnormal or if there is evidence of dehydration. Primigravida in particular often settle quickly on admission to hospital without any specific treatment being given and this would appear to support the view that an emotional factor is present.

Normal leucorrhoea is increased during pregnancy and as the quantity varies from one woman to another, the patient herself may be the best judge of whether the discharge is normal or abnormal. Any vaginal discharge which is thought to be abnormal because of its quantity, its colour, or its smell, should be cultured and examined microscopically. Pruritus vulvae, usually caused by *Candida albicans*, can be severe and distressing. The intense itching associated with it is described as being more distressing than pain and it may be aggravated by attempts made by the patient to ease the itch. These can involve the application of antiseptic creams or undiluted liquid antiseptics or sitting in water which contains a strong disinfectant. *Candida albicans* affects particularly the vulva and the lower third of the vagina and swabs should be taken from these regions. Occasionally, pruritis vulvae and the vaginal discharge may be caused by *Trichomonas vaginalis* which may be suspected on speculum examination by the appearance of the discharge (cream colour and 'frothy') and the inflamed cervix which is surrounded by pus. A swab and a smear from the cervix will show the presence of trichomonas and an additional swab should be taken from the cervical os and sent immediately, in a transport medium, to the laboratory as occasionally, a gonnoccocal infection may also be present. Nystatin ointment and pessaries dramatically relieve pruritis due to *Candida albicans*. Trichomonal infections are best treated in pregnancy by metronidazole which should be taken orally by both the patient and her husband. A swab should be taken after the course of treatment has been completed (7 to 10 days) and the patient should be warned not to stop her treatment prematurely when her symptoms are relieved; to do so can result in a recurrence of the infection. The health visitor should advise the patient on the care of the vulval area and warn her against over-vigorous cleansing or the use of strong antiseptics or disinfectants.

Emotional lability is more common in the pregnant patient than at other times, and often little attempt is made to recognise anxiety and even less to treat it. The primigravid patient is particularly prone to anxiety because of her lack of knowledge about childbirth, which is often compounded by the exaggerated tales of well-meaning friends and relatives. The anxiety is generally non-specific, whereas in the multiparous patient there can be a not unnatural anxiety or fear that the baby may be born with some abnormality. Anxiety is best alleviated by discussion and the doctor should make sure that the patient is allowed the opportunity to air any problems or worries that she may have and that problems are considered seriously with adequate explanation and reassurance. In this respect the continuing support that the midwife and the health visitor can give is invaluable. Tranquillisers are generally not required, although if insomnia is present and particularly in the third trimester, a hypnotic (temazepam 10–30 mg) may be necessary. No woman should arrive in the labour room tense or anxious, or exhausted through lack of sleep.

Episodes of *unhappiness and weeping* are not uncommon in the early months of an unplanned pregnancy or in the later months of any pregnancy. Again, this problem is usually amenable to sympathetic understanding, particularly if given by the husband and the family, but the health visitor and occasionally the social worker may have to be involved. True depression, however, is best managed in consultation with the psychiatrist. In every case the important factor is that the patient needs someone to whom she can talk in a quiet and unhurried way, which is not always possible during a normal consulting session.

Low back pain is not uncommon, particularly in the later stages of pregnancy. The pain often radiates into the groins and is usually due to strain of the vertebral ligaments with spasm of the surrounding muscles. The pain can be persistent and distressing and tends to become worse towards evening. It is eased by lying down, particularly on a firm surface, and advice may be given to the patient to a place a firm board under the mattress. Simple analgesics such as paracetamol will ease the pain. A prolapsed disc lesion which was prsent before pregnancy can become particularly acute. The patient should be confined to bed for about 2 weeks with the mattress supported by a firm board. As with the carpal-tunnel syndrome the condition is aggravated by the salt and water retention which occurs in pregnancy and a short trial of a thiazide diuretic, can produce a considerable improvement. Both the prolapsed disc lesion and the carpal-tunnel syndrome usually improve spontaneously following delivery. Admission to hospital may be necessary if a home-help is not available or if there are no relatives who can help with the housework and can look after the patient at home. It should be remembered that the admission of the patient to hospital, for any reason, may mean that arrangements have to be made to care for the family.

Pain over the symphysis pubis and in the sacro-iliac joints is common in the later stages of pregnancy and tends to be aggravated by prolonged standing or walking. Simple measures such as explanation, advice, and analgesics will be sufficient to relieve any discomfort or anxiety that the patient may have. Pain under the costal margin can be troublesome from about 36 weeks until term and is due to pressure from the fundus, particularly when the patient is sitting. Reassurance as to the cause of the problem is sufficient.

ABNORMALITIES OF PREGNANCY

During the routine ante-natal examination the uterus may be found to be larger or smaller than is expected. The dates of the last normal period should be re-checked, remembering however, that women often have difficulty in remembering the exact date of the last period. If there is doubt as to the maturity of the fetus or if an abnormality such as a multiple pregnancy or dysmaturity is considered possible, re-examination by ultrasonography should be arranged.

If a patient is found to have antibodies, either to the rhesus or ABO groups, the ante-natal care should be discussed with the obstetrician. Amniocentesis is required if the antibody titre rises to more than 1 in 8 and this procedure is usually carried out between the 25th and the 32nd week of gestation depending upon the titre. Following the delivery the family doctor is responsible to ensure that any rhesus negative patient who is at risk of sensitisation is given anti-D gammaglobulin.

In *congenital rubella* the persistence of the virus causes damage to the fetus in a high proportion of cases and the most vulnerable organs are of the heart, eye and ear. The incidence is difficult to estimate but in one survey intra-uterine death associated with congenital rubella was twice that of the control group and the infant mortality rate was 76.5 per 1000 live births compared to 25.8 per 1000 in the control group. The risk to the fetus diminishes as the pregnancy advances. If infection occurs in the first month there is a 61% chance of the fetus being affected. Comparable figures for the second and third months are 26% and 8%.

After the first trimester there is still an appreciable risk to the fetus, particularly of deafness, and because of the high risk of the baby being born with congenital defects, termination should be considered if the mother develops rubella at any time during the first 3 months of pregnancy.

Exposure to rubella can occur in two ways — the single contact with a patient known to have rubella, and the continuing exposure to infection in the home, especially when one or more children have the illness in the prodromal infectivity period. In young children the typical rash of rubella may be absent and it is then difficult to diagnose the infection on clinical grounds. A mother who is in early pregnancy may then be unaware that she has been exposed to the infection. The exposure to rubella, or rubella-like illnesses occurring in a pregnant patient must be recognised at an early stage if laboratory studies are to allow a definitive diagnosis to be made. When rubella is suspected, two specimens of serum should be taken — the first as soon as the illness is suspected and the second 15 days later.

Vaccination against rubella is available for 13-year-old school-girls. Such schemes were introduced in the expectation that the number of women who reach child-bearing age unprotected against rubella would steadily fall. A recent study from Glasgow (Gilmore et al 1982) however showed that 11.7% of women aged 13–21 years (mean age 17 years) who were eligible and offered rubella immunisation at the age of 13 were still susceptible to the infection. The corresponding figures for males, who had not been included in the school-based rubella immunisation programme, was 15.6%. Clearly in the practice in question the number of young women remaining susceptible to the rubella had not been reduced by the immunisation programme. The authors concluded that the immune status towards rubella of all girls should be checked at the age of 15 years so that as many as possible could be rendered immune before leaving school. This is clearly a potentially beneficial responsibility of the general practitioner. It is worthwhile establishing the immune status of all patients before they become pregnant and to arrange vaccination if they are found to be susceptible, particularly for those who work with children such as nurses and schoolteachers. It is obviously important to ensure that vaccination is not given to patients who are in early pregnancy as the teratogenic potential of the vaccine strains is not known. An immunological pregnancy test should therefore be done *before* vaccination is given and pregnancy should be prevented in the 8 weeks following vaccination.

It will obviously be difficult to arrange that all women of child-bearing age are screened, and the ante-natal clinic provides a useful catchment area. Screening for rubella antibodies is therefore a routine part of the first ante-natal visit even for those patients known to have been vaccinated in the past. Patients who are found to be immune can be reassured that they are not at risk to rubella, those who are susceptible should be warned of the need to avoid contact with rubella, and arrangements should be made to vaccinate them in the immediate post-partum period. Pregnancy can be prevented at this time by the use of Depo-Provera intramuscularly. There is evidence to show that passive immunisation using low-titre immunoglobulin in a dose of 750 mg is of little value. High titre immunoglobulin does prevent viraemia and other signs of infection and therefore presumably reduces the chance of congenital rubella infection.

Bleeding is a common problem in the first trimester of pregnancy and may be confused with an abnormal period. It is usually possible to confirm the presence of a pregnancy by vaginal examination at about 8 weeks after the first missed period. If there is any doubt or if the duration is less than 8 weeks, a pregnancy test may be helpful. The patient with a threatened abortion can be managed at home provided that the relatives are willing and able to give the care that is advised and the district nurse or midwife should visit the patient daily. The patient should be kept in bed and not allowed up until 3 days after the bleeding stops. The patient should be admitted to hospital if the bleeding is heavy or continuous or if cramp-like abdominal pain develops.

When the abortion is incomplete the patient should be given 0.5 mg of ergometrine intramuscularly and admitted to hospital. The family doctor should be satisfied that the patient is fit to travel and if there is any evidence of shock an intravenous infusion of saline should be set up before the patient is moved from the home. An abortion that is complete can normally be managed at home, and the patient should not be allowed to return to her normal activities for at least 7 days. A missed abortion can be confirmed by ultrasonography and should be dealt with in hospital. Any type of abortion occurring before the 12th week is likely to require evacuation of the uterus and the patient should be sent to hospital after resuscitation, if this is required. Abortions after this date are usually complete and if so can be managed at home. Ergometrine should be given intramuscularly in a dosage of 0.5 mg. The patient's haemoglobin should be checked following an abortion and an adequate course of iron given if there is evidence of anaemia.

Anti-D immunoglobulin: any patient whether rhesus negative or positive should be given 50 μg of anti-D immunoglobulin within 3 days of having an abortion.

A patient who is rhesus negative and who delivers a viable child should be given 100 μg of anti-D immunoglobulin. Two days later the mother's blood should be checked for the presence of fetal cells (Kleihauer Test). If fetal cells are present a further 100 μg of anti-D immunoglobulin is given and the mother's blood rechecked within a further 2 days.

Very occasionally the Kleihauer Test indicates that there has been a large infusion of fetal cells and up to 400 μg anti-D immunoglobulin may be required.

Ectopic pregnancy is a difficult problem both to the general practitioner and to the specialist but fortunately is relatively rare. There has been an increase in the incidence of ectopic (tubal) pregnancy with the growing popularity of tubal ligation as a means of contraception. There will be a history of amenorrhoea but perhaps little other indication of a pregnancy. The external bleeding is usually slight in amount and is generally accompanied by lower abdominal pain. A history of dizziness or faintness is a useful clue to an ectopic pregnancy. It is usually difficult to palpate the tubes on vaginal examination due to the pain and tenderness felt by the patient. The advice of a gynaecologist should be sought whenever this diagnosis is suspected. Once the fallopian tube has ruptured there is usually no difficulty in making a diagnosis but resuscitation of the patient may be necessary before she is moved to hospital. The help of the flying squad may be required if emergency infusion of saline is not sufficient to maintain an adequate blood pressure. It should be remembered that ectopic pregnancy can occur in a patient who has been fitted with an IUCD.

Ligation operations, even those performed as long as 10 years previously, can be complicated by an ectopic tubal pregnancy.

A *hydatidiform mole* should be suspected when the growth of the uterus is not as expected, and particularly when this is associated with bleeding occurring at about 22 to 24 weeks or when signs of pre-eclampsia occur in the early pregnancy. The presence of a mole can be suspected if an immunological pregnancy test is positive in high dilution, and confirmed by ultrasonography. The patient should be admitted for specialist care. Patients who have had a mole require close supervision for about 2 years following delivery and should be discouraged from becoming pregnant again for about 1 year. An oral contraceptive can be safely used for this purpose.

Abnormal presentations of the fetus can usually be corrected and managed by the general practitioner. The patient should be referred to a specialist if any difficult is experienced in correcting the position or if the fetus reverts to the abnormal presentation after the 36th week of pregnancy.

Every woman has the right to ask to be considered for *termination* of a pregnancy. It should be clearly understood that the practitioner's responsibility is to advise on the best form of care and certainly not to sit in moral judgement, and the opinion of the patient herself and her family should be sought and respected. The doctor should be aware of his own attitudes to termination, and as with alcoholism, self-poisoning and sexual deviation, must prevent these attitudes from distorting his judgement. When there is doubt about the decision or if the doctor has difficulty in making an objective assessment, a second opinion should be sought. The attitudes of general practitioners and specialists may be influenced by moral and religious factors which affect the decision that is given, and this can be one cause of the variation that exists from one area of the country to another. This difference in attitude is understandable but its resulting influence on the availability or otherwise of termination can cause dissatisfaction in the community and as such, should cause concern to the medical profession.

The decision as to whether to recommend the termination of a pregnancy should only be made when all the physical, psychological and social factors that may be relevant are known. It may often be necessary to ask the advice of the health visitor or the social worker whose knowledge of the family dynamics may be more complete than that of the doctor. The decision is an important one and it is best if the family doctor and the specialist discuss it face to face, rather than to rely on the inadequate information contained in a referral letter.

The family doctor's decision should be made known to the patient and her family but it should also be explained that the gynaecologist may not hold the same opinion and that the signatures of two doctors are required by law before a termination can be carried out. There is no place for referring a patient to a gynaecologist after leading her to believe that the termination will automatically be performed. Similarly, it is not right to leave the full responsibility of the decision to the specialist: the family doctor must firmly state his own recommendation.

The after care of the patient who has an abortion or a termination is often neglected. She should have a complete post-natal examination 6 weeks after the abortion at which time advice can be offered on family planning. This is best done with the co-operation of the health visitor. The patient should remain off work for 4 weeks and any emotional problems which occur should be managed with sympathetic understanding and support.

Women who are refused termination require considerable support during the pregnancy by the family doctor, the health visitor and the social worker. There is no justification in refusing termination and then leaving the patient and her family to their own devices. The patient has usually asked for a termination in the belief that her problems were so great as to make the pregnancy un-

acceptable. The termination of a pregnancy should not be made conditional on the patient agreeing to be sterilised. This decision should be considered dispassionately on its own merits. Conversely, termination cannot be allowed to become an acceptable form of contraception.

POST-NATAL CARE

GENERAL CONSIDERATIONS

The care of the mother and her new baby is not complete until she has fully recovered — physically and psychologically — from the birth process and until her care of her child has reached a happy, confident and competent level. Indeed it could be said that the general practitioner's responsibility for the new family which began during or before the ante-natal period does not end with the post-natal examination but merges into the continuing care of the growing child and his family.

Whereas in ante- and intra-natal care the focus of responsibility moves steadily with time towards the obstetrician and the hospital, the reverse holds true for post-natal care. The midwife has the responsibility to supervise the wellbeing of mother and child and a professional duty to visit the family at least twice daily until the third day and daily thereafter until the 10th day. From then onwards the health visitor assumes the midwife's duties reflecting the importance of this stage in the change of the mother's needs from those of practical nursing to those of maintenance of health and promotion of good mothering skills. The general practitioner is responsible for the medical supervision of the post-natal period for 14 days, but in reality his interest and involvement assumes an ongoing nature as befits his role of family doctor. In many ways this time limit of 14 days also implies that the needs of mother and child are substantially different in the days before and subsequent to this date.

Although the responsibilities of the general practitioner will be described under fairly specific headings, and although the time of responsibility — 14 days — implies that he has a different role before and after this date, in reality his care should be holistic with but a difference in emphasis at different stages that is dependent on the needs of mother and child. There is also likely to be some overlap between the responsibilities of midwife, health visitor and doctor — or at least a perception of overlap — or of neglect of a responsibility on the assumption that it is in the province of another: in this as in any other example of team or shared care it is worth establishing and maintaining close co-operation with others so that comprehensive and complete care can be achieved.

CLINICAL CONTENT OF POST-NATAL CARE

Complete involution of the uterus and the return towards normality of the birth passages can be expected by the 14th–21st day following the birth and the clinical care of the patient in this early stage thus focuses on this process and on the early recognition and effective treatment of the most likely threat — infection. In most instances the lochia steadily diminishes in blood content and volume to become absent by 3 or 4 weeks: slight vaginal discharge however frequently persists up to the time of the first menstruation. Signs of infection include pyrexia and malaise, an increase in the volume of the lochia, the return of fresh vaginal bleeding and a change in the odour of the lochia. Severely ill patients in whom there is a risk of sudden profuse post-partum haemorrhage should be admitted urgently to hospital: the less ill patient can be looked after at home being treated with a broad spectrum antibiotic in full dosage (for example amoxicillin 500 mg t.d.s. for 10 days), which should be given immediately after a swab of the discharge has been sent for bacteriological examination and the antibiotic changed if the sensitivity patterns of the pathogen indicate that this is necessary. Urinary tract infection — the other and more common infection — can be recognised and treated in the normal way. By the time of discharge from hospital — usually between the 6th and 10th day following delivery for a first time mother — the perineum will have healed or be healing normally and seldom requires any further attention.

The breasts require care and attention in the early weeks until satisfactory breast feeding has been achieved or until suppression of lactation and involution of breast tissue has been completed. The common problems include cracking or fissuring of the nipple or areola and breast abscess which can follow the appearance of a fissure. These complications are generally due to improper fixation of baby to the breast resulting in the infant chewing with his gums on the nipple or immediate surrounding area of the areola. Fissures will normally heal quickly and naturally if the breast is rested and the milk expressed from it at the time of each feed. Frank infection will require systemic antibiotic therapy with again the breast being rested. Suppression of lactation — either because of persistent infection or maternal wishes — can be achieved with bromocriptine 2.5 mg daily for 2 days then 2.5 mg thrice daily for 14 days.

The monitoring of the state of the lochia, the progress of any perineal wound and the state of the breasts is usually the responsibility of the midwife who will bring any problem to the doctor's attention. It is preferable however if the doctor also pays attention to these areas whenever he visits his patient.

The formal post-natal examination usually takes place when baby is almost 6 weeks old and should include an assessment of the health of both mother and child. The physical examination should concentrate on ensuring that the mother's health has returned to normal — with an absence of vaginal discharge, the re-establishment of menstruation, the healing of any vaginal tear or episiotomy and the return of normal tone to pelvic and abdominal muscles. The blood pressure should be checked and if found to be raised the appropriate follow-up, investigation and treatment plan should be commenced. The urine should be tested for protein and sugar and sent for bacteriological culture. The haemoglobin estimation should be made and any anaemia found should be corrected. This is also an appropriate time to take a cervical smear — if not done during the ante-natal period — and to restart or initiate contraception in those patients who wish family planning. Rubella immunisation should be given — after a pregnancy test has been returned as negative, and under contraceptive cover — to those mothers who were found to be non-immune at the start of the pregnancy. It is important to check that sero conversion has occurred following this post-natal immunisation.

Of as much importance is the need to assess the emotional state of the mother and to identify any problems she may be experiencing with her family or her new baby. Since the health visitor will be intimately involved in the management of such problems it is best if she is present during this part of the post-natal examination.

An increasing number of general practitioners now include some form of preschool developmental screening as a routine part of their child care provision and the 6-week examination of the mother provides a good starting point for such preventive child care. The physical examination of the baby and the developmental tests appropriate to the 6-week-old infant are detailed in Chapter 8 (pp. 102–103).

THE PSYCHOLOGICAL WELLBEING OF THE MOTHER

Many mothers experience what for them are unexpected and wholly unwanted feelings of heightened emotion and tearfulness in the early puerperal period: this is however a normal biological consequence of childbirth and usually responds to explanation and support. These feelings however can persist and perhaps become more pronounced if the patient's general condition is aggravated by fatigue or worry or by a feeling of not being able to cope adequately with her family, the home and the new baby. As much attention should therefore be paid to ensuring that the mother is getting adequate help in the home, that she is able to have 'her feet up' rest in the afternoon and adequate sleep at night.

Certain other circumstances can adversely affect a

mother's psychological health during the puerperium. The most obvious of these is when the child was unplanned and perhaps unwanted: the mother's rejection of her child is usually covert but in extreme instances can lead to an abandonment of any response to the baby's needs. In contrast the late child of a previously childless older couple or the child born after a number of previous abortions can become the focus for increased maternal affection and concern that can manifest through exaggerated anxiety about any apparent departure from normal in the baby's behaviour. The mother who previously seemed only just able to cope with the day by day problems and demands of husband and home may find herself out of her depth with the added responsibility of a child. The need that then arises for sustained additional support from health visitor and doctor should have been anticipated and built into the management plan for the puerperium. It is important that the doctor does not resort to anxiolytic or antidepressant drug therapy in these circumstances: of much more value to the long-term psychological health of the mother is education and constructive support to allow her mothering skills to become fully and competently developed.

True puerperal psychosis is a rare complication, occurring in only two of every 1000 births, and can only be predicted with any certainty if the patient has been known to have had one or more psychotic illnesses prior to the pregnancy. The presentation is as in any psychotic illness except that the symptoms occur most suddenly with a heightened intensity. The condition is usually acute in onset with marked agitation, visual or auditory hallucinations, perplexity and disturbances of the conscious state. This illness constitutes a psychiatric emergency and the advice of a specialist with regard to home treatment or hospital admission should be sought.

It is an important philosophy that post-natal care is simply one aspect of a continuum of care that can be viewed as beginning with the adult patient, preceding through the ante- and post-natal period to the care of the child and thus of the future adult. Only in general practice can such a continuum become a reality and where the doctor has such a potential to affect the health — or the illness — of successive generations.

REFERENCES

Gilmore D, Robinson E T, Gilmour Harper W, Urquhart G E D 1982 Effect of rubella vaccination programme in schools on rubella immunity in a general practice population. British Medical Journal 284: 628–630

Hartley R M, Velez R, Morris R W, D'Souza M F, Heller R F 1983 Confirming the diagnosis of a mild hypertension. British Medical Journal 286: 287–288

Robinson E T, Barber J H 1977 Early diagnosis of pregnancy in general practice. Journal of the Royal College of General Practitioners 27: 335–338

Social Trends 1981 HMSO, London

Child health and general practice

It might seem obvious that health care for children of necessity develops in response to the morbidity specific to the society served, and must alter in response to changing priorities. History shows that this is not always so. Social paediatric research in developed countries highlights the increasing significance of psychological and developmental problems as the classical serious physical disorders of childhood decline; problems which in the past have received less attention and too often scant resources. A number of government reports and reports from academic institutions in the United Kingdom and United States emphasise the early detection and management of such problems, preventive health care, and the equitable distribution of comprehensive services for all children.

Table 7.1 lists the main obstacles to good health care. Primary care and the family doctor are considered to have a fundamental contribution to make to the effective and strategic development of these services (Table 7.2).

The purpose of this chapter is to outline some of the ways in which this contribution is being and might be made.

Perhaps the most important development in child health in recent years has been the understanding that the care of children is a partnership between family doc-

tors, community medicine, nursing, and hospital clinical services. Of crucial importance in providing effective child care is the need for responsibilities to be clearly defined and for information to be sensibly and appropriately shared. The emphasis on the community care of children, particularly of the handicapped, does make major demands of general practice. Amongst the consequences is an increasing involvement of family doctors in giving advice about service developments, and in contributing to undergraduate and postgraduate education.

CHILDHOOD MORBIDITY

Studies of general practice in Britain show that about 30% of the work of family doctors is concerned with children. A considerable proportion of this concerns minor and self-limiting morbidity (Table 7.3).

There is perhaps a danger of regarding much of this minor morbidity as insignificant and unworthy of follow-up, although many of the common communicable diseases have a small but very definite risk of serious complications.

The prevalence of major continuing disabilities in any given practice is small. Few general practitioners are likely to encounter children with rare metabolic or neurological disorders, but with advances in therapeutics and rehabilitation many children with disorders such as cystic fibrosis are now surviving into adolescent and adult life and will need the continuing help of their family doctors.

Of some considerable importance are those less esoteric problems of childhood which may have a considerable significance for the future health and social and educational achievements of the child. One study (Bassett 1981) (Table 7.4) revealed a considerable disparity between the recorded and surveyed prevalences of certain continuing disorders of childhood.

Few children die at home but childhood mortality and its consequences on family life are part of the experience of every general practitioner. Table 7.5 shows the major causes of death in a group of 43 children dying over a 7-year period. More than half of these deaths, in the final

Table 7.1 Obstacles to preventive and longitudinal child health care

1. Unequal distribution of manpower and resouces
2. Complex administration, planning. Poor records and communication
3. Ineffective, inappropriate and poorly organised services
4. Inappropriate use and abuse of services
5. Inadequate training

Table 7.2 The case of primary care

1. G.P., H.V., District Nurse in right place at the right time
2. Knowledge of local health and social problems
3. Greater expertise of childhood problems — improving training of G.Ps., H.Vs
4. Health Centre, building programmes allow better practice zoning in areas of high population density

Table 7.3 Childhood morbidity patterns

Condition	% Consultations by children	% All consultations
Respiratory disorders	32	47
Infection/Parasitic illness	15	55
Disorders of CNS	12	44
Symptom/Ill-defined problems	10	31
Skin disease	9	36
Accidents, poisoning, violence	5	25
Mental health problems	4	11

(Adapted from Stark, Bassett, 1975)

Table 7.4 Recorded and actual prevalence — some problems of children

Problem	Recorded prevalence/1000	Surveyed prevalence/1000
Behaviour disorder	15	80
Learning problems	—	33
Visual acuity defect	13	81
Squints	10	31
Amblyopia	5	26
Partial sight	1	3
Colour blindness	—	11
Chronic recurrent middle ear disease	7	10
Partial hearing loss	3	15
Major disorders CNS	4	8
Speech disorders	4	14
Mental handicap	2	13
Long term orthopaedic disorders	3	8
Congenital heart disorder	—	8
Skin disorders (mainly eczema)	5	31
Undescended testicle	3	16

Table 7.5 Causes of death in 43 children (0–14 years) in a Scottish New Town

	Male	Female	Total
Perinatal and neonatal			
Malformations	4	4	8
Prematurity and complications	5	1	6
Infection	4	1	5
Post neonatal			
Malformations	0	4	4
Infection	8	2	10
'Cot death'	1	1	2
Home trauma/poisoning	0	3	3
Road traffic accidents	0	3	3
Non-accidental injury	0	1	1
Appendicitis	0	1	1

analysis, might be considered as avoidable, 33% being due to congenital malformations or associated with prematurity and 51% to infection, accident, poisoning or violence. Such deaths of course provide a very major challenge to even the most supportive systems of health and social services.

MORBIDITY WITHIN THE FAMILY

It almost seems unnecessary to remind ourselves that a child's health and wellbeing and that of his family are interdependent. Some idea of the dimension of family health problems in relation to children can be gleaned

Table 7.6   Continuing health and social problems in families of children (> 6 months)

Social class	%			
	I–II	III	IV–V	All
Active health problems	44	63	89	65
Active social problems	7	13	39	17
Co-existing health/social problems	4	9	25	11

from Table 7.6 which shows the extent of continuing health and social problems in a randomly selected cohort of about 400 children. An analysis of the continuing health problems of these families reveals that mental health disorders account for 29%, with anxiety and depression and alcohol problems predominating. It should be axiomatic that the assessment of any child in sickness or in health is incomplete without considering that of the entire family. It is a cause for some concern that while about 4% of children in Central Scotland will have a parent (fathers 3:1 compared with mothers) with cardiovascular disease, 47% will have a first degree relative with ischaemic heart disease and 29% with hypertension compared with only 14% and 12% for diabetes and chronic renal disease. Preventive medicine begins in childhood as much for these disorders as for the communicable diseases.

The importance of family health and wellbeing will be referred to again when considering learning and behavioural problems in childhood.

ORGANISATIONAL ASPECT OF CHILD CARE IN GENERAL PRACTICE

The organisation of child care in general practice continues to be a matter of considerable debate. The differing circumstances of rural practice, sparse populations, urban development and inner city areas require different solutions. Nevertheless there are two guiding requirements:

1. That children should have ready access to acute and continuing medical care at all times.
2. That children should have equal access to all preventive medical services.

Family medicine in making a commitment to total child care must facilitate both. To begin with there must be an equitable distribution of family doctors with good practice facilities and adequate ancillary support. Whether in rural or urban practice it is necessary to adopt a systematic approach to child care which makes an economic use of nursing and ancillary services and has clearly defined responsibilities and good communication. Next no procedure should ever be delegated unless the persons in-

structed have the professional sanction and expertise to do so. Whether the Primary Care Team consists simply of the general practitioner, his district nurse, midwife and an attached health visitor, or a large multidisciplinary group, good child health practice can only proceed on such a basis.

Group practices can organise child care in several ways; commonly individual general practitioners assume a total responsibility for preventive and non-specialised clinical care of children. In many the responsibility for preventive child health services is delegated to community child health clinical medical officers. A third approach which has been proposed suggests that within group practices one doctor with additional training and expertise in child health undertakes a general supervisory responsibility for all the child health services provided by the group. Such an approach should not interfere with the general responsibilities of individual doctors for individual children and their families. When group and health centre practices serve a large number of children rationalisation of services can lead to an economical use of medical and nursing time. Although the principal beneficiaries are children, greater opportunities result for teaching and research. A list of those involved in Primary Care Teams serving large group and health centre practices and of the services currently available from many of these is shown in Table 7.7.

It has been argued that the co-ordination and assessment of the Primary Care Teams' preventive services should be a responsibility of community medicine, leaving the family doctor to deal with the day to day management of clinical problems. Several large group practices have general practitioners with a specific interest in child health who are prepared to co-ordinate and develop the services of children served by their practices. How this is done is illustrated schematically in Tables 7.8 and 7.9. Whatever approach practices choose to adopt, and there are certainly no absolutes, none must infringe the principle that care for children should be as personalised as it is for their parents.

The complexity of legislation relating to child health and social welfare, the variety of professions involved and ever changing social conditions have resulted in changing demands of family doctors and of their relationships to other professions. Issues of confidentiality can lead to

Table 7.7   Personnel involved in Primary Care Teams and services currently available

Medical	
General Practitioners	— General medical service
(Vocational trainees)	Care of handicapped
	Screening — immunisation
Visiting Consultants	— Specialist assessment — paediatric, psychiatry, orthopaedic, etc.
Clinical Medical Officer	— Screening — immunisation
	Review and ascertainment of children with special needs
Nursing	
Health Visitor	— Preventive care — health education
	Promotion and involvement in screening — immunisation
	Well baby clinics
	Home visiting — ascertainment of needs
Practice nurse	— Minor treatment service
	Product assistance with immunisation
	After care of children discharged from surgery
Visiting paediatric nurse	— Follow up children discharged from hospital — liaison with community services
Midwife	— Responsibility for neonate to age of 10 days
Therapists	— Orthoptics
	Physiotherapy
	Speech therapy
Clinical psychologist	— Management of behaviour problems
	Management of phobic illness
	Assessment of specific problems of learning and development
	Liaison with educational psychologist
Social worker	— Assessment and ascertainment of needs
	Counselling of parents and children
	Supervision of children and families at risk, or at request of Courts

Table 7.8   The organisation of a general practice child health service

1. Establish practice referral system and define responsibilities
2. Establish clinical and ancillary support
3. Establish case review system with colleagues with appropriate social work/education liaison
4. Identify G.P. with paediatric interest and appropriate training
5. Define child population
   a. Age/sex register
   b. Immunisation and screening call-up system
   c. Implement child health record (A4, POMR, etc.)
   d. Develop data retrieval system
   e. Implement handicap continuous morbidity register

Table 7.9   The functions of the G.P.(P)

1. To advise on and oversee paediatric practice
2. To provide a first line consultative service for colleagues and team
3. To ensure effective immunisation and screening
4. To provide formal/informal day to day clinical advice to colleagues
5. To maintain a record of handicapped children/specialist problems in the practice
6. To provide a practice liaison with education/social work
7. To provide advice to local voluntary and statutory bodies
8. To assist/conduct teaching and research at local level and at regional level

conflict but doctors have to accept that other professions have ethical codes just as strict as their own. The interests of children are paramount even more so when this involves their safety and security or possibilities of criminal activity towards them.

THE PRIMARY CARE TEAM AND CHILD CARE

The visiting consultant
Present health service policy encourages the development of peripheral consultative services which involve specialists in the community and primary health care of children. Several advantages arise when children are seen on domiciliary consultation, or at practice based clinics. Parents and child do not have to travel great distances, on occasion at great expense. Unnecessary delay, investigation, and hospital admission can all be avoided and parents, child and family doctor have the benefit of an immediate authoritative opinion without an intermediary.

The health visitor
In Britain, historically and by definition, the health visitors' functions are largely concerned with maternal and child health, although these are now being considerably expanded to include the care of the elderly. Their work is concerned with:

1. Promoting the immunisation of children and encouraging defaulters to complete immunisation schedules.

2. The promotion of developmental screening in which they may be actively involved.

3. Advice to mothers about general health and child care.

4. Facilitating access to health and social services.

5. Liaison with specialised nursing services and with other nursing disciplines involved in child care.

6. Involvement in the health and welfare and hygiene of children in schools.

7. Assuming responsibility as the 'named person' for handicapped preschool children. The 'named person' as defined in the Warnock Report is proposed as that person to whom the parents of handicapped children can turn to for day to day advice and support.

8. Advice to local community, voluntary and statutory authorities about child care in their own communities. Health visitor attachment to primary care teams and to individual practices has proved highly effective and avoids communication lapses, which can be particularly important when non-accidental injury of children is suspected.

The practice nurse
As much as half of the work of practice nurses may be concerned with children. Most of this will be concerned with skin disorders, minor trauma, dressings and advice about minor illness. There are other ways in which they prove invaluable notably in assistance with immunisation. With training they are more than competent to undertake simple investigative procedures such as audiometry and tuberculin testing. Practice nurses may be privately employed by family doctors or seconded by health authorities. In either circumstances responsibility for their clinical work with children rests with the individual general practitioners concerned who must be satisfied that any procedure is appropriate, safe and within the experience and competence of the nurses involved. In some areas children discharged from hospital on complex treatment or requiring specialist nursing procedures will be followed up at home by a hospital based paediatric nurse who can liaise with community and practice nurses. This has proved particularly useful for children with chronic disabilities, is reassuring to parents and child and may reduce the need for frequent hospital consultations.

THE G.P. AND THE SCHOOL CHILD

It is a statutory responsibility of the National Health Service to ascertain the health status and special medical requirements of school children. With an increasing emphasis on early education this, in association with social work, is being extended to cover nursery schools and children in the first 3 years of life. School medical services play a most important part in the immunisation of children against rubella, tuberculosis and tetanus. It has been suggested that much of the non-specialised work of school health should be incorporated into primary care. In some areas where practices and schools serve the same, usually geographically well-defined populations, this has proved eminently practicable. The advantages of such an approach are that:

1. Children and families are well known to the practices.

2. Continuity of care is ensured.

3. Duplication of effort and unnecessary procedures are avoided and referral for specialist opinion is simplified.

4. The common interest of family doctors and teachers in the welfare and achievement of children can be mutually enhanced and misunderstandings avoided.

Some practices which include a general practitioner with an interest in such work are already undertaking school health duties on a sessional basis.

CHILD HEALTH SOCIAL WORK IN GENERAL PRACTICE

There are many developments and changes relating to the care and safety of children and in the rights and entitlements of married partners. These may involve family doctors in several ways and an understanding of the principles involved is essential. There has been a parallel development in the responsibilities of social work services and of health visitors reflected by an expansion in their numbers and in the whole or part-time attachment of workers to group practices and health centres. Speed of access and the avoidance of communication problems are the outstanding benefits of such attachments: much of the professional antipathy and misunderstandings which exists between medical and social work can be avoided and a better understanding of each other's professional responsibilities results. Some problems arise out of misconceptions and unrealistic expectations of each other. One reason for this may be that doctors with their individual executive authority can, without reference, treat and investigate — in other words be directive; whereas social workers must perforce work in an hierarchical system often with quite severe constraints on material resources and above all must not be seen to be directive, unless their clients are under some form of court supervision. The common concern of attached social workers and health visitors with the social wellbeing of parents and children is a potential area of conflict which must be and can be quite easily avoided.

Although an over-simplification, family doctors' need for social work assistance and his legal obligations will in general relate to:

1. Deprivation of children and their families, particularly when health is affected.
2. Children at risk to physical ill-treatment or emotional and sensory deprivation.
3. Maladjusted children or children with intellectual handicap.
4. Children received into statutory care by local government authorities.

Differences in the legal system and organisations of social work in the United Kingdom affect the way in which these problems may be handled. In Scotland for example a system of children's Hearings conducted by Reporters deal with problems concerned with children under the age of 17 who are, for example, psychologically, sexually or physically at risk, as well as with most children accused of statutory offences. There are undoubtedly times when the separate interests of child and parents may make a doctor hesitant to present evidence to social work and legal authorities. In some instances this can be resolved by honest discussion with the parents who, not infrequently, welcome such an approach and will 'so to speak' make a clean breast of things, and sanction disclosures of their problems, in a desire to seek help and resolution of their difficulties. Legal and social work proceedings relating to children and families should ideally always be held in camera and only in exceptional circumstances should there be any public disclosure of the proceedings. When difficulties arise doctors should seek legal advice from their defence union before submitting written or oral evidence. It goes without saying that a written record of the circumstances and event pertaining to any child is essential.

Family doctors may be required to examine children received into and discharged from statutory care or to examine children being placed for adoption. Another requirement includes the assessment and examination of adults seeking to adopt children or those concerned with child care — play leaders, child minders are obvious examples.

ALLOWANCES

Several allowances are available for disabled children and children with special needs. It is necessary for the family doctor to be aware of these and to advise parents of their availability. In addition doctors may be required to provide medical information in support of claims and in the clinical assessment of disabled children. These allowances principally concern:

1. Attendance allowance — payable to children over the age of 2 who require more or less constant supervision with, for example — toileting, feeding, dressing and washing.
2. Mobility allowance for children so profoundly disabled as to be unable to walk any significant distance.
3. Family income supplement for children with special nutritional, heating, and clothing requirements, for example, assistance with the purchase of washing machines. (The Family Fund is administered on behalf of the government by the Joseph Rowantree Trust and will also provide grants of this nature).

VOLUNTARY AGENCIES

A large number of voluntary agencies and charitable trusts exists for children with different disabilities or for children in distress and need. Generally speaking they will provide:

1. Material or financial assistance.
2. Holiday or respite care.
3. Opportunities for children and families to meet each other and share and learn from their individual experiences.
4. Counselling.
5. Fund raising for research and development.
6. Pressure on statutory authorities for improvements in the levels of financial support and an improvement in the services available for the disabled.

While most parents of disabled children are aware of the various agencies that can help they may seek the support and advice of their family doctors. Information about the statutory and voluntary services available for children with special needs is most easily obtained by contacting local social work departments, or hospital social workers. Many social work authorities publish an annual directory of services; health visitors prove another invaluable source of information.

CHILD HEALTH RECORDS

The Child Health Record has two important functions; it should be on the one hand a working aid in clinical management, treatment, and preventive health care, and on the other a source of reliable information for epidemiological and research purposes. Good records are the foundation of good child care. The Child Health Record should ideally satisfy the following requirements:

1. It should be structured to allow for the recording of developmental progress and immunisation procedures, and present salient information at a glance.

2. Adopt a systematic approach to the recorded clinical narrative which should nevertheless leave room for the inclusion of statements made by children and parents.

3. Incorporate the health visitor narrative.

4. File records, reports and abstracts in a sequential manner.

Developments in microcomputers and data recording in general practice are moving fast and have been encouraged by recent DHSS grants to some practices introducing microcomputing. Other systems of data handling not dependent on computers exist. (The subject of medical records and information systems is dealt with elsewhere.) Some thought must be given however to the codification of disorders of childhood for example, whether or not to use the British Paediatric Association modification of International Classification Disease or the Wonca system devised for primary care (also based on the international classification). For general practice, given the prevalence of the more esoteric disorders of childhood the Wonca system is recommended.

The development of a systematic approach to records undoubtedly leads to better patient care and communication within the practice. Immunisation rates and attendances at developmental screening sessions can be improved considerably. Audit of child care becomes practicable while a valuable contribution can be made to local and national information systems. General practice is still a largely untapped source of important information about child health.

REFERENCE

Bassett W J 1981 Child and family health in a Scottish new town. Health Bulletin 39: 7–20

RECOMMENDED READING

Apley J, Ounstead C (eds) 1982 One child. S.I.M.P., Heinemann Medical Books, London. (An elegant review of some of the many circumstances affecting children, their families, their achievements and the quality of their care)

Miller F J W, Court S D M, Knox E G, Brandon S (eds) The school years in Newcastle-upon-Tyne (1952–62). Churchill Livingstone, Edinburgh. (A classic of social paediatric research being a further contribution to the original 1000 family study)

Hart C (ed) 1982 Child care in general practice. Churchill Livingstone, Edinburgh. (Written by G.Ps. for general practice. This book presents the challenges of child care for general practitioners with useful contributions on the organisation of care of children in general practice as well as their clinical management)

Mitchell R G (ed) 1980 Child health in the community. Churchill Livingstone, Edinburgh. (This is an authoritative standard reference on community child care clearly set out, well written, and easily read)

Clinical paediatrics and the general practitioner I

EXAMINATION TECHNIQUES

The art of child care is not to underestimate children but to see things with the perspective of childhood. Children are amongst our most discerning and perceptive critics. Whatever the viewpoints of parents or indeed doctors, a child must be approached with respect, confidence and empathy. No matter how young, speak to the child in the language of childhood. Whenever possible hear his story in his own words. This said, taking a history of childhood problems demands careful questioning of parents, discarding the influences of folk lore, imprecise symptom description and avoiding over-eagerness to ascribe symptoms to unlikely causes. To give examples — teething does not cause fits nor does infestation with worms, while diarrhoea and vomiting must be accurately defined as indeed must be such ill-defined statements as 'the child is burning up'. Caution is required in the acceptance of parental diagnosis notably with exanthematous infectious diseases. In essence keep an open mind and do not be guiled into a too ready and too facile an acceptance of proffered diagnoses.

Children are sensitive to the demeanour, stature, voice and appearance of their doctor. Speak to the child face to face, eye to eye, explaining what your wishes are and demonstrating what you intend to do. Show the child the stethoscope and the auroscope and constantly reassure. If it is necessary to inflict discomfort then say so but in a reassuring way which will enlist the child's co-operation and minimise this discomfort. With gentleness and explanation few children will resist examination and many will enjoy it. Even so, some protesting children will need to be restrained. Before doing so start with those parts of the examination procedure which are least threatening leaving to the end examination of ear, nose and throat, the genitals and rectum.

Never strip a child naked for examination unless it is absolutely necessary. Respect his or her modesty and examine him whenever possible in close proximity to his mother or preferably sitting on her knee.

PRACTICAL PROCEDURES

Reluctance to inflict discomfort on children sometimes deters family doctors from resorting to parenteral treatment or investigative procedures. Given suitable explanation and understanding children can be very co-operative and forgiving. Fortunately most practical procedures required of family doctors are not difficult and are few in number.

BLOOD SAMPLING AND INJECTIONS

In older children blood can be taken from the antecubital vein without restraint; in infants and small children it is advisable to use restraint by wrapping them in a blanket exposing only the site of venepuncture. With instruction and experience blood can be taken from other sites including the femoral vein. In babies adequate samples can often be obtained by heel stab using the anteromedial fleshy part of the heel. After cleaning with surgical spirit apply a very fine film of sterile vaseline, prick the heel firmly with a sterile disposable lancet and 'milk' the heel so that blood collects in large globules which can be easily collected in appropriate containers (laboratories will advise). If all that is required is a simple estimation of haemoglobin the use of the American Optical Company haemoglobinometer is to be recommended, this providing a cheap on-the-spot estimation. Intramuscular injections in infants and small and thin children should be given in the outer and upper quadrant of the buttock or occasionally in the lateral aspect of the thigh and never in the arm. This site is painful for the child, local reactions are not always so well contained and there is a risk of damage to the radial nerve.

BACTERIOLOGICAL SPECIMENS

Stool cultures
Faecal samples are best collected fresh, if necessary from

the infant's napkin, and should be sent in the appropriate sterile container. This is particularly important if stools are to be examined for cysts. If stools are very fluid and difficult to collect then a rectal swab may suffice provided this arrives at the laboratory fresh or is sent in a suitable 'transport' medium.

Nose and throat swabs

Swabs of the nose and throat should be obtained gently but firmly and in the case of tonsillitis with slight pressure on the tonsils so that exudate may be obtained from the tonsilar crypts. Swabs should be sent to the laboratory either fresh or in Stuart's Medium. Per nasal or supra-laryngeal swabs may be sent for examination if pertussis is suspected although many bacteriologists would prefer a Bordet Cough Plate.

SKIN SWABS

Again swabs from the skin or conjunctivae should be sent in a transport medium. If lesions are very dry and exudate cannot easily be obtained on a dry swab the answer is to dip the swab into sterile water, saline or preferably Stuart's Medium and then swab the lesion. Skin scrapings for mycological examination are obtained by gently stroking the infected lesion with the edge of a clean microscope slide.

Urine

Reliable midstream specimens of urine can be obtained from school children after cleansing of the perineum or penis with soap and water. Specimens may be voided directly into a sterile container or into a pot or pan that has been washed out and sterilised with boiling water and then cooled, the urine being subsequently transferred to the specimen container. In infant males a clean catch urine may be obtained by gently supra-pubic pressure soon after a feed has been given. Alternatively it may be necessary to use an adhesive disposable plastic bag which can be fitted over the penis or vulva. Urine so obtained may be contaminated and unless growths are significant and are accompanied by a large number of leucocytes, culture results must be treated with caution.

While specimens of urine can be stored in a refrigerator overnight ideally they should be sent to the laboratories as soon as possible after being obtained. Culture of freshly obtained urine on dip slides incubated for a period of 12 hours can provide a semi-quantitative estimate of Gram negative infections and have proved useful in child population screening or in areas with difficult access to laboratories.

Urinalysis

Analysis of urine using test strips is as for adults. Caution must be shown in interpreting results of tests for ketone since these readily appear in the urine of any febrile or fasted child. Test strips can be used on wet napkins but again results must be treated with caution, particularly with regard to albumen since this test may be influenced by a number of chemical substances and detergents used in cleaning the napkin.

TUBERCULIN TESTING

A variety of commercially available single unit tuberculin tests are now available. Their reliability has been questioned and many prefer to use Heaf testing or intradermal Mantoux testing, neither procedure being particularly difficult. The results of Mantoux tests are read 24 hours and 48 hours and Heaf tests 4–7 days after being carried out, positive results being indicated by erythema and induration.

SKIN TESTING

Skin testing for allergens may be carried out by patch or prick testing using extracts of a number of possible allergens, the results being compared with controls. In general terms the place of skin testing in very small children is somewhat restricted.

PRESCRIBING FOR CHILDREN

The therapeutic armamentarium necessary for the management of childhood illness is quite modest. Prescribing for children need cause no anxieties if certain principles are observed:

1. Infants, like the elderly, have physiological limitations on the efficiency with which they metabolise and excrete some drugs.

2. Dosage tolerances may be very limited and in the case of certain drugs, such as anticonvulsants, side-effects can be expected if these are exceeded. Blood levels of such drugs should be monitored.

3. Paradoxical effects may occur, notably with such drugs as phenobarbitone which may cause hyperactivity and aggressive behaviour, diazepam which does the opposite of tranquillise and amphetamines and ephedrine which may sedate.

4. Symptomatic treatment of minor illness seldom if ever requires the use of powerful analgesics, anti-emetics or anti-diarrhoeals.

5. The range of anti-microbial drugs required in general practice can be severely restricted to erythromycin ethyl succinate, co-trimoxazole, phenoxymethylpenicillin and a broad spectrum penicillin such as ampicillin or amoxycillin. Other anti-microbial agents should

be used with discrimination and ideally only after bacteriological evidence indicates their need.

6. Psychotropic drugs are very seldom necessary except perhaps in older children and adolescents.

7. No drug should ever be prescribed without an explanation as to why and advice about its proper use, potential dangers and safe custody. This advice, age permitting, should also be given to the child.

It is true that the treatment of many childhood ailments has to be symptomatic and at times empirical. Much can be achieved by good nursing including such measures as tepid sponging and a liberal intake of fluid in a febrile illness, but it should not be forgotten that children do experience pain, myalgia and all the symptoms which adults experience. Children are as entitled to symptomatic relief as are their parents. Do not hesitate in recommending the use of paracetamol or soluble aspirin in the relief of symptoms associated with many childhood infections such as otitis media. Sensible explanation to a parent and child can do much to avoid an unnecessary prescription but time-honoured practices and public expectations die hard and practicalities may dictate that a bottle of medicine is required. Indeed sometimes it can help, particularly decongestants for the catarrhal child while the syrup vehicle of many preparations probably has a demulcant effect on inflamed oro-pharyngeal mucosa. The rule should be that the preparation must be safe and inexpensive. There is evidence which suggests that with explanation the demand for medicines for self-limiting disorders may be reduced.

The decision to use anti-microbial drugs requires a great deal of commonsense. Pragmatism enters into the decision. It is by no means always possible or indeed sensible to await bacteriological proof of organism sensitivities before starting treatment with antibiotics. Many other determinants influence the doctor's decision to prescribe these. Poor physique such as handicaps, particularly when associated with respiratory disorders, poor nutrition, possible contact with pertussis, recurrence of otitis media or severe measles. Several formulae exist for the calculation of drug dosages in children but for practical purposes appropriate doses are indicated on all drug data sheets and in prescribing references such as the British National Formulary, now published at regular intervals. A list of the commonest drugs used in treating children in general practice is given in Table 8.1. Those listed in capital letters are considered useful for 'the doctor's bag'.

DEVELOPMENTAL SCREENING AND IMMUNISATION

DEVELOPMENTAL SCREENING

Developmental screening of children is based on the assumption that given the processes of growth, physiological and psychological maturation and the ability to adapt, the early detection of deviations and abnormalities may lead to their correction or at least modification. The screening of the new born for certain metabolic disorders such as phenylketonuria and congenital hypothyroidism has resulted in their early biochemical correction, with most rewarding results. Sceptics suggest that most serious problems of childhood present at birth and are readily detected at this time, but this denies the existence of many physical problems which can be seen outwith the neonatal period; to give but a few, the 'missed' or 'late' congenital dislocation of the hip, visual and hearing problems, squints and rarely serious neurological, orthopaedic and cardio-respiratory disorders. Criticism on the grounds of cost effectiveness has been advanced, but personal experience suggests that of the important problems of early childhood as many as 6% may be picked up by screening. The exigencies of general practice and concern with acute illness and the care of the chronic sick and disabled may, some suggest, leave little time for the luxury of developmental and population screening, but for the average general practitioner it is likely that screening would involve more than one and a half hours to two hours per fortnight.

Although what follows is a discussion of the screening of children from birth to school entry at the age of 5, growth and development continue until the epiphyses fuse and adulthood is reached. Every contact with the child should prompt the thought 'how is he or she doing — growing well, keeping active and progressing at school and happy at play?' Screening is concerned with four areas of development:

1. Physical growth
2. Sensory development
3. Motor development
4. Language and social skills

The techniques of screening are well described in a number of references and are simple and easily learned. They do not involve sophisticated examination or equipment and are practicable in any consulting room or in the child's home. Tests of hearing of infants and small children and the exclusion of squints are relatively easy. The testing of visual acuity can be done but its necessity and value in the preschool child has recently been questioned although squints must be recognised as early as possible.

There are a number of caveats about the interpretation of findings of developmental screening, which must recognise the influences of:

1. Pre-term delivery.
2. Ethnic differences in the rates of development of motor, social and language skills.
3. Acute illness.

Table 8.1 Basic formulary of common substances use in treating children in general practice. (Drugs in capital letters useful for 'Doctor's bag'.)

Drug	Usual format	Dosage	Main indication
Respiratory			
Terbutaline	Aerosol inhaler	250 μg 4-hourly as needed	Asthma
SALBUTAMOL	Aerosol inhaler	100 μg 4-hourly as needed	Asthma
	Inhaled powder	200 μg 4-hourly as needed	Asthma
Aminophylline	Oral slow release tablets/syrup	100 mg 12-hourly	Asthma
Sodium cromoglycate	Inhaled powder	20 mg 8–12-hourly	Prophylaxis asthma
Ketotifen	Oral syrup/tablet	1 mg 12-hourly	
Alimentary			
Dicylomine HCl	Syrup	5 mg 1–6 minutes before feeds	Infant colic
Aluminium OH/			
Magnesium oxide/	Mixture (Paed)	2.5–5 ml 1–6 minutes before feeds	
Dimethicone			
Danthron	Liquid	12.5–25 mg Bedtime	Constipation
Dioctyl-sodium	Elixir	25–50 mg 3 times daily	
Sulpho succinate			
Bisacodyl	Suppository	5 mg rectally in morning	
Infections			
PHENOXYMETHYL PENICILLIN	Syrup/tablet	62.5–250 mg 6-hourly	Gm +/− penicillin sensitive organisms
BENZYL PENICILLIN	Injection	300 mg 6-hourly	Gm +/− penicillin sensitive organisms
Amoxycillin or ampicillin	Syrup/capsules	62.5–250 mg 6-8 hourly	Sensitive Gm +/− infections
ERYTHROMYCIN ETHYLSUCCINATE	Syrup/tablets	125–250 mg 6-hourly	Gm +/− when penicillins contraindicated
COTRIMOXAZOLE	Suspension/tablets	120–240 mg 12-hourly	Gm +/− infections — particularly urinary
Nystatin	Suspension	1 ml (100 000 u) 6-hourly	Oro-pharyngeal candidiasis
Analgesics			
SOLUBLE ASPIRIN	Tablet	75–300 mg 4–5-hourly	Mild-moderate pain — febrile illness (avoid under 1 year of age)
PARACETAMOL	Syrup/tablet	125–500 mg 4–6-hourly	Mild-moderate pain — febrile illness (avoid under 1 year of age)
Indomethacin	Suspension/capsule	12.5–25 mg 6–8-hourly	Joint rheumatic disorders
Nefanamic acid	Suspension/capsule	50–100 mg 6-hourly	Joint rheumatic disorders
Chloral hydrate	Elixir	30–50 mg/kg (max 1 g) (In divided dosage — 4–6 hourly)	Short-term sedation/use in sleep disorders
Trimeprazine	Syrup	3 mg/kg	Short-term sedation/use in sleep disorders
Prochlorperazine	Syrup/tablets	5 mg (8-hourly children over age of 6 years)	Antiemetic/prophylaxis against migraine
Anti-allergics			
CHLORPHENIRAMINE	Syrup/tablets	1 year — 1 mg 12-hourly 5 years — 2 mg 8-hourly 6 years — 4 mg 8–12-hourly	Hay fever and acute allergies
	Injection	10 mg	IM in case of severe acute allergic reactions
Clemastine	Tablets/syrup	0.5–1 mg 12-hourly	Seasonal long term prophylaxis — hay fever/asthma
ENT			
Ephedrine HCl 0.5 — 190 solution	Nasal drops	2 drops/spray 4–6-hourly	Nasal catarrh
Triprolidine/Pseudo Ephedrine preps.	Syrup	2.5–5 ml 8-hourly	Catarrhal upper respiratory disorders
Brompheniramine/ Phenylephrine preps.	Syrup	2.5–5 ml 8-hourly	Catarrhal upper respiratory disorders
Dioctyl-sodium sulphosuccinate	Ear drops	2 drops 8-hourly	Removal of wax from ears

Drug	Usual format	Dosage	Main indication
Nutrition			
Sodium iron edetate	Syrup	30–60 mg 12-hourly	Iron deficiency anaemia and in prophylaxis anaemia
Ferrous sulphate mixture B.P.	Mixture	30–60 mg 12-hourly	Anaemia in pre-term infants
'Abidec'	Drops		
Children's Vit. drops (DHSS)	Drops	0.3–0.6 ml daily	Children at risk to dietary deficiency Vit. D prophylaxis in pre-term and low birth weight infants
SODIUM CHLORIDE/ DEXTROSE POWDER	Powder	Reconstituted in 200 ml water	Oral fluid replacement in diarrhoeal illness
Hormones			
HYDROCORTISONE	Injection	100 mg	Emergency treatment — asthma, severe allergy, cardio-respiratory collapse, meningococcaemia
PREDNISOLONE	Tabs. 5 mg	Variable 5–20 mg 4-hourly	Exacerbations of asthma allergy or problems requiring long term steroid therapy
Insulin preparations	Various preps. standard u100 strength from 1983	Variable	Diabetes mellitus
Combined oral contraceptive	Tablets	Low oestrogen 30 μg	Juvenile/early adolescent menorrhagia
Anti-convulsants			
Phenytoin	Tablets/capsules	From 50 mg/day	Major epilepsy
Sodium valproate	Enteric coated tablets/syrup	From 200 mg/day	Major/complex epilepsies
Carbamazepine	Tablets/syrup	From 100 mg/day	Partial epilepsy — temporal lobe
Ethosuxamide	Capsules/syrup	From 500 mg/day	Petit mal (monitor blood levels of each to achieve control and avoid toxicity)
Diazepam	Injection	5 mg/ml IV/rectal	Administer slowly rectally in small children/IV older until control of status is obtained
Poisoning			
PAED. IPECACUANHA EMETIC MIXTURE	Mixture	14 mg/10 ml single oral dose	Acute poisoning — DO NOT USE with Hydrocarbon if corrosive poisons suspected
Activated charcoal	Effervescent granules	5–10 g/100 ml single oral dose	Drug poisoning, e.g. anti-depressants
Skin preparations			
Hydrocortisone	Ointment/creams	0.1–2.5%	Eczemas/contact dermatitis
Betamethazone	Ointment/creams	0.1%	Moderate severe eczemas as above
Clobetasol	Ointment/creams	0.05%	Severe exacerbations eczemas as above
Emulsifying	Ointment	—	Skin cleansing
Benzyl Peroxide	Creams/Gels	5–10%	Acne
Icthammol	Ointment/creams	5%	Soothing broken skin — Eczemas
Gamma Benzene Hexachloride	Lotion	1%	Scabies. Pediculosis
Malathion	Lotion	1%	Pediculosis capitis
Cetrimide	Solution	1%	Skin cleansing
Ophthalmic			
CHLORAMPHENICOL	Ointment/drops	1% & 0.5%	Conjunctivitis
Antazoline	Drops	0.5%	Allergic conjunctivis

4. Interruptions in domestic and social circumstances such as when mother is in hospital or the birth of a new sibling.

5. The phenomenon of developmental dissociation, for example when truncal and upper limb motor developments proceed faster than that of the lower limbs.

Some of these may be associated with apparent or transient delays or regressions in development which in an overall sense are not necessarily significant. Overhasty predictions have to be avoided and serial assessments and expert paediatric opinion sought before firm opinions are given.

Reference has been made to the minimal equipment required. This should include:

1. 1 doz. 2.5 cm cubes of different colours, including red, blue, green and yellow.
2. Paper and crayons.
3. A small bell or high frequency rattle.
4. A centimetre tape measure.

5. A good auroscope.

6. Reference growth charts for head circumference, weight and height for infants and older children. A useful inexpensive aid is the Cole slide rule calculator based on Tanner-Whitehouse standards from 0–19 years (Castlemead publications).

7. A reliable stadiometer and, if available, a measuring board suitable for the measurement of infants and toddlers up to about the age of 3 years (a suitable measuring board can be made simply by fixing a 1 metre long brass measuring rod to the side of a smooth board with a fixed head end and moveable foot board, small children always being measured supine).

8. One or two simple picture books.

Several screening protocols have been published, each with their merits and demerits. The most important thing to remember is that screening is an art, albeit a simple one, and it is trends over a period of time that matter and not 'one off' findings.

Optimal timings have been suggested for developmen-

Table 8.2   Basic attributes and checks at developmental screening

Age span	
1st Week	Adequancy of performance and feeding ability
	Exclusion of congenital anomalies
	Screening for phenylketonuria (PKU) and congenital hypothyroidism
	Bonding
6 weeks	Response to mother — smiling — gaze fixation
	Stilling of cry in response to voice — quality of cry
	Symmetry of primitive reflexes
	Abnormalities of muscle tone
	Exclusion of congenital dislocation of hip and undescended testes
6–10 months	Social responses — babbling — smiling
	Hand eye regard — early manipulative ability
	Gross motor control — Head control — ability to sit with support and take weight on legs — crawling
	From 8–9 months — early attempts to walk
	Feeding self with a biscuit or drinking from a cup
	Bisyllabic vocabulary — da da, etc.
	Check for undescended testes
	Exclude squints and check hearing
18 months–2 years	Extension of social skills — recognition of parts of body or of dress. Responds to questions and simple instructions.
	Involvement in social and constructive play and immitative behaviour
	Check of hearing — exclude squints
	By 2 years ensure child is walking
	From about 2 years control of anal sphincters
3–3½ years	Explorative play — expanded language with simple sentence structure and free conversation.
	Listens readily to stories
	Immitative behaviour well established. Feeding self without difficulties
	Progressive control of bladder and anal sphincter
4–4½ years	Running and climbing
	Active, Social, imaginative play. Uses crayons, drawing materials. Speaks freely in sentences
	Check speech — vision and hearing
	Bladder and bowel control established
	Check males for undescended testes
At each examination	Each assessment should include measurement of height, weight and up to 2 years — O.F.C.
	Physical examination should include a check of dental state of children over 3 years
	Review general behaviour and parental difficulties.

tal screening and indeed selective screening has been advocated for children with defined perinatal hazards, episodes of illness with possible sequelae, or children socially at risk or otherwise disadvantaged. With experience developmental screening is possible and practical at any time in the first 5 years of life but in general terms is recommended in the first week of life, at 6 weeks, at 6–10 months of age, 18 months to 2 years of age, 3–3½ years and 4–4½ years. In brief outline the points to be established at each examination are detailed in Table 8.2.

IMMUNISATION

Children in the United Kingdom are routinely offered immunisation in their preschool years against diphtheria, pertussis, tetanus, poliomyelitis and measles. From about the age of 10 until leaving school immunisation against rubella, tuberculosis and booster immunisation against tetanus and poliomyelitis is available. With the exception perhaps of BCG and to a smaller extent rubella (more often than not given at school), the routine immunisation of preschool children is recommended as part of the preventive medical services offered by family doctors. Some general practitioners prefer to arrange the entire immunisation programme for their child patients. The child immunisation schedule commonly operated in the United Kingdom is detailed in Table 8.3.

Recent controversy about the safety of pertussis immunisation did little to help the promotion of an already declining uptake of immunisation procedures. The reappearance of epidemic pertussis in 1978 and 1982 and the recommendation of the Joint Committee on Vaccination and Immunisation has done much to redress the balance and immunisation rates once again are beginning to improve.

There are few contraindications to the active immunisation of children against diphtheria, pertussis, tetanus and poliomyelitis. At present the absolute contraindications against pertussis and measles immunisations are given as:

1. Existing neurological impairment or abnormality.
2. Epilepsy, or epilepsy in a first degree relative.
3. A major reaction or undue irritability as a result of a previous injection containing pertussis antigen.
4. Parental wishes after due consideration and advice.

Temporary contraindications include:

1. Current acute illness, e.g. with a communicable disease.

Table 8.3 Routine immunisations available to British children

Diseases	Vaccine type	Dose and route	Optimum timing of administration
Diptheria	Toxoid } Aluminium Hydroxide		
0.5 mls by deep subcutaneous injection			
3 months			
Tetanus	Toxoid — Adsorbed	or	5 months
Pertussis	Killed *Bordetella pertussis*	IM	9 months (Boosted by Diph/Tet. at 4–5 years)
Alternative			
Diphtheria	Toxoid } Aluminium Hydroxide	0.5 mls IM	As above
Tetanus	Toxoid — Adsorbed	SC	Boosted at 4–5 years Tetanus Toxoid at 12–15 years
Poliomyelitis	Strains — Live attenuated strains Types 1. 2. 3. (Kidney cell cultured)	Oral 3 drops	3 months, 5 months, 9 months 4–5 years with DPT or DT Boosters as above at 12–15 years
Measles	Schwarz strain — live attenuated (Egg cultured — freeze dried)	0.5 mls IM or SC	During the second year of life
Rubella	RA27/3 or Cenderhill strain — freeze dried (Rabbit kidney/human diploid cell cultured)	0.5 mls IM or SC	To girls of 10 years of age
Tuberculosis	BCG (Freeze dried)	Intradermal over deltoid insertion 0.05 mls for babies otherwise	At birth to 'at risk' neonate or after Tuberculin testing to negative reactors (NB Tuberculin reaction may be suppressed in children suffering recent exanthematous illness, e.g. Chickenpox, Measles — Repeat test after 6 weeks)

2. Prematurity when timing of the immunisation programme must make allowance for the gestational age of the infant at birth.

3. Immunological compromise in children with hypogammaglobulinaemia or those on immuno-suppressive drugs for leukaemia or other reasons.

The immunisation of an immunological comprised child with for example measles vaccine should be accompanied by the concurrent administration of specific measles immunoglobulin and in any event best done only after expert advice.

SOME PRACTICAL POINTS

Call up procedure

Figure 8.1 outlines one procedure for the call up of children for immunisation screening. Such a programme lends itself particularly well to management by computer and high rates of attendance can be achieved. Although the optimal timing of immunisation procedures is given in Table 8.3, a practical approach has to be adopted to defaulters who may have to be immunised as and when they present. It is better to have the immunisations irregularly spaced than not done at all. Repeated rescheduling is neither practicable nor desirable since some children can in such circumstances receive too many doses of vaccine!

The procedure

After due discussion and explanation parents should be

asked to sign consent to the procedure on their child and all immunisations should be documented and a record card given to the mother. These are often provided free of charge by health authorities or by vaccine manufacturers. Vaccine expiry dates should always be checked, batch numbers recorded and unused vaccine discarded at the end of the session (single unit doses of vaccine will be made available by health departments in Scotland and the need for multi-dose vials avoided).

Up to school entry the arm should be avoided as an injection site. Injections of vaccine should always be given by deep subcutaneous or intramuscular injection with the exception of BCG which is given intradermally.

Reactions

While major reactions are exceedingly rare, 1/1000 adrenalin solution should always be available for injection in the event of anaphylaxis. More commonly reactions are mild; occasionally infants are somewhat fretful during the next 12 to 24 hours and require the administration of paracetamol syrup. Care must be taken to avoid ascribing the symptoms of a coincidental minor virus infection to immunisation procedures. Less commonly children may appear to have a convulsion or to be unusually distressed; observation in hospital may be advisable and subsequent doses of trivalent vaccine or pertussis vaccine avoided. Minor morbilliform illnesses may follow measles immunisation but serious reactions, such as sub-acute sclerosing panencephalitis have not been observed with live attenuated measles vaccines. Infection with wild measles

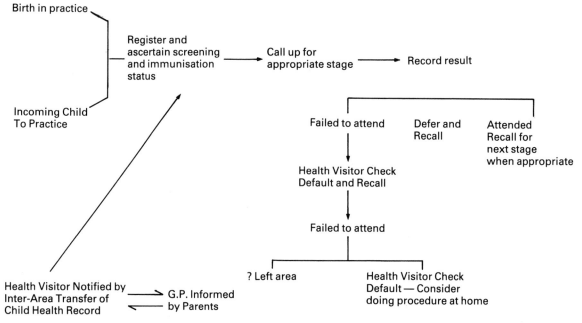

Fig. 8.1 Call up procedure for child immunisation and screening

virus on the contrary is associated with a significant risk of meningo encephalitis, febrile convulsions and EEG abnormalities.

Most reactions to immunisation are local, consist of erythema and induration and most commonly follow the too shallow injection of the aluminium hydroxide adsorbed vaccines. Occasionally a sterile abscess may result requiring incision. Generally speaking small children under the age of 5 who have been actively immunised against tetanus do not require booster injections of tetanus toxoid for injuries. If it is considered essential to give children boosters in such circumstances than adsorbed tetanus toxoid should be avoided and simple non-adsorbed toxoid used.

Children not previously immunised against whooping cough may if their parents wish and there are no specific contraindications be given mono-component pertussis vaccine. The use of this vaccine in unprotected children is recommended up to the age of 6 years.

Unimmunised children: three doses of 0.5 ml pertussis vaccine by subcutaneous or intramuscular injection at intervals of 1 month.

Children already given one dose of diphtheria/tetanus vaccine may be given one dose of pertussis vaccine and this followed up by the use of two doses of trivalent diphtheria/tetanus/pertussis vaccine.

Children already given two doses of diphtheria/tetanus vaccine may be given two monthly-spaced doses of pertussis vaccine followed up by one dose of trivalent diphtheria/tetanus/pertussis vaccine.

Immunisation against cholera, smallpox, typoid and hepatitis B. Doctors may be occasionally asked to immunise children travelling to the tropics against these diseases. Caution has to be shown particularly with small infants and in general terms immunisation should be avoided in infants under the age of 1 year. The advice of the appropriate community health authority should be sought.

THE FAMILY DOCTOR AND THE NEONATE

The basis for the successful care of the new born lies in anticipating problems. Looked at from the point of view of the unborn child, there are certain circumstances which suggest possible troubles ahead (Table 8.4) and certain conditions which are required at the time of birth (Table 8.5).

A precise diagnosis of neural tube defects is becoming possible very early in pregnancy using ultrasonic scanning and several chromosomal and genetic disorders can be detected by amniotic fluid cell culture and histochemical analysis.

ANTE-NATAL CARE

The health education component of ante-natal care with its emphasis on good nutrition, physical fitness, the avoidance of the hazards of alcohol and smoking and the routine prescription of iron and folic acid do much to ensure good fetal growth. Not enough emphasis is placed on vitamin D intake particularly in Asian women living in northern climes. Neo-natal hypocalcaemia, poor enamelisation of the primary dentition and infantile rickets are possible consequences for infants born to women with inadequate vitamin D intake. DHSS vitamin D tablets should be routinely prescribed, certainly during the autumn and winter months.

Considerable attention is paid to physical illness, cigarette smoking and alcohol abuse and a poor home environment as risk factors for the neonate, but often of

Table 8.4 Some ante-natal predictors of risk of children

Genetic and metabolic	Autosomal recessive; cystic fibrosis
	Autosomal dominant; achondroplasia, neuro-fibromatosis
	Sex linked; Duchenne muscular dystrophy
	Sex chromosome; Turners syndrome (XO), Klinefelters syndrome (XXY)
	Numeric/structural e.g. Downs syndrome — trisomy 21, 21/translocations. Deletions and partial deletions etc.
Maternal Social	Socio-economic deprivation
	Mothers <19 years >40 years of age
	Poor nutrition — (Vit. D. deficiency in Asian immigrant)
	Smoking
	Alcohol and drug abuse
Medical	Chronic disease, e.g. diabetes — renal disease — cardio-respiratory disease
	Infection — rubella, cytomegalovirus, tuberculosis, syphilis
Psychiatric	Rejection or denial of pregnancy
	Apathy
	Established or recurrent depression
	Rejection of or violence towards mother in her childhood by her own parents
Mental handicap	(Psycho-social factors may also involve fathers equally putting an infant at risk)

Table 8.5 Some basic requirements for the safety of the neonate

1. Anticipate troubles. If in doubt deliver in hospital. Transfer early even if labour has commenced.
2. Ideally do not confine primigravida at home.
3. Do not confine at home unless:
   a. Proper midwifery services are available.
   b. Basic resuscitation equipment is available, e.g. neonatal airways and mucous aspirators.
   c. Hypothermia can be avoided.
   d. Transfer facilities exist to take ill babies to a special care unit.
   e. Vit. K and naloxone HCl (Narcon) is available (preferably avoid Pethidine/Promazine/Promethazine as maternal sedation and analgesia).
4. After delivery:
   a. Promote bonding immediately or as soon as possible. (Ideally put infant to the mother's breast immediately after birth).
   b. If infant has to be sent to a special care unit ensure mother as access to her baby at all reasonable opportunities.

much more serious import are those sometimes 'soft' psychological predictors which suggest the possibility of bonding failure or even of outright injury to the new born infant. The family doctor's early suspicions and help with these may be of crucial importance to mother and baby.

The delivery

After oropharyngeal aspiration and any immediate resuscitative measures — ensuring, for example, a patent airway and the establishment of regular respiration — the baby should be wrapped in a warm towel and given as soon as possible to the mother. Babies of mothers sedated with opiate derivatives may experience difficulty in establishing respiration which can be reversed by a single intramuscular injection of naloxone HCl (Narcan) in a dose of 60 μg per kilo (maximum dose 200 μg).

Very low birth weight or pre-term babies, those born with major congenital malformations and those showing evidence of respiratory distress or recurrent apnoea should be transferred at once to special care facilities (preferably with the mother). Care should be taken to avoid hypothermia by wrapping the baby's limbs and trunk head in sterile gamgee and if available aluminium cooking foil exposing only the face. Most special care units and ambulance authorities have available pre-heated portable incubators with an oxygen supply, and these should be requested at the time the baby's admission to hospital is being arranged.

Jaundice

Jaundice commonly causes mothers a lot of anxiety. Usually this is mild in degree, the serum bilirubin level generally not exceeding 170 mmol/1, most of this being unconjugated bilirubin. The commonest explanation for this is physiological immaturity of the hepatic enzyme systems in a low birth weight or pre-term infant, but it is also common in breast-fed babies. There are several serious and rare metabolic and anatomical causes of prolonged and progressive jaundice in the newborn but haemolytic disease due to rheusus incompatibility is becoming much less common. Occasionally babies can become quite jaundiced because of ABO incompatibility or the more rare occurrence of congenital haemolytic anaemia (hereditary spherocytosis). Jaundice in the acutely ill newborn should also lead one to suspect a septicaemic illness and pyelonephritis. Congenital hypothyroidism is an important cause when jaundice is accompanied by slow feeding. Jaundice accompanied by poor feeding, vomiting and failure to progress always demands urgent investigation. In a vigorous, alert and thriving infant, especially when breast fed, all that is required is reassurance and careful observation.

Bowel upsets

Vomiting

Feeding difficulties apart, vomiting may occur because of gastro-intestinal anomalies, acute infections and intracranial lesions. The vomiting of bile stained material should always be regarded as indicating small bowel obstruction until otherwise proved. Coffee grounds vomiting may occur with hiatus hernia or pyloric stenosis, while apparent vomiting associated with respiratory embarrassment should suggest possible tracheo-oesophageal anomalies. Pyloric stenosis, commonest in males, most often shows between the 10th and 14th day of life although sometimes later, and is associated with the classical triad of projectile vomiting, visible gastric peristalis and a palpable pyloric mass, with the secondary features of constipation and water and electrolyte imbalance — dehydration, and in the early stages, alkalosis. Unexplained and repeated vomiting in an unwell baby or one who is losing weight demands investigation in hospital.

CONSTIPATION, DIARRHOEA AND BLOOD IN THE FAECES

Constipation and diarrhoea are terms which must be defined and should be used when, on the one hand the faeces is hard, inspissated and associated with dyschezia, or on the other with the passage of frequent watery faeces. Both may be associated with the passage of blood; in the case of constipation with a fissure-in-ano and in diarrhoea with dysenteric infection or rarely intussusception. Green staining of the faeces with bile pigments may occur in both constipation and diarrhoea and in itself is not significant. Failure to pass meconium within 24 hours of birth may be due to ano-rectal malformations or to plugging with inspissated meconium in cystic fibrosis. Careful examination of the abdomen and the anus should exclude any serious anomaly. Simple constipation is best managed by giving water between feeds while diarrhoea, if mild, can be managed by resting the gut and introducing a graduated feeding routine over the next 24 hours starting with plain water or paediatric dextrose/saline solution (Diorylate). Meleana or the passage of large amounts of fresh blood in the stool in the first 5 days or so of life requires the exclusion of haemorrhagic disease of the newborn and the administration of 1 mg of Vit.K1.

Fits and crying

The cry of hunger and for attention is instantly recognised by mother, is familiar to most and readily stilled by meeting the baby's needs. There are three situations which should arouse a doctor's suspicions: when a mother complains that her baby is unusually quiet or has become so, when her baby seems to be unduly irritable, in pain or distress or is inconsolable, and when the cry has changed in quality. While there may be little basis for anxiety and all that is required is some adjustment in feeding or the treatment of infantile colic these features may be the earliest signs of developmental delay or of more sinister neurological problems. Expert assessment and follow-up is indicated. A shrill cry, especially when associated with abnormalities in posture, possible fits or an increase in fontanelle tension and in occipital-frontal head circumference, demand urgent hospital admission. Apparent twitching or neuromuscular irritability in the first week of life may indicate transient neonatal hypocalcaemia and hypomagnesemia and is usually self-limiting. Twitching may occur with hypoglycaemia and should be suspected in the first 48 hours of life in dysmature term infants born at home. The diagnosis can readily be confirmed by finding a destrostix blood glucose reading of less than 2.2 SI units per 100 ml on a heel prick sample. This is easily corrected by supplementary feeds of 5% dextrose solution.

ANOMALIES

Major anomalies are usually self-evident and require the immediate transfer of an affected baby to the appropriate special paediatric unit. Those such as talipes equinovaris or congenital dislocation of the hip which are not life threatening, require orthopaedic treatment and appropriate splintage. Occasionally infants with congenital cardiac or pulmonary anomalies but without overt clinical signs or murmur may suddenly deteriorate at home and go into cardiac failure. The signs of neonatal cardiac failure are tachycardia, tachypnoea and hepatomegaly, distress on feeding and cyanosis. Peripheral oedema is not a feature of a cardiac failure in early infancy.

Commoner are those minor anomalies and blemishes which cause a great deal of maternal anxiety. Included are those such as accessory auricles, nipples, extra digits and skin tags, most of which require no immediate action and can be subsequently referred for cosmetic surgical treatment. Capilliary and cavernous haemangiomata commonly show centrifugal regression in later infancy and only rarely require treatment. Extensive lesions and large pigmented and hairy moles will later require the expert attention of dermatologists and plastic surgeons. A large capilliary haemangioma in the distribution of one trigeminal nerve should keep in mind the possibilities of Sturge Weber syndrome and will require periodic review.

Downs syndrome due to Trisomy 21 or translocation chromosomal defects is the commonest congenital anomaly found at birth. The characteristic facial appearances and hypotonia do not usually present much diagnostic difficulty. Once the diagnosis has been confirmed there should be no delay in informing the parents and the necessary long-term supportive measures should be set in motion.

THE HANDICAPPED CHILD

Most major handicapping disabilities are recognised at or about birth and are associated with congenital abnormalities of the central nervous system, musculo-skeletal system, the heart, kidneys and other organs, or are metabolic in nature. Nevertheless, it is wrong to consider handicap purely in such terms, and necessary to recognise that children with less commanding problems may be as severely disabled. The essential point is to consider handicap in functional rather than diagnostic terms. Thus the child with sensory and emotional deprivation or with poorly controlled asthma may in the long-term be as or more disadvantaged as is a favourably placed child with a neurological defect. In the United Kingdom proposals in new educational legislation for handicapped children suggest a 'record of need' to which parents and children have access of right, and which is concerned with looking at a child's disability in functional terms.

THE RECOGNITION OF HANDICAP

Albeit the recognition of most major handicaps occurs at or about birth, family doctors need to be alert to those disabilities which may arise at any time as a result of poor social circumstances, trauma, serious episodic illness such as meningitis, or occasionally from more obscure causes. Severe regression in development may, for example, herald some of the more esoteric metabolic neurological diseases or other serious brain disorders.

ADVICE

Much of the counselling and advice given to children and parents will be by professionals involved in multidisciplinary care. The family doctor has much to contribute and should be involved from the outset. Parents may have difficulty in following or interpreting information given to them at the time of diagnosis. They may be given differing advice and conflicts can occur which require reconciliation and explanation. Although genetic counselling is most often given by a geneticist or paediatrician the family doctor with a long-standing knowledge of the family should be involved. Genetic counselling is much more than a bald statement of statistical odds and while it should be informative and cautioning it must never be seen to be dogmatically proscriptive.

Over the years the doctor's advice will be sought on many issues concerning allowances, ability to travel, schooling, play, future work and marriage. The parents of badly handicapped children will have particular worries about the long-term future when their child leaves school, when so often much of the statutory support seems to cease or become less evident. Real anxieties exist about what will happen to the handicapped child or person in the event of death of the parents. Marital tensions, divorce, anxiety and depression are all common in the families of handicapped children and may be so severe that formal psychiatric referral and marriage guidance may be required. One important relief that family doctors can arrange is respite care for the profoundly disabled child so that parents and siblings can go off on holiday from time to time or otherwise socially relax.

Management of the child

The specialised management of handicaps apart, the routine needs and the treatment of episodic illness are the responsibilities of the child's family doctor. Some general practitioners may undertake the role of family doctor to residential schools for the handicapped. In the management of the handicap itself the family doctor, practice nurse and health visitor can be of great assistance. Examples of the sort of help needed include:

Changing dressings, appliances and catheters.
Prescribing and obtaining aids and appliances, for example incontinence pads or pants.
Monitoring treatment compliance and control, for example anticonvulsant levels and the control of diabetes mellitus.

An involvement in the specific management of disabilities can reduce clinic attendances and sometimes avoid the need for residential schooling. Difficulties which can sometimes occur in obtaining more specialised aids and drugs, should be discussed with the appropriate specialists and arrangements made for their supply either from hospital or community child health sources.

Clinical paediatrics and the general practitioner II

SIGNS AND SYMPTOMS OF CHILDHOOD ILLNESS

When is a child really ill as opposed to having a minor acute and unpleasant disorder which will resolve in a few days? Time and experience tell but there are general clues which can prove helpful.

APPEARANCE AND COLOUR

In many ways the roseate appearance of a protesting febrile child is reassuring. By contrast the recent onset of skin pallor, poor skin turgor and central or peripheral cyanosis always signify serious illness. Generalised purpura suggests the possibilities of acute leukaemia or of septicaemic illness.

CRYING AND UNCONSCIOUSNESS

Consciousness may vary from the coma and stupor of acute catastrophic illness to the heightened awareness and angst of a child dying from serious disease, or suffering from a reversible disorder such as acute asthma. Babies, infants and small children express their fears, pain and distress by crying and the cry of an ill child can be most revealing. Most ill children can be consoled, but seriously ill children may hardly protest or have an unusually shrill cry. Children with minor illness do not moan, whimper or scream inconsolably, and these features must always be regarded as significant.

POSTURE AND MOVEMENT

Posture and movement, or the lack of it, may be informative: a child, for example, in a state of actual or impending circulatory failure for any reason, infection or otherwise, will lie inert and unresistant. Opisthotonus occurs with meningitis but also in babies and children with intra-cranial haemorrhage. At its worst a decerebrate posture may be adopted with the head severely retracted and the arms and legs fully extended.

Children with abdominal pain due to gut or visceral injury, or severe colic, will lie with their knees drawn up onto their abdomen and are distressed by movement. Limb movement will be restricted or absent with acute bone or joint infection or trauma, the infected limb adopting the position of maximal comfort.

SMELL

A good sense of smell can be a useful aid to diagnosis such as in detecting the characteristic smell of acetone on the breath of a child with diabetic keto acidosis. There is also a characteristic fetor in the breath of children with acute appendicitis while an unpleasant and hard to define odour is associated with severe gastroenteritis. The sense of smell may also be useful when dealing with children suspected of swallowing domestic hydrocarbons such as paraffin or cleaning agents. These may give off a definite aroma either around the mouth or in exhaled air.

RESPIRATION

Children with respiratory distress from whatever cause will sit up in bed and lean forward supporting themselves on extended arms. The accessory muscles of respiration will be used and intercostal recession will be evident. Pneumonia is classically associated with a pronounced expiratory grunt and asthma with wheezing, although in severe asthma this may not always be evident. Pertussis will be accompanied by its characteristic whoop although this is not exclusive to this infection. Croup is invariably associated with a harsh, brassy, dry cough. The immediate stridor, choking and cough of upper airways obstruction due to a foreign body may disappear as it moves into one of the bronchi, stridor is then replaced by wheeze, or after a silent period by harsh cough and evidence of atelectasis and infection in the affected lung segment. While also present in older children with airways obstruction, respiratory distress in babies is accompanied by tracheal tug and by subcostal and intercostal recession. Rapid respiration, while predominantly a feature of respiratory and cardiac disease, is also present in shock and metabolic disorders, notably renal failure, diabetic keto acidosis and salicylate poisoning, when it is typically pauseless and deep.

PAIN

In infancy and early childhood the severity and nature of pain can only guessed at by the amount of distress shown. As children grow their ability to describe and localise pain improves, but in the early years a 'sore head' may reflect the pain of otitis media, tonsilitis, dental abscess or any condition of the head or neck. Only careful examination by a process of exclusion can define what is meant. Migraine, even in the early juvenile years, is not uncommon and often goes unrecognised. A strong family history of this disorder, the periodiccity of headaches and an association with vomiting or complaints of disturbed vision should alert one to this possibility. In general practice the relief of most childhood pain requires little more than soluble aspirin or paracetamol and perhaps mefenamic acid but it is important to give a regular and adequate 4-hourly dose until symptoms have abated. If it is necessary to give relief for severe pain to a child who has to be moved in difficult or time consuming circumstances, an injection of diamorphine should be considered.

COUGHING AND WHEEZING

The commonest cause of a cough is an upper respiratory tract viral infection. Coughing either reflects the need of the respiratory tract to expel excess tracheo-bronchial secretion or the irritant effect on inflamed mucosa of external stimuli such as cold or dry air. Although the primary protective function of coughing should be explained to parents and the child, the use of soothing demulcant syrups and hot drinks do much to ease discomfort. In general cough sedatives are not indicated in childhood but decongestants containing pseudoephedrine or phenylephrine can give some symptomatic relief to catarrhal children. Persistent night coughing unassociated with respiratory infections should alert one to the possibilities of asthma when treatment should be directed towards dealing with the trigger mechanisms responsible, and the administration of appropriate bronchodilators. Typically, the harsh brassy cough of croup begins late at night and is eased by humidifying the child's room with steam.

Wheezing with viral bronchiolitis often due to respiratory syncytial virus (RSV) is common between the ages of 9 months and 2 years. Although many doctors will prescribe an antibiotic the most useful thing to do is to keep the child in an environment of warm, humidified air. The distressed infant showing intercostal recession should be admitted to hospital, particularly if poor social circumstances prevail. About 30% of children with recurrent wheezing will give a past history of repeated lower respiratory tract infections and there seems little doubt that such infections are of aetiological significance in asthma. 80% of children with asthma will start wheezing in the first 4 years of life. Recurrent wheezing in children should be regarded as asthma and parents so informed. Appropriate prophylaxic measures should be introduced along with specific management. Antibiotics are seldom necessary and the diagnosis of wheezy bronchitis should be avoided. The management of asthma in childhood has been simplified by the development of inhaler therapy with ß$_2$ adrenoceptor agonists and prophylaxis with inhaled sodium cromoglycate and beclothemazone. The prolonged administration of oral ketotifen may prove useful in the prevention of asthma and provides a useful alternative to sodium cromoglycate when difficulties are being encountered in the use of this substance. The use of sodium cromoglycate may be associated with wheeze, caused by the inhaled vehicle for the drug. If this occurs an inhalation of a ß$_2$ agonist should precede inhalation of sodium cromoglycate.

SORE EAR AND SORE THROATS

Sore ears and sore throats, next to coughs, are the commonest complaints of childhood. Only about one in 10 of sore throats are likely to be due to bacterial infection with a haemolytic streptococcus. The majority are due to a variety of different viruses which include myxo viruses, picornoviruses, reoviruses, herpes, EB virus and adenoviruses. A definitive diagnosis on the basis of clinical inspection alone is by no means reliable although the whitish-grey haemorrhagic exudative tonsilitis of anginose infectious mononucleosis has a fairly characteristic appearance, and the classical follicular tonsilitis and peritonsillar abscess due to a haemolytic streptococci should not cause too much difficulty. Otitis media is simple to diagnose when there is purulent exudate and a perforated ear drum or the drum is bulging and fiery red. Difficulties arise with children when the drum fails to show its glistening light reflex, is lack-lustre or slightly pink.

Faced with a late night visit and having to make a decision as to whether or not to use an antibiotic perhaps the best guidelines are pain, fever and systemic upset. It is not unreasonable to prescribe penicillin or a broad spectrum antibiotic (not a tetracycline). Ampicillin should not be given when the possibility of infectious mononucleosis exists because of the association of this antibiotic with unpleasant rashes.

All children with earache and evidence of middle ear infection should be reviewed some weeks after treatment and attention paid to the child's hearing. Many children will recurrent upper respiratory tract infection and earache go on to develop secretory otitis media and partial hearing loss. This may often be detected by the mother, or at school, and a conductive hearing loss can be demonstrated in the older child by tuning fork tests or by audiometry and tympanometry. The common association of partial hearing loss, earache and catarrhal respiratory symptoms have given rise to a number of different treatment routines which include systemic decongestants, myringotomies, grommet insertion and adenoidectomy. The common occurrence of catarrhal respiratory disorders between the ages of 18 months and 6 years coincides with a period when children start going to nurseries, schools and otherwise extending their social experience. At the same time they are actively developing immunological mechanisms to cope with a whole gamut of infective agents and allergens; this has given rise to the very apt American description of these disorders as being part of the 'First Grades Syndrome'. Most parents can be reassured that their child will improve with time and that little is required other than symptomatic treatment. There is no doubt however that a very few with recurrent hearing loss and evidence of allergy or of recurrent pain and infection in the middle ear will require specialist referral and that to some tonsillectomy and adenoidectomy may prove beneficial.

SOME ABDOMINAL PROBLEMS

Colic is common between the ages of 2 and 16 weeks causing distress to the infant and sleepless nights for the parents. Several reasons have been given for infantile colic but it would seem not unreasonable to suppose that this is due to aerophagy associated with over-eager feeding or bad feeding technique. Although said to be less common in breast-fed babies, it most certainly occurs. Treatment consists of correcting feeding difficulties and the administration of dicyclomine 10 to 15 minutes before each feed. Outside of infancy the commonest causes of colicky abdominal pain are constipation and gastrointestinal infections and occasionally parasitic infestation with, for example, ascaris lumbracoides.

There are some children who from an early age complain of recurrent peri-umbilical pain often accompanied by effortless vomiting to such an extent that they develop quite pronounced ketonuria. The term 'periodic syndrome' has been used to describe children showing these features. Examination usually shows little apart from perhaps some evidence of weight loss and occasionally

quite definite dehydration. Affected children are afebrile and usually remarkably little concerned by their symptoms although typically their distressed, over-solicitous mothers will be seated by the bedside with the sickness bowl at the ready. Treatment should be concerned with defusing a tense situation and reassuring the child and mother that all will soon be well. A liberal intake of sweet drinks should be encouraged on the basis of little and often. Occasionally a single injection of intramuscular prochlorperazine may help to break the cycle of vomiting. Less often, when the child is very dehydrated or the situation is out of hand, admission to hospital is required.

Acute appendicitis, next to trauma and elective ear, nose and throat surgery, is the commonest reason why children are admitted to hospital for surgery. It is uncommon under the age of 5 when it is notoriously difficult to diagnose and when the typical signs of central abdominal pain lateralising in the right iliac fossa are not always present. Rectal examination will usually demonstrate tenderness in the right iliac fossa although this may be absent if the inflamed appendix is retro-coecal. A number of conditions can mimic appendicitis, particularly adenoviral infections which are associated with enlargement of the mesenteric lymph nodes and occasionally with the complication of intussusception.

Henoch-Schonlein syndrome may present with quite severe abdominal pain preceding the onset of the typical anaphylactoid purpura which appears in the buttocks, extensor aspects of the lower legs and sometimes on the shoulder and neck. Cyclical abdominal pain is not uncommon in pubertal or adolescent girls and may be associated with ovulation or may occasionally be premenstrual. Ovulatory pain — Mittelschmerz — is typically mid-cycle, unilateral and transient in nature. In boys abdominal pain may be associated with testicular injury or infection and is usually felt in the central abdomen. It is important to remember that central abdominal pain may be a presenting symptom of diabetes.

Diarrhoea

Diarrhoea is usually infective in nature and if bacterial may be accompanied by blood and mucus. The history of the illness will usually make the diagnosis evident but careful examination is always required to exclude the rare possibilities of intussusception, bleeding Meckel's diverticulum and ulcerative colitis. Acute infective diarrhoea is best treated by resting the gut and by introducing graduated feeding and a liberal intake of fluid. It is wise to caution parents about the dangers of an excessive intake of plain water with the dangers of water intoxication, or of incorrectly constituted saline solutions. Antibiotics and diphenoxylate are not recommended in the routine management of acute diarrhoea in childhood. After a bout of infective diarrhoea some infants and toddlers go on to develop prolonged symptoms with rather offensive and sour-smelling stools. This is probably associated with transient dysfunction of gut enzyme systems and carbohydrate intolerance, and may be helped by the temporary use of milk free diets or of milk substitutes. Another common problem is infant toddlers diarrhoea — 'peas and carrots' syndromes — which probably reflects increased motility of the gut and can be helped by increasing dietary fat intake.

Persistent troublesome diarrhoea from early infancy associated with failure to thrive and recurrent respiratory infections should alert one to the possibilities of cystic fibrosis, while diarrhoea occurring from about the age of 9 months associated with fatty, offensive stools, a distended belly and failure to thrive may suggest coeliac syndrome. Cystic fibrosis is readily diagnosed in hospital by the finding of elevated sweat sodium levels and coeliac disease by the finding of sub-total or total villous atrophy on jejunal biopsy.

URINARY INFECTION IN CHILDHOOD

The presentation of urinary tract infections and their significance depend on the age at onset of symptoms, the site of infection and the extent of renal parenchymal damage. In babies and infants signs and symptoms may be non-specific and a diagnosis may be reached only after a screen for infection which includes urinalysis. At this age urinary tract infections are equally as common in boys as in girls and in both must always be regarded as significant and in need of investigation. After infancy, urinary tract infections become predominantly a problem of girls and unusual in boys in whom they should always be investigated.

Although population screening has shown about 2% of girls to have asymptomatic bacteriuria only a few will have symptoms suggestive of urinary tract infection. The presentation of urinary tract infection may range from frequency, dysuria and strangury to loin pain and tenderness, fever, rigor and vomiting.

The onset of urinary incontinence in a previously continent child should always prompt microscopy and culture of the urine. Clinical examination must include inspection of the external genitalia for evidence of poor hygiene — vulvitis and inflammation of the external urethral orifice — and in boys balinitis. Treatment with co-trimoxazole or ampicillin, should be started in advance of the results of a midstream urine culture.

How far should investigation be taken in children who have proven urinary tract infection? Certainly it is always indicated when attacks are recurrent or if there are clinical features of loin pain suggesting kidney inflammation. It may be that the routine, careful examination and follow-up of children with urinary tract infections will reveal those girls who, in adult life, will have renal problems in pregnancy or might eventually become hypertensive and at risk of chronic renal failure. Advances in urological investigation using DMSA scanning and ultrasound have made this much less speculative or difficult than in the past with only minimal radiation exposure on DMSA scanning. Excretion urography and micturating cysto-urethography may demonstrate vesico-ureteric reflux but if by school entry DMSA scanning has not demonstrated renal cortical scarring then surgical intervention is probably not required. Nevertheless the urine should be monitored at regular intervals and symptomatic and asymptomatic bacteriuria treated with the appropriate antimicrobial. Although the diagnosis of urinary tract infection is not as a rule difficult, protein and leucocytes may appear in the urine, in acute appendicitis and salpingitis. Haematuria may occur in acute urinary tract infections. The diagnosis of the much less common condition of acute haemorrhagic nephritis is readily confirmed by urine microscopy demonstrating tubular casts, sterile urine culture and a history of sore throat within the previous fortnight with elevated antistreptolysin titres (ASO).

THE REPRODUCTIVE SYSTEM

In boys only two problems need to be mentioned. The first, undescended testes, should be recognised early and at routine examination. The testes are very retractile in early childhood, but in a warm room can easily be persuaded into the scrotum. Children with undescended testes should be referred for surgical opinion as soon as discovered and certainly before the age of school entry. The second problem is that of torsion of the testicle. This is commonly mistaken for the very much more rare condition of epididymo orchitis and is an indication for urgent referral for emergency surgery.

Vaginal bleeding may occur in the first week of life in female infants and is associated with falling levels of transferred maternal oestrogens. Breast hypertrophy in the neonate can occur in both sexes under the influence of maternal oestrogens and is self-limiting, only rarely being complicated by acute bacterial infection. Vaginal discharge in children may result from poor hygiene or occasionally a monilial infection following the administration of a broad spectrum antibiotic. More commonly a mucoid discharge is found at the time of puberty and may be accompanied by slight brownish cyclical staining. Even before the onset of the menarche at about the age of 12, some girls will show pronounced breast development, one breast development sometimes in advance of the other. This asymmetry and the appearance of the breast bud in young children may cause parents undue anxiety.

The commonest menstrual problems of girls in their early adolescent years are dysmenorrhoea and occasionally severe menorrhagia and polymenorrhoea. This is best managed by the cyclical administration of a combined oestrogen/progestogen preparation such as one of the oral contraceptives, or the progestogen norethisterone. True precocious puberty is seldom seen in general practice and many normal girls regularly menstruate from about the age of 10. Failure to menstruate by the age of 16 should be investigated.

ACCIDENTS IN CHILDHOOD

Between 40 and 60% of children will have had an accident at some time or other. Nearly half of all accidents consist of simple contusions and lacerations while about 10 to 20% will involve long bone fractures. Thereafter in order come, head injuries, burns and scalds, and accidental poisoning. Despite public concern about environmental hazards the commonest place of injury is the child's own home. It is almost certainly true that far too many children are referred and admitted to hospital for minor accidents which might be better dealt with at home or by their own doctor. The following guidelines may help.

SERIOUS INJURIES

Basic resuscitation may be required including the use of external cardiac massage and mouth-to-mouth respiration. Severely injured children should be removed as soon as possible to hospital, which should be given advance warning of the child's imminent arrival. Severely injured children needing to be moved from remote areas or from difficult terrain may need sedation with diamorphine (0.1 mg/kg).

SUSPICIOUS CIRCUMSTANCES

Clear evidence which suggests criminal assault should be brought to the attention of the police authorities without delay. Clinical examination may suggest non-accidental injury with finger bruising in the region of the arms, shoulders, head and neck, bruising consistent with punching about the face and linear bruising of the buttocks and thighs with the use of belts and sticks. Stupor and coma with dilated pupils, retinal haemorrhage and profound hypotonia suggests serious and violent head injury. Discreet punched out burns may be caused by lighted cigarettes. A new variant in the spectrum of non-accidental injury includes poisoning with a variety of drugs and even intoxication with water. Whenever non-accidental injury or assault is suspected a child must be admitted to hospital forthwith and consideration given in

due course to obtaining a place of safety order. In view of likely legal proceedings it is essential that the family doctor documents in considerable detail his findings and his action.

LACERATIONS

Simple short lacerations are best cleaned with 1% cetrimide solution and sutured without local anaesthesia. Some lacerations, particularly those of the face and forehead, heal well if the wound edges are opposed and maintained in position with adhesive sterile strips (steristrips). Lacerations which are thought to be possibly disfiguring or associated with damage to deeper structures such as tendons require proper debridement and referral for expert surgical attention. Deep penetrating injuries may require exploration under general anaesthesia and should also be referred to hospital. Children not immunised against tetanus should be given a full course of tetanus toxoid and if more than 5 years has elapsed since their last immunisation a booster dose of simple non-adsorbed toxoid should be given.

BURNS

Simple scalds and blistering should be cleaned with sterile saline or 1% cetrimide solution. Blisters which have burst should be trimmed and removed; those intact should be left alone. Dressing of the burned area with a mixture of liquid paraffin and chlorinated lime/boric acid solution (Eusol) proves soothing and promotes rapid healing. An alternative to this is to dress the lesion with tulle gras overlaid with swabs soaked in 0.2% nitrofurazone solution. Burned fingers should be dressed separately.

FOREIGN BODIES

Small beads in the ears can be removed by gentle aural lavage and no attempt should be made to remove these with forceps; objects which are larger and impacted should be removed in hospital. Foreign bodies in the nose can often be successfully dislodged by promoting sneezing or occasionally by asking the child to blow the nose. Unless easily removed by turning a child upside down and firmly slapping the back, children who have inhaled foreign bodies should be referred at once to hospital. Despite their sometimes alarming appearance, the majority of small objects such as pins and toys which are swallowed pass harmlessly through the gastrointestinal tract to be expelled a day or two later. Occasionally girls with frequency and dysuria or an offensive vaginal discharge will be found to have a foreign body in the bladder or vagina.

POISONING

Children with a clear history of swallowing a corrosive poison such as ferrous sulphate or an alkali such as sodium hydroxide should be admitted to hospital without the administration of emetics. Emetics should not be given to children who have swallowed hydrocarbons such as paraffin or petrol because of the dangers of their inhalation with consequent serious lung injury. Provided there has been no undue delay in the doctor being told of the accident, the administration of children's ipecacuana mixture or alternatively an adsorbant charcoal mixture, may prove very effective in eliminating the toxic substance. The longer the delay the less effective is gastric lavage, which is probably best carried out in a hospital casualty departmnt. It is not uncommon for toddlers to swallow their mother's oral contraceptive pills. These, apart from causing some degree of nausea and occasionally sickness, cause no real problem.

Fortunately the vast majority of children who swallow potentially noxious substances come to very little harm and many can safely be treated at home. Useful guidance can be obtained in the United Kingdom from the Regional Poisoning Centres in Edinburgh, Belfast, Cardiff, Dublin and London.

SOME COMMON INFECTIOUS DISEASES OF CHILDHOOD

Any review of childhood illness in general practice would be incomplete without some comment on the common epidemic infectious diseses, measles, rubella, chickenpox, mumps, pertussis, and some viral diseases.

MEASLES AND RUBELLA

The features of classical measles are unmistakable. After an 8 to 14 day incubation period there is often a prodromal illness characterised by a transient erythematous rash and greyish spots on the buccal mucosa (Koplik's spots). This is followed in about 3 days by a maculopapular rash which commences at the hairline proceeding distally and regressing with recovery in the same order leaving brownish staining of the skin and, in severe cases, fine desquamation. During the acute phase of the illness there is gross upper respiratory catarrh with moist cough, conjunctivitis and photophobia. Naturally acquired measles confers life-ling immunity and the disease is very rare before the age of 6 months, due largely to passively transferred maternal measles antibody. The differential diagnosis is between drug rashes, rubella, ECHO 4, 9, 11, 16, 19 virus infection and Coxsackie A5, 9, 10, 16 and B3, 5 virus infection. Drug rashes tend to be accompanied by itch, lack the typical progression of measles and if anything last longer. The rash of rubella is much more discreet and conjunctivitis and systemic upset are absent, while typically there is posterior auricular lymphadenopathy. The maculopapular rash of ECHO and Coxsackie viral infections can be confusing and probably accounts for some 'second' attacks that parents report, but with these infections the prodromal illness is usually mild and sometimes accompanied by diarrhoea and vomiting. Conjunctivitis and upper respiratory catarrh are not features but an aseptic meningitis is a not unusual complication. The common complications of measles are otitis media and lower respiratory tract infections. Many children undoubtedly show transient EEG abnormalities and some have febrile convulsions in the acute phase of the illness. A very few develop meningo-encephalitis and an even smaller number sub-acute sclerosing panencephalitis. It is very unlikely that the family doctor will ever see these complications.

Anti-microbial treatment is justified when the general state of the health is poor or there is evidence of a specific secondary infection such as otitis media.

The diagnosis of rubella does not as a rule cause problems but ECHO 9 and 19 virus infections and Coxsackie A5, 10 can produce mild discreet maculopapular rashes which can be confusing. Another illness of presumed viral aetiology which can sometimes cause problems is roseola infantum. This is a mild febrile illness of infancy sometimes accompanied by catarrhal symptoms; the disappearance of fever is accompanied by a transient maculopapular rash. The illness is very short lived with little, if any, constitutional upset.

Rubella is a trivial minor illness and its positive diagnosis is important only in the sense that its transmission to a non-immune woman in the first trimester of pregnancy carries a definite risk of fetal damage. When it is important to make a specific diagnosis of an exanthematous viral illness paired sera, taken at an interval of 10–14 days between samples, should be submitted for viral antibody studies.

MUMPS

This myxo viral illness has an incubation period of 14–21 days, can be extremely mild in nature and indeed almost completely asymptomatic. Typically a child will complain of pain in one or both sides of the face, become feverish, and by the next day will have a swollen face due to enlargement of the parotid glands and in about 10% of cases the submandibular glands. The glands are tender to palpation and the orifice of the parotid duct may take on a somewhat pouting prominent appearance. The illness is generally mild but can be complicated by meningitis and mild pancreatitis with abdominal pain. Both complications are unpleasant but not serious. Epididymo orchitis is very rare before puberty. Another rare but important complication is the development of acute diabetes mellitus which is permanent and insulin dependent.

CHICKENPOX

This common illness caused by the varicella virus develops after an incubation period of 12–16 days. It typically begins with a few lesions in the hair and some on the palate, but the skin over the trunk is most densely affected. Lesions appear in crops and go through stages of macule, papule, vesicle and pustule although in clinical practice most children present in the vesicular stage. An unpleasant but relatively mild condition, it is only serious in children who are immunologically compromised or suffer from thrombocytopenia. In such circumstances hospital admission for specialised treatment with immunoglobulin and anti-viral drugs is required. Treatment at home is symptomatic, keeping the skin as clean as possible and dealing with any secondary infection. The time honoured remedy for soothing the skin is calomine lotion. Severe pox lesions will produce scars, particularly if there is secondary infection. Evidence of a previous infection can often be revealed by finding linear white scars on the skin of the trunk. The disease is not difficult to diagnose although Coxsackie A16 virus infection can produce vesicular lesions on the hands, feet and palate — 'hand, foot and mouth disease'. Molluscum contagiosum due to an unrelated pox virus can cause small unbilicated nodular lesions affecting the arms, legs, face and thighs but spares the hands and feet. Lesions are uniform in nature and generally not profuse, and are easily managed by puncturing and expressing their contents. It is usual to apply pure phenol to the cavity of the lesions although this must be done with great care and precision.

ORAL HERPES

Primary herpetic stomatitis due to herpes virus type 1, largely occurs in childhood and is a miserable condition. After a short non-descript illness of a day or two, vesicles appear in the mouth and on the lips and gums. These soon rupture leaving shallow ulcers accompanied by inflammation and swelling. Severe infection may be accompanied by cervical lymphadenopathy and by the constant drooling of saliva which can be lightly tinged with blood. Treatment is symptomatic; paracetamol syrup may relieve some of the pain and distress. Oral nystatin is not

indicated and neither is an antibiotic. Children with poor general health, in poor social circumstances with parents who cannot cope may require admission to hospital for nursing care.

Primary herpetic stomatitis usually runs a short course with considerable improvement after about 7 days but oropharyngeal ulceration may not completely disappear for a further week or two. Occasionally a thumb or finger sucking child may transfer the virus to a finger and produce localised inflammation and swelling — the so called 'herpetic whitlow'. This does not require antibiotic treatment. The commonest oropharyngeal viral disease confused with herpetic stomatitis is herpangina due to coxsackie virus but in this disease lesions tend to appear in the posterior aspect of the oropharynx whereas herpes virus affects the anterior aspect. The condition is sometimes confused with oral candidiasis (thrush) but this is uncommon in older infants and children and can be readily confirmed on microscopy of scrapings of the white mycelial deposits on the tongue and mucosa. The condition responds rapidly to oral nystatin or 0.5% aqueous gentian violet solution.

PERTUSSIS

Whooping cough (pertussis) occurs at any time of the year but can appear in epidemic proportions. Controversy over the rare complications of immunisation has overshadowed the very real morbidity and mortality associated with this miserable illness. Infants in the first 6 months of life are most seriously at risk when apnoea associated with paroxysmal coughing may result in severe hypoxic brain damage or death.

Caused by *Bordetella pertussis* and para pertussis the illness begins with a prodromal catarrhal phase lasting a few days, which is then followed by paroxysmal coughing which can last for many weeks before it gradually abates. Not uncommonly in the acute phase children will develop sub-conjunctival haemorrhage but the major complication is patchy atelectasis and in some children the development of bronchiectasis.

The diagnosis of whooping cough is usually made clinically although adeno viral and RSV infection may produce a clinically indistinguishable illness. A positive diagnosis can be made during the first 2 weeks by culture of the offending organism obtained by pernasal swabbing but in the later stages serological testing may be required. During the acute phase of the illness the peripheral blood will show evidence of lymphocytic response with lymphocyte counts which may be very considerably raised.

Cotrimoxazole and erythromycin are indicated in the treatment of the acute phase of the illness and the prophylactic administration of these drugs to unimmunised siblings is considered advisable particularly if they are under the age of one year.

EXCLUSION PERIODS FROM SCHOOL

Doctors may be asked by parents or schools for advice about the exclusion from school of children with communicable diseases. To a large extent this depends on the clinical progress of individual patients. It is by no means always practicable to enforce the isolation of children in poor social circumstances but Table 9.1 gives some general guidelines for the exclusion of children from schools and nurseries.

SOME MEDICAL PAEDIATRIC DIFFICULTIES

In urban areas with ready access to hospital, seriously ill children can be admitted in a very short space of time. Even so family doctors must be prepared to deal with emergencies and do as much as possible to ensure a child's safe and quick arrival in as good a condition as possible. Children living in remote areas may need to be 'air evacuated' and ambulance authorities should be properly briefed as to the seriousness of the emergency so that adequate life support equipment and expert help can be provided for the journey. In this country the common medical emergencies doctors are most likely to face are acute diabetes mellitus, status epilepticus, acute asthma, fulminating infection and septicaemia. A few words need also to be said about the doctor's responsibilities in the event of being called to see a child who has died unexpectedly.

DIABETES MELLITUS

Diabetes mellitus may begin at any time and is not uncommon in the first year of life. It has become increasing-ly evident that viral infection from coxsackie or mumps virus may precipitate the onset of acute diabetes in a child with a genetic predisposition to the disorder. HLA antigen typing may offer a means of detecting children with a family history of diabetes who may be at risk, with the possibilities of immunisation against specific viral conditions thought to be of aetiological importance. The onset of diabetes mellitus in children constitutes an emergency with a serious risk of the rapid onset of keto acidosis. No attempt should ever be made to investigate the problem at home or as an out-patient, and the child should be admitted to hospital without delay. Diabetes may present with bedwetting in a previously continent child but, more common are features of thirst and polyuria, and gradually, as keto acidosis intervenes, abdominal pain, dehydration and air hunger. Urinalysis will demonstrate gross ketonuria and glycosuria and acetone can usually be detected in the breath.

Diabetic children with acute febrile illnesses may show ketones in the urine without glycosuria. It is essential that in such circumstances the child's routine dose of insulin is given as usual and more often than not supplementary doses of soluble insulin will be required.

Hypoglycaemia unlike keto acidosis is sudden in onset and accompanied by pallor, sweating, loss of consciousness and occasionally twitching and frank convulsions. Intravenous glucose will correct the hypoglycaemia but this may be difficult to administer. An alternative is to give an intramuscular or deep subcutaneous injection of 0.5–1 mg of glucagon which will usually restore blood glucose to satisfactory levels within a few minutes. The cause of the hypoglycaemic episode should then be identified and remedied.

CONVULSIONS

About 2.5% of children in the first 5 years of life will have a convulsion associated with a febrile illneess and a similar percentage of the general propulation will have

Table 9.1   Exclusion periods from schools/nurseries for infectious diseases

	How long transmissible	Exclusion from school
Chickenpox	From 5 days before rash to 6 days after last appearance of vesicles	From onset until days after appearance of last vesicle
Measles	From onset of symptoms until 4 days after appearance of rash	Until recovery but not less than 4 days after appearance of rash
Mumps	From 7 days before onset of symptoms until parotid submandibular swelling subsides	Until recovery but not less than 7 days from onset of symptoms
Rubella	From 7 days before to 4 days after the appearance of the rash	4 days from onset of rash
Pertussis	From 7 days after exposure to infection to 21 days after onset of paroxysmal cough	21 days from onset of paroxysmal cough

epilepsy. Generalised convulsions assoociated with a febrile illness are usually short lived, lasting only a minute or so but occasionally can become prolonged. Occasionally children with major epilepsy may go into prolonged seizures. Because of the serious consequences of cerebral hypoxia and the risk of a permanent hemiplegia it is essential that convulsions be terminated as soon as possible. Intravenous or rectal diazepam has largely superceded the parenteral injection of paraldehyde and phenytoin. Intravenous diazepam is usually given in a dose of 0.25–0.4 mg/kg and is rapidly effective. It does however carry the risk of short-lived respiratory arrest which can usually be dealt with my mouth-to-mouth ventilation using, if available, a small airway. A good response can be also obtained by the administration of diazepam rectally in a dose of 0.5 mg/kg, the preparation used being the intravenous form of drug which can be easily administered using a 1-ml syringe gently introduced into the rectum. Considerable argument exists about the need for admission of hospital of children with febrile convulsions but if a seizure has been of any duration and the child's general condition is unsatisfactory, for example with possible aspiration into the lungs, then admission should be sought. Other circumstances which influence the decision to admit include poor social circumstances and parental distress.

About one-third of children with febrile seizures will have a recurrent seizure and many now advocate the routine prophylactic administration of sodium valproate until a child reaches the age of 4 or 5 years. Seizures occurring after the age of 5 should always be regarded as epileptic until proved otherwise.

ACUTE ASTHMA

Prevalence rates for asthma vary considerably but about 3–6% of children suffer from the disorder. For a common illness which is eminently treatable it has an unacceptable mortality which is almost entirely preventable. Part of the problem lies with the reluctance of doctors to make the diagnosis and to recognise that the key to successful management is the effective use of inhaled β_2 adrenoceptor agonists, good prophylaxis and careful regular review. It is however a disorder in which treatment compliance can be notoriously poor and one in which even with meticulous attention to detail patients can get into difficulties and become non-responsive to bronchodilators. The end result is gross airways obstruction, hypoxia and respiratory failure. This may happen progressively over many hours or a day or two, but can happen even more dramatically in a very short space of time — minutes rather than hours. While wheezing is the characteristic signature of asthma, severe asthma may be present with a silent albeit over-inflated chest. Cyanosis may be more readily detected in the lips, ear lobes and finger nails while the face may be quite pallid. Rapidly increasing tachycardia is an ominous sign. Some chest physicians advocate a policy of open access, self-referral to hospital of patients in difficulties and this undoubtedly has saved lives. Such a policy is not always practicable and some would argue that it is not the answer to the problem of optimal patient management. Whatever the merits or otherwise of this argument family doctors must be able to provide on the spot assistance to any child in difficulty even if hospital admission is to be arranged.

The first thing to do is to ensure that inhaler therapy is available and is being used effectively. It is surprising how often acute attacks can be quickly terminated by the proper administration of inhaled salbutamol or terbutaline. Many practices now have available for emergency use portable nebulisers which can be used with terbutaline and salbutamol. Salbutamol respiratory solution which is perhaps the most commonly used preparation comes as an 0.5% solution and can be given at the rate of 0.03–0.05 ml/kg 4-hourly, the solution being appropriately diluted with saline before use. Some parents of young asthmatic children prefer to use this routinely rather than an aerosol or inhaled powder (rotacaps) but this can only be agreed to on the basis that instructions for the use of the nebuliser are carefully followed and that the child is kept under proper review. Parents should also be cautioned that failure to respond rapidly to the nebuliser is an indication for further treatment and that medical attention must be sought at once. It is inadvisable to give intravenous aminophylline to small children at home and especially dangerous to give this to children already being given oral slow release preparations of aminophylline and theophylline. Children requiring admission to hospital should be sent in an ambulance with oxygen available and should be propped up on pillows. If they have to travel any distance an intramuscular injection of 100 mg hydrocortisone is advisable and many would give this whatever the circumstances. The place of oral steroid therapy in acute asthma is hotly debated, some paediatricians holding the view that oral steroid therapy should only be commenced in hospital. If a child appears to be adequately oxygenated and home circumstances permit it is reasonable to start oral prednisolone with an initial dose of 40 mg gradually reducing this over a period of 7 days and then stopping the drug. Response to treatment can be judged on the basis of a reducing respiratory rate, ease in respiratory effort and falling pulse rate. Failure to respond adequately to vigorous treatment withhin a period of 6 to 12 hours justifies hospital admission.

Oral bronchodilator drugs and antihistamines have no place in the management of acute asthma and antibiotics are only indicated if there is evidence of infection.

SERIOUS INFECTION

Serious life threatening infection calling for instant recognition and action occurs seldom in general practice. There are three situations which the family doctor must recognise. These concern acute osteitis and septic arthritis, meningococcaemia and fulminating gastroenteritis. The interval between the onset of often vague and misleading symptoms and critical illness can be extremely short, especially so in infancy.

Acute pyogenic bone and joint infection is characterised by sudden onset high fever, rigor, intense pain and localised tenderness over the infected site. Evidence of a superficial progenic skin lesion in the form of a boil or furuncle may be present. The illness is septicaemic and *Staphylococcus aureus*, the usual pathogen, can be isolated on blood culture. Antibiotics should not be given at home and until such time as blood has been taken for culture. Whenever the suspicion arises of septic bone or joint infection admission to hospital should be requested.

Acute meningococcal meningitis may begin after a prodromal mild and nondescript upper respiratory upset. The classical features of neck stiffness and opisthotonos accompanied by haemorrhagic rash do not present great diagnostic difficulties but in infancy the illness can be much more insidious in its onset and neck stiffness may be absent. A bulging tense fontanelle indicating raised intracranial pressure will however be present. Meningococcaemia will progress rapidly to peripheral circulatory failure and profound shock. Called to a shocked child with a rash and features suggesting this possibility the doctor must assume that infarction of the adrenal is imminent (Waterhouse-Friderichsen syndrome) and immediately administer 100 mg hydrocortisone — preferably intravenously — and 300 mg intramuscular benzyl penicillin. This is especially important if transfer to hospital is likely to involve any appreciable time. It is imperative that parents and siblings have their carrier status checked by culture of throat swabs and are given prophylactic antibiotic therapy — currently rifampicin is recommended because of meningococcal resistance to sulphonamides.

An acute fulminating gastro-intestinal infection can be due to a variety of enteropathogens, viral and bacterial. Severe hyperosmolar dehydration and metabolic acidosis can develop with amazing rapidity. The infected child appears apathetic and listless with poor skin turgor and is sunken eyed. In infants the fontanelle will be depressed. Diarrhoea may not always be very apparent but gentle digital examination of the rectum will be accompanied by the profuse expulsion of fluid on withdrawing the examining finger. No attempt should ever be made to give oral rehydration or antibiotics and admission to hospital for intravenous rehydration and biochemical monitoring is mandatory.

SUDDEN DEATH IN INFANCY

The family doctor may be called to the home of an infant who has been found dead, or be informed by a hospital casualty department or ambulance authority of an infant being found 'dead on arrival'. The doctor's duties are several, dealing not only with the immediate circumstances and distress, but also with the long-term help which families will need.

About 0.5% of a group of parents studied by the author reported a cot death — a figure similar to other reported studies. The term 'cot death' is used to describe deaths in which antecedent prodromal symptoms can be elicited after careful questioning and in which subsequent post mortem study will often indicate a definable cause of death. The term is also used to describe a second group of infants in whom no antecedent symptoms exist and in whom no definable cause of death may be found. Studies of explained cot deaths have shown a clear social class correlation with a decline over a period of years in the numbers being reported. Death in the second group seems to be related to some inherent defect of respiratory control with the sudden development of apnoea during sleep. These deaths seem to be unrelated to social class and relatively constant in their frequency of occurrence. There is a definite risk of subsequent infants being similarly affected. In an attempt to avoid this, studies of apnoea monitoring are being carried out in a number of centres. Parents wishing to consider the use of an apnoea monitor should be referred to a paediatrician for advice and in the United Kingdom may get useful help from The Foundation for the Study of Infant Deaths, 23 St Peter's Square, London W6 9NW.

What may be termed the 'avoidable' group of deaths present a challenge to general practice which has often been criticised for failure to recognise the potentially serious situation, and for failing to follow up children who might be at risk. Improving organisation of primary medical care services will undoubtedly help but even so some infants will die unexpectedly from fulminating illness or for other reasons, no matter how well services are organised and how expert the care provided. Called to the home of a dead infant the family doctor's first duty is to confirm the fact of death and to help the distressed parents. It is then necessary to find out the circumstances leading to death and to inform parents that this must be reported to the Crown authorities. In England, Wales and Northern Ireland this is the Coroner and in Scotland the Procurator Fiscal. Both may be informed directly or through the agency of the local police. The infant's body cannot be removed and a death certificate issued without legal authorisation. Family doctors must be aware of the possibilities of non-accidental injury and in any event will be required to give a statement of their findings and actions to the Crown authorities.

These formalities apart the doctor's main concern will be with the distressed parents and family and in dealing with the complex emotional reactions which can include hostility towards colleagues, guilt and anger and all the subsequent effects of bereavement. Above all it is important to try and offer as accurate an explanation as possible for the cause of death and to give whatever reassurance one can about the possible risks to other children in the family, or for any future children that may be born.

BEHAVIOUR AND LEARNIING

'Train up a child in the way he should go and when he is old he will not depart' — *Ecclesiastes* 22(6).

In Western society as life-threatening physical illness has disappeared or has been mastered greater attention has been focused on problems of behaviour and learning. They are common, important, preventable and manageable. For the most part they are determined by the private world and general social circumstances of the individual child. Family doctors are well placed to help in their prevention, early recognition and management. Only rarely in a lifetime of practice will a doctor see a child with psychotic illness or one whose problems are caused by structural or metabolic brain disease. A study by the author of 400 randomly chosen children showed that the principal worries reported by mothers concerned behaviour, learning and bedwetting (Table 9.2). Behaviour problems in the context of this study included any serious continuing problem and excluded minor problems of early childhood. Enuresis was non-organic in nature and defined as occurring in children over the age of 5 years. To add perspective 25% of families had a continuing problem affecting mental health; 20% of these concerned chronic anxiety and depression, and alcohol abuse. A somewhat subjective assessment of maternal stress suggested that 10% of mothers were severely stressed (20% in social class IV/V) and about 5% showed little, if any, interaction with their child. Chronic or recurrent unemployment, alcohol abuse, heavy cigarette smoking, marital breakdown and family disruption, low income and bad housing are the chief determinants which interact to provide the circumstances in which children will fail socially and educationally. A major part of health care in the future must be concerned with helping parents and their children to cope with stress and in ensuring their access to all appropriate resources.

Leaving generalities aside only a few aspects of a large canvas can be covered:

Problems of infancy
The over-active child
Enuresis and encopresis
Anxiety, depression and maladjustment
Problems at school

PROBLEMS OF INFANCY

Sleep
Children do not develop a regular adult sleep pattern until about the time of school entry and, given the chance, will sleep as and when they need to. Many infants and toddlers with poor sleep patterns and attention-seeking night waking, will sleep well if a settling ritual is introduced. Disturbing influences such as television should be avoided and a bedtime bath and story should be given at the same time each evening. Attention-seeking behaviour should be firmly ignored. Sometimes, and for a period of 1 to 12 weeks, a sedative dose of chloral hydrate or trimeprazine may be given at bedtime but the continuing or recurrent use of these drugs should be avoided. Despite common fears and attitudes, settling a restless infant at night in the parent's bed is quite reasonable and may help the child to go off to sleep quickly, soon to be returned to his or her cot.

Breath holding
Many children express their ill-humour by breath holding and go blue in the face sometimes even falling unconscious and twitching. Incidents often happen in response to some minor injury or upset. Parents can be reassured that nothing serious will happen and that future incidents should be firmly 'ignored'. Breath holding attacks should be distinguished from 'white attacks' which are also benign and due to transient vagal mediated asystole in response to minor injury, and from momentary lapses in consciousness due to minor epilepsy.

Feeding — fads and food refusal
These are best dealt with by a firm approach which avoids the use of bribes and informs the child that nothing will be given until the next meal is due.

Tantrums
Naughtiness, biting, spitting and socially unacceptable behaviour is best dealt with by the 'time out' technique which excludes the child from company, television and other desirable comforts for a short period, and allows return on the basis of good behaviour. Healthy children soon learn and understand social conventions. They are quick to exploit differences in approach and consistency

Table 9.2   Problems experienced by mothers

Problem	% Mothers expressing anxiety	Prevalence/1000
Behaviour	18	80
Learning	8	33
Enuresis	8	80

in handling by both parents is essential. Spanking by parents, almost universal, is not psychologically damaging when controlled and modest in nature.

THE HYPERACTIVE CHILD

The hyperactive child by definition has a very limited attention span and is constantly restless. This behaviour is not infrequently accompanied by destructive and aggressive tendencies. Between the extremes of restlessness and inattentiveness and unacceptable aggression is a wide spectrum of disturbed behaviour. Quite commonly hyperactive children have serious learning problems and visuospatial perceptual difficulties. Some are undoubtedly intellectually handicapped. Occasionally hyperactive children show no regard for common dangers and tend to wander away from home or school. There are several reasons for hyperactivity and more than one may operate in any patient. Minimal cerebral dysfunction with incoordinate motor development and specific learning problems and intellectual handicap often feature but commoner by far is the hyperactivity of children from psychosocially disturbed families.

The investigation and management of hyperactive children is a matter of paediatric neurologists and clinical psychologists, but family doctors will be involved in treating the rest of the family. Occasionally amphetamines or methylphenidate (Ritalin) may benefit the child who has an organic basis for his disorder. They are of no value when the problem is sociopathically determined. Benzodiazepines and phenothiazines are of no value.

ENURESIS AND ENCOPRESIS

The age at which sphincter control is achieved varies widely and is in part culturally determined. Although often diagnosed before the age of 5 years, the term enuresis should not be applied until after the age of school entry by which time the majority of children will have achieved control of their bladders. Certainly for practical purposes lack of control thereafter proves a problem not only to the child and parents but also to the school. It is usual to describe enuresis as being primary, that is sphincter control has not yet been achieved, or secondary, to imply incontinence reappearing in a child who has been continent for some time. All children irrespective of the type of enuresis should be carefully examined to exclude an obvious genito-urinary malformation while urinalysis and culture should also be done. Some children previously continent may start bed-wetting as a result of a urinary tract infection or occasionally because of the onset of acute diabetes mellitus. Unhappiness arising out of events at school, home or at play is most likely to predispose to enuresis. The problem is often compounded by ridicule and by unsympathetic handling at home or at school and not infrequently by the adoption of harsh punitive measures by the parents.

The management of younger primary enuresis begins with explanation to parents and advice about protecting the mattress with plastic sheeting. An incentive training programme using star charts and modest rewards for dry days and nights should be explained to the child who should be asked to keep his own progress chart. Parents need to be advised that rewards should be modest and frequently spaced and that a child's concept of time is a fairly constricted one. Above all patient and perseverance are required. Older children respond well to battery operated buzzers and pads which are activated at the onset of micturition. There have been a number of advances on the design of such alarms which are becoming quite modestly priced. However when alarms are not readily available a short trial of imipramine 25–50 mg at bedtime will undoubtedly help, but relapses are common when this is withdrawn. Imipramine if used must be prescribed on the basis that its cardiotoxicity and need for secure safekeeping is explained to the child's parents. It should not be prescribed for children under the age of 7 years. The successful management of enuresis above all depends on the enthusiasm of the therapist and the family doctor who may succeed in helping the child for no other reason than by providing the necessary enthusiasm which parents cannot find.

SOILING

Faecal incontinence due to chronic diarrhoeal illness or to fluid faeces bypassing scyballa in a loaded colon, must be distinguished from voluntary defaecation into the pants or in inappropriate places and circumstances. Hirschsprungs disease and megacolon are rare but important anomalies which can cause overflow incontinence. This may also occur however as a result of stool withholding in an attempt to avoid the painful defaecation which can occur with a fissure-in-ano. The assessment of the problem of soiling always requires proper clinical examination including digital examination of the rectum.

True encopresis is much less common than enuresis and always signifies some serious psychological or psychosocial problem within the family which must be identified and corrected. The management of the bowel itself includes a high fibre diet and the occasional evacuation of the bowel with suitable enemata or bisacodyl suppositories. For a time an evening dose of danthron or dioctyl sodium sulphosuccinate may help to establish regular bowel evacuation. When the problem is very severe and refractory it may be necessary to admit the child to hospital for a period of toilet training. Given such circumstances referral to a child psychiatrist may be necessary.

ANXIETY, DEPRESSION AND MALADJUST-MENT

Anxiety and depression are commoner in children in their juvenile years than is sometimes supposed. Specific phobic states concerning doctors, dentists, spiders and other nasties present a relatively straightforward challenge which can be very effectively dealt with by referral to a clinical psychologist. Severe anxiety and depression, an altogether different matter, may present in a rather unobtrusive way with a quiet, withdrawn, reticent, fearful or tearful child who may be restless at night and in whom school performance will be deteriorating. Alopecia areata, nail biting and mannerisms are not uncommon and occasionally hair can be pulled out in large quantities. Children in their early teens may make more dramatic gestures by tentative wrist cutting or by parasuicidal overdosing.

Sociopathic behaviour including stealing, solvent and alcohol abuse and abusive threatening behaviour, while obviously unacceptable and disruptive, can have a more favourable prognosis than chronic anxiety and depression.

Many of these problems will present at school and will be referred by school authorities to child guidance departments and some children showing evidence of sociopathic behaviour will be referred for psychiatric opinion as a result of legal intervention. The family doctor's contribution more often than not, is to deal with the problems of the rest of the family. In childhood anxiolytics and antidepressants are seldom needed.

RECOMMENDED READING

Developmental screening
Egan D F, Illingworth R S, McKeith R C 1969 Developmental screening 0–5 SIMP, Heinemann, London

Immunisation
Immunisation against infectious diseases HMSO, Published by DHSS, SHHD, Welsh Office
Dick G 1978 Immunisation. Update Books, London

Genetic counselling
Harper P S 1981 Practical genetic counselling. John Wright & Sons, Bristol

Clinical paediatrics
Forfar J O, Arneil G C (eds) 1984 Textbook of paediatrics, 3rd Edn. Churchill Livingstone, Edinburgh

Diseases in the cardiovascular system

Diseases of the cardiovascular system are responsible for 14% of all consultations in general practice, but they account for more than 50% of the deaths. These conditions become prevalent with increasing age but their effect on the patient and his family can be quite devastating if they occur at a younger age. In general practice 21% of all consultations are for chronic long-term illness and diseases of the cardiovascular system form a significant part of that workload. In a year a general practitioner with a list of 2500 patients will see 10 patients with acute myocardial infarction, 30 patients with chronic cardiac failure, 100 patients with high blood pressure, 50 patients with coronary artery disease, 20 patients with cerebrovascular disease, and one patient every 5 years with congenital heart disease.

Deaths from ischaemic heart disease can have catastrophic effects on the middle aged at a time when personal and financial commitments are considerable. Within a practice of 2500 patients there will be three deaths each year in the age group 45–64 years and one death every 3 years in those under 45. Ischaemic heart disease is responsible for 44% of all male deaths in the age group 45–64 years. In general practice three diseases of the cardiovascular system are responsible for the majority of the consultations: coronary heart disease, hypertension and congestive cardiac failure.

SYMPTOMS OF CARDIAC DISEASE

CHEST PAIN

The commonest cardiac symptom presenting to the general practitioner is chest pain which to the patient usually means an association with the heart however vague the symptom may be. The patient's previous experience with a relative with heart disease, or a friend at work sustaining a myocardial infarction promotes a degree of anxiety which can lead to the patient seeking an earlier consultation and in some cases seeking repeated consultations for trivial symptoms. In their symptom survey Dunnell & Cartwright (1972) found that 5% of the

population studied had suffered chest pain in the previous 2 weeks. There was no difference in incidence between men and women and the symptom seemed to be equally common at all ages. A study of a rural practice in Warwickshire (Hull 1969) showed that 2% of new consultations were for chest pain and that these were commoner amongst patients in the lower social classses. A similar study in London (Morrell et al 1971) found that chest pain was the predominant symptom in 3% of patients and in less than half the doctor was able to make a definite diagnosis. This study showed that the incidence of new complaints of chest pain was 37.3 per 1000 practice population each year. These figures suggest that the general practitioner will be faced with a patient with chest pain about twice during a week but these will only be a fraction of those in the community suffering from this complaint.

In the history it is important to determine the site of the pain, whether it radiates, what precipitated the pain in the first instance, and if anything relieves it or makes it worse. Are there any accompanying symptoms? Does the patient give any verbal or non-verbal clues? It is important to note whether the patient is anxious and whether the pain is accompanied by breathlessness. Is it related to movement of the neck or the limbs or to straining of any of the chest muscles? Further questions should be asked to exclude respiratory or alimentary causes for the pain. The general practitioner's main difficulty is in differentiating between cardiac pain and pain which arises elsewhere. In studies which have been carried out in general practice more than half of the patients who present with chest pain will suffer from musculoskeletal pain; cardiac disease is responsible for only about 20% of patients who present with chest pain.

DYSPNOEA

Dyspnoea is one of the most difficult symptoms to evaluate in practice and in assessing it the general practitioner has to take into account the patient's age, his general physical condition and the amount of exercise he normally takes. In addition breathlessness can be influenced by such factors as obesity and smoking or it may just be the result of a head cold or a symptom of an anxiety neurosis. True cardiac breathlessness first appears on exertion and gradually progresses until it is present at rest. Dyspnoea is a subjective symptom but by closely questioning the patient it is possible to assess its severity objectively. If orthopnoea is present — breathlessness when the patient is lying flat — there is an increased likelihood of it having a cardiac origin. Severe cases have a tendency to paroxysmal nocturnal dyspnoea: the patient wakes in the early hours of the morning gasping for breath.

The elderly may be breathless and accept this as being part of the ageing process and as a result may present with more florid symptoms of longer duration. In the elderly, dyspnoea appearing for the first time is usually significant of a serious organic cause.

OEDEMA

Oedema is another manifestation of cardiac disease but may simply be due to prolonged standing or be secondary to varicose veins. Pressure with the thumb at the ankle will displace the fluid and leave a small pit. When the patient is confined to bed the oedema can occur in the sacrum or the thighs.

OTHER SYMPTOMS

Palpitations — the patient being aware of his heart beating is usually secondary to anxiety but can be a symptom of an arrhythmia. A cough — particularly a nocturnal cough — can be a symptom of cardiac failure in the elderly. The patient often does not realise the significance and the seriousness of coughing up clear fluid. Syncope, anorexia, nausea, vomiting and tiredness can all be associated with heart disease but these symptoms in general practice are non-specific and give little lead to the ultimate diagnosis. When taking a history it is most important to obtain the patient's cardiovascular risk profile and an adequate family history relating to cardiac problems. The patient's height and weight should be checked and a note made of his alcohol consumption and the number of cigarettes smoked.

CONGESTIVE CARDIAC FAILURE

CAUSES

Cardiac failure is a disease of the elderly and 90% of patients suffering are over the age of 60. It usually occurs as a secondary phenomenon to coronary heart disease,

hypertension or chronic obstructive airways disease or rarely valvular disease of the heart. It can also be secondary to atrial fibrillation in the context of underlying coronary heart disease. One of the skills of the general practitioner is to make an early diagnosis of life threatening conditions. This is particularly important in conditions such as cardiac failure.

SYMPTOMS

Dyspnoea is the earliest symptom becoming first noticeable going upstairs, progressing and then being present at rest. The patient may ultimately be unable to lie flat and suffer from paroxysmal nocturnal dyspnoea. This is usually accompanied by a cough and there may be haemoptysis. Peripheral oedema can occur in the ankles, or sacrum if the patient is in bed, and in severe cases ascites or a pleural effusion can develop.

SIGNS

On examination cyanosis may be noticed in the lips, cheeks or hands. The jugular venous pressure is elevated. Oedema is obvious and there is often an enlarged and tender liver. On palpation there are signs of left ventricular enlargement and the presence of triple rhythm and basal crepitations confirms the diagnosis.

MANAGEMENT

The management of cardiac failure poses particular problems and affects the patient's lifestyle. A housewife may be unable to cope with her home and family but every effort should be made to make her home environment as suitable to her physical state as possible. Relatives or a home help can be of assistance with heavy tasks and a move to a ground floor flat in an area of shops can make all the difference to the patient's independence. The social work department can deal with many problems before a crisis arises. The knowledge that the patient may not be able to look after her family can cause a mother considerable worry but if a doctor understands this then be measures taken to organise help at a time of crisis can constitute a valuable therapeutic measure. A man should be kept at work as long as possible thus maintaining financial security and preventing demoralisation. If possible he should get a lighter job within the firm but the patient may not be keen on this because of reduced income and status. If he is confined to the house then he should increase his recreational activities and the help of an occupational therapist can be helpful in this area. In an elderly patient cardiac failure may be only one of many pathologies present — osteoarthritis or diverticulitis — and the patient may be taking multiple therapy. This can cause further confusion and tablets may be taken in the wrong dosage. The patient should be seen regularly either by the doctor or another member of the practice team.

The majority of patients with cardiac failure are treated at home and those who need referral to hospital are usually in the younger age group where failure is secondary to an arrhythmia, if the patient lives in poor social circumstances or if the condition is refractory to treatment. The patient should rest and if working, should stay off work. In the initial stages most of the time should be spent either in a chair or in bed. If the patient spends longer in bed than is required there is a significant danger of him developing deep venous thrombosis. Advice is required about diet. If obesity is present a restriction of calorie intake is required and there should be some limitation of salt intake.

DRUGS

In the initial stages a potent diuretic should be used, such as frusemide 40 mg or bumetanide 1 mg daily. A single dose of each is given in the morning and the diuresis is complete within a few hours. The majority of diuretics used in the treatment of heart failure work by reducing the reabsorption of sodium from the loop of Henlé and the proximal part of the distal tubule. In the less dramatic patient or when there has been an adequate response to a more potent diuretic a thiazide diuretic is usually all that is required. Although thiazides vary in terms of potency and duration of action there is little to choose between the different preparations in terms of effectiveness. The patient's potassium level must be assessed before commencing treatment, although potassium supplements will usually only be required with prolonged diuretic use or in the elderly. In elderly patients where compliance may be a problem there is a case for a combined preparation. Occasionally the oedema will be resistant to the common diuretics due to secondary hyperaldosteronism and an aldosterone antagonist such as spironolactone 100 mg daily is worth trying.

Before the advent of powerful diuretics, digoxin was the mainstay of treatment as its use results in increased myocardial contractility, promotes the efficiency of cardiac contraction and thus a decrease in the ventricular end-diastolic volume. The improvement in cardiac performance is followed by an improvement in renal function giving a secondary diuretic effect. Digoxin depresses atrioventricular conduction and so reduces the ventricular rate. Diuretics should always be used as first line treatment in cardiac failure. The only real indication in the community for digoxin therapy is the presence of atrial fibrillation. In this situation an initial dose of 0.5–1 mg is given and the maintenance dose is usually 0.25 mg daily.

Digoxin toxicity is a particular problem if the patient has hypokalaemia; any patient who is being started on digoxin therapy requires serum potassium monitoring before commencing the therapy and at least a monthly reappraisal in the initial stages. The commonest side effects of digoxin are nausea and vomiting and a pulse rate of under 60/min will confirm that the symptoms are a manifestation of digoxin toxicity. Arrhythmias are the most serious side-effect with ectopic beats being the commonest: if unrecognised these can progress to the more serious ventricular arrhythmias or complete heart block. Prolonged diuretic therapy can cause hypokalaemia and, when thiazides are used, can induce diabetes mellitus or gout. These side effects are more pronounced in the elderly.

Until recently the treatment of cardiac failure was restricted to the agents already mentioned but vasodilators which produce an improvement in cardiac performance have been introduced recently. Vasodilators act by one of two methods: by arteriolar dilation which reduces both peripheral vascular resistance and left ventricular pressure at systole and results in improved cardiac output, or by venous dilation which results in the dilation of capacitance vessels, an increase in venous pooling and diminution of the venous return to the heart thus decreasing left ventricular and diastolic pressure. Symptoms of heart failure are therefore relieved. There are three main groups of drugs and they would normally be used under hospital supervision in cardiac failure. The nitrates act predominantly by venous dilation; hydrallazine acts predominantly by arterial dilation; prazosin and sodium nitroprusside produce both arterial and venous dilatation. In hospital, combinations of these drugs would be required and such measures would only be used in the most severe cases.

LEFT VENTRICULAR FAILURE

One of the most dramatic situations which the family doctor has to deal with is the sudden presentation of acute pulmonary oedema. The patient is wakened from sleep, is choking and gasping for breath with a dry repetitive cough and a white frothy sputum which is often blood stained. He is anxious, pale, sweaty and cyanosed. On examination there is a rapid pulse; often a triple rhythm at the apex, pulsus alternans and basal rales on chest examination. If he is not already sitting up he should be put in that position, given 5 mg of cyclomorph intravenously and 10 mg intramuscularly. This should be followed by 40 mg frusemide intravenously and if there is evidence of bronchospasm the patient may benefit from the intravenous injection of 250 mg aminophylline, given slowly over 5 minutes. Once this initial treatment has been carried out and the patient has improved the doctor can then consider further management and whether this should take place at home or in hospital.

CORONARY HEART DISEASE

AETIOLOGY

There is no one single cause but a variety of factors are implicated.

RISK FACTORS

Most important are cigarette smoking, raised serum cholesterol, hypertension, and the genetic make-up of the individual. The relationship with smoking is particularly relevant under the age of 45 and those who smoke 25 cigarettes per day increase their chances of dying from coronary heart disease ten-fold. A smoker is twice as likely to have a coronary as a non-smoker. An increase in the cholesterol level to above the normal range of between 5.8 and 7.75 mmol/1 is said to increase the risk of myocardial infarction three-fold. A blood pressure over 160/95 increases the risk of coronary thrombosis 2.5 times in men and 3 times in women. The presence of diabetes mellitus in males doubles the risk whereas in females it increases it five-fold. Obesity, a stressful lifestyle and the oral contraceptive have also been implicated.

PRESENTATION

The clinical presentation of angina is typically of retrosternal or left sided chest pain which is gripping, tight and radiates to the neck, the jaw and the left shoulder, into the left or right arm, the epigastrium or through to the back. It can be precipitated by exercise, emotion, a heavy meal and cold. If the causative factor is removed then the pain usually settles within 5 minutes. The patient gives non-verbal cues in this situation by holding his clenched fist over the pain or showing the distribution of the pain by his opened hand (Figs. 10.1 and 10.2). The pain can be accompanied by dyspnoea, by fatigue or palpitations. There may be evidence of an aetiological factor, e.g. xanthoma, but usually there are few physical signs and the diagnosis is principally made from the history. The presence of exertional pain which responds promptly to glyceryl trinitrate is a reliable confirmation of diagnosis. The ECG can be normal in up to 50% of patients so little reliance can be placed on a negative result. The principal ECG findings in angina are depression of the ST segment

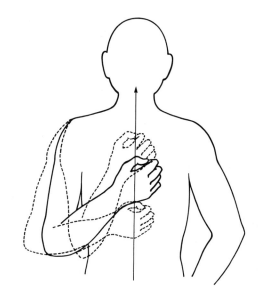

Fig. 10.1 Non-verbal communication of anginal pain

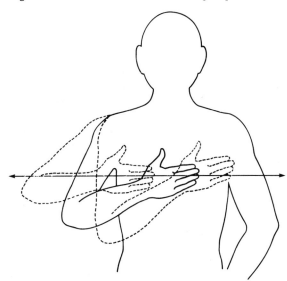

Fig. 10.2 Non-verbal communication of anginal pain

with progressive flattening and then inversion of the T wave, or a previous myocardial infarction or left bundle branch block. A chest X-ray is another worthwhile investigation. This can be normal but it could also show evidence of pulmonary oedema or of left ventricular hypertrophy with the cardiothoracic ratio increased to above 50%. If further diagnostic tests are required the patient should be referred to hospital. Studies (Fulton et al 1972) which have been carried out in general practice have shown that of patients with angina 47% develop stable angina, 37% become pain free and 16% become unstable.

MANAGEMENT

The patient requires advice about his lifestyle and should be advised to reduce his walking speed or give up leisure activities which provoke pain. Ideally his situation at work should be such that activity does not provoke pain and that there is no additional danger to the patient if he should have an attack of angina pectoris. This immediately excludes such occupations as driving, particularly of heavy goods vehicles (HGV), working at heights, operating moving machinery or work where it is impossible to avoid heavy manual labour. The question of the suitability of the type of work should be fully discussed with the patient and the importance of this should be stressed. Any change of employment thought necessary should be discussed with the patient and the factory doctor; the help of the industrial medical advisory service may be required. The patient's home conditions are important, particularly if there are flights of stairs to climb or if he has to walk up a hill on his way home. It may be difficult to arrange a move but if this is required every effort should be made to arrange it through the local housing authority.

The management should include reduction of any risk factors present and specific anti-anginal therapy. Patients should be encouraged to give up smoking or if this is impossible to reduce their intake to under 10 a day. Hypertension if present should be treated vigorously and beta blockers are particularly useful as they are therapeutic in both conditions. It is still thought that the serum cholesterol level should be reduced through dietary means although the preventive value of this measure is now being questioned. It is however important to keep weight to a reasonable level and the patient should be encouraged to take exercise. If diabetes mellitus is present particular attention should be paid to its management.

DRUGS

Glyceryl trinitrate is still the cornerstone of traditional drug management and should be taken both symptomatically whenever the patient develops chest pain, and prophylactically. Long-acting nitrates are now being used increasingly in the UK but the development of the beta-blockers has been the major advance in the medical management of angina pectoris. Their main action is to reduce myocardial oxygen demand by reducing not only the heart rate during the exercise but also the force of contraction of the muscle myocardial fibres thus conserving oxygen.

Beta-blockers have been shown to improve exercise tolerance in most patients with angina. The dose should be increased until symptoms settle or until the resting pulse rate is 55–60/minute. If the patient has any history of chronic obstructive airways diseasse it is preferable to use a cardioselective beta-blocker.

The calcium antagonists are being increasingly used in the treatment of angina. They reduce cardiac work and oxygen demand during exercise, and cause peripheral and coronary vasodilation. Nifedipine is the product most widely used but some care should be taken if verapamil is used with a beta-blocker as there is a risk of precipitating cardiac failure. Patients who have angina pectoris often have a marked psychological overlay and there may be a case for mild sedation with one of the benzodiazepines.

When patients are on established therapy for angina pectoris it is important that this is maintained: if it ever requires to be stopped this should be carried out gradually. If treatment is stopped suddenly the patient can have a rebound effect and the angina can become worse. Patients whose angina cannot be controlled with standard management should be referred to a physician for further advice. Other patients who should be referred are those under the age of 50 and those who suffer from increasingly severe pain. Coronary arteriography is indicated if surgery is contemplated or if the site of the lesion requires to be specified. The results of coronary bypass surgery have been encouraging.

UNSTABLE ANGINA

The group of patients with unstable angina is particularly worrying in general practice and can cause a great deal of anxiety to the doctor: because of the unpredictable outcome of this form of angina an urgent medical outpatient appointment should be arranged with a cardiologist. A study in Teeside (Colling et al 1976) of nearly 2000 patients with myocardial infarction showed that 20% of those who survived gave evidence of new or worsening angina in the days or weeks before the infarct. This study has suggested that there is a higher incidence of chest pain the month before myocardial infarction than occurs in the normal population.

MYOCARDIAL INFARCTION

In myocardial infarction the distribution of pain is similar to angina pectoris but it is more severe, lasts for more than 30 minutes, is accompanied by sweating and nausea and the patient is often pale and vasoconstricted. When the patient is seen at home the general practitioner should check the pulse, decide whether or not an arrhythmia is present, measure blood pressure aand exclude the presence of cardiac failure. The triad of breathlessness, tachycardia and a third heart sound is often indicative of impending cardiac faulure. The diagnosis of myocardial infarction is made from the history with confirmation from ECG and cardiac enzymes.

MANAGEMENT

The introduction of coronary care units was responsible initially for a drop in mortality of between 10 and 20% due to the control of life-threatening arrhythmias. There has been no further improvement in mortality rates due to two main reasons, firstly the high mortality from pump failure and secondly the delay before the patient is admitted to the coronary care unit. Only 2% of patients are normally seen within the first hour. Few patients are in a coronary care unit within 2 hours of the onset of pain. Pantridge in Belfast (Pantridge & Geddes 1967) was able to reach 28% of his patients within the first hour and showed the value of early care. Of patients who die of a myocardial infarction 25% do so immediately or within 15 minutes, 15% die in the next 45 minutes and 10% in the second hour. Thus 50% of all patients who are going to die do so within the first 2 hours and it is during this time that the general practitioner's role is vital. Several studies have highlighted the controversy of whether patients who sustain a myocardial infarction should be managed at home or in hospital. It is now felt that if the general practitioner can provide initial coronary care in the patient's home, and admit patients of high risk to hospital, then whether the patient stays at home or is sent to hospital can be based on a number of objective criteria (see below). Although many general practitioners are reluctant to accept this responsibility, competent care is well within their capabilities. It is most important that the doctor gets to the patient quickly, gives adequate analgesia and remains with him until he settles down and his clinical condition stabilises. The patient must be given sufficient analgesic to relieve pain: a small amount should be given intravenously with the remainder being given intramuscularly.

DRUGS

Diamorphine is the drug of choice: the dose is 10 mg with half being given intravenously and half intramuscularly. If this does not relieve pain a further 5 mg of diamorphine should be given intravenously or intramuscularly 10 minutes later. Cyclomorphine can also be given — 5 mg intravenously and 10 mg intramuscularly — and this combination often reduces the incidence of sickness. If the patient is having frequent ectopics (a compensatory pause after a normal beat with a frequency of more than one in six normal beats) a dose of lignocaine should be given intravenously (1 mg/kg) and a similar dose intramuscularly. Atropine 0.6 mg intravenously is indicated if the heart rate is slower than 60 beats per minute and if this is accompanied by hypotension. If there is evidence of cardiac failure, 20–40 mg of frusemide should be given intravenously. The early deaths in myocardial infarction are usually due to an arrhythmia found in over 90% of patients within the first 6 hours and thereafter becoming less common.

MANAGEMENT

Patients who die in coronary care units do so secondary to pump failure. Other compliations of myocardial infarction are an extension of the infarct, pericarditis or a pulmonary embolism. Systemic emboli can also occur.

The choice of where the patient should be managed is particularly difficult in general practice as most doctors have had experience of a patient who seemed ideal for home management but who died suddenly 2 hours later. It is difficult in this situation for relatives to accept that the best care was given. Each case must be judged on its own merits but certain factors influence the decision of whether to treat the patient at home or in hospital. In general he can be treated at home if his attitude and that of his relatives is favourable, if he has a stable cardiac rhythm, if he is first seen 2 hours and particularly 12 hours after the onset of pain, if he is aged over 60, if there are no signs of cardiac failure, if he has a systolic blood pressure above 100 mmHg, if the journey to hospital would be long and if he lives in good social circumstances. When a patient is kept at home the general practitioner should wait for up to 2 hours until the pain has been relieved and the clinical situation has settled and then make a further visit later that day. Thereafter the frequency of visiting will depend on the patient's clinical condition.

The patient who is best suited to management within a coronary care unit is the one who has an unstable rhythm, particularly ventricular extrasystoles, and when a bradycardia persists which has not responded to treatment with atropine. Hospital management is also indicated if the patient is seen within 2 hours of onset, if he is below the age of 60 and particularly if under 45, if cardiac failure is present, if he is hypotensive with a systolic pressure below 100 mmHg, if the pain persists despite adequate analgesia and if there is a previous history of either myocardial infarction, diabetes mellitus, a lipoprotein abnormality or a family history of ischaemic heart disease. Poor social circumstances are also a justifiable reason for admitting the patient to hospital. These are mainly medical guidelines but the final decision is often related to the patient's attitude and that of his relatives.

If a patient with myocardial infarction is to be managed at home there must be continuity of care with the out-of-hours work for that patient being covered by doctors from the practice or by a doctor who is familiar with the patient's condition. There must be good communication between the doctor and other members of the practice team such as the district nurse who may be involved. If there are no complications the patient should be mobilised as soon as possible and advice about risk factors should be given at an early stage. It is important that a cardiac neurosis does not occur and positive information should be given early about such factors as smoking, sexual intercourse, driving, working in the garden and returning to hobbies and work. A positive approach leads to a much better response from the patient. The aim should be that the patient returns to his normal employment but if this is not possible, for example, a public service vehicle driver, contact with the medical employment advisory service is mandatory at an early stage.

CARDIAC REHABILITATION

The main indicator of successful rehabilitation after a coronary is return to work and this process should start when the patient is first seen after myocardial infarction. 80% of survivors eventually return to work without special measures with a higher proportion if it is the first infarct and if the patient is under the age of 60. Most physicians consider that the majority of patients with mild infarcts can return to work within 2 months if they have a light job and 2 weeks later if work is more physical. In reality only 50–60% are back at work after 3 months and it is thought that there is a considerable amount of unnecessary and prolonged invalidism. Underlying psychological factors are likely to be the main reason for delay but there can also be physical complications. It is very important that the mild uncomplicated case should not be cosseted.

Certain occupations, for example an airline pilot, are obviously incompatible with a return to work after an infarct. Within social classes 4 and 5 patients are more likely to have arduous work and are thus less likely to be given part-time work: delay in this group can be expected. A successful return to work should be presented to the patient as the prime target from the start of the illness. The annual sickness rate for patients with cardiac disease is only 9 days each year and this fact should be appreciated by employers. It is of advantage for the patient to visit his employer when recovery is advanced to demonstrate how well he is and to give some idea of his future expectations. A good employer will usually make extensive adjustments in work to suit the return of a man who has done well for him. Patients with psychological problems, physical disabilities and inappropriate jobs should be identified early and properly assessed so that a special programme for each, perhaps including vocational training, may be arranged. Doctors should consider

facts and assess reasons carefully before allowing incapacity to go beyond 10–12 weeks. Where there is some difficulty, a trial of work or a cardiological opinion should be sought.

HYPERTENSION

Fry (1974) in his practice found the incidence of hypertension over a 20 year period to be 15% of adults over 30. The diagnostic criteria used was a persistently raised (on three or more occasions) diastolic pressure of 100 mmHg or more. The incidence increased with age and was more frequent in women in the older age groups. In the same 20-year period only 10 cases of malignant hypertension were discovered. Blood pressure is distributed in the population in a smooth bell-shaped curve and it follows from this that very high levels are rare.

INCIDENCE

Population studies among middle-aged people demonstrate only a very small number with a very high risk of complications. In the Renfrew study (Hawthorn et al 1974) only 0.5% of men and women aged 45–64 had a diastolic pressure of 130 mmHg or more. The Renfrew study also demonstrated that 5% of the population had a diastolic pressure of 110 mmHg or more: this is the group which forms a major part of the family doctor's workload. When these figures are transferred to an average general practice of 2500 the general practitioner will have two patients in the 45–64 age group with severe hypertension (diastolic above 130 mmHg), 24 with moderate (diastolic 110–129), 180 with mild (diastolic 90–109): 328 of his patients will be normotensive.

THE RISK

Data published 30 years ago by Life Insurance Companies has demonstrated that the life expectancy of an individual is directly proportional to the level of his blood pressure and is closely related to a single casual reading. Data from Insurance Companies and population studies have defined the extent of risk of complications from varying levels of blood pressure. All have demonstrated that there is no level which can be regarded as safe. A 35-year-old male with a casual blood pressure reading of 150/100 has a 16 year reduction in his life expectancy. Hypertension can be considered to be a state of graded risk rather than a clinical diagnosis. The height of the blood pressure is the most important risk factor in the development of stroke. In addition, blood pressure is a prime risk factor in relation to coronary heart disease and sudden death. Patients with an elevated blood pressure have a two to three times greater risk of having a fatal heart attack, are three to five times more likely to have a stroke and six times more likely to have cardiac failure than is a normotensive patient. The level of blood pressure rises with age and at any particular level the risk is less severe for women than for men. The height of the blood pressure is an important predictor of vascular complications at any age.

There has been some controversy as to the benefits of treatment of hypertension but there is now firm evidence that patients with a diastolic blood pressure above 115 mmHg who are adequately treated have a reduced rate of complications and mortality. Studies in the United States (Hypertensive Detection and Follow-up Co-operative Group 1979) of patients with diastolic blood pressure between 90 and 114 mmHg have shown significant reductions in mortality and in the incidence of stroke after 5 years of treatment and organised recall. In Western societies — in contrast to underdeveloped countries — blood pressure rises with age and a diastolic pressure of more than 90 mmHg is said to be present in 20% of 40–50 year olds and in about 50% of the population over the age of 70. The aetiology is multifactorial and many factors have been implicated: excess weight, inheritance, salt intake, acidity of drinking water and stress. It should be remembered that hypertension is an asymptomatic disease and is either found at routine examination or when the patient presents with one of its complications.

SCREENING

Clinical studies have demonstrated that hypertensive patients who receive anti-hypertensive therapy develop fewer complications than those who are untreated. Furthermore, amongst treated hypertensives the degree of blood pressure control rather than the initial severity is the most important predictor of outcome. The quality of medical care and follow-up are therefore of prime importance in preventing complications.

PRESENT STATE

In the United Kingdom only half of the patients in the population have had their blood pressure checked and as hypertension is asymptomatic only 50% of those with the condition have been detected. Of those detected only half are receiving treatment and only half of those have attained an adequate level of blood pressure control. Thus of the total number of hypertensive patients in the population only about 12.5% are receiving satisfactory care: there is the great scope for improvement. A study in general practice in Edinburgh (Fulton 1979) showed that

two-thirds of general practitioners felt that they should be screening for hypertension although only a small number were actually doing so. A random sample (Heller & Rose 1977) of 697 patients aged 20 and above in London general practices showed that only 24% had had their blood pressure checked in the previous 5 years and 39% of the hypertensives detected in this way had not been followed up. A study in two London teaching hospitals (Heller & Rose 1977) showed that 32% of general outpatients had had no blood pressure check and 38% of the hypertensives who were discovered had not been followed up.

CRITERIA FOR SCREENING

In any community the resources available are not equal to the needs of the patients and priorities have to be decided. In deciding the criteria for screening, the disease must firstly be a common hazard to health, secondly, it should be easy to detect and thirdly, worth treating at an early stage.

Hypertension fits each of these criteria. It is a hazard to health, particularly for those with a diastolic pressure above 110 mmHg. A large proportion of heart attacks and strokes are sustained by people who have blood pressures in the mild hypertensive range and there is evidence that early treatment does confer benefit in terms of preventing complications. Special epidemiological screening units are certainly able to detect large numbers of previously undiagnosed hypertensives and with special effort can reach 80% of the eligible population. This could be regarded as the optimum way but it is extremely expensive and is of no value unless there is systematic follow-up which represents an even greater potential for spending.

In the United Kingdom primary health care is based in general practice with the hospital providing back-up for selected cases. Clinics with a responsibility for screening and follow-up could lead to a third branch of clinical medicine. Screening should be a continuous long-term process since individuals with normal and borderline levels will need to be rescreened at different intervals. Casual screening has been tried in the United States using blood pressure measuring devices in supermarkets and department stores. The evidence has shown that those who use such devices have had their blood pressure measured by a doctor and are merely checking the findings, and that those who have never had their blood pressure checked do not think the machines are for them. There is of course an anxiety factor in borderline cases.

Occupational screening might seem to be worthwhile for new employees and as an annual examination for executives. This approach however has made little impact: employers are not keen, there are problems of confidentiality, those attending clinics may miss promotion as they may be unable to cope with the additional strain and there could be reduced productivity as a result of attending clinics.

It now seems that hypertension should be detected using a case-finding mode within general practice. Most general practitioners work in groups and over 90% of their patients will consult at least once over a 3-year period. If all pateints in the target age group have their blood pressures checked when attending the surgery for any reason screening would be achieved without the need for setting up special units. The general practitioner can do the screening himself or he can arrange for the practice nurse to take blood pressures routinely on all patients who present. It is important there should be standardisation of technique and Korotkoff Stage V — the disappearance of sound — is now taken as the correct diastolic reading. Screening that is carried out in general practice allows adequate follow-up of both identified patients and defaulters.

THE PATIENT FOUND TO HAVE HYPERTENSION

HISTORY

When a patient is found to have hypertension an attempt should be made to find any aetiological factors, assess the probable prognosis and decide on therapy. In taking the history it is important to ask about renal and cardiac symptoms, past renal history, and any family history of cardiovascular disease. Note should also be made of any recent deterioration in eyesight.

EXAMINATION

Physical examination should include the blood pressure recorded with the patient sitting and standing. Unless the blood pressure exceeds 120 mmHg diastolic several baseline readings should be obtained before treatment is started; three readings at weekly intervals is the usual practice but some authorities advocate six since treatment will be lifelong. Physical examination should exclude Cushing's syndrome and a renal bruit should be listened for. Any renal enlargement should be noted and the femoral pulses should be examined for evidence of delay or poor volume. Other points to note include the presence of xanthelasma, the grading of optic fundi, signs of left ventricular hypertrophy and the presence of cardiac failure.

COMPLICATIONS

The complications of hypertension are due to two main effects:

1. Persistently raised intra-arterial pressure giving rise to cardiac and renal failure and to stroke.
2. Exacerbated and accelerated artherosclerosis giving rise to ischaemic heart disease and peripheral vascular disease.

It is also useful to consider complications with reference to the target organs affected:

1. Renal: chronic renal failure.
2. Cardiac: ventricular hypertrophy, left ventricular failure, angina and myocardial infarction.
3. Cerebral: cerebral haemorrhage and thrombosis, transient ischaemic attacks, subarachnoid haemorrhage and hypertensive encephalopathy.

INVESTIGATIONS

Over 90% of patients with raised blood pressure have essential hypertension and only a small proportion have a potentially correctible cause. All patients should have a urine sample examined for sugar, protein and culture, an estimation of blood urea and electrolytes, an ECG, chest X-ray, full blood count and ESR. The young — that is under 40 years of age — require a creatinine clearance and an IVP. Those with a diastolic pressure greater than 130 mmHg may require further investigation and it is probably best for the young patient and those with very high pressures when first found to be referred to hospital for full investigation and treatment.

WHO IS TREATED

It is important at an early stage to decide which patients should have treatment. Treatment should be offered if there is any evidence of target organ damage, for example fundal grade II changes (reduction in the arterial calibre and nipping at the arterial venous crossings), or if there is a strong family history of ischaemic heart disease when complications are three times more likely. All patients under the age of 65 years with a blood pressure in excess of 180/110 mmHg must be treated and it is advisable to treat those pressures exceeding 115/95. Treatment should also be given t
blood pressure exceed

MANAGEMENT

In the treatment of a:

ERRATUM

Page 130, column 2, line 40
115/95 should read 155/95

more than in any other illness it is most important to form a rapport with the patient and the general practitioner is ideally placed to do this. It is essential to explain fully to the patient why he is being treated for an asymptomatic disease with tablets which can have side effects. The overweight patient should bring his weight to within 10% of the calculated ideal weight, cigarette smoking should be stopped and if anxiety is a significant factor, behavioural modification or relaxation can play a part.

Drug therapy should be as simple as possible, with treatment being taken once daily when possible and with the drug that is associated with fewest side effects. Side effects are usually dose related and it is better to use another agent to produce the desired hypotensive effect rather than to reduce the dose of the offending drug and allow the pressure to rise. It is customary to start either with a thiazide diuretic or with a beta-blocker. The beta-blocker is preferred in the younger patient, especially if angina pectoris is present while the thiazide diuretics tend to be the drugs of choice in the elderly, especially if there is evidence of congestive cardiac failure. If the patient fails to respond to either of these drugs a combination of both will control the blood pressure in 75–80% of patients. The addition of a third line drug, for example a vasodilator, an alpha-blocker or a CNS-acting drug, will control a further 15%. The patient should be referred to a specialist hypertensive clinic if there is difficulty controlling the blood pressure using these groups of drugs and if poor compliance is not the reason. A diuretic can take 2 to 3 weeks to act so it should be tried at least for 4 to 6 weeks. A simple thiazide, such as bendrofluazide 5–10 mg, is the treatment of choice. Side effects include potassium loss, which is usually of little clinical significance, urate retention, impotence and impairment of glucose tolerance. Beta-blockers produce a reduction in blood pressure within a few days. A small dose is given to start with gradually increasing the dose every 7 days. Propanolol, a non-selective beta-blocker, is used initially in a dose of 80 mg increasing to a maximum of 320 mg. The dose regimes of cardio-selective beta-blockers are as follows: atenolol: the minimum dose is 50 mg with a maximum of 200 mg; metopropolol: the dosage range is 100–300 mg. The side effects of beta-blockers include lethargy, disturbing dreams, peripheral vascular disease, cold extremities and, especially with the non-selective beta-blockers, cardiac failure and bronchial constriction can be precipitated. In a step care approach a vasodilator is usually the third line drug: hydrallazine commenced in a dose of 25 mg b.d. and gradually increased to a maximum of 200 mg. Side effects include GI tract symptoms, palpitations, headache and an SLE-like syndrome. Another third line drug is prazosin. The first dose can cause severe hypotension so initially 0.5 mg should be given at bedtime then 1 mg b.d. increasing the dose by 1 mg every 2 or 3 days. The daily dose can vary

from 2–30 mg and there are few side effects. This drug should never be stopped suddenly as a rebound hypertensive effect can result.

Methyldopa acts centrally, stimulating receptors in the brain stem and thereby decreasing sympathetic activity. The commencing dose is 250 mg b.d. and this can be increased to 2 g daily. It can cause drowsiness, dry mouth, nasal congestion, general malaise, impotence, diarrhoea and a positive Coomb's test.

The general practitioner in the initial stages should see his patient with hypertension every 2 weeks but after blood pressure control this period can be reduced to 2 months. Compliance is one of the most important factors and a great deal of support should be given to the patient at each visit. The rationale behind treatment must be constantly explained with great care.

ATRIAL FIBRILLATION

Atrial fibrillation can occur in up to 10% of the elderly and ischaemic heart disease is the usual underlying cause although thyrotoxicosis is an important and often missed aetiological factor. In the middle-aged fibrillation can be secondary to rheumatic mitral valve disease or pulmonary embolism. The pulse is totally irregular and digoxin is used to reduce the ventricular rate. An adult should be given 0.25 mg b.d. for a week after which the dose is reduced according to the clinical response. The ventricular rate should not fall below 60 beats/minute. The elderly should be started on a dose of 0.125 mg b.d. and with a maintenance dose of 0.0625 mg b.d. The potassium status of the elderly must be checked before starting therapy: the toxic effects of digoxin are accentuated in the presence of hypokalaemia.

CARDIAC MURMURS

Few new patients are now seen with valvular heart disease but cardiac murmurs are not infrequently heard during routine examination. The correct assessment of murmurs requires constant practice and few general practitioners are in a position to obtain this. The results of modern surgery are encouraging and accurate diagnosis and assessment are now of utmost importance: any patient with a cardiac murmur should be referred for a full cardiological assessment.

RAYNAUD'S SYNDROME

Mild Raynaud's syndrome, when fingers become 'dead' and white in cold weather as a result of arterial spasm, is commonly seen in general practice. The symptoms may only last for minutes or may persist for hours. The spasm is followed by pain and flushing of the affected fingers as the circulation returns. Any primary disease or underlying cause such as a collagen disease should be identified and treated, and protection from the cold is obviously indicated in all patients. Vasodilator drugs may be tried but the results are disappointing. The more severe cases should be referred to hospital where newer drugs or surgical techniques can be tried.

INTERMITTENT CLAUDICATION

Intermittent claudication is common in practice and five new patients are seen with this condition each year. The characteristic history is of cramp like pain which is felt in the calf on exercise and which comes on at progressively shorter distances. After resting the pain disappears. On examination there is often an absence of arterial pulsations in the leg. In studies carried out in general practice improvement seems to occur spontaneously in 40%, in 40% the symptoms remain unchanged and only 20% are benefited by operation. It is important to test the urine as intermittent claudication can be a complication of diabetes mellitus and in the elderly, its presenting symptom.

The patient must be given advice about his condition, informed about the value of exercise and the deterioration caused by infection: prevention of sepsis is of great importance, for example cutting of toe nails. If there is any evidence of a break in the skin the patient must know to seek attention immediately either from the chiropodist or the general practitioner.

PULMONARY EMBOLUS

Pulmonary embolus is seen by the general practitioner on three occasions each year. The predisposing factor is deep vein thrombosis as a result of a period of prolonged bedrest, or phlebitis. It can occur as a complication of myocardial infarction. The condition is more common in women than in men, mainly because of the increased likelihood of varicose veins and the use of the oral contraceptive. It has a sudden onset and usually presents with chest pain: other presenting features are cough, haemoptysis and a fever. Patients should be referred urgently to hospital. Long-term oral anticoagulants may be given to prevent further venous thrombosis in the legs, and this fact should be prominently displayed in the patient's GP record.

VARICOSE VEINS

Varicose veins are a common finding in general practice.

They occur five times more commonly in women than in men. They are the result of prolonged standing and commonly appear after pregnancy. The distended superficial veins are obvious, the aching pain is worse after standing, especially when the varicosities are small, and there is often discolouration or irritation of the skin which can precede ulceration. Varicose eczema, ulceration, thrombophlebitis and deep venous thrombosis are all complications of simple varicose veins but the treatment will often be determined by the cosmetic effect which will influence the patient's choice of the long-term management of her condition.

PREVENTION OF HEART DISEASE

There is now an increasing awareness of the role of prevention in the management of cardiac disease.

CIGARETTE SMOKING

Cigarette smoking promotes atheromatous and thrombotic changes in arteries and probably facilitates arrhythmias. Male doctors who stopped smoking between the age of 34 and 55 reduced their mortality from coronary disease by half within 5 years compared to doctors who continued to smoke. The effect of stopping smoking on coronary mortality is relatively quick: about half the eventual benefit is reached within 1 year of stopping. The degree of risk relates closely to the number of cigarettes smoked. Smoking appears to have an important synergistic effect with the oral contraceptive pill increasing the risk of both coronary disease (20-fold at 35 cigarettes a day) and subarachnoid haemorrhage. Smoking also accelerates occlusive peripheral arterial disease, particularly in diabetics.

There is good controlled evidence that straightforward personal advice against smoking given by general practitioners is effective in stopping smoking for a year or more in about 5% of cigarette smoking patients aged 16 or more consulting for any reason (Russell et al 1979). The potential yield from this procedure were it applied by all general practitioners would be more than half a million ex-smokers each year.

HYPERTENSION

High arterial pressure is an important risk factor for stroke, heart failure, coronary disease and peripheral arterial disease. Stroke, left ventricular failure, ruptured aorta, renal and retinal damage can be almost eliminated by bringing the diastolic pressure down to below 90 mmHg. Case finding for hypertension has been carried out successfully in general practice and this seems to be the way ahead. It is equally important that control of known patients with hypertension (a diastolic blood pressure above 100 mmHg) is ensured by planned follow-up and active recall.

LIPIDS

The abnormalities of lipid metabolism are associated with increased risks of arterial disease but there is no conclusive evidence that changes in diet can alter these risks. All authorities are agreed that the first aim of treatment of any hyperlipidaemia is the attainment of an ideal weight.

OBESITY

Obesity is a visible and intelligible target. Reduction in weight in association with regular exercise has some protective effect against arterial disease. It may be of greater value as part of an all round programme for improvement of fitness and enjoyment of life: on its own it may be of little importance.

DIABETES MELLITUS

There is a marked association between diabetes mellitus and the premature development of arterial disease. Known diabetic patients should be adequately controlled and those at high risk of diabetes mellitus, for example a family history, should be periodically screened for the disease. In the United States active steps have been taken in the prevention of heart disease and while over the last few years there has been a reduction in the number of such patients there is no definitive evidence as to any particular factor being responsible. One recent report has advocated the use of beta-blockers in the prevention of further coronary incidents in patients who have had a myocardial infarction and the preliminary results are encouraging.

REFERENCES

Colling A, Dellipiani A W, Donaldson R J, McCormack P 1976 Teeside Coronary Survey. British Medical Journal 2:1169

Dunnell K, Cartwright A 1972 Medicine takers, prescribers and hoarders. Routledge and Kegan Paul, London

Fry J 1974 Common diseases. MTP Medical Publications, Lancaster

Fulton M et al 1972 Natural history of unstable angina. Lancet 1:860

Fulton M et al 1979 The management of hypertension — a survey of opinions among general practitiones. Journal of the Royal College of General Practitioners 29:583

Hawthorn V M, Greaves D A, Beevers D G 1974 Renfrew Hypertension Study. British Medical Journal 3:600

Heller R F, Rose G A 1977a Current management of hypertension in general practice. British Medical Journal 1:1442

Heller R F, Rose G A 1977b Current management of hypertension in hospital. British Medical Journal 1:1442

Hull F M 1969 Social class consultation patterns in rural general practice. Journal of the Royal College of General Practitioners 18:65

Hypertension Detection and Follow-up Co-operative Group 1979 Journal of the American Medical Association 242:2562

Morrell D C, Gaga H C, Robinson N A 1971 Symptoms in general practice. Journal of the Royal College of General Practitioners 21:32

Pantridge J F, Geddes J S 1967 A mobile intensive care unit in the management of myocardial infarction. Lancet 2: 271

Russell M A H et al 1979 Effect of general practitioner's advice against smoking. British Medical Journal 2:231

Respiratory illness

INTRODUCTION

Respiratory illness is one of the most important and challenging areas of general practice. It is important because it causes one-third of new consultations and nearly a quarter of all consultants. It is challenging because it is the area of clinical work where referral to hospital is least common and in which hospital experience therefore is least related to the presentation of disease in the community setting.

Throughout this chapter two themes will recur and intermingle. The first is the need for the doctor to discuss the clinical medicine of the field in terms of signs and symptoms rather than diseases. Aetiology and pathology must always be important background considerations, but these are normally predicted on a probability basis rather than proposed or confirmed on the basis of the conventional hospital investigative approach. The second theme relates to behaviour — behaviour of patients and of doctors — and its implications for the way illness is organised, presented and managed in general practice.

During the last two decades the debate over whether general practice was principally a branch of physical or of behavioural medicine has had a salutary, even if at times divisive, effect on the discipline. In some fields physical issues are clearly of paramount importance as are the psychological and social ones in others. Respiratory illness is common, normally short-lived, but is potentially serious, apparently well-defined and researchable. Inevitably, too, it is likely to coincide with domestic stress, whether as cause or effect. Thus it has rightly been the substrate for many of the recent and continuing debates about standards of clinical care and about balancing of art and science in the making of clinical judgements.

The first part of this chapter discusses some general principles; the second section examines the presentation and management of both the more common and less common illnesses of the respiratory tract. Whether the general or the particular should be read first is a matter of choice; what is certain is that neither can be fully understood in isolation from the other.

SECTION I — GENERAL PRACTICE

Incidence and prevalence

Various diary-card studies have shown that the symptoms of acute respiratory infection — nasal catarrh, sore throat and cough — are amongst the most prevalent complaints experienced by the public. Estimates of the proportion of those minor illnesses which come to be presented to doctors vary from one in four to one in 20 (Horder & Horder 1954, Banks et al 1975). The best known lists of frequency of presentation of common illnesses (Fry 1977, British Medical Journal 1974) suggest that one such illness is presented each year for the first 6 years of life and one every 2 years thereafter. This equates with a figure of one illness presented for 10 experienced. Practices which dissuade patients from presenting minor self-limiting illnesses, whether by repute or with notes on self-care of minor illness for issue to patients, will see less and the prescribing habits of doctors will also influence workload as discussed below.

The chronic chest illnesses of asthma and chronic bronchitis have a lower incidence but, because of their essentially drawn-out natural history, a higher prevalence. Perhaps one child in 10 (boys more than girls) have a wheezy variant of the catarrhal-child syndrome and at least a quarter of these go on to have asthma in one form or another in adult life.

Chronic cough is an invariable sequel to regular cigarette smoking at the 20-a-day level and merges inexorably with chronic bronchitis as defined by the MRC. Estimates of prevalence are necessarily approximate but may well exceed 20% of adult males in some areas.

In contrast, lung cancer, although by far the commonest cancer in the United Kingdom, has an incidence of perhaps three patients per doctor per year. With the short life expectancy prevailing, its prevalence is also low. Tuberculosis remains a condition to keep in mind and occurs with a not dissimilar frequency.

Presenting features

Cough is the most common acute symptom presented being the main complaint in half the illnesses seen and a component of three-quarters. Sore throat forms the main symptom in a quarter of illnesses and is a component of half. 'Colds' presented early will be dominated by a sore throat which, by the fourth or fifth day, will be replaced by cough. Nasal catarrh overlaps both symptoms and is less commonly presented as a major feature. Sore ears dominate in 10% of illnesses, mainly in children and often in children whose parents have been sensitised to the problem through past experiences. Purulent sputum often co-exists with a cough — especially in smokers — and is often the main reason for consultation for persisting symptoms at between 7 and 14 days after a cold or flu-like illness.

On the basis of clinical examination, abnormal chest signs are found in around one patient in five (usually rhonchi) and the divide of upper to lower respiratory infection of about four to one is usually accepted as normal. Patients complaining of sore throat often have remarkably little to see in the way of redness and pus on tonsils is more noticeable for its absence than presence. Most sore ears can be seen as related to inflamed eardrums — and the eye of hope or faith probably heightens the correlations found.

Cough is again the most common persisting symptom to present, usually with negative clinical findings, even when the sputum is purulent. Breathlessness — except associated with wheeze in asthma, chronic bronchitis or its variants — is rather uncommon and a cause for anxiety. Croup causes much anxiety although usually relatively easily treated. Haemoptysis, perhaps the classic symptom of serious respiratory illness, is also uncommon and, even when present, has a serious basis in only about one patient in 20. Pain is usually due to tracheitis or simply to the muscular strain of coughing; true pleuritic pain is again unusual.

Reasons for consultation

Although the natural history of the respiratory illnesses of general practice is reasonably easily described and relatively predictable, the proper use of both drug and non-drug treatments requires not only knowledge of but also understanding of the reasons why patients consult. Many of the reasons are clinical and obvious, but some of the most significant and most amenable to change are behavioural.

Children

Consultations about children reflect anxiety of parents. Usually the anxiety is understandable, particularly in those 'catarrhal' children in whom one illness seems to follow another with no apparent break or improvement in sight, and often it is justifiable. Management of the illness on a physical basis provides short-term relief. Long-term relief requires education and information for the parents as well as demonstration of the place of

symptomatic as well as specific treatments. The presence of fever is a major reason for asking help and the presence of cough is another. Fever is usually an early feature of a respiratory illness whereas cough, as well as starting early, tends to persist. Cough disturbs, particulary at night, and disturbs the parents often as much as the patients. Both parents and children may thus need to be seen as patients. A major reason for consultation is the expectation that drugs will be prescribed (antibiotics and cough mixture) and the belief (of doctors as well as parents) that they help. Management which does not take account of these expectations and beliefs represents incomplete medicine.

An unwell child also creates tension in the home and easily precipitates domestic disharmony or brings it to the surface. A relatively minor physical illness may also be the last straw in the often fragile balance between coping and not coping — whether with illness in parents or grandparents or in the multitude of financial, employment and relationship problems that reflect normal family life. The involvement of the doctor may be a request for help with these or, if not a request, an opportunity to practise the wider implications of family medicine. These issues have been discussed elsewhere (Howie & Bigg 1980); they can easily be exaggerated, and equally easily minimised. It is probable that as many as a quarter of children's respiratory illness consultations are precipitated by behavioural problems and that in perhaps half of these, the physical illness requires less attention than the reasons underlying the consultation.

Younger adults

Again excluding those consultations for obvious clinical illness, and those where the physical illness masks emotional difficulty, there are at least three issues of significance which determine consulting behaviour. The first is habit (based on family attitudes to minor illness and to the place of doctors in its management) and lack of consideration of the implications for the health service of consultation for minor, self-limiting, and self-treatable illness. Many young adults present with a few hours of sore throat or malaise, having tried nothing or only a couple of aspirins and expect a cure. Unfortunately many of these patients are given medication rather than health education and the problem is perpetuated. In the same vein, calling colds 'flu' has meant that when influenza does strike many patients over-react, understandably contrasting the level of malaise with what they had come to expect as typical of this condition.

The second important issue is the need for legitimisation of illnesses whether for employment, domestic or other purposes. Society has created this difficulty and doctors should sympathise when, for example patients (often State employees) are caught in the trap of having to produce certificates to confirm claims of ill-health. If the doctor can anticipate such a request he can avoid wasting time, for example, by writing a prescription for an unnecessary and unwanted medication.

The third issue to watch for is the early stage of chronic bronchitis. Young adults who consult regularly (or even sometimes only occasionally) with persisting cough and sputum include an excess of cigarette smokers. Chronic bronchitis has no offficial starting point and this kind of presentation is again an ideal opportunity for practising preventive medicine. Once again, if the picture is recognised quickly, more time can be made available for its effective handling.

Older adults

The issues mentioned above all apply again but in more resistant forms. The new dimension is of course the possible added contribution of cardiac sequelae. The reason for separating older from younger adults in this sub-section is to highlight how age changes the probabilities of behavioural and pathological reasons for consultation away from the first and towards the second.

Aetiology and pathology

It is easy to forget that general practice, like all clinical disciplines, is based on the long-established ground rules of general pathology. Although each symptom has its special conditions which vary with age, sex, environment and the like, most illnesses can be classed as inflammatory, degenerative, vascular, neoplastic and so on. Each pathology has its pattern of natural history and the sciences of diagnosis and therapeutics are based on making the most accurate and rapid assessment of the morbid process affecting the patient. A diagnosis is made by plotting the development of separate items of information (symptoms, signs, investigations in particular) as a graph against time, and matching the patterns against known groupings of information and time scales. Most infections develop relatively rapidly but less fast than many vascular lesions; tumour has a slower development; some conditions are intermittent, while others relate to behavioural or environmental factors. The difficulties of making management decisions in respiratory illnesses encountered in general practice usually arise because the clinical history is either minimal ('4 hours of sore throat') or non-specific ('aches and pains all over'), because examination is so often negative, and because the results of investigations are not available. Thus the need to know about — and to understand — pathology and its probabilities in terms of both incidence andd natural history.

The common pathology is inflammation and infection is the main cause or aetiology. In most parts of the respiratory tract the vast majority of infections are viral. There is a disappointingly low correlation between clusters of signs and symptoms and individual viruses, and even the correlation between exudate on tonsils and B-haemolytic streptocci is only about one in three. Other inflammatory lesions, such as chronic bronchitis, are non-infective and can mostly be attributed to smoke and other inhalants; viral infection can be added and secondary bacterial infection can then supervene. Each variant has its own range of presentations and natural history. The serious pathologies include tumour (uncommon as a proportion of respiratory illness but common as a proportion of tumours) and this may be primary or secondary and so on. Also potentially serious are the obstructive airway diseases which are special to the respiratory system and the less common and thus easily overlooked conditions such as embolism, pneumothorax and inhaled foreign bodies. Again the important knowledge is that implied by awareness of pathology and the important skill is the ability to recognise when the natural history which is seen to be unfolding is not explained by or in keeping with initial clinical assumption. Time becomes the most useful clinical investigation available and listening and observation the key investigative techniques.

Space limits the full detailing of the pathologies and their causes; what is required for all consultations is an awareness of the general principles outlined and how to blend undergraduate knowledge of pathology, postgraduate experience of medicine in hospitals and new experiences of the illnesses of general practice. Ability to cope with the new, the unexpected or the puzzling bears a direct relation to understanding the fundamentals of basic medical training.

Management

It is all too easy to equate management with drug prescribing. Respiratory illness predominates during the winter and peaks of incidence and pressure of work often coincide. Understandable anxiety to consult as quickly and as positively as is compatible withh reasonable care easily leads to the tendency to end a consultation by using a medicine. Such a decision assumes three judgements; firstly, that pathology capable of being usefully alleviated by medication is present and is the main or a significant reason for the consultation; secondly, that where the drug is prescribed to prevent further work due to reconsultation either because of worsening or non-improvement of the illness, the real consequence is a conditioning of both doctor and patient to the ritual of medication when next ill (Howie & Hutchison 1978); and thirdly that the side-effects of medication are indeed not themselves as considerable as the symptom to be treated.

As well as ending a consultation by prescribing or certification (in some ways a procedure governed by similar considerations) an important range of self-help and educational options are available. Some are so obvious that they are overlooked; salicylates help pain, malaise and pyrexia; tepid sponging, especially in the young and elderly, lowers fever; avoidance of smoking helps at any time; steam inhalation is a splendid expectorant and hot drinks wonderfully soothing for coughs and sore throats. Patients with colds spread them at work and should use common sense and stay at home when their contribution to productivity is likely to be lower than their capacity to promote an epidemic. Patients with 'flu should accept they will feel *very* ill for several days and, if really afflicted by an even moderately nasty strain, are more likely to be off work for 2 weeks than for one.

Very occasionally management means referral — one patient in 100 — or investigation or even a fundamental reappraisal of environmental problems at home or at work. Much more often follow-up or reassessment after sufficient time to allow the pathology of an illness to declare itself is the best management, combining as it does rational clinical practice with opportunities for both patient and doctor education.

Self-help

No management suggestions should ever be proposed without asking what the patient has tried for himself. It is unusual to find that any effective action has been taken. Most of the common symptoms can be helped by aspirin, hot drinks, rest and inhalation and by a recognition of doctor and patient of the expected natural history of the illness. A course comprising a total of two aspirins, one steam inhalation (the steam is the effective medicant and not the proprietary drops or crystals so often added to a pint of fluid whose minimal output of vapour lasts only seconds before the temperature falls too low to help) or one day's abstinence from cigarettes, is the norm rather than the exception. Advice on smoking may well be best aimed at the ill patient with at least short-term motivation to stop, and like all health education, it should be administered with conviction. There is evidence to suggest that health education should be supplemented by written material and a variety of hand-outs relating to self-help of minor respiratory symptoms have been described and found to be effective (Anderson et al 1980).

In the same way, many patients may already have been advised by the local pharmacist. Pharmacists play an important part in management of minor illness and normally fulfil their role with wholly professional responsibility and skill. They know the values of the placebo and of the symptomatic remedy and often know their 'patients' as well as the doctor does. It does nothing for relationships between pharmacists and doctors, nor does it recognise the pharmacist's role in the medicine of the community to be dismissive or critical of suggestions he may have made. Pharmacists usually become able to gear their advice to what they know are the beliefs and policies of their local doctors and a new partner or trainee misses out if he fails to establish good working links with his local pharmacist early in his time in a practice.

Antibiotics

Two groups of drugs merit some general comments in their own right. The first is antibiotics. About 35 million prescriptions are written for antibiotics each year by general practitioners (the commonest drugs prescribed outside the 'repeat prescription' system) and 80% of these are given for respiratory illnesses, these mainly being new acute episodes. On the surface the variation rather than the consensus of prescribing policies is most striking with doctors prescribing antibiotics to about half the respiratory illnesses they see. This average balances some doctors who prescribe antibiotics for all or nearly all respiratory illnesses and others who prescribe for a quarter or even fewer. The main reasons for this variation lie in the issues identified in the first paragraph of this chapter. The 'illness' indications for antibiotic use are relatively few and are described in the relevant parts of the next section. The behavioural realities, reflecting habit, belief and expectation of doctors and patients, dominate. It is not necessarily bad medicine to be influenced by these but it is sloppy practice not to recognise them when they are the main influences on clinical decisions (Howie 1976).

There are relatively few occasions when the relatively safe and relatively well-tried antibiotics will not cover a patient's needs. Oral penicillin V is (almost) universally effective against streptococci and pneumococci and ampicillin or amoxycillin is effective against haemophilus. Erythromycin doubles-up for patients allergic to penicillin and oxytetracycline is effective in acute exacerbations of chronic bronchitis. The usual reason for an antibiotic not working is that it is being used to treat a viral illness where it is not indicated. The next most common reason is that it is not being taken properly — compliance remains an important problem, as much the responsibility of poor doctoring as of misguided patients!

Preparations to relieve cough

It is appropriate to end the section on general principles by looking briefly at preparations prescribed to relieve cough. Although given only half as frequently as antibiotics they are prescribed even less consistently by general practitioners. In truth, the case for or against their efficacy remains unproven. It is true that there is little firm evidence of their efficacy in the routine respiratory illness, but equally this could simply mean that appropriate ways of demonstrating real benefit remain elusive. It is well known that public belief in their efficacy is substantial; although few doctors take them themselves many admit to prescribing them for their children. Many of the behavioural issues behind decisions to present an illness or on how to manage it can be parried by using this form of medication. In other words a cough may reflect illness in itself or precipitate or be an excuse for presenting emotional or relationship problems; the prescription of a cough mixture may be a token of support, or an attempt to provide real relief, or a cheaper, safer and more dependable placebo than an antibiotic.

Behavioural issues have been one of the two themes of this section. The other theme was the identification of aetiology and pathology, often initially proposed on the basis of probability and substantiated or restated after a period of observation or a trial of therapy. Three principal pathologies cause cough and most proprietary medications aim at one or more of these. The first is inflammation, the second is allergy and the third is obstruction, whether due to tumour, bronchospasm or foreign body. As a secondary problem, cough interferes with sleep and tires both sufferers and carers. Most remedies include one of three active constituents — antihistamines, which may reduce inflammatory exudate or allergic reactivity or promote sleep; antispasmodics or sympathomimetic drugs which may also reduce inflammatory exudate or promote relaxation; and sedatives such as pholcodine or opiates which reduce the responsiveness of the cough reflex and may be particularly valuable in the cough of neoplastic illness.

Just to avoid creating a feeling of false tidiness to the field of respiratory symptoms, cardiac failure is a particularly important and treatable cause of cough in the elderly — easily overlooked as the primary precipitating event may often be an apparently straightforward respiratory infection. Again, the approach outlined above, geared to recognising and responding to unexpected or unexplained patterns of natural history or presenting symptoms, brings together the mix of knowledge and skills, applicable to so much of general practice illness but so well exemplified in the illness of the respiratory system.

SECTION 2 — THE ILLNESSES

The aim of this section is to describe the presentation and management of the commoner and the more serious of the respiratory syndromes with which the general practitioner has to deal. The text concentrates on those aspects of clinical medicine not usually emphasised in conventional textbooks and should be seen as complementary to rather than a replacement of basic undergraduate or 'hospital' teaching. Classification, as has already been emphasised, is difficult. However, the separation of acute from chronic illness is reasonably easy and some illnesses can be separated for their potential to threaten life. Finally some comments are made on the problems posed by epidemics.

ACUTE ILLNESSES

Sore throat

Although not the commonest presentation of acute re-spiratory illness, 'sore throat' is probably the most controversial because of the debate over the merits and risks of prescribing antibiotics for its treatment. Patients fall into two main groups — young to middle-aged adults who complain of the *symptoms* of sore throats, and children, usually under 6 years of age, who are presented by their mothers as fevered, generally unwell, off their food or suffering from the cold and found to have inflammation of the throat as the major abnormality. In both presentations the symptoms are usually of hours rather than days duration. Particularly in adults, the level of constitutional upset is often low. The clinical separation of 'viral' throats from 'bacterial' throats is not reliable in the individual case, but the group of patients with pus on their tonsils, tonsillar adenopathy and fever (often high if present at all) contains an excess of streptococcal throats when compared with the group of patients without these symptoms but having the more general catarrhal symptoms of the common cold. The young adult patient with cheesy exudate on the tonsils may well have glandular fever (in which case he must *not* receive ampicillin which almost invariably produces a macular rash) and, although venereal disease and diphtheria may be the 'sore throat' worries of tomorrow and yesterday, most general practitioners will have seen neither and can only hope to recognise them accurately if they do present.

The controversy over whether to use antibiotics is one of the most important in general practice medicine because it represents a microcosm of the difficulties which face the general practitioner as a prescriber in so many fields of his work. The debate has clinical and behavioural facets. Even although oral penicillin (the only drug of choice unless patients are allergic to it in which case erythromycin is usually chosen as an alternative) only reduces the duration of an average streptococcal tonsillitis by about 1 day in five, almost all doctors would regard the spotted tonsil as a normal indication for therapy. The risk of quinsy is certainly worth minimising although it appears that *at present* and in at least the United Kingdom, the antibiotic treatment of sore throats makes no contribution to reducing the risk of subsequent development of nephritis (Taylor & Howie 1984) or rheumatic fever. If the aim of treatment is to clear the throat of streptococci as against simply treating the clinical findings, a 10-day course is needed as the majority of throats will be recolonised by streptococci by 1 month following a course of either 5 days or 7 days. However, streptococci cause no more than a third of sore throats and pus on the tonsils is much less common than most doctors think. Much debate on whether to treat the generality of sore throats on a blind basis is doomed to being inconclusive because of the difficulty of comparing groups within and between published trials. It does not seem to matter too much. If the case for treating severely inflamed throats is as marginal as the literature now suggests, the clinical case for treating throats which are only moderately red must be negligible. Difficulty may be caused when illnesses are presented so early in their natural history that projection to the eventual maximum pathology is made difficult. Often it is only the accompanying level of malaise or its absence that will guide the decision. On the other hand, sore throats which have lasted for several days without proceeding to manifestly severe pathology cannot realistically be expected to respond to antibiotics. When penicillin is used, high blood levels are rapidly obtained after oral use; intramuscular penicillin is painful, almost all recorded anaphylactic deaths have followed this mode of administration and its use can only rarely be necessary.

Patients with sore throats usually try aspirin before consulting, but often give up after one or two doses have failed to effect cure. The best basis of treatment is several days of salicylates, hot drinks and an effective attempt to inform the patient of the expected development and duration of his illness.

Cough

At some times of the year, cough may seem to be the only symptom of which patients complain. Out of the multiplicity of syndromes in which it occurs, several recur with some regularity. If generalisations can be made, it would be that when cough is associated with wheeze or difficulty in breathing and situation is potentially serious and should be watched carefully. However, when cough is not accompanied by much in the way of malaise, physical examination will nearly always reveal little or nothing and it will usually prove to be a self-limiting symptom, capable of being adequately managed with advice and health education.

One of the commonest presentations of cough falls between these opposites and is mainly found in young children, often in their early years of school life. The presenting complaint is of several days of cough, mainly at night and following an apparently simple cold. The main features of note are the negative findings on examining the chest and a mother who seems anxious to persuade the doctor that the child, although seemingly well now, was far from well during the night. It is important to take a careful history and worth looking through the past notes. Many of these children end a bout of coughing at night by wheezing and often the notes refer to eczema or other skin problems and show recurrent episodes of respiratory illness, often including croup. Whether these 'catarrhal' children should or should not be regarded as in a group which overlaps asthma is not yet clear, but they often appear to respond well to a few days on salbutamol syrup and the appropriate use of steam inhalations. This course of action may provide sufficient reassurance to both mother and doctor to prevent the recourse to antibiotics

to which such consultations so often eventually lead.

Possibly the next commonest situation is the young to middle-aged adult who complains of persisting productive cough, again after a routine cold, and whose sputum is usually described as yellow or green. The patient is otherwise well and once again physical examination is normally unhelpful. In particular, the chest is clear. A substantial majority of these patients smoke and indeed a patient who smokes 20 or more cigarettes a day can expect a 50% excess of morbidity to follow any respiratory infection. Many patients will already have tried a proprietary cough mixture and it is worth checking on this before recommending one — a course which although never proven to help has never been proven not to help! The main point to make is that although the presence of purulent sputum is usually regarded as an indication for antibiotic use, there is good evidence that antibiotics do not improve the natural history of the syndrome (Howie & Clark 1970, Stott & West 1976).

The third common 'cough' problem is that seen in the baby of under a year old. Most such illnesses are no more than mild colds ('snuffles') and the fact that the baby does not look ill and is probably feeding reasonably (apart from difficulty due to nasal blockage which is easily helped by ephedrine nose drops) is reassuring. Warning signs are an increase in respiratory rate, the use of accessory respiratory muscles, pallor, irritability and complete loss of interest in feeding. Again the chest is often clear but this may be seriously misleading and a doctor faced with a baby showing any of these signs should pay close attention to the avolution of the illness. Hydration is important and the baby should be nursed in a warm and, if possible, humid atmosphere. Penicillin (62.5 mg/5 ml strength) is advisable, whether as a prophylactic or a therapeutic measure, and the mother should pay close attention to the evolution of the illness. matter of priority. It is wise to be willing to see any baby whose mother is unhappy about it. Pneumonia can present remarkably non-specifically and cot-deaths have an unconfirmed association with mild respiratory symptoms. No-one is guilty or blamed for looking and not finding, but not looking — whether or not justifiably — precipitates guilt and blame which last forever. Advice and reassurance should be based on the best available evidence rather than on guesswork.

At the other end of the age scale, cough in the elderly can also be mischievously non-specific. Acute infection of the coryzal and influenzal type merges all too easily with the typical acute bronchitis or pneumonia where the significance of a cough is all too easily under-rated by patient and doctor. Such a patient may be only moderately breathless and slight cyanosis is easily missed in the elderly in a poorly lit bedroom. The physical signs in the chest are however diagnostic and again penicillin is normally the drug of choice. Chest pain is a less prominent feature than often imagined and usually central chest tightness is what is described. When pain is located it will usually be pleuritic and a codeine-containing preparation will help relieve pain and suppress the cough. The co-existence, or even dominance, of congestive cardiac failure may confuse and explain unexpectedly delayed recovery; it is treated as normally.

In the 10–20% of illnesses where cough is associated with chest signs — rhonchi, or fine or course crepitations — the patient is usually clearly unwell. Malaise is normal, fever is often present and the sputum which is eventually produced is purulent. Again a feeling of chest tightness is usually more prominent than actual pain and breathlessness is probably more noticeable as a sign than a symptom. Penicillin and steam inhalation form the best basis for treatment. Many of these patients may have a tendency to either asthma or chronic bronchitis; in which case a broad spectrum penicillin becomes the preferred treatment, and bronchodilator therapy may have to be introduced or increased. Again many patients are smokers, and an event of this kind is an ideal springboard for an attempt to stop this habit.

In short 'cough' is a part of many illnesses, some well described in standard textbooks, others more the domain of the general practitioner. Problems are created when the acute symptom begins to blend with the chronic illness, and serious pathology often presents first as an acute and unremarkable illness which then persists. Doctors must advise patients how the natural history of their illnesses should develop and outline the circumstances under which they should consult again.

And don't forget that inhaled foreign bodies also present as coughs!

Earache

Whether coincidentally or causally, the availability of antibiotics and the decline of acute mastoid infections are realities of modern general practice. However, acute otitis media is still a common illness, most prevalent between the ages of 2 and 7 years. The most common overt presentation is at night when the child wakens in pain and obvious distress. The child has often been noticed to have a cold and may seem hot and to be flushed. The child may hold his sore ear, complain of headache or keep pulling at the offending ear lobe. If a request to visit such a child is made, it is worth advising the mother to sit the child up and give a hot drink; often the worst of the crisis is thus resolved before the doctor arrives. The doctor should practise examining ill children carefully because otherwise drums may be difficult to see in just those children in whom a direct view is most wanted. The diagnosis is usually easily confirmed in the symptomatic child and indeed, even if the drum is not seen because of wax or difficulty in gaining co-operation, it is reasonable to infer the diagnosis from the history. Occa-

sionally a bulging pus-filled drum is seen; in a toxic child this will occasionally justify referral for myringotomy — a preferable procedure to uncontrolled rupturing of the drum.

The basis of management is antibiotic therapy — ampicillin or amoxicillin is recommended for the first 6 years of life, penicillin itself thereafter — together with an attempt to decongest the eustachian tube and allow drainage. Various suggestions for achieving this include antihistamine, ephedrine nasal drops and inhalation of steam. Many acute infections recur, particularly in catarrhal children; for them nightly antihistamine should be tried for a period of 2 months.

Chronic secretory otitis media (glue-ear) follows a proportion of acute infections and should be suspected when hearing loss after an acute episode does not resolve within 2 to 3 months. In severe cases the drum is indrawn, vessels can be seen and a fluid level noticed. Often, however, there is little to see and the presence of fluid is almost impossible to confirm or exclude on clinical grounds. Although the risk of hearing loss is well known, few children are in fact followed up 'properly' after acute ear infection. Whether the fault lies in parents or doctors or both is debatable but the problem is one requiring solution; it provides an admirable opportunity for a trainee who wishes to leave a useful contribution behind after his or her practice year.

The other presentation of acute otitis media is as an incidental finding in a pyrexial, vomiting or non-specifically ill child, usually under 3 years of age. Often the diagnosis is made on the basis of no more than slight bilateral pinkness of the drums and the accuracy of the diagnosis is at best subjective and often clearly questionable, being used as a justification rather than a reason for prescribing antibiotics.

Repeated recurrent episodes raise the question of the need for adenoidectomy — but not tonsillectomy.

Hoarseness

As an acute symptom hoarseness often intervenes between the 'sore throat' and 'cough' stage of an otherwise non-specific respiratory infection. There are two main presentations, one seen in the adult and one in the young child. In the adult the symptom is mainly of loss of voice and the implications are annoying rather than serious. Often the throat is or has recently been sore or there is an annoying dryy cough and perhaps some tightness in the chest. As often as not, the patient consults because the symptom is interfering with ability to work. Resting the voice and inhaling steam is the treatment of choice and its effectiveness generally astonishes patients. Patients in whom the symptom does not resolve within 3 weeks should be investigated, particularly when the symptom does not seem to have been related to a recent infection.

In children the symptom is relatively common and

often a cause for concern. Those children who seem most at risk are those who later go on to develop the asthma/eczema syndrome and even during their first year of life, the association between these different facets of syndrome may be evident. The illness is often associated with an epidemic of respiratory syncytial virus and experience suggests that these epidemics are most commonly found early in the winter. An infant may go to bed with an apparently minor cold only to wake around midnight with the typical stridor of 'croup'. The diagnosis is often possible over the telephone and treatment by steaming can be started while the doctor is travelling to the call. Two different appearances can be found. When the baby looks flushed there is usually not too much to worry about, and once again the response to kettles of steam is as dramatic as it is reassuring. The child is often fevered but usually, although apparently having some difficulty in breathing, its chest is clear. On the other hand the baby with croup who is found to be pale and 'flat' constitutes a worrying emergency. A quiet chest may indicate respiratory difficulty rather than normal function and there is every justification in considering hospital admission. The fact that rapid recovery in a steam tent is the usual outcome should not be seen as a reason for not referring when in doubt. There is debate in paediatric circles over whether it is safe to examine the throats of children with croup in case of the presence of epiglottitis. The sensible compromise seems to be to conduct a careful exploration of the mouth and throat, taking greater than usual care not to struggle to obtain a good view. Although conventional teaching is against the use of antibiotics, they are widely used in hospital and, balancing their relatively high safety margin against the serious consequences of a pneumonia or haemophilus epiglottitis, seem defensible when there is any anxiety. Ampicillin or amoxycillin — using the starter pack to initiate quick treatment — is the option of choice.

Sinus problems
Sinusitis is a diagnosis made frequently by some doctors and rarely by others; involvement of the sinuses is a common accompaniment of upper respiratory tract infection although a firm diagnosis is dependent on eliciting pain on tapping the area over the affected sinus. The diagnosis is one that is frequently adopted by patients to describe the generalised congestion of the common cold but true sinusitis is characterised by acute localised pain which is worse in the morning and occurs as a sequel to an otherwise uncomplicated episode of coryza. Relief is obtained by establishing drainage of the secretions and once again this is best achieved by steam inhalations. The decision to use antibiotics is influenced by the severity of the symptoms, by toxaemia, and the presence or absence of a muco-purulent nasal discharge, but also varies to some extent with the prescribing habits of the

doctor. Penicillin itself is the first line treatment.

Episodic sinus pain may be associated with the congestion of the turbinates that is a feature of allergic rhinitis and a therapeutic trial of local or systemic antihistamines may be of value. Topical disodium cromoglycate (Intal) has so far proved to be less effective in the prevention of this condition than in preventing bronchial asthma. Persistent or recurrent episodes of sinusitis that are not associated with coryza should suggest the possibility of defective drainage of the sinus due to nasal polyps; specialist referral is indicated in these cases.

EPIDEMIC ILLNESS

Most winters bring a spell during which an epidemic — either of the ill-defined viral illnesses which are a common denominator to all the symptoms described in the last section, or of the more specifically epidemic illnesses — disorganises normal working and introduces stresses and strains which hazard normal medical care. Because of the often massive increase in demand and workload, sometimes aggravated by a partner or oneself also succumbing to the prevailing illness, several real risks are introduced. These include the inadequate follow-up of unrelated illnesses and problems, the tendency to generalise about the particular illness which is prevalent and thus to miss recognising serious variants, and the tendency to diagnose and prescribe by telephone. In addition, fatigue easily leads to irritability and the consequent risk of the kind of unhappy disputes with patients, either face-to-face or more often on the telephone, which sour long-term relationships, and more immediately, the work of the next hour or so. Reception staff are also subjected to greatly increased pressures from both patients and doctors and again the working relations within the practice are subjected to important pressures.

The commonest illnesses presenting this way are the respiratory syncytial virus outbreaks in children, which have already been referred to, and influenza in adults. Influenza usually attacks during the second half of the winter and epidemics vary substantially in the morbidity they cause. Generalisation either between or within epidemics is dangerous although inevitably necessary to an extent. Of course the problem is compounded by the fact that an epidemic creates its own momentum and all 'colds' become 'influenza'. The changing of self-certification regulations is likely to help control many of the problems outlined in this section and will allow doctors to concentrate on patients most ill or most at risk. Doctors need to recognise a few truths about influenza: it causes a much more acute short-term illness than most patients and many doctors expect — but its course is usually self-limiting and only requires symptomatic treatment; even young and normally fit patients may become dangerously ill very quickly and great care has to be taken to be sure of making as few mistakes as possible; the elderly are greatly at risk but young children relatively immune; those with serious chronic illness are also at risk and should be treated at the first sign of attack with a broad spectrum antibiotic — these patients should, of course, be offered prophylactic immunisation each autumn despite the restricted effectiveness of this in the face of the mutating nature of the influenza viruses.

In children, measles and whooping cough are illnesses which in theory should belong to the past. Each presents a variation of the same clinical problem — the diagnosis is easy to make during an epidemic when it is high in the differential diagnosis of otherwise non-specific respiratory illness. Not much needs be said here about the clinical patterns of these illnesses. Measles is an acutely discomforting illness characterised by coryzal symptoms and a painful cough, both of which usually precede the often extensive macular rash, photophobia and conjunctivitis of the typical illness. Otitis media and chest infection are common sequelae to be treated on their own merits, but otherwise treatment is symptomatic. Cough may persist for several weeks and parents should be warned of this. Occasionally children develop a variety of croup and less frequently encephalitis; both are serious illnesses and it is the prevention of the second in particular that makes the case for immunisation increasingly difficult to resist.

Whooping cough has been the subject of much recent debate. Like measles, it is an irregularly recurring epidemic disease which when mild is relatively harmless but when present in a more severe variant is always unpleasant and occasionally dangerous. The case for immunisation seems stronger than that against, but when patients or relatives express serious anxieties these should always be respected. It is, of course, always easier to come to terms with individual 'non-conformers' when the vast majority of patients are being protected, as the risks of being unprotected are then greatly reduced. The thoroughly distressing cough of established whooping cough is unfortunately not helped by antibiotics nor by the atropine-containing remedies which are often recommended. It is possible that erythromycin in the early, almost pre-symptomatic, stage may modify or abort the illness and probably reasonable to prescribe it to unprotected infants who are close contacts of a suspected case.

CHRONIC ILLNESS

The two main chronic or recurring illnesses of the respiratory tract are, of course, asthma and chronic bronchitis. The conditions, although similar in producing cough and difficulty with breathing as their main symptoms, have substantial differences in both their natural history and their susceptibility to treatment. The standard teachings on aetiology and pathology are assumed to be known to the reader and this section of the chapter aims to complement rather than repeat basic undergraduate information on clinical presentation, differential diagnosis and management.

Asthma

Much is made of the old adage that 'all that wheezes is not asthma'. Modern thinking might emphasise the possibility that a great deal that does not necessarily wheeze may also be a reflection of allergic airways disease and should be thought about under the same heading. The traditional patient with asthma has a history of recurrent coughing illnesses — often including croup — in early childhood, often a family history of allergy, and often a tendency to have had various eczematous and other allergic illnesses in early life. Often wheeze does not become a part of the picture until 3 or 4 years of age and the ability to separate the allergic from the infective element in the production of acute exacerbations may require a mixture of shrewd observation and suspicion on behalf of parents and doctors. The fact that asthma has been so substantially underdiagnosed in the past reflects unnecessary reticence by doctors to use the term and discuss its implications with patients and parents. Now that such effective medication is available an altogether franker and healthier relationship is becoming the norm — to everyone's benefit.

The most important pitfall to avoid is the failure to think of the diagnosis. Recurrent night cough is a particularly common presentation and the absence of physical signs next morning a notorious trap. Exposure to animals (dogs, cats and horses in particular) is often related, and of course pollen, plants and the house dust mite are frequently mentioned culprits. Much debate has been given to the contribution of psychological problems in the exacerbation of asthma attacks; being asthmatic must itself generate anxiety for patients and relatives and the separation of the emotional from the physical is probably as impossible as it is invidious. Even if it is only because of the ready response of asthmatic symptoms to appropriate medical treatment, it seems reasonable to regard the usual 'extrinsic' asthma of childhood (or starting in childhood) as a physical illness with psychological implications rather than the reverse.

Investigation and referral are not routinely required but often helpful where exacerbations seem likely to be frequent, when response to treatment is disappointing or when episodes are severe enough to require consideration of acute admission. Above all, continuity of care is desirable and so often this is hard to find in group practices and outpatient clinics. The harm done by conflicting opinions and advice is rarely recognised by those responsible. Desenitisation seems generally disappointing as well as potentially dangerous. (Severe seasonal asthma is probably better treated with a depot steroid by injection.) Patients and relatives should be informed of the generally favourable outlook, although made aware that the tendency to be allergic is probably a life-long reality. In particular children embarrassed by the very common exertional dyspnoea should be encouraged to use an inhaler prophylactically (either cromoglycate or salbutamol) and their attention can be drawn to the many stars of the sports field whose problems have been shown to be manageable.

The onset of asthma between adolescence and the middle thirties is uncommon, and the frequent difficulty in identifying allergens and the normally poorer response to drugs which control allergy-induced asthma suggest that a different aetiology — possibly emotional — may contribute to the illness. After the age of 35 the incidence of bronchospasm rises and the distinction between 'pure' asthma and developing chronic bronchitis may be difficult. The prognosis, and risk to the patient, are similar in both categories of illness and so formal distinctions between the two syndromes are less important than the need to plan a programme of management and to check its effectiveness after establishing baselines of pulmonary function. Use of the peak flow meter both in the surgery and at home helps planning and monitoring of treatment. This applies equally to patients with asthma and chronic bronchitis

Although allergic lung disease of occupational origin (such as 'bird fancier's lung' and byssinosis) has a different presentation, these causes should always be borne in mind when bronchospasm is encountered for the first time in middle-aged adult patients.

Since the first edition of this book was written, there has been a constructive move to the more positive use of inhaled bronchodilators and various methods ('spacers', 'rotahalers' and 'nebulisers') introduced to help. Oral salbutamol causes unacceptable tremor and is probably only useful as a night-time medication in small children. The commonest reason for treatment failure is improper use of the inhaler and doctors should check repeatedly that inhalers are being used properly. Patients can be encouraged to monitor their own respiratory function and titrate their treatment accordingly. The conditions under which they should seek advice (usually failure to respond quickly to previously successful regimes) must be made clear. Earlier use of intermittent courses of steroids is another sensible trend in management; prophylaxis with cromoglycate seems successful in many cases but is surprisingly unpopular with many patients (the new inhaler may help this) and many never seem to grasp that its use must be in advance of expected problems rather than as a treatment once wheeze is present.

Given adequate checks that repeat prescriptions are not being over-requested, with careful attention to education of the patient, most asthma sufferers can be helped to see their condition as a 'health problem' rather than as a 'chronic illness'.

Chronic bronchitis

In contrast with asthma, chronic bronchitis is an illness of adult life, largely created by man himself, resistant to anything other than symptomatic treatment and likely to be progressive unless the patient can be effectively motivated to avoid its cause.

The pathology is worth restating as it draws attention to the need for the earliest possible detection of what will otherwise become an inexorably progressive disease process. The basic lesion is destruction of normal ciliated respiratory epithelium by noxious agents (usually industrial fumes or cigarette smoke), and its replacement by mucus-producing epithelium — in which ssecondary bacterial infection readily becomes established — and fibrous tissue. The condition is dangerous because it develops insidiously and because its determinants are often apparently unavoidable (industrial) or part of a truly addictive and superficially pleasurable social habit (smoking). The habit is usually well established in the patient's early adult life and seen by the patient as unbreakable by the time symptoms develop. The doctor's first opportunity to help is when presented with the typical persistant productive cough at the end of an otherwise routine viral respiratory illness. Patients who present with this picture contain a substantial excess of confirmed heavy smokers; to prescribe antibiotics and cough mixtures is not only useless but a distraction from the real issues — that the symptoms are the early ones of what in effect becomes a terminal illness, and that the remedy lies substantially in the patient's own hands. One of the recurrent faults of compiling problem lists is the tendency to devalue the importance of repeated consultations with minor respiratory illness. This is perhaps the prime example of the importance of early diagnosis and positive health education.

Normally the doctor's involvement is during an acute infective episode of the slowly progressing continuous illness. Breathlessness is usual (another concern is the rapidity with which chronic bronchitics come to accept poor lung function as 'normal'), wheeze often prominent and the chest full of added sounds audible without the need to use a stethoscope. Broad spectrum antibiotics are normally given and seem to work reasonably well in the early stages of illness although in the later stages they often appear to give more side-effects than benefits. Steam inhalation is the only really effective mucolytic agent although most patients like to have a proprietary cough mixture prescribed — the basis of any benefit which is obtained has not been established! Although there is often very little measurable response to inhaled bronchodilators, most chronic bronchitics believe they help and should be prescribed for them. Various long-acting aminophyllines can also be tried although there is some anxiety over their safety when combined with ß-stimulant drugs. The aminophylline suppository at night in the patient with more severe disease is often valuable.

Several more contentious issues should be considered. Firstly, it seems reasonable to provide established sufferers with their own supply of antibiotics (a tetracycline is the safest) with instructions to start a course in the early stages of a cold or flu-like illness (chronic bronchitics should be immunised against the anticipated epidemic influenzal strains each year in September or October). Secondly, patients who fail to respond to normal active therapy should be considered for a short course of oral steroid — say 30 mg prednisolone on day one, reducing to 5 mg by day six and continuing at that level up to perhaps day 10. (Persistent failure to respond suggests a need to think of an added dimension — for example cardiac failure or malignancy.) Lastly, comes the issue of the provision of domiciliary oxygen. Apart from the risks of fire involved, home oxygen is both inconvenient and expensive and present thinking is more against than in favour of its use. It would seem reasonable practice to suggest that this measure be used as an extreme resort and normally on the recommendation of a specialist colleague.

The social and psychological implications of severe chronic bronchitis are substantial. Many with labouring jobs have to accept that they cannot continue working and those living up stairs may become prisoners of their illnesses. In times of high unemployment and in parts of the country where suitable housing is at a premium, the doctor can often do very little that is effective. He can, however, always support. The last dilemma is over what to do about the seriously ill late-stage sufferer who is still smoking. Evidence suggests that it is always beneficial to be an ex-smoker — but at what point does the potential benefit outweigh the loss of perhaps the only effective solace for the consequences of a life-time habit?

MAJOR ILLNESSES

The commonest of the major illnesses are the more severe or more acute forms of the infective or obstructive illnesses already described. Acute infections include croup, epiglottitis and viral and bacterial pneumonia; acute asthma and acute exacerbations of chronic bronchitis form the second group but, of course, many of the most dangerous illnesses result from combinations of the two pathologies. The dangerous features include the potential for rapid deterioration from an apparently routine illness to a potentially fatal state, the problem of giving patients and relatives clear enough information on what to report without creating too much alarm in routine cases, and the fact that most serious illnesses are coincident with the heavy workload of epidemics, when tiredness in the doctor or pressure of new calls, can all too easily prevent the doctor spending as much time with the family as he might do normally.

These conditions apart tumour, tuberculosis, pneumothorax, pulmonary embolism and the inhaled foreign body are the unusual but dangerous conditions that the doctor in general practice continually fears but seldom (or rarely) meets. Once again the pathology, presentation and management is described in standard undergraduate texts and the conditions are usually easily recognised as out of the usual and serious; only a few general points are appropriate here.

In cases of both tuberculosis (still more prevalent than often realised) and tumour, the greatest problem is the recognition of when the chronic cough so often present before the onset of these conditions has in fact changed its significance and become part of a new disease process. Repeated X-ray examination often does no more than cause anxiety and waste resources, and its benefits are dubious for most cancer sufferers although of supreme value for those who have contracted tuberculosis. Frequently the earliest opportunity to make a diagnosis is during an apparently routine respiratory infection. Improvement after antibiotic therapy can be misleading and it is either unexpected delay in recovery or the early onset of a new bout of symptoms that gives the first clue. Advice to patients on what to report (for those with acute or chronic illness in particular) should thus include not only delay in recovery but also apparent relapse. Haemoptysis is often the first sign of serious pathology — although probably 95% of haemoptyses have an innocent basis — and great care has to be taken over its assessment and follow-up. Finally care must be taken not to be misled by reported normal X-ray findings. All too many patients who were diagnosedd as having lung cancer have in fact been recently X-rayed without the lesion — although presumably present — being identified.

No chapter no respiratory illness in general practice would be complete without emphasising the ease which the inhaled foreign body can be missed as a cause of persisting unexplained chest illness. The patient is usually a young child who does not or cannot give a proper history; delay is caused by not thinking of the diagnosis and resentment often caused by the doctor apparently failing to respond to the parent's insistence that something unusual is wrong.

OVERVIEW

The general practice medicine of the respiratory tract provides an excellent model for thinking about general practice medicine in its totality. The differentiation of the physical and behavioural elements of illness requires both knowledge (of probabilities) and skills (of winning patient trust at consultations) which at the same time are distinct from and complementary to those of specialist practice. Investigation plays a relatively small part in routine practice (only occasional throat swabs; almost no sputum cultures; some chest X-rays; and occasional paired sera to search for confirmation of illness such as mycoplasm, psittacosis and so on) and referral to hospital either in an emergency or on an out-patient basis is unusual enough (less than once in 100 new consultations) to emphasise the very different experience which generalists and specialists gain and use.

At the same time the basic teaching of undergraduate pathology and clinical method remains the foundation on which to build. Management can only be chosen and evaluated against an understanding of the natural history of symptoms and syndromes and the significance of patient expectation and doctors' concessions to it is substantially greater outside rather than inside hospital.

Because of these realities and because the illnesses of the respiratory tract seem so often to divide between the categories of being self-limiting or patient-induced, the skills of health education and the promotion of preventive medicine are particularly relevant.

This chapter has aimed to reflect the ideas, values and attitudes which these concepts imply. That this has sometimes been at the expense of clinical or therapeutical detail reflects partly that such detail is readily available elsewhere, but partly that 'correct' decisions on management still often (perhaps too often) remain negotiable between the patient and his doctor.

REFERENCES

Anderson J E, Morrell D C, Avery A J, Watkins C J 1980 Evaluation of a patient education manual. British Medical Journal 281:924–926

Banks M H, Beresford S A A, Morrell D C, Waller J J, Watkins C J 1975 Factors influencing demand for primary medical care in women aged 20–44 years; a preliminary report. International Journal of Epidemiology 4:189–195

British Medical Journal 1974. Antibiotics and respiratory illness: Editorial. British Medical Journal 3:1

Fry J 1977 The content of practice. In: Fry J (ed) Trends in general practice, Royal College of General Practitioners

Horder J, Horder E 1954 Illness in general practice. Practitioner 173:177–187

Howie J G R 1976 Clinical judgement and antibiotic use in general practice. British Medical Journal ii: 1061–1064

Howie J G R, Bigg A R 1980 Family trends in psychotropic and antibiotic prescribing in general practice. British Medical Journal 280:836–836

Howie J G R, Clark G A 1970 Double-blind trial of demethylchlortetracycline in minor respiratory illness in general practice. Lancet ii:1099–1102

Howie J G R, Hutchison K R 1978 Antibiotics and respiratory illness in general practice: prescribing policy and workload. British Medical Journal 2:1342

Stott N C H, West R R 1976 Randomised controlled trial of antibiotics in patients with cough and purulent sputum. British Medical Journal 2:556–559

Haematology

INTRODUCTION

Haematology is particularly satisfying in general practice; unlike some other specialties, it gives the family doctor unique opportunities for diagnosis, treatment and follow-up. Given enthusiasm and close co-operation with the local laboratory, most problems can be solved without referral to the haematologist but connection is vital. Obviously, physical examination is as important in blood disease as in disorders of other systems, but it can often be misleading. The colour of the conjunctiva, the lips, the palms, or the appearance of the tongue are seldom good guides to the degree of anaemia, and never to their cause. Spoon shaped nail deformities, when present, are indicators of iron deficiency — but their absence guarantees nothing. The only way to reach an accurate diagnosis, upon which rational treatment of any blood disorder can be based, is to use the laboratory. Prescribing iron empirically as a 'tonic', without a routine screen, is inexcusable in modern practice.

The information available from simple routine blood testing is extensive and Table 12.1 gives some idea of the diagnostic range. Most laboratories can report routine haematology tests in a day or two: this is almost always adequate for the general practitioner's needs. Doing one's own haemoglobins and films is not only time-consuming — it will be less efficient unless one has considerable experience in clinical haematology. The ESR is the exception to this rule; the Westergren tube method is inexpensive and practical and can provide a quick guide to the diagnosis or progress of an illness. It is particularly helpful in distinguishing between organic and psychological illness when a raised ESR will indicate the need to identify an underlying organic cause.

THE ANAEMIAS

Tiredness, weakness and dyspnoea are the clinical complaints of the anaemic patient — as they are of those who

Table 12.1 Requirements for routine haematological investigations (with acknowledgement to R.D. Eastham)

Sequestrene blood (4 ml)

White blood count	$7.5\pm3.5 \times 10^9/1$	
Mean cell volume	85 ± 8 fl	
Mean corpuscular haemoglobin	29.5 ± 2.5 pg	
Platelets	150–$450 \times 10^9/1$	
	Men	*Women*
Red cell count	$5.5\pm1.0 \times 10^{12}/1$	$4.8\pm1.0 \times 10^{12}/1$
Haemoglobin	15.5 ± 1.5 g/dl	14.0 ± 2.5 g/dl
Haematocrit	0.47 ± 0.07	0.42 ± 0.05
Reticulocytes	2%	

Erythrocyte sedimentation rate (Westergren 0.9 mm/hour)
Plasma viscosity 1.5–1.72 centipoises
Paul-Bunnell test (infectious mononucleosis)
Rose-Waaler screen test (rheumatoid arthritis)
C-reactive protein screen (non-specific acute inflammation)
Plasma fibrinogen
Haemoglobin electrophoresis
Sickle cell screen
Direct Coombs' test
Red cell folate
Malarial parasites
Sugar water test for PNH screen (paroxysmal nocturnal haemoglobinuria)
Glucose-6-phosphate dehydrogenase

Clotted blood (4 ml)
Serum vitamin B_{12}
Serum iron
Serum TIBC (total iron binding capacity)
Serum ferritin
Serum folate
Cold agglutinins
Autoantibody screen, including:
   antinuclear antibodies
   parietal cell antibody
   intrinsic factor antibody
   plain muscle antibody
   mitochondrial antibody
   thyroid antibodies (various)
Antenatal serology

Citrated blood (2 ml)
Plasma clotting factor screen
(ESR — Westergren)
British Comparative Ratio (prothrombin ratio)

are depressed or anxious although severe anaemia is rarely missed and the clinical picture is obvious. Minor degrees of anaemia are very much more common and are often overlooked in patients whose main complaint is loss of wellbeing. It is too easy to persuade oneself of a psychological basis for a patient's complaints when a blood test would reveal a haemoglobin in the region of 10 or 11 g%.

Iron deficiency is by far the commonest anaemia in Britain (Samson 1982) followed by vitamin B_{12} and folate deficiency and then by the anaemias associated with chronic diseases. Immigrant communities may have special problems; thalassaemia may occur in Asians and Greeks, and combined B_{12} and iron deficiency anaemias may be found in vegetarian Indian patients. Clinical indications of iron deficiency include angular stomatitis, koilonychia and, occasionally, dysphagia. A smooth tongue and neuropsychiatric changes are a feature of the illness in two-thirds of patients with megaloblastic anaemias (Shorovon et al 1980); 40% of patients with vitamin B_{12} deficiency have peripheral neuropathy. Folate deficiency is more often associated with an affective disorder. One patient in four with B_{12} or folate deficiency has organic mental changes — often dementia, which is reversible with the correct treatment. Vitiligo and premature greying may suggest pernicious anaemia (Samson 1982).

Clinical suspicion of anaemia must always be confirmed by a blood count, remembering that normal haemoglobin levels vary with both age and sex by as much as 4 g/dl so that 'anaemia' may be over-diagnosed in children and in women if they are expected to have the haemoglobin of men (Table 12.2). Haemoglobin levels do not fall with increasing age and are the same in healthy old people as in young adults.

Once a low haemoglobin level confirms a diagnosis of anaemia, the next most important index is the mean corpuscular volume (MCV). A low MCV suggests iron deficiency, a thalassaemia trait or an anaemia of chronic disease. A high MCV indicates deficiency of B_{12} or folate, or one of the macrocytoses with a normoblastic marrow. The last combination is found in liver disease or in hypothyroidism. The commonest cause of unexplained macrocytosis is excessive alcohol consumption and MCV

Table 12.2 Normal haemoglobin levels (with acknowledgement to D.M. Samson)

Age	Haemoglobin g/dl
Birth	14.5–19.5
8/9 Weeks	9.5–12.5
1 Year–Puberty	10.5–13.0
Puberty	11.5–15.0
Adult female	11.5–16.5
Adult male	13.5–18.0

estimations are thus a useful measure of continuing alcohol intake (Wu et al 1974). Drug-induced macrocytic, normoblastic anaemias include those due to phenytoin, phenobarbitone, mysoline and oral contraceptives. Anaemia with a normal MCV suggests acute blood loss but these diagnostic indicators are not definitive. When B_{12} or folate lack is combined with iron deficiency or a thalassaemia trait, the MCV may well be normal. Anaemia with a normal MCV may also be the first sign of a haemolytic anaemia, of myeloproliferative disorders or of neoplastic marrow infiltration.

IRON DEFICIENCY ANAEMIAS

Once it is suspected from the blood count, the diagnosis of iron-deficient anaemia should be established by measuring the serum iron and total iron binding capacity (TIBC). In adults, the cause is almost always chronic blood loss, usually from menorrhagia or gastro-intestinal lesions. Regular consumption of irritant proprietary drugs is the commonest reason for the latter. Dietary iron deficiency is hardly ever the sole reason for anaemia, but it may occur at periods of high risk, such as the first year of life, during the pubertal spurt in growth, during pregnancy, and in old age.

In children
Anaemia is often suggested by mothers as an explanation for poor appetite, tiredness and irritability in 'faddy' children under 5 years old. It is rarely the true cause. If they are found to be anaemic, then an underlying reason should be sought: renal disease, malabsorption, and diabetes, although unlikely, are among the differential diagnoses. Palpation for enlarged lymph glands and spleen — for the very rare possibility of a leukaemia — should, of course, be routine.

True iron deficiency in preschool children usually suggests a grossly mismanaged diet and this possibility must be closely explored. Mothers who allow copious 'junk foods' and sweets destroy the child's appetite for normal food. Some immigrant families restrict children to milk for the first 2 years of life — a diet grossly lacking in iron. On the whole, however, fatigue in an otherwise normal child is simply due to lack of sleep. Advice about the correct time to put him to bed is far more helpful than iron or vitamin supplements. Once at school, children are even less likely to be anaemic; it is virtually confined to the 'latch-key' child whose rushed, inadequate breakfast is followed by a lunch of crisps and sweets, and whose mothers are ignorant of the value of iron-containing foods.

In women
Three-quarters of the cases of anaemia in practice are in

women of child-bearing age. In 80% it is linked with heavy periods. Pregnancy further drains the body's iron reserves and can intensify folate deficiency. With the regular attendance of women at ante-natal, family planning and cytology clinics, and at blood donor sessions, most anaemias are picked up on routine testing, and can be corrected quickly. The Blood Transfusion Service notifies family doctors when would-be donor haemoglobins are below 12.5 g/dl. Most find refusal of their blood for transfusion something of a shock, but as their level is usually above 12, they can be reassured and, if necessary, checked again in the following month.

All initial examinations in any pregnancy should include a haemoglobin estimation. Experts argue about the value of prophylactic iron and folic acid throughout pregnancy, but, on balance it seems to be a sensible and inexpensive prophylaxis. If, initially, the haemoglobin is normal, then further tests need only be done at 28 and 36 weeks. A first haemoglobin around 10 g/dl or below makes further investigation essential. Rarely, such a low haemoglobin is the result of a folate deficiency which is intensified by the growing demands of the fetus. The objective is for the woman to reach full term with a normal blood count but it is also important to repeat the count at the post-natal visit.

In men

Significant anaemia in men demands a full investigation. Blood loss from haemorrhoids, peptic ulcer, gastro-intestinal drug reactions and colonic lesions are the most common reasons. The medical history may provide the clue when it is important to enquire about old tuberculosis or renal disease. Urinary examination for blood, regardless of a negative history, is necessary and rare causes, such as lymphomas and leukaemias, should be borne in mind.

In the elderly

Iron deficiency anaemia is commonplace in the elderly and particularly so in those living alone. Poverty and neglect together with deteriorating physical and mentaal health can combine to produce an inadequate diet so that a view of the kitchen is as important to the diagnosis as a physical examination, or the patient's response to questions about eating habits. The Health Visitor or District Nurse can be invaluable in assessing and managing the problems of these patients of which the anaemia is usually only one.

MANAGING ANAEMIA

The management of anaemia has three objectives: treatment of its cause, reversal of the anaemia, and replacement of the iron stores. Oral iron almost invariably achieves the last two. Parenteral iron does not raise the haemoglobin faster than oral iron and should be reserved only for those genuinely unable to tolerate iron tablets. Slow release preparations release the iron beyond the duodenum — the site of maximum absorption — and so they may not be as efficient as the simpler ferrous sulphate, fumarate or gluconate.

This last factor must be weighed against the advantages for patient compliance of tablets taken only once each day. Patients are much more likely to continue with a single tablet than with thrice-daily doses over months, and toddlers who may take the brightly-coloured sugar-coated tablets of simple iron preparations for sweets, rarely make the same mistake with the slow-release preparations. Successful therapy is marked by a rise in haemoglobin of about 1 gram per week. Treatment should be continued for 3 months after the blood picture has returned to normal in order to replace iron stores.

Managing pernicious anaemia may be left largely to the District Nurse after the initial, usually dramatic, response to cyanocobalamin. The nurse's monthly injection should be supported by a 6-monthly check by the doctor. This implies the need for a system for long-term follow-up and for 'chasing' defaulters.

RARER HAEMATOLOGICAL PROBLEMS

Few practices are without one or two cases of rare haematological disease. Among them are bleeding disorders, haemoglobinopathies and the leukaemias and lymphomas. Although they may arise only rarely in a medical lifetime, they should not be forgotten in the differential diagnoses of any anaemia.

BLEEDING DISORDERS

Excessive bleeding after injury may be more common than is generally recognised. A group of 'mild bleeding disorders' which are less severe than classical haemophilia, Christmas disease or von Willebrand's disease was recognised in 1980 and may affect 1 patient in 2000 (Beck 1980). The clue to their diagnosis is unexplained bruising or untoward bleeding after trauma, surgery or childbirth. Hepatic, renal or drug-induced diseases exacerbate such tendencies. There are no simple diagnostic laboratory tests, but patients who protest that they bleed more than others should be taken seriously and especially when surgery (such as tonsillectomy) is being considered. Points to look for are bruises which are palpable, or larger than a 50-pence coin, which occur in the absence of sufficient injury or which are distributed evenly over the body surface, rather than in localised areas. Recurrent persistent nose bleeds which last for more than an hour should also raise suspicions. In women, menorrhagia may be the only sign.

Suspicion of even a minor bleeding disorder should mean referral to the haematologist, who will then decide on further referral, where necessary, to a specialised haemophilia centre. Such referral is essential for all the more serious bleeding disorders, such as haemophilia, Christmas disease and von Willebrand's disease. British patients are fortunate that self-treatment with Factor XIII and Factor IX at home has been pioneered in this country.

THALASSAEMIA TRAIT

Thalassaemia trait produces a blood picture very similar to that of iron deficiency anaemia. In Greek and Indian patients, the common form is ß-thalassaemia, in which the haemoglobin is only moderately reduced — never below 10 g/dl. The MCV is much lower than the haemoglobin would suggest however and is typically between 60 and 70. The red cell count is normal or even high. Serum iron and TIBC are both normal, and the diagnosis is confirmed by finding abnormally high HbA2 with or without HbF levels. Recognising a ß-thalassaemia trait is important for two reasons. Firstly, the patient avoids being treated unnecessarily and uselessly with iron. Secondly, the diagnosis should lead to genetic counselling and testing of the marriage partner. Ante-natal diagnosis of the fetal state can be offered at 18 to 20 weeks gestation. The ∝-thalassaemia trait is commoner in other Asians and in Chinese and is less severe. The only feature is often microcytosis with a normal haemoglobin (Walford 1977). Even homozygous ∝-thalassaemia is mild in its effects although relatively more severe in Chinese patients.

POLYCYTHAEMIA

The plethoric middle aged man whose complaints of headaches, dizziness, tinnitus, visual problems, itch and gout are seemingly explained by an initial finding of hypertension may need a little more attention — and a full blood count. Primary polycythaemia is easily missed but there are clues to the true cause of this host of symptoms. Among them are dusky mucous membranes, injected conjunctiva, hepatomegaly and splenomegaly. The last is important because it differentiates primary polycythaemia rubra vera from the polycythaemia that is secondary to lung disease. The haemoglobin is between 18 and 24 g/dl and the red cell count well above $8 \times 10^9/l$ (Goldstone 1982). The white cell count is raised above 15 $\times 10^6/l$, and may sometimes be at levels that are suspicious of leukaemia. The ESR is very low, often below 1

mm/hour; serum uric acid is usually raised and the symptoms may be those of gout.

Stress polycythaemia, on the other hand, is the result of a raised haemoglobin and packed cell volume, but with a normal red cell mass and low plasma volume It is common in heavy smokers and drinkers, in hypertension and anxiety states, and in patients taking long-term diuretics. It is not a benign condition and carries the same risk of morbidity and mortality from thrombosis as does polycythaemia rubra vera.

The therapeutic objective in polycythaemia rubra vera is to lower both haemoglobin and haematocrit. Simple repeated venesection remains the treatment of choice. Phosphorus-32 therapy is useful in the elderly; it is probably not as leukaemogenic as once thought. Proper control of polycythaemia is vital because it extends the median survival from the time of diagnosis from 2 years to 14 years (Goldstone 1982). Thrombosis and haemorrhage are the usual causes of death, especially when the haemoglobin is high before elective surgery. One in four patients with primary polycythaemia eventually dies of acute myeloid leukaemia or myelofibrosis.

WHITE CELL DISORDERS

Primary disorders of the white blood cells are relatively uncommon in practice. Low white cell counts are rare, except as a consequence of other diseases or cytotoxic drug therapy. In fact in general practice, drugs are the commonest cause of neutropenia (Summerfield 1982). Apart from the cytotoxic drugs those most often implicated include phenylbutazone, chloramphenicol, gold salts, meprobamate and tolbutamide. The continuing popularity of phenylbutazone despite its known toxicity is difficult to understand because there are many alternatives. Family doctors are unlikely to see a case of primary lymphocytopenia in a lifetime of practice; the hereditary immunodeficiency syndromes which have been described are all very rare.

Lymphocyte numbers do fall to very low levels, however, in myasthenia gravis, sarcoidosis, Hodgkin's disease, herpes zoster, collagen diseases and in drug reactions, all of which are disorders of immunity. The effect is to make the patient susceptible to severe secondary infection. This danger is likely to be of increasing significance to the general practitioner as more and more patients are sent home from hospital on effective immunosuppression. The resulting combination of neutropenia and lymphocytopenia lays the patient open both to overwhelming infection and to second malignancies. The new malignancy rates in transplant recipients is higher than normal, yet their graft survival depends on the immune suppression which has presumably left them open to the risk of neoplasms. Very great care has to be taken of the patient on long-term cytotoxic and steroid immunosuppression. Weekly visits from the nurse and appointments with the doctor at intervals of no more than 1 month at the best of times are essential. The patient, the family and the nurse should be aware of the early signs of infection, and they should be acted on promptly and appropriately. Close co-operation with the local laboratory for culture of swabs and other specimens is vital.

LEUKAEMIAS AND LYMPHOMAS

The dawning realisation that a young patient may have acute leukaemia or Hodgkin's disease is very hard to face. Fortunately, the average doctor has to do so only once in about 5 years for each of these devastating diseases. The fear of leukaemia is uppermost in the minds of many parents of sick children, and almost always it is easy to dispel such fears very quickly and completely. Yet doctors must remain alert to the possibility whenever it remotely arises. A blood test which establishes an early diagnosis can make all the difference to eventual survival.

The management of all leukaemias and lymphomas is rightly in the hands of specialist units, but the family doctor's duty is not finished once early referral has been made. The family depends on their 'own' doctor for information, guidance and support so that he must therefore keep abreast of all that is happening and be able to answer the many questions of the understandably anxious and unhappy parents or spouses. Explanation must be based on the doctor's judgement of their understanding, but the use of euphemisms and the display of spurious optimism is wrong. People are well aware of the reputation of leukaemia and Hodgkin's disease and it is best to be honest in discussing the diagnosis.

Now, such discussion can be tempered with some hope. The parents of children with acute leukaemias can be encouraged that complete remissions can be achieved in 80%, and that 5-year survival rates in good health are very high, and still rising (Summerfield 1982). In the months after their child leaves hospital in remission, the parents will call on the doctor for every minor health upset. The doctor must be happy to visit, to check for recurrence, and to reassure the parents where he can. Similar support must be given to the patient with lymphoma. The 5-year survival is around 50% so that the patient, usually a young adult, may be given a cautiously optimistic prognosis (Summerfield 1982). As the disease progresses, however, the family must have considerable support from doctor and nurse. The ability of the spouse to cope with the final illness and the adjustment afterwards must be finely judged. It is at such times that the doctor can fulfil most completely his roles of physician and friend to the whole family.

REFERENCES

Beck E A 1980 Mild bleeding disorders. Seminars in Haematology 17:292
Goldstone A H 1982 Polycythaemia. Practitioner 226: 72–76
Samson D M 1982 Impaired erythropoiesis. Practitioner 226: 45–57
Shorvon S D, Carney M W P, Chanarin I, Reynolds E H 1980 The neuropsychiatry of megaloblastic anaemia. British Medical Journal 281:1036–1038
Summerfield G P 1982 Disorders of leucocytes. Ibid. 59–69
Walford D M 1977 Annotation: thalassaemia in the UK. British Journal of Haematology 35:347–350
Wu A, Chanarin I, Levi A J L 1974 Macrocytosis of chronic alcoholism. Lancet i: 829–831

RECOMMENDED READING

Bloom A L, Thomas D P 1981 Haemostasis and thrombosis. Churchill Livingstone, Edinburgh
Hardisty R M, Weatherall D J 1974 Blood and its disorders. Blackwell Scientific, Oxford
Symposium on Haematology. Published in the Practitioner, January 1982

Gastro-intestinal problems in general practice

Diseases of the digestive tract are normally described in terms of their anatomical site. In general practice, however, patients of different ages present with symptoms which are causing them concern when the age of the patient is often an important pointer to the diagnostic probabilities which need to be explored. The five symptoms which cover most of the conditions encountered in practice are pain, nausea and vomiting, diarrhoea, constipation and jaundice. In this chapter the common causes of these symptoms will be discussed in four age groups: children up to the age of 4 years, older children (5-15 years), adults, and patients over the age of 65. Although this can be a useful method of classification it is artificial in that diseases are not generally age specific. The diagnostic process in general practice is based on probabilities and in deciding on them the age of the patient is an important factor.

YOUNG CHILDREN

PAIN

Colic
Most mothers of babies aged from 0–6 months will report one or more episodes of colic. It is important to find out precisely what the mother means by this term. The most common description is of an attack that occurs in the evening following a feed when the baby appears to be fretful, draws up his knees and cries or screams. The attack which can last from a few minutes to several hours may be punctuated by brief periods of sleep and is usually accompanied by audible abdominal borborygmi and the passage of wind. Some babies are more liable to these attacks than others.

Theories about the cause of colic include air swallowing, gulping the feed, bottle-fed babies with too small or too large a hole in the teat, and more recently breast-feeding mothers who drink too much cow's milk. None of these theories are firmly established. Frequent attacks can cause a great deal of distress and anxiety to the mother which in turn is communicated to the baby thus worsening the situation. In such instances the mother

may require considerable support from the health visitor and the general practitioner. Any likely cause should be identified and remedied, the benign outlook should be stressed — attacks will almost certainly cease once mixed feeding has been established — and dicyclomine hydrochloride 5 mg 15 minutes before a feed will help to alleviate the attack.

Intestinal obstruction

Intussusception
The characteristic age for intussusception to occur is between 5 and 9 months. A previously well child suddenly develops an attack of severe abdominal pain associated with screaming, drawing up the legs, and pallor. There is usually associated vomiting and on examination a palpable mass may be felt somewhere along the line of the colon. On rectal examination — performed carefully with the fifth finger — the rectum is usually found to be empty apart from some blood-stained mucus. Urgent referral to hospital is indicated.

Strangulated inguinal hernia
This should be obvious on examination. The danger of strangulation of an inguinal hernia is greater in infants under 2 years of age than at any other time. Any infant with an inguinal hernia however benign it appears should be referred for early herniorraphy.

NAUSEA AND VOMITING

Simple regurgitation
Simple regurgitation is very common and must be carefully distinguished from true vomiting which can have a much more serious consequence in the young child. It is more likely to occur with overfeeding with milk or fluid foods but beyond that the only explanation seems to be that 'some babies do and others don't. Mothers of those who do should probably be advised to reconcile themselves to milk stained clothing at least until their baby reaches his or her first birthday. Since the likely cause is overfeeding the mother should be

advised to give smaller quantities of milk at more frequent intervals.

Hiatus hernia

Deciding when simple regurgitation is due to a possible hiatus hernia can be difficult. In the latter condition the quantities vomited are likely to be larger, and the vomiting more likely to occur when the baby is lying down rather than when he is being winded. The vomit may also contain streaks of blood as a result of a secondary oesophagitis. Chronic bleeding may in its turn give rise to iron deficiency anaemia and there may be a more general failure to thrive. Confirmation of the diagnosis by barium swallow is seldom necessary and only if the quantities vomited lead to failure to thrive or to dehydration. Treatment consists of nursing the baby in a propped-up position and thickening the feeds with Gaviscon Infant Sachets. The condition will with time resolve.

Pyloric stenosis

Characteristically pyloric stenosis occurs in male infants between the age of 2 and 6 weeks. The most important diagnostic feature is projectile vomiting of large amounts of milk shortly after a feed. In addition the baby is constipated and will usually have visible gastric peristalsis. When the diagnosis is suspected hospital admission for surgical treatment should be arranged with some urgency.

Acute infection

Vomiting is very commonly a symptom that can accompany any acute infection in children under the age of 5. It has a wide variety of possible causes (Table 13.1). A concise history together with a careful physical examination of the child and treatment of the underlying infection will usually result in a cure.

DIARRHOEA

Gastroenteritis

A transient episode of diarrhoea in an otherwise well child is usually due to dietary changes. This should be easily distinguished from gastroenteritis, which is the frequent passage of watery stools often but not always in

Table 13.1   Common causes of vomiting

Acute otitis media
Acute gastroenteritis
Lower respiratory tract infections
Onset of appendicitis
Intestinal obstruction
Urinary tract infections
Meningitis

Table 13.2   Enteropathogenic organisms

Rotavirus
Echoviruses
Coxsackieviruses
Parvo viruses
Escherichia coli
Campylobacter fetus
Shigella spp.
Salmonella spp.

association with vomiting in a child who is obviously unwell. The causative organism may be any one of a wide variety of enteropathogenic organisms (Table 13.2). Although rotavirus infections usually start with an upper respiratory tract infection and Shigella infections usually give rise to bloody diarrhoea, identification of the organism on the absence of symptoms is unreliable. Culture or electron microscopy of a fresh specimen of stool is the only reliable method. This however is a counsel of perfection and it is acceptable to reserve stool culture for those cases with prolonged or severe symptoms and where infection seems to be spreading through a family or an institution. The main danger of gastroenteritis is dehydration which can develop rapidly and with serious consequences in the infant. The physical examination should therefore concentrate on assessing the degree of hydration and treatment consists of maintaining an adequate fluid intake. All milk and solid food should be withdrawn for at least 24 hours, with water or fruit juices being given as a substitute. When the parent is an infant or less than 6 months of age the parents should be supplied with sachets of sodium chloride and Dextrose oral powder. The contents of a sachet when dissolved in 200 ml of boiled water provide a suitable replacement fluid which should be given in small frequent feeds. If the child is improving after 24 hours, half strength milk feeds should be introduced followed by full strength milk the next day. If there is no improvement admission to hospital should be arranged.

When there is pressure to prescribe, Kaolin mixture will probably do least harm, although evidence suggests that even Kaolin will prolong the period of excretion of the infecting organism and thus delay recovery. Antibiotics, because of the dangers of cross resistance and because most of the infections will be viral, and Lomotil, because of its anticholinergic side effects, are both positively contraindicated.

Chronic diarrhoea

Toddler diarrhoea

This usually occurs in the second year of life and consists of the passage of loose stools containing recognisable food particles. It is thought to be due to failure to chew food and, despite the diarrhoea, weight gain is invariably adequate. The child's mother should be given an explanation and reassured that this form of diarrhoea is of little consequence.

Post-infectious diarrhoea

The degree of diarrhoea can persist for up to 2 weeks following an episode of gastroenteritis. The diarrhoea is not usually as fluid or as frequent as that due to the infection and children with this condition are irritable rather than unwell. Weight is usually fairly well maintained and attention to fluid intake is clearly important. The cause is believed to be a lactose intolerance secondary to damage to the intestinal villi resulting from the infection. Temporary withdrawal of milk from the diet is usually all that is required in treatment.

Malabsorption

Coeliac disease and cystic fibrosis should be excluded in any child with chronic diarrhoea whose weight falls below the 3rd centile. Although uncommon in any individual doctor's list of patients the importance of any chronic disease in childhood lies not simply in the specific treatment but in the more comprehensive management that the child and his family require. As an example of this it is worthwhile considering the management of coeliac disease in some detail.

Coeliac disease is due to an intolerance of the gluten component of wheat and rye flour. It only presents after the child has been weaned from milk onto cereal foods: the most florid cases will therefore present at the age of 6 months but a more sub-acute form of the disease may develop at any age.

The symptoms of florid coeliac disease are anorexia and irritability, weight loss and the appearance of loose, offensive and bulky stools. Marked wasting of the gluteal muscles with an excessively protuberant abdomen, give the unmistakable appearance. In addition to evidence of weight loss the poor absorption of food may be associated with anaemia or vitamin deficiencies.

The slowly developing sub-acute form is more difficult to recognise. The symptoms so markedly present in the severe case are less obvious, but irritability, fatigue and abnormal stools are usually prominent features. The steatorrhoea may present as an apparent constipation despite three or more motions each day, and a child may be brought to the doctor with the story that his underpants are always soiled or offensive. If the condition first appears at school age, the fatigue and irritability may be attributed to the strains of a day at school. For these reasons the parents of the child with a story of developing coeliac disease may only seek help when the condition has been established for months or even years.

When coeliac disease is suspected, the free fat content of a 5-day stool collection should be measured. This investigation should be arranged when the child is at home or on holiday from school, as a complete collection is necessary. The investigation will only show whether there is a steatorrhoea present and hospital investigation is necessary to determine the precise aetiology.

The long-term treatment of the condition is a diet from which all gluten-containing foods have been excluded. In the more severe forms of the disease, anaemia may have to be corrected with iron or folic acid, and vitamin supplements may be necessary. It is always difficult to decide for how long the diet should be continued and this is a question which parents will ask. In the more florid cases, the patient may need to continue on the diet into adult life: in those who present in later childhood, it may be possible to try a normal diet after adolescence and to watch for the return of symptoms and to repeat the jejunal biopsy after the patient has been on normal food for several months.

The diagnosis of coeliac disease is always dependent on a complete investigation in hospital, and the initial dietary advice, which is so important to the treatment, must always be given by a trained dietitian. Most hospitals will issue the mother with comprehensive lists of foods which are allowed and which are prohibited, together with recipes and advice on baking with gluten-free flour. While it will be obvious to most mothers that such foods are bread, cakes and biscuits are prohibited, there is a wide range of foods which, although apparently innocuous, contain flour. Many soups and tinned meats are thickened with flour, while some sweets contain flour or are coated with it during manufacture. The mother should be advised to join the Coeliac Society which can provide a comprehensive list of food manufacturers together with lists of their products which are gluten-free. Certain such foods can be given on prescription — gluten-free flour, bread, biscuits, macaroni and spaghetti — and the booklet from the Coeliac Society also contains the names and addresses of bakers who make gluten-free bread. During the first few months of the diet it is important that the child does not think he is different from the rest of the family and that he is not continuously faced with his brothers and sisters eating foods which he previously liked and which are now forbidden to him. It is helpful to the child if others in the family also reduce, or exclude, gluten-containing foods during the early months: later, foods containing flour such as bread, cakes, biscuits and puddings can be slowly re-introduced for the rest of the family.

The parents should take time to repeatedly talk to the child about the importance of his diet and he should be encouraged to look up his booklet to find out for himself what foods he is allowed. With explanation and encouragement many children can be very strict with the diet and it may be that the sense of wellbeing which they feel once they are established on the diet encourages even young children of 6 or 7 years to persist with it.

Deviations from the diet are inevitable from time to time and parties at friends' houses, presents of food from well meaning relatives, or simply just the attraction of a forbidden food, mean that lapses will occur. Unfortunately the time lag before the effects appear of even small quantities of gluten can be very variable, and the mother may learn to expect the child to become fatigued, irritable or off his food for some days or even a week or two after the flour-containing food has been taken. The mother should be warned that these lapses are liable to occur and she should be alert to this possibility.

Once a child has been established on his diet he should be reviewed at yearly intervals by the family doctor. The absence of symptoms and the opinion of the mother both on the child's general health and the strictness of the diet, are the most important factors to consider. The child's height and weight should be entered on paediatric percentile charts at each review consultation as a continued intolerance of small amounts of gluten in the diet may only show as a degree of retardation of growth. If it is suspected that the condition is not fully controlled, the stool fat estimation should be repeated and the mother and child should be seen again by the dietitian. Thereafter the health visitor should keep a watching brief on the family and continue to advise on the dietary regime prescribed.

CONSTIPATION

Mothers of young babies may express concern that the baby appears to strain or cry on defaecation, and attribute this to constipation. Straining is usually a normal reaction, but if it appears excessive or the cry is one of pain rather than of distress, true constipation or a fissure-in-ano should be suspected. Young infants may readily become constipated, passing infrequent hard stools, in warm weather when their fluid intake is less than is required. Many mothers do not realise that milk-fed infants also require water and that four or five additional water 'feeds' may be required during the summer months.

Fissure-in-ano can usually be suspected by the way in which the child screams when passing a motion, and can be confirmed by a gentle examination of the anus. The pain of fissure-in-ano is severe and persists after the motion has passed: the pain is such that the child will not infrequently resist defaecation and a secondary constipation can compound the problem. Treatment consists of softening the stool with a preparation such as liquid paraffin BP and by the use of a local anaesthetic gel applied to the anal canal prior to each feed.

There is a wide variation in the normal frequency of defaecation. If this is a cause of concern, stool frequency can usually be increased by the addition of a small amount of sugar to milk feeds or in children who have been weaned by the addition of more fruit and vegetables to the diet.

JAUNDICE

Physiological jaundice of the newborn

Jaundice in a newborn infant is caused by a temporary deficiency of the enzyme glucuronyl transferase which reduces the rate of conjugation of bilirubin. Jaundice appears after the first 24 hours and reaches its peak on the fourth or fifth day. Thereafter it quickly disappears. If the baby is clearly unwell, fretful or listless and off his feeds, a major infective illness such as pyelonephritis or septicaemia should be suspected. These conditions are potentially serious and their investigation and treatment requires urgent admission to hospital.

CHILDREN OF SCHOOL AGE

PAIN

Appendicitis

Appendicitis is the most important acute illness in this age group and is suspected in more cases than are proved by operative treatment. The classical presentation of central abdominal pain which later shifts to the right iliac fossa is uncommon: the more usual finding is of central abdominal pain with tenderness on palpation in the right iliac fossa. The signs of localised peritonitis in this site usually develop at a later stage; while they are of diagnostic value in the hospital, they may be absent when the primary diagnosis is sought. It is usual for the doctor to be called within 4 to 12 hours of the child becoming ill and to find little other evidence other than systemic upset and toxaemia. In these circumstances central abdominal pain that is steady and persistent should suggest appendicitis. It is also important to remember that a retrocaecal appendix may simply present with abdominal pain and what is described as diarrhoea.

The decision about admission to hospital must be made on the assessment of each patient; there can be no simple rule of thumb. Hospital admission is mandatory in those cases where the clinical evidence allows a definite diagnosis to be made but when the child is less ill and the doctor has carefully considered and rejected appendicitis as the most probable diagnosis, the patient can be nursed at home with a fluid diet. If this course is adopted, frequent return visits are necessary and the progress of the child should be kept under continual review. The parents should be given clear instructions about the expected course of the illness and should be told that the doctor should be called urgently if the child's condition deteriorates or if the pain stops only to restart a few hours later. If, for example, the first call to the patient was received during the morning, another visit should be made that afternoon and again in the evening.

Hospital admission will be indicated if the child's condition deteriorates, if the doctor is not fully satisfied with the progress by the time of the evening visit, or if no improvement is found 24 hours after the illness started. The diagnosis of appendicitis is difficult in hospital and the results of appendicectomy reflect this difficulty. It is important for the doctor in practice to err on the side of safety by tending to admit his patient early rather than late in the course of the illness.

Periodic syndrome

At least 10% of children in this age group suffer from recurrent abdominal pain. The pain is usually felt in the centre of the abdomen and is often associated with vomiting and headache. It rarely lasts more than 12 hours. The commonest cause is stress at home or at school and a familial factor is also involved because there is a high incidence of similar complaints, and of migraine, in the parents, usually the mother, and in the siblings of these children.

The parents' main concern is that there is something physically wrong with the child. It is therefore important to perform a thorough physical examination in order to reassure them. The only mandatory investigation is microscopy and culture of a urine specimen as urinary tract infection can occasionally cause similar symptoms. The urine should also be tested for sugar since in this age group abdominal pain can be a presenting symptom of diabetes. Management should be directed at removing or alleviating the cause of stress. The identification of a stressful factor, and the measures that should be used to alleviate the problem should be considered with the co-operation of the school as well as the parents. A follow-up study of children with this condition showed that one-third continued to have recurrent abdominal pain in adult life, one-third developed recurrent headaches — usually of a migrainous type — and one-third were completely free of symptoms.

NAUSEA AND VOMITING

Episodic attacks of upper abdominal pain associated with nausea and vomiting and caused by dyspepsia become more common after the onset of puberty. The majority of cases are precipitated by stress and the degree of illness or the frequency of recurrence of these episodes will also be increased if the child is permitted to use them as a means of escape from the causal situation by over-sensitive parents. The time of onset and the duration of symptoms are usually clearly related to the onset or anticipation of stress which may be a dislike or fear of school, a home in which tension and disagreement are common, or an unwelcome evening activity which is forced on the child by the parents. If a causal factor is identified, it is important that sufficient time is spent with both the child and his parents to enable each to understand clearly the possible origin of the symptoms. The action which the doctor advises will obviously depend on the nature of the problem but in the majority of instances full explanation and discussion with the family will be all the therapy that is necessary.

The incidence of peptic ulcer is much lower in children than in adults but this possibility should be considered if stress appears to be a factor in the illness, when there is a family history of dyspepsia and when there appears to be a relationship between the onset of symptoms and the intake of food. The psychological factors which are present to a lesser or greater degree in all adult patients with peptic ulcer are usually present in a more simplifiied form in the younger patient. It is not uncommon to find that the patient has an obsessive tendency towards his school work or his play, that he sets high standards for himself, and becomes excessively anxious in his attempts to reach and maintain them. It will not be possible to alter the young person's personality, but the doctor may be able to modify it through discussion and by encouraging him to adopt less rigid standards. This psychotherapy will be an adjunct to more specific treatment on more conventional lines. Dietary advice will only be needed if the diet is markedly abnormal: it will usually only be necessary to ensure that regular meals are being taken and that they do not contain any foods which the child has found to upset him in the past. An antacid should be taken midway between each meal and on occasions referral for investigation and appropriate therapy for a proven peptic ulcer should be initiated.

Psychogenic nausea

Nausea and vomiting is frequently part of the periodic syndrome, but vomiting without abdominal pain may occasionally be due to emotional causes. The management is the same as that for the periodic syndrome.

DIARRHOEA

Acute enteritis

There is an increased likelihood that infection may be due to one of the enteroviruses or to excessive or incautious eating, or occasionally to Shigella or Salmonella infection. More social contacts outside the home increase the opportunities for contracting infection. Transmission of infection is usually by the faecal–oral route and hand-washing after defaecation is often overlooked. Since the condition is likely to be self-limiting within 2 to 4 days little active treatment is required. If the degree of diarrhoea warrants therapy simple Kaolin BP can be given to reduce the fluidity of the stool: diarrhoea accompanied by significant abdominal pain should be treated with diphenoxylate hydrochloride (Lomotil) 5 mg three times daily (13–16 years).

CONSTIPATION

Encopresis

Encopresis is persistent and volitional faecal soiling. It must be distinguished from the overflow incontinence due to intrinsic bowel dysfunction which occurs in Hirschsprung's disease and congenital megacolon, both of which are characterised by gross faecal retention and colonic dilatation. Children with encopresis may be constipated and impacted with faeces but this is more often due to them holding the stool rather than anorectal disease although a fissure-in-ano can be a complicating factor.

The disorder may prove more difficult to manage than enuresis, with which it often co-exists, and usually indicates some profound disturbance of the child/parent relationship which may have begun in an innocent way with, for example, a short separation from the mother such as occurs with admission to hospital. Encopresis usually indicates a profound sense of insecurity in the child and its presence means that this feeling, resulting from physical or emotional rejection or deprivation, is of long standing. The symptom may also be the child's way of obtaining attention: his previous attempts clearly having brought him none of the affection and security that he requires.

Many children can be competently managed by their family doctor, particularly when the causes are simple and not too intractable. When the cause is obscure and deep-seated the expert attention of a child and family psychiatrist may be required. The nature of the disorder should be explained to both parents and the absolute necessity of a common policy of management agreed. Initially it may be necessary to empty the bowel with enema and gentle purgatives but their prolonged use may only intensify the problem so they should be discouraged. The use of tricyclic antidepressants is not indicated.

ADULT PATIENTS

PAIN

Hiatus hernia

Reflux oesophagitis commonly presents with heartburn as its main symptom, frequently with an associated reg-urgitation of 'water brash' but seldom with abdominal pain. It is a common and troublesome symptom during late pregnancy and can be controlled satisfactorily by an antacid such as Mucaine which contains a local anaesthetic. The patient can be reassured that her 'indigestion' will not last beyond the pregnancy. Reflux oesophagitis caused by a true hiatus hernia is most common in the older patient and requires a different therapeutic approach. Initially, the symptoms come and go and the patient gradually alters her eating habits and treats herself with proprietary antacids in an attempt to control symptoms. The diagnosis is seldom in doubt but the differentiation between oesophagitis and angina can sometimes be difficult because both may be provoked by a heavy meal and by exercise; in the elderly patient the two conditions may co-exist. Electrocardiogram taken both before and after exercise is of help in excluding angina as a cause of the patient's symptoms. The initial stage of treatment should include advice on the avoidance of postures which induce reflux, together with an antacid after each meal and a milk drink last thing at night. An important aspect of management is to take a careful dietary history and to ensure that the control of symptoms is combined with a balanced dietary intake: the patient's own attempts at treatment may mean that her diet has become unsatisfactory in the period prior to the consultation. Haemoglobin estimation should also be made; in addition to dietary problems a slightly persistent blood loss from the oesophagitis may have been present for some time before the patient seeks advice.

If these simple measures are not sufficient to relieve symptoms, the presence and type of hiatus hernia should be established by a barium swallow and advice should be sought on the question of surgical treatment. Surgery is a major procedure for the elderly patient and should be considered only when other treatments have failed to control the symptoms. Cardiovascular or respiratory complications may exclude operative treatment and more conservative measures will then have to be continued indefinitely. It is important to remember that the elderly patient frequently has several co-existing medical problems and that dyspepsia may be aggravated by the treatment of other conditions. Pain in the joints and muscles are common in the elderly and are often treated with aspirin or other proprietary analgesics without the doctor being aware of their consumption unless he specifically asks about it. It must also be remembered that aspirin is sold in many guises and is taken for a variety of reasons. Once the diagnosis is established, arrangements should be made to review the patient at regular intervals and frequent appointments will be necessary until symptoms have abated. Thereafter the patient should be seen every 3 months to ensure that she remains well or that her diet is adequate both in quality and quantity and that anaemia does not develop.

Duodenal ulcer

Males are affected with duodenal ulcer four times more frequently than are females, and the annual incidence of new episodes is between 4 and 5 per 1000 patients at risk. The onset is generally between the ages of 20 and 40 years, although younger teenage patients and older patients can obviously develop the condition. There is a peak incidence in new illness in the winter and early summer months.

The natural history of duodenal ulcer is important from the point of view of management. In 60% of patients the symptoms persist for between 5 and 10 years before resolving, usually never to return. A fifth of patients will continue to have recurrent debilitating attacks and are clearly candidates for surgical treatment. Of the remaining fifth, approximately one-sixth (3% of all patients) perforate and the remainder (17% of all patients) will have one or more episodes of bleeding.

It can sometimes be difficult to differentiate between true peptic ulceration and 'ulcer type dyspepsia' in which no radiological or endoscopic evidence of ulcer will be found. It is likely that the two conditions represent different ends of a spectrum of illness since some 50% of those with 'ulcer type dyspepsia' will be found to have a peptic ulcer within a further 5 years.

One of the most important characteristics of peptic ulcer is its periodicity: symptoms occur for between 1 and 3 weeks then resolve and there is remission for a period of 3 to 4 months before the symptom reappears. The pain of peptic ulcer is usually clearly localised, by one finger, to the epigastrium and during the acute phase, tenderness in this area can also be elicited. Nocturnal pain is another valuable diagnostic feature: waking the patient from sleep at between 2 and 3 a.m. but quickly responding to a milky drink or an alkali. Nausea and vomiting are variable in degree and appetite is usually well maintained. The patient may be of an anxious or worrying kind — familial or occupational stress may be identified — but whether the anxiety is cause or effect is open to question. Finally there is frequently a family history of the condition.

Ideally X-ray or endoscopic proof of the presence of an ulcer should be obtained before management is begun. This however is a counsel of perfection and it would seem rational to adopt a two stage approach. The initial step is to attempt to change any provoking lifestyle factors — of which cigarette smoking and alcohol are important — and to correct any grossly irregular dietary habits. The addition of a simple antacid taken midway between meals and last thing at night, will allow many patients to become symptom-free.

Should this simple regime fail and treatment with the more specific H_2-receptor antagonists be contemplated it is as well to refer to patient for barium studies, or preferably for endoscopy. Other indications for investigation include the patient with a markedly atypical history, the older patient in whom neoplasia may be suspected and when the differentiation between peptic ulcer and gall bladder dyspepsia proves difficult. Specific treatment consists initially of an antacid: if this is unsuccessful those with proven ulcer should be prescribed cimetidine 200 mg three times daily with 400 mg at night or ranitidine 150 mg twice daily. Both of these drugs produce gastric hypochlorhydria as a result of their H_2-receptor blocking action. Ideally they should be used in full dosage for 4 to 6 weeks then stopped. Should symptoms recur within 4 weeks the initial dose should be repeated and the patient should be put on a maintenance dose of cimetidine 400 mg at night for a further 3 months. In a proportion of patients symptoms will again recur and it is tempting to consider long-term suppressive therapy with the night-time dose of cimetidine. There is doubt however as to the safety of long-term use of H_2-receptor blocking drugs and it is probably wise to consider surgical treatment should the second step of treatment prove ineffectual. Patients who develop complications such as bleeding, perforation or pyloric stenosis will obviously require admission to hospital for the consideration of surgical intervention.

Gastric ulcer

The onset of gastric ulcer is at a later age than that of duodenal ulcer — between the ages of 50 and 70 years. The natural history is similar to that of duodenal ulcer although the incidence of complications is less frequent: bleeding will occur in 10% of patients and perforation in 1%. Because of its later age of onset investigation by endoscopy — so that a biopsy can be taken if an ulcer is found — is mandatory. This is most important since the symptoms of a gastric ulcer — although similar to those of duodenal ulcer — are more non-specific, since the age of onset also coincides with that of gastric cancer, and because the dyspeptic symptoms of both conditions will be helped by antacids and thus delay the diagnosis in the case of cancer. The specific treatment of gastric ulcer, despite its being associated with normal or low acid concentrations rather than with hyperchlorhydria, is as for duodenal ulcer.

It is important to remember that dyspeptic symptoms — vague or concise — that seem to occur in relation to pay day or to weekends can be an early presentation of an alcohol problem.

Gall bladder disease

Controlled studies have demonstrated that dyspepsia, flatulence, bloating and fatty food intolerance bear very little relationship to gall bladder disease. The pain of acute cholecystitis is usually felt in the right hypochondrium and is accompanied by nausea, vomiting and fever. If there have been previous similar episodes of pain or if the pain radiates to the shoulder or subscapular region, the diagnosis is strengthened.

Clinical examination reveals local tenderness in the gall bladder area. The finding of a leucocytosis with a raised alkaline phosphatase and a low grade hyperbilirubinaemia is useful supportive evidence for the diagnosis.

Most attacks will settle with bed rest, analgesics and an antibiotic which should cover Gram negative organisms. The diagnosis should later be confirmed by cholecystogram. If gall stones are demonstrated the patient should be referred for elective cholecystectomy. Attempts to dissolve gall stones with drugs have so far proved disappointing.

Attacks which fail to settle within 48 hours or in which frank jaundice develops should be referred for admission to hospital. Progressively severe obstructive jaundice suggests that the stone has become lodged in the common bile duct. The emergency treatment of gall bladder colic involves an analgesic and antispasmodic: pethidine 25–100 mg IM and atropine sulphate 0.4–1 mg IV.

Acute pancreatitis

Acute pancreatitis is a condition which varies widely in severity. The two most important conditions which are associated with it are higher than average alcohol ingestion — and acute pancreatitis frequently follows a particularly heavy drinking bout — and the presence of gall stones. The basic lesion is intrapancreatic activation of the proteolytic and lipolytic enzymes of the pancreas causing autodigestion with inflammation of pancreatic tissue. This may be relatively mild giving only slight upper abdominal pain, alternatively disabling pain may radiate through into the back to be accompanied by nausea and vomiting. Occasionally severe fulminant pancreatitis may give rise to circulatory collapse with consequent renal, cardiac and ventilatory failure.

The clinical appearance is often non-specific but the diagnosis can be established by estimation of serum amylase which is invariably highly elevated. Severe cases will require admission to hospital but mild cases may settle at home with analgesics and fluids only by mouth.

IRRITABLE BOWEL SYNDROME

This common disorder appears to be due to an exaggerated colonic response to psychological stress which results in either hyper- or hypomotility, particularly of the sigmoid colon. Hypermotility and spasm are manifested by pain and constipation, the latter because the faecal bolus cannot pass the spastic area. Hypermotility without spasm is associated with diarrhoea since the colonic contents are not retained for long enough for normal water absorption to occur.

The classical symptoms are therefore lower abdominal pain relieved by defaecation, alternating constipation and diarrhoea and the passage of small calibre stools. These symptoms obviously mimic those due to more serious disorders and clearly if either diarrhoea or constipation is the predominant symptom investigations must be arranged to exclude a neoplastic cause of this altered bowel habit. When the patient first presents it is mandatory to complete a rectal examination and to arrange for sigmoidoscopy and barium enema. If these are normal, and intermittent symptoms, usually related to stress, persist without obvious signs of physical deterioration, then the diagnosis can be considered as established. The long-term use of bran or other faecal bulk-forming agents such as methyl cellulose granules helps to reduce the number of attacks. Abdominal pain in association with diarrhoea will usually respond to codeine. The patient should be strongly reassured about the benign origin of the symptoms and attempts should be made to identify and correct any causative stress factor. It is unusual however to find any aetiological factor, the condition is most commonly found in those whose personality inclines towards anxiety, and regular and repeated consultations should be planned so that the patient can be given the supportive reassurance that they so commonly require.

NAUSEA AND VOMITING

Alcohol

The manifestations of excessive drinking can be multiple and protean. Good anticipatory care involves the recognition of the problem before the onset of irreversible organ damage. A high index of suspicion and good records which may reveal a recurring pattern of illness are the general practitioner's instruments of detection. The young or middle-aged man who presents on a Monday evening requesting a sick note and complaining of nausea, vomiting and epigastric pain should always be asked about his alcohol intake. If this is more than an average of four pints of beer per day he should be advised that continuation of this pattern of drinking will almost certainly affect his health (see ch. 25).

Women usually take greater steps to conceal or even deny their drinking habits. If excessive drinking is suspected objective confirmation can be obtained by finding a high mean corpuscular volume and a raised level of gamma-glutaryl transferase (GT).

Diarrhoea

Food-poisoning

The three most frequent causes of this group of illnesses are the contamination of food with organisms of the salmonella group, with *Clostridium welchii* and with staphylococcal toxins. Food is affected when there is a lack of hygiene on the part of persons engaged in preparing food; in the case of salmonella a common source of infection is from food handlers who are themselves recovering from an infection and who are still excreting the organism. A further mode of infection is the contamination of frozen, prepared food such as chicken or other poultry; inadequate thawing before cooking can mean that the bird's body cavity acts as an incubator for organisms that are already present. Raw unpasteurised milk is also a not uncommon source of epidemic outbreaks of salmonellosis. Cooked meats and other foods which are partially reheated are liable to infection with *Clostridium welchii* whilst staphylococcal toxins are more commonly transmitted in cream and other prepared milk products. The clinical presentation of food poisoning is dependent on the nature of the infecting organism. Staphylococcal toxins induce an intoxication (not an infection) of sudden onset which is characterised by vomiting and abdominal cramps which precede the onset of diarrhoea. The illness begins from 2 to 6 hours after the ingestion of the contaminated food. *Clostridum welchii* infection has a rather later time of onset — about 10–12 hours — and begins with severe abdominal colic which is followed by diarrhoea. Nausea and vomiting may be absent. Infection with salmonellae has a longer incubation period — normally 12–13 hours. Diarrhoea is a marked feature and this is associated with nausea and vomiting. Typhoid and para-typhoid fevers have still longer incubation periods (1–10 days and 1–3 weeks respectively) and the possibility of these conditions should be considered if the incubation period for an outbreak of food poisoning appears to be longer than 1 or 2 days.

Stool cultures should always be obtained and all cases of infection reported to a community medicine specialist. The number of persons affected may be much greater than those seen by any one doctor and the source of infection may be difficult to identify unless a detailed epidemiological picture is established. This is particularly important when the source is a person working in a restaurant or canteen when repeated minor epidemics can spread over a wide area.

The treatment of patients with an illness caused by staphylococcal toxins includes a high fluid intake and symptomatic relief from the diarrhoea and pain through the use of Kaolin or Lomotil. Where the infection is thought to be from salmonella cotrimoxazole is the treatment of choice. Any treatment given should be continued for 24 hours after a symptomatic recovery has taken place. Patients whose employment involves handling food should not be allowed to return to work until three consecutive stool specimens have been reported as free from infection.

Foreign travellers
Patients who have returned from an overseas trip usually suffer from no more than the transient diarrhoea which affects many people following a change of environment and food. More exotic diseases however should be considered and should be excluded by examination of a fresh stool specimen for ova, cysts and parasites. The commonest abnormal finding is giardiasis which should be treated with metronidazole 400 mg three times daily for 7 days.

Chronic diarrhoea

Ulcerative colitis
Ulcerative colitis is a relapsing and remitting chronic inflammatory disorder of the colon. Its aetiology is unknown but the major symptoms are diarrhoea which contains blood and mucus, abdominal pain, fever and weight loss. The extent of bleeding and of diarrhoea is variable, ranging from several semi-formed stools per day to the frequent passage up to 20 times daily of liquid stools with blood and pus. 94% of patients have rectal involvement. A presumptive diagnosis can therefore be made by the general practitioner who performs a proctoscopy and discovers inflamed and friable rectal mucosa.

All patients with this condition should be referred for specialist supervision in order to confirm the diagnosis by biopsy, discover the extent of the disease in the colon, and decide whether an ileostomy with total procto-colectomy should be performed in order to remove the future dangers of toxic megacolon and the increased incidence of carcinoma of the colon.

In mild cases an acute attack will usually respond to treatment with loperamide hydrochloride or codeine phosphate to reduce bowel motility and hydrocortisone retention enemas to reduce inflammation. Sulphasalazine 500 mg four times daily is helpful in maintaining remissions but as in any other chronic debilitating disease a considerable amount of support needs to be afforded to the patient.

Crohn's disease
Crohn's disease is a non-specific granulomatous disease which more commonly affects the small bowel but can also involve the colon. Its aetiology is unknown. It presents in a similar fashion to ulcerative colitis but there is an absence of bleeding although the other symptoms of diarrhoea, malaise and abdominal pain are present. Crohn's disease is characterised by an increased incidence of fistula formation and peri-anal and peri-rectal abscesses. Referral to a specialist is necessary to confirm the diagnosis and to construct a treatment plan which will usually involve a combination of medical and surgical approaches.

Post-gastrectomy diarrhoea
Increased stool frequency often with frank diarrhoea is a

common result of gastric surgery. It can result in malabsorption of iron, vitamin B_{12} and folic acid with a consequent anaemia. In addition there may also be malabsorption of calcium presenting as osteomalacia or osteoporosis. Patients who have had gastric surgery should be identified by their general practitioner and screened annually with a full blood count, serum iron, serum B_{12}, serum folate and serum calcium, phosphate and alkaline phosphatase estimations.

CONSTIPATION

The belief that a regular daily bowel movement is important for health is widespread, resulting in large scale use of laxatives. It is important that the general practitioner has a rational approach to the problem when he is asked to advise about constipation.

There are three groups of laxatives:

Bulk-forming drugs which relieve constipation by increasing faecal mass which stimulates peristalsis. Advice about a high-roughage diet and the use of unprocessed bran is often successful. Alternatively one of the proprietary preparations of methyl cellulose granules may be helpful.

Stimulant laxatives act by increasing intestinal motility. The most commonly used stimulant laxatives are bisacodyl, danthron and standardised senna preparations. When abused they can precipitate an atonic nonfunctioning colon and hypokalaemia. They are best reserved for those patients who have analgesic induced constipation.

Faecal softeners act by maintaining a volume of fluid in the bowel by osmosis. Lactulose is the most commonly used agent in this group.

JAUNDICE

Acute hepatitis
Hepatitis A (Infectious hepatitis) is the usual cause of jaundice which follows a 7–10 day period of general malaise with anorexia in a young adult. The causative virus is usually either ingested in contaminated food or spread through the faecal–oral route. The incubation period varies from 4–6 weeks. Investigations will reveal a leucocytosis with elevated bilirubin, mildly elevated alkaline phosphatase and greatly raised aminotransferase.

Treatment consists of bedrest during the acute phase with a 3-month abstinence from alcohol. Most patients will have recovered within 6 weeks although general malaise with depression may persist for some time after this. It is advisable to repeat liver function tests at least 3-monthly intervals until they show normal readings. In the great majority of patients the test will become normal

within 3–6 months: a few however will show evidence of permanent parenchymal damage to the liver and will progress towards hepatic insufficiency. In these patients any further hepatotoxic drugs — such as alcohol — must be carefully avoided.

Hepatitis B (serum hepatitis) is associated with the presence of Australia-antigen. There is a high prevalence in the Far East, in the West it is more common among the sexually promiscuous, drug addicts and those subjected to multiple transfusions or tattooing. This pattern reflects its mode of transmission which is usually through sexual contact or from blood or blood products. The incubation period is approximately 3 months. The onset is more insidious than in hepatitis A but investigations reveal the same pattern apart from the presence of Australia-antigen.

A significant proportion of sufferers may develop fulminant hepatic failure or progress to chronic liver disease. Those who recover are frequently carriers of the disease and can be identified by the persistent presence of Australia-antigen.

Chronic hepatitis
The commonest cause of chronic inflammation of the liver progressing to cirrhosis is alcohol. It is usually diagnosed when the patient presents with complications of the disease; bleeding, jaundice, ascites or neurological disturbance. The other physical features to look for are spider naevi, liverpalms, clubbing, splenomegaly, loss of body hair and in males gynaecomastia and small testes. Liver function tests will usually be abnormal but confirmation of the diagnosis depends on liver biopsy. Management consists of treatment of the complications and prevention of progression of the disease by a total avoidance of alcohol.

PATIENTS OF 65 YEARS AND OVER

PAIN

Gastric ulcer
Gastric ulcer is more common in this age group. It is estimated that as many as 20% may be asymptomatic only coming to light when complications such as perforation or bleeding occurs. In the other 80% there is a variable clinical picture. It differs from that found with duodenal ulcer in that the pain is usually less localised and more diffuse, rarely occurs at night and may be aggravated rather than relieved by food. Non-specific symptoms such as anorexia, nausea and a vague bloating feeling are common.

The diagnosis should be established by barium meal or endoscopy. The second method allows a biopsy to be taken in order to exclude malignant disease. Treatment is with cimetidine or rantidine in full dosage for 6 weeks. A repeat barium meal or endoscopy should be performed after 8 weeks to check that the ulcer has healed.

Intra-abdominal cancer

Incidence rates increase logarithmically with age, the disease being rare before the age of 40.

Oesophagus

Predisposing influences appear to be alcohol, smoking and possibly diet. The major presenting symptom is anorexia with increasing dysphagia for solids. The diagnosis can usually be established by a barium swallow and should be confirmed by endoscopy and biopsy.

Stomach

There are marked geographical variations in the incidence of gastric cancer which suggests that some unidentified dietary factors are important in its aetiology. The commonest clinical manifestations are anorexia with weight loss, poorly localised epigastric discomfort and a sensation of fullness or bloating which is aggravated by meals. By the time they begin to cause symptoms most gastric cancers are fairly advanced. This is the main cause of a 5-year survival rate of only 10–20% after surgery. The only way to improve prognosis is through early detection. This is frequently difficult but a good rule is that any patient over the age of 50 years who develops dyspeptic symptoms for the first time should be assumed to have a gastric cancer until investigations have proven otherwise.

Pancreas

Because of its location, cancer of the pancreas is a very difficult diagnosis to establish with certainty. The predominant symptoms are constant upper abdominal pain which radiates through to the back and is relieved by leaning forward, and loss of weight. Jaundice due to partial or complete obstruction of the common bile duct is frequently painless and steadily progressive. Confirmation of the diagnosis may have to await exploratory laparotomy. The prognosis is appalling as it is estimated that only 10% of cases are operable at diagnosis and that of these only 5% survive for 5 years.

Caecum and colon

Tumours in the caecum are papilliferous and rarely cause obstruction because the caecum is patulous. They usually present late with anaemia, weight loss, a palpable mass and often secondary deposits in liver. Tumours in the colon are usually annular giving rise to partial or complete obstruction with altered bowel habit. The best method of early diagnosis is a high index of suspicion with early investigation. Attempts at screening by regular testing of faecal occult blood has so far been disappointing. Surgery is the treatment of choice and the overall 5-year survival is approximately 50%.

Rectum

Tumours of the rectum are theoretically amenable to early diagnosis as there are early specific symptoms: bleeding, rectal urgency, pain and soiling. Diagnosis in a number of cases can also be confirmed by digital examination and proctoscopy. The danger is that the symptoms may be attributed to pre-existing haemorrhoids and a rectal examination may thus not be performed.

Diverticular disease

The incidence of colonic diverticula increases exponentially with age in Western populations. They are far less common in African populations. This is thought to be due to the fact that a low fibre diet predisposes to segmental muscular hyperactivity causing high intraluminal pressures with resulting diverticula. Patients with diverticulosis are either asymptomatic, or have complaints parallel to those in the irritable bowel syndrome and should be treated similarly. Occasionally diverticulitis develops with acute inflammation as a result of faecolith impaction. The clinical picture is similar to left sided appendicitis with sudden onset of pain and tenderness in the left iliac fossa which is associated with fever and leucocytosis. Most patients will respond to rest with fluids only by mouth and treatment with a broad spectrum antibiotic such as ampicillin. A few patients develop pericolic abscesses or even a perforation with general peritonitis and they will obviously require referral to hospital. A less common complication of diverticulosis is sudden, profuse painless rectal bleeding.

Ischaemic colitis

In the elderly sudden onset of severe abdominal pain with rectal bleeding and diarrhoea may be due to thrombosis or embolism of the mesenteric vessels.

NAUSEA AND VOMITING

With the high incidence of intra-abdominal cancer in this age group it is not surprising that one of the commonest causes of nausea and vomiting is terminal illness due to cancer. Treatment with either chlorpromazine or prochlorperazine is usually helpful. Chlorpromazine provides more sedation than prochlorperazine: both of them are available as either tablet, syrup, injection or suppository. If the vomiting is thought to be due to delayed gastric emptying, metoclopramide may sometimes be more useful.

DIARRHOEA

Carcinoma of the rectum has already been dealt with as have the infectious causes. One cause which may be misdiagnosed is spurious diarrhoea due to overflow from faecal impaction.

CONSTIPATION

Faecal impaction in this age group is a common problem. Poor muscle tone and reduced physical activity result in decreased frequency of bowel movements. This, on occasions, allows a large dry faecal mass to build up which the patient is then unable to evacuate. Overflow diarrhoea may occur around this faecal mass. In addition pressure on the bladder neck may cause incontinence or retention of urine, and some vulnerable elderly people with impaction become acutely confused.

Treatment consists of removal of the faecal mass by manual removal or phosphate enemas. Once this has been accomplished the aim should be to achieve regular bowel movements in order to prevent recurrence. Stimulant or osmotic laxatives are usually required as bulk producing agents in combination with a low fluid intake may cause rapid relapse. Rare cases which do not respond to this approach require regular suppositories or even weekly enemas.

JAUNDICE

Two causes, hepatic secondary deposits from cancer of the bowel and obstruction of the common bile duct due to carcinoma of the head of the pancreas, have already been mentioned. Drug induced jaundice should not be overlooked. The commonest offenders are phenothiazines such as chlorpromazine or thioridazine.

Endocrine disease

Endocrine disease in the community is uncommon but once a diagnosis has been made the care required in the management of these disorders is lifelong. The general practitioner is unlikely to meet more than one or two new cases of pituitary or adrenal disease in a lifetime but thyroid disease and diabetes are relatively more common. The management of both can be shared between the general practitioner and his specialist colleagues depending upon the individual case. Despite the low incidence of these disorders, they will make demands upon the general practitioner's time that are out of proportion to the numbers of patients involved.

Problem solving is the essence of general practice, and, in many situations, making a diagnosis is of secondary importance. In endocrine disease a diagnosis is essential and should not only be based on clinical findings but also requires laboratory confirmation.

THYROID DISEASE

The diagnosis of thyroid disease is not easy because the symptoms of both over and under secretion by the thyroid can mimic much more common and less specific conditions. The apathetic and elderly patient who has lost interest in life in general may be suffering from hypothyroidism; the nervous and excitable girl of 20, apparently in an anxiety state, may have an excess of thyroid hormones in her circulation.

TESTS FOR THYROID FUNCTION

An accurate measurement of hormone levels is essential in the diagnosis and management of thyroid disease.

Physiology

The hypothalamus synthesises thyrotrophic-releasing hormone (TRH) which stimulates the anterior pituitary to synthesise thyroid stimulating hormone (TSH) and release it into the general circulation. TSH acts upon the thyroid causing it to synthesise and subsequently release from the gland into the general circulation the two thyroid hormones Thyroxin (T4) and Tri-iodothyronine (T3). These hormones circulate in an inactive form bound mainly to Thyroxine binding globulin (TBG); only very minute quantities are non protein bound and metabolically active. The tiny quantities of active hormones exert a negative feedback upon the anterior pituitary so that in hyperthyroidism the circulating TSH levels fall and in hypothyroidism TSH levels rise.

Normal values

1. Serum Thyroxine (T4): The normal range of serum T4 levels varies in different laboratories and each laboratory establishes its own norm.
2. Serum Tri-iodothyronine (T3): The normal range in adults is between 1.0 and 2.0 nmol/l (0.65–1.70 μg/ml).
3. Thyroid Stimulating Hormone (TSH): Normal levels are up to 6 mU/l.

THE EFFECT OF DRUGS AND PREGNANCY ON THYROID FUNCTION

Oestrogens including the oral contraceptive pill increase the circulating Thyroxine binding globulin (TBG) resulting in higher levels of both thyroid hormones but in their relatively inactive protein bound form. Estimations of the hormones are, therefore, misleading in such patients.

Increased oestrogen production during pregnancy similarly increases the circulating TBG resulting in higher levels of both thyroid hormones, especially T4. The method used to assess thyroid function during pregnancy is to measure the free T4 level either by an estimation of the free thyroxine index or by a free T4 assay.

Thyroid enlargement, fatigue, heat intolerance, varying degrees of anxiety and emotional upset are often found in normal pregnancy and can easily be confused with hyperthyroidism.

Drugs that reduce the plasma levels of thyroid hormones are salicylates, lithium and phenylbutazone.

Hypothyroidism

Hypothyroidism may be defined as a condition which results from suboptimal circulating levels of one or both thyroid hormones (Evered 1976). It is one of the most rewarding and satisfying conditions for the general practitioner to diagnose and manage.

Incidence and aetiology

In a survey in the United Kingdom symptomatic hypothyroidism was found in 1.1% of the adult population; 1.9% of females and 0.2% of males (Tunbridge et al 1975). In an average practice of 2500 it was found that five persons with hypothyroidism consulted annually (Fry 1979). Tunbridge found that the disease was associated with autoimmune thyroiditis in 80% of cases and was a consequence of destructive treatment to the thyroid in most of the remainder. Other causes were rare but included the use of antithyroid drugs and drugs which interfered with thyroid function such as iodides which are a common constituent of cough medicines.

Overt hypothyroidism

In the well established case the disease is easily recognised especially if the patient is being seen for the first time or has not consulted the doctor for some months. The patient, most often female, may complain of both physical and mental lethargy. On questioning she may admit to cold intolerance, weight gain, constipation and anorexia. On examination there will be dryness of the skin, coarseness of the hair and, in many cases, infraorbital puffiness and oedema of the wrists and ankles — the classical signs of myxoedema.

The voice may be hoarse, the pulse slow and there may be a delayed ankle jerk. The thyroid gland is often impalpable. Despite these striking clinical features there must be few experienced general practitioners who have not been mortified by the realisation that he has been witnessing one of his patients gradually developing hypothyroidism over several months before the diagnosis was made.

Mild hypothyroidism

Mild degrees of the disease are often difficult to spot. The clinical features are frequently non-specific and the physical signs subtle and slow to develop. The diagnosis must always be kept in mind, especially in the elderly and if there is a family history of thyroid disease. The use of a patient summary card acts as a reminder that the patient may have had destructive treatment to the gland in the past and it may also record a family history of thyroid disease. To miss hypothyroidism in a patient who has had a thyroidectomy years previously can be a source of embarrassment. Frequently the only symptoms are a lack of energy and a general loss of interest in life. Psychiatric complications, especially depression, are not uncommon; agitation, delusions and hallucinations (the so-called myxoedematous madness) are encountered more rarely. The only physical signs may be a slight infraorbital puffiness.

Laboratory diagnosis

1. The TSH is always raised in hypothyroidism, substantially in overt failure and significantly in mild. If the TSH is within normal limits a diagnosis of hypothyroidism due to primary thyroid disease can be excluded.

2. The T4 level is usually diminished in hypothyroidism but it may be just within the lower limit of the laboratory's normal range. The T4 is not as reliable a test as the TSH in the diagnosis of hypothyroidism, especially in the elderly when other disease, especially of a chronic nature, can cause a reduction in thyroid hormone levels.

Infantile hypothyroidism and cretinism

The recognition of infantile hypothyroidism is very important because of the consequences of the disease upon the physical and, more especially, the mental development of the child. It is not apparent at birth because the hormones cross the placental barrier. Failure to thrive, feeding problems and constipation should alert the doctor to the possibility of thyroid failure. An early diagnosis can prevent cerebral damage and the development of true cretinism.

Management

Replacement therapy using Thyroxine (T4) is the method of choice. The aim is to restore the TSH to normal using the minimal dose of T4. It must be stressed to the patient that he or she will require to take thyroxine for the rest of their lives.

The diagnosis of the disorder including laboratory findings must be clearly documented in the patient's records. 50 μg of T4 is given daily for 2 weeks increasing to 100 μg daily in a single dose for a further 6 weeks when blood should be taken for estimation of TSH and T4.

If the patient is symptom-free, no longer shows signs of hypothyroidism and if the laboratory results are within normal limits, the daily dose of 100 μg is maintained. Annual review should be undertaken mainly to confirm patient compliance.

If either symptoms or signs, or both, persist the daily dose of thyroxine should be increased to 150 μg and the patient reviewed in 3 months. Further TSH and T4 estimation should be performed and if these are within normal limits and the patient free from symptoms and signs the dosage can be reduced to 100 μg daily and a further review undertaken in 3 months when adjustment can be made according to clinical and laboratory findings.

Thyroxine should always be given in a single daily dose

so that the risk of patient non-compliance is reduced. The majority are controlled on 150 μg daily, some on 100 μg and only a few require 200 μg. If symptoms of hypothyroidism persist on 200 μg daily the patient is probably not taking the drug as instructed.

In the elderly, especially those suffering from ischaemic heart disease, cardiac side effects such as palpitations or angina or even heart failure may occur before the symptoms and signs of the disorder are eradicated. In such cases propranolol 20 mg three times a day, or some other beta-blocker, should be prescribed and increased according to response. In a small number of cases hospitalisation may be necessary.

Once the optimal dose of thyroxine has been established it is likely that the dosage can be maintained indefinitely although, theoretically, the degree of failure in autoimmune thyroid disease could increase and a larger dose of thyroxine be required. In such cases an annual estimation of TSH and T4 is indicated.

Hyperthyroidism

Hyperthyroidism may be defined as those clinical conditions which result from an increase in the circulating levels of one or both thyroid hormones and at least 99% of cases are associated with Graves disease or nodular goitre (Evered 1976).

Incidence and aetiology

In a survey in the United Kingdom the incidence of newly and previously diagnosed cases of hyperthyroidism was between 1.2 and 1.7% giving a prevalence rate of 21–27/1000 females and 1–2/1000 males (Tunbridge et al 1975). In an average practice of 2500 it was reported that a total of four patients with hyperthyroid disease consulted annually (Fry 1979).

The aetiology of Graves disease remains obscure but currently it is thought to have an immunological basis (Evered 1976, Hall et al 1980). Hyperthyroidism due to excessive ingestion of thyroid hormone in a patient being treated for hypothyroidism is probably not recognised sufficiently (Clark 1982). Patients taking more than 200 μg thyroxine daily may display symptoms of hyperthyroidism.

Clinical picture

In the well established case the recognition of the disorder is easy. The patient, most frequently a woman, presents in a nervous and often agitated state, jittery and fidgety. She may complain of increased anxiety and on questioning admits to intolerance of heat and loss of weight. Frequently there is a fine tremor of the outstretched fingers and the palms are sweaty. There is a tachycardia with a full and bounding pulse. Eye signs are an important feature with swelling of the eyelids, conjunctival oedema which often causes irritation and possibly exophthalmos and lid retraction. In Graves disease the thyroid is frequently symmetrically enlarged but in a small proportion of cases the thyroid appears to be normal. In some cases there is a stystolic bruit over the gland. In toxic nodular goitre the thyroid enlargement may be considerable but eye signs are usually absent. In the younger patient the most difficult diagnosis is the differentiation of hyperthyroidism from an anxiety state, especially if thyroid enlargement is absent.

Presentation of hyperthyroidism in the elderly can be misleading. The disease frequently presents with cardiovascular symptoms and signs such as palpitations, angina or even heart failure. Atrial fibrillation is a frequent finding. Failure to respond to the usual therapy for these conditions should alert the doctor to the possibility of the disorder.

Laboratory diagnosis

A clinical diagnosis must always be confirmed by the laboratory because the treatment of the disease, no matter which method is chosen, is not without risk.

1. *Thyroid hormones.* Hyperthyroidism usually results in raised levels of both thyroid hormones. T4 toxicosis occurs in 95% of cases but it is wise to request a T3 estimation in order to pick up the remainder. The latter most frequently occurs in patients who relapse after thyroidectomy or antithyroid drugs and in toxic nodular goitre.

2. *TSH response to TRH.* If hyperthyroidism is suspected, especially in elderly patients, and hormone levels are found to be at the upper limit of laboratory normal, it is wise to ask for the TSH response to an injection of 200 μg of TRH. Euthyroid patients reveal a rapid increase in TSH; hyperthyroid patients show no such increase.

Management

Three methods of treatment are available, antithyroid drugs, partial thyroidectomy and radioactive iodine. All cases of hyperthyroidism will respond in some measure to antithyroid drugs. The only method available to the general practitioner is the use of antithyroid drugs combined with a beta-adrenergic blocking drug such as propranolol. Natural remission of the disease or relapses can occur during treatment and it is probably preferable for the general practitioner to manage cases of hyperthyroidism in collaboration with a specialist colleague.

The drug of choice is carbimazole (Neo-Mercazole) in a dose of 10 mg four times a day spaced throughout the waking day for 4 to 8 weeks depending upon response, an assessment of which is made mainly upon clinical grounds based upon the improvement in the symptoms and signs of the disease. At this stage laboratory tests can be misleading. Complications of drug therapy are relatively uncommon. At the outset the patient must be warned of the rare complication of agranulocytosis, and the possible occurrence of drug rashes. If the latter appears or if mouth ulcers occur the patient must be told to stop the drug immediately and attend her doctor.

In the early stages of treatment the distressing symptoms of hyperthyroidism, tachycardia, sweating and tremor can be mitigated by the use of propranolol. As the effect of carbimazole increases, the beta blockade can be discontinued. Once the patient is euthyroid the dose of carbimazole is reduced to 10 mg daily and maintained for at least 1 year or possibly two. Some physicians combine the maintenance dosage of carbimazole with thyroxine 0.15 mg (Evered 1976). If, during or after treatment with antithyroid drugs, there is a relapse, specialist referral is indicated so that surgery or treatment with radioactive iodine may be considered depending upon the age of the patient and the clinical findings.

DIABETES MELLITUS

INCIDENCE AND AETIOLOGY

Diabetes mellitus is the commonest endocrine disease in the United Kingdom. Surveys have reported a prevalence of 1–1.5% of whom about half were previously undiagnosed (Redhead 1960). Most of the unknown cases were of the non-insulin dependent type formerly known as maturity-onset diabetes. In an average sized practice of 2500 it was reported that in any year there were two to four new cases of diabetes diagnosed and 15–20 diabetic patients consulting (Fry 1979).

Diabetes is no longer regarded as a single entity but as a syndrome whose essential characteristic is hyperglycaemiia and consequent glycosuria. The hyperglycaemia may occur only after the intake of carbohydrate and there may be no symptoms. If the hyperglycaemia persists however the quantity of glucose lost through the kidney increases giving rise to polyuria, thirst and weight loss. The causative mechanisms of the syndrome have as yet not been clearly defined (Hall 1980).

PRESENTING SYMPTOMS AND SIGNS

Symptoms occasionally develop rapidly over several hours but in the large majority of patients, especially in the older age groups, the onset is insidious; indeed, there may be no symptoms whatever.

The classical presenting features are:

1. Thirst, polyuria and tiredness
2. Weight loss
3. Recurrent skin sepsis and boils
4. Pruritis vulvae or balanitis
5. Deteriorating visual acuity

6. Glycosuria
7. Ketocidaemia

Testing for glycosuria

In certain circumstances testing for glycosuria is essential:

1. The patient who complains of symptoms suggestive of diabetes.
2. Urinary symptoms: frequency, dysuria, nocturia, enuresis.
3. Recurrent skin infections, pruritis vulvae, balanitis, and foot ulcers.
4. Unexplained tiredness and apathy.
5. Eye symptoms, deterioration of visual acuity.
6. In the middle aged and elderly: angina, claudication and neuritic pain in the limbs.

Routine screening for diabetes in general practice is unrewarding and should be confined to selected peak risk groups (Redhead 1975):

1. Those of 50 years and over.
2. Those with a family history of diabetes.
3. Women who have had a baby of 4.5 kg (10 lb) birth weight or over.
4. Women who have had six or more children.
5. Women who have had four or more unexplained stillbirths.
6. Women who have shown excessive weight gain in pregnancy.

DIAGNOSIS

Frequently the symptoms and signs are so clear-cut that a confirmation of the diagnosis can be made by taking a random blood sugar. A level in excess of 11 mmol/l (200 mg/100 ml) clinches the diagnosis. In a fasting patient a level of 8 mmol/l (140 mg/100 ml) is diagnostic (Keen 1981).

If the results of either of these investigations is borderline or if there is any other indication such as glycosuria in pregnancy, a 2-hour blood sugar screen is indicated. The patient is given a loaded oral dose of 75 mg of glucose 2 hours before taking a single blood glucose estimation. If this value is less than 6 mmol/l (110 mg/100 ml) the patient is normal. When the 2-hour value is above 12 mmol/l (215 mg/100 ml) the diagnosis is diabetes. Values between these two limits indicates impaired glucose tolerance (IGT) and requires a full oral glucose tolerance test. Interpretation of this test is generally based on criteria suggested by Jarrett & Keen (1976) (Table 14.1).

Table 14.1   Oral glucose tolerance test: 75 g glucose load

	Venous whole blood	Capillary whole blood
For the diagnosis of diabetes mellitus		
Fasting	>7.0 mmol/l (126 mg/100 ml)	>7.0 mmol/l (126 mg/100 ml)
2 hours after glucose	>10.0 mmol/l (180 mg/100 ml)	>11.0 mmol/l (198 mg/100 ml)
With at least one intervening value	>10.0 mmol/l (180 mg/100 ml)	>11.0 mmol/l (198 mg/100 ml)
To define impaired glucose tolerance		
Fasting	<7.0 mmol/l (126 mg/100 ml)	<7.0 mmol/l (126 mg/100 ml)
2 hours after glucose	>7.0 mmol/l (126 mg/100 ml)	>8.0 mmol/l (144 mg/100 ml)
With intervening values	<10.0 mmol/l (180 mg/100 ml)	<11.0 mmol/l (198 mg/100 ml)

Classification

In the past the syndrome was divided into juvenile onset diabetes and maturity onset diabetes. Generally this classification was practical but in a minority of cases it could be misleading. Maturity onset diabetes occurring in the young is rare but not infrequently the insulin dependent form of diabetes, indistinguishable from juvenile onset diabetes because of the relative acuteness and rapidity of onset in some cases, can occur in patients of mature years with potentially serious consequences.

A classification of diabetes mellitus was devised by the Medical and Scientific Section of the British Diabetic Association (1978), which divided primary diabetes into the insulin dependent type (IDDM Type 1) and the non insulin dependent type (NIDDM Type 2) which it then subdivided into the obese and non-obese. Other conditions listed in the classification are gestational diabetes, in which the disorder is first recognised in pregnancy and remits thereafter, and impaired glucose tolerance which should not be regarded as normal. Long-term follow-up of these patients has shown that annually 2–4% of patients with impaired glucose tolerance develop unequivocal diabetes (Keen 1981). It is therefore essential that the defect should be carefully documented in the patient's records, preferably on a summary card.

The two clinical syndromes of diabetes have hyperglycaemia as their common characteristic but are strikingly different in many respects. Type 1 cases are usually diagnosed before the age of 30 years; in these patients the onset is rapid, they became ketotic without treatment and almost invariably require insulin. Complications of diabetes are common in later years. Type 2 cases are usually middle-aged or older, the onset is insidious, ketosis is rare, they respond to diet alone or to oral hypoglycaemics and only very rarely require insulin.

Complications of diabetes

For many years it was believed that if the diagnosis of diabetes was made early and treatment commenced the complications of the disease could be prevented or postponed (Joslin et al 1946). Experience over the past 30 years has not confirmed this hypothesis and complications are common even in the apparently well controlled diabetic. The incidence of complications is thought to increase in the presence of persistent hyperglycaemia even of moderate degree.

Diabetic retinopathy

In the United Kingdom 14% of all new registrations of blindness in patients aged 30–64 years are due to diabetes and diabetes is the commonest cause of blindness in this age group. As many as 80% of diabetics suffer from retinopathy within 15–20 years from the diagnosis (Kohner 1981). Approximately 2% of all diabetics are registered as blind (Clark 1980).

Early clinical diagnosis of retinopathy is important because it is possible to prevent further deterioration by tighter diabetic control (Clark & Duncan 1978). Clinically retinopathy is classified as background, maculopathy, proliferative and advanced. Background retinopathy produces no visual symptoms and it is wise to make an ophthalmological assessment as soon as a diagnosis of diabetes is made. Many experts consider that a specialist ophthalmologist should make a yearly assessment of all cases of diabetes. This puts an enormous burden upon the ophthalmological services and a clinician who undertakes the management of diabetes must be able to recognise background diabetic retinopathy so that when it is diagnosed a specialist ophthalmological opinion can be sought. Even a slight deterioration in visual acuity is a danger sign in a diabetic.

The more advanced degrees of retinopathy are now treatable in some measure but early recognition is of paramount importance.

Diabetic neuropathy

Neurological complications of diabetes usually take the form of a sensory neuropathy of the glove and stocking variety, more commonly the latter. It occurs in long-term diabetics, is more common in men and is irreversible. Autonomic neuropathy is relatively rare but can be unpleasant causing diarrhoea, postural hypotension, impotence and other manifestations of autonomic disturbance.

The diabetic foot

Disorders of the foot in diabetes which can ultimately result in gangrene are caused by a combination of factors: vasculitis, trauma, infection and neuropathy. The slightest trauma should be treated seriously and the patient warned to consult his doctor even with a lesion that he might consider to be trivial. Regular chiropody and early chemotherapy have resulted in a decrease in the incidence of gangrene.

Diabetic nephropathy

The warning sign of diabetic nephropathy is proteinuria which should call for an immediate tightening of diabetic control. Once persistent proteinuria has been established the progress of diabetic nephropathy is relentless and cannot be halted.

Management of diabetes

The clinician and chemical pathologist can assess the disturbance of carbohydrate metabolism with varying degrees of success. Patient understanding of his disorder is frequently a key factor in successful management but even the well controlled patient frequently develops complications as described above.

The aims of treatment are:

1. To maintain the blood sugar as near normal as possible.
2. To prevent or delay complications.
3. To enable the patient to lead as normal a life as possible.
4. To educate the patient to the limit of his mental capacity so that he has the knowledge and motivation to provide for his own care.

THE ROLE OF THE GENERAL PRACTITIONER

In 1971 Malins & Stuart stated that most of the 500 000 diagnosed diabetics in the United Kingdom were referred to diabetic clinics at least once and the vast majority continued to attend the clinics regularly. Patients had come to rely upon the clinics for the regular care of the disease so that the general practitioner had largely ceased to take an interest in their problems and in diabetes in general. Diabetic clinics were thus overburdened with a heavy load of routine work. Malins & Stuart and their staff of the Birmingham General Hospital diabetic clinic combined with four general practitioners in an experiment in shared care which proved to be of benefit to the patient, to the general practitioner and to the diabetic clinic.

In recent years other workers have reported successful shared care schemes (Thorn & Russell 1973, Hill & Upton 1981, Saunders & Ruben 1981). Such schemes depend upon the willingness of all those involved in primary and secondary care to work together as a team; the hospital consultant with his specialist nursing staff often including a liaison sister who will visit the patient at home, the dietitian, the clinical pathologist, the general practitioner, health visitor, chiropodist and in many cases the ophthalmologist.

In group practice consideration should be given to the establishment of a clinic within the practice. A practice of four doctors might have as many as 80 diabetics on the list and therefore a monthly clinic could be organised by the partner with a particular interest in this disorder. Visits by the hospital consultant to the general practitioner clinic on a regular basis have been found to be helpful and clinical meetings and discussions at the hospital clinic enhance co-operation. Hill & Upton (1981) in the shared scheme in Poole have devised a Co-operation Record Book which contains not only useful information for patients but allows all those actively concerned in the management of the patient to record and communicate one with another.

Shared care is particularly useful in non-insulin dependent diabetics who account for 50% of the average hospital clinic attendances. Many well controlled insulin dependent patients may also attend their general practitioner and only attend the hospital clinic occasionally, thus allowing the specialist more time to deal with the difficult cases.

Initial stabilisation

Patients with Type 1 diabetes are frequently stabilised in hospital but there are some clinicians who advocate initial stabilisation of IDDM at home (Bridgman 1981). Type 2 diabetes can be stabilised by the general practitioner without referral to hospital but the very essence of shared care is that all cases of diabetes should receive the benefit of all the facilities available, such as a dietitian, a chiropodist and a structured educational programme which is available in some centres (Hill & Upton 1981).

The insulin dependent diabetic will have the acute illness controlled under specialist supervision by the use of short acting insulins and thereafter a basic dosage regime established. Injection technique and experience of hypoglycaemia are arranged. Dieting principles and urine or blood testing are taught and explained.

The non-insulin dependent cases are given a target weight and instructions about diet. If the target weight is achieved and the disease is still uncontrolled, oral hypoglycaemic agents may be necessary. Urine testing is taught.

Follow-up

The aims of follow-up must be:

1. To achieve good diabetic control.

2. To detect complications.
3. To be certain that patients attend regularly according to their requirements.

If patient care is being shared between general practice and the hospital clinics it is important that these aims should be monitored and in particular that patients are not lost to follow-up, probably the most frequent failure in any scheme especially when several agencies are involved. The combined regular review of patients by both the diabetic clinic and the general practitioner are essential if these aims are to be achieved.

As the maintenance of normoglycaemia is the most important factor in the prevention of complications, the introduction of portable machines to measure whole blood glucose levels makes it possible for the more intelligent patients to attain more consistently normal glucose levels. Stickland & Wales (1982) have reported favourably on the performance of a reflectance photometer (Glucometer, Ames Division, Miles Laboratories), but other testing methods are available utilising a printed colour scale, which do not require the use of a meter and these have proved to be of value. Although less accurate they are less expensive.

For the less intelligent and for the patients who cannot afford to purchase a meter, the introduction of the Glycosolated haemoglobin (GHb) determination is available in many centres. This test correlates the mean blood glucose during the previous 4 to 6 weeks and provides a more meaningful measure of plasma glucose levels than the random blood sugar estimation. The GHb should be used at 3-monthly intervals when attempts are being made to improve control. Under normal circumstances a yearly estimation is useful.

Planned long-term care
The frequency of consultation and whether it will be with the general practitioner or at the diabetic clinic depends upon the stability of the disorder, the presence of complications and the intelligence of the patient, but the requirements are similar:

1. Duties performed by nurse before the doctor's consultation:

Weight
Urine — glucose, protein, ketones
Blood pressure — at least yearly
Visual acuity — at least yearly, more frequently if there has been deterioration in vision, in long-standing cases and in those of middle age and over
Blood sugar and glycosolated haemoglobin

2. Doctor's consultation:

Subjective — General health
— Specific symptoms — hypoglycaemia, visual disturbance, foot problems, paraesthesia
Objective — Review of patient's urine or blood charts
— Data provided by the nurse
— Examination of CVS, nervous system, eyes, feet and injection sites
Action — Depending upon findings, adjust diet, insulin dosage and treat complications and if necessary refer for specialist advice.
Plan — Date, time and place of next appointment
— Record the salient points onto the patient's records and, if shared care is being undertaken, onto a co-operation card.

REFERENCES

Bridgman J F 1981 Management and stabilisation of insulin dependent diabetics at home. Update 23: 1543
Clark B F 1980 Treatment of diabetes. Update 21: 1311–31
Clark B F, Duncan L J P 1980 In: Alstead S, Girdwood R H (ed) Textbook of medical treatment, 14th edn. Churchill Livingstone, Edinburgh.
Clark F 1982 Thyrotoxicosis. Practitioner 226: 1364: 197
Evered D C 1976 Diseases of the thyroid. Pitman Medical, London
Fry J 1979 Common diseases, their nature, incidence and care, 2nd edn. M T P Press, Lancaster
Hall R, Anderson J, Smart G A, Besser M 1980 Fundamentals of clinical endocrinology, 3rd edn. Pitman Books, London
Hill R D, Upton C E 1981 Care of the diabetic in the community. Medicine International 1: 8–105
Jarrett R J, Keen H 1976 Hypoglycaemia and diabetes mellitus. Lancet 2: 1009
Joslin E P, Root H F, White P, Marble A, Bailey C C 1946 Treatment of diabetes mellitus, 8th edn. Lea and Febiger, Philadelphia
Keen H 1981 The nature of the diabetes syndrome. Medicine International 1: 8 334
Malins J M, Stuart J M 1971 Diabetic clinic in general practice. British Medical Journal iv: 161
Medical Advisory Committee of the British Diabetic Association 1978. Draft Memorandum regarding diagnostic criteria for diabetes
Redhead I H 1960 Incidence of glycosuria and diabetes in a general practice. British Medical Journal 1: 695
Redhead I H 1975 In: Hart C R (ed) Screening in general practice. Churchill Livingstone, Edinburgh
Stickland M H, Wales J K 1982 Blood glucose determination: the use of a new reflectance photometer. Practitioner 226: 1364 271
Saunders J, Ruben A 1981 Diabetes — the St Thomas' district approach
Thorn P A, Russell R G 1973 Diabetic clinics today and tomorrow: mini clinics in general practice. British Medical Journal 11: 534
Tunbridge W M G et al 1975 Thyroid diseases in an English community. In: 7th International Thyroid Conference. Excerpta Medica, Amsterdam
Working Party of the Royal College of General Practitioners 1962 A diabetes survey. British Medical Journal 1: 149

Genito-urinary problems in women

INTRODUCTION

Gynaecology is no longer specifically a branch of the surgical art. With the shift of emphasis towards diagnosis and prevention medical gynaecology is fast emerging, and is increasingly relevant to good general practice. Progress in the fields of endocrinology, radiotherapy, chemotherapy, and early screening for cancer has banished the mutilating surgery of the past.

The practitioner with an average list of patients can expect around 400 consultations of a gynaecological nature per annum (Lloyd 1976). Much is heard of the frequency with which patients with gynaecological complaints are referred to out-patient clinics. Perhaps it could be interpreted that the doctor is too busy to provide adequate care, but many practitioners do not think they have the necessary facilities available for the investigation and treatment of gynaecological problems. Emphasis nowadays is on larger group practices and the numbers of patients with similar problems become such that special clinics can be organised, with appropriate nursing assistance — for example ante-natal, family planning and gynaecological. In the smaller group practices, the numbers of patients with gynaecological problems may not merit a separate structured clinic, but many practitioners find it an advantage to allocate a consulting session with longer appointments, to facilitate a detailed examination with nursing assistance.

HISTORY-TAKING

For the accurate diagnosis of gynaecological problems, as in other areas, the most important evidence is produced by the history (Jeffcoate 1970), with confirmatory evidence being sought through speculum and bimanual examination. It must always be remembered that the discussion of private and intimate matters in gynaecological problems is an ordeal for the patient who may well have thought long and hard before presenting herself at the surgery. The response to the embarrassed and anxious patient needs to be sympathy, tact and understanding if the history obtained is to be comprehensive and meaningful.

A systematic approach to a gynaecological history is best. Figures 15.1a and 15.1b show the proforma used in Craigshill Health Centre, Livingston, with standard headings in a systematic layout, so that no significant points are missed. From personal knowledge or practice records, background information concerning the patient is available which will often be helpful in completing the clinical picture.

The patient should be allowed to express herself freely. This will give her confidence, and allow the doctor to make an assessment of the patient's own priorities relating to her symptoms — whether they be gynaecological or otherwise. With increasing experience, attention can then be focused on what is seen as the essence of the problem — be it gynaecological, psychosomatic, or even psychosexual.

THE EXAMINATION

THE NURSE

For a detailed gynaecological examination, adequate nursing assistance and proper equipment are essential. The nurse in attendance (whether a practice nurse, or a member of the community nursing team) is invaluable during a gynaecological assessment. She has primarily a supportive role for the patient, to assist with undressing, and preparing her on the couch for the examination. While so doing she can explain the procedures involved, check on the equipment required (such as the choice of speculum, the spatula for taking a cervical smear, or the fixative medium) and at the same time exert a reassuring influence on the patient. This role is of inestimable value as a chaperone and in allowing the patient to relax. The nurse can also complete the preparation and labelling of any culture medium bottle, slide or containers and laboratory forms that may be required for blood tests.

CRAIGSHILL HEALTH CENTRE

Date: **Patient's Name & Address**
Hospital No.:
Health Centre No.:
Age   Parity   L.M.P.   E.D.D.

Present Complaint
MSWD   Religion   Menarche   Menopause
Infertility   —   Primary   —   Secondary   —   Voluntary   —   Involuntary

Gynaecological Symptoms
Menstrual Cycle   :   Dysmenorrhoea   :
Menorrhagia   :   Vaginal Discharge :
IM Bleeding   :   Colour
PC Bleeding   :   Blood Staining   :
PM Bleeding   :   Odour   :
Hormone Therapy :   Pruritis Vulvae   :
Contraception   :   Dyspareunia   :

Gynaecological History

Urinary Symptoms
Frequency :   Urgency :   Loin Pain :
Dysuria   :   Stress Incontinence :   Ureteric Colic :
Nocturia   :   Haematuria :

Previous Medical History   Allergies :   Current Drugs :
TB: UTI: Operations :
Blood Transfusions: Last Chest X-ray:

A **Previous Obstetric History**

Family History

Social History
CVS   Angina   Oedema   Dyspnoea
RS   Cough   Smoking   Bronchitis
GIS   Appetite   Weight   Dyspepsia
                             (Gain/Loss)

Examination
Appearance   Build   Breasts
Hair Distribution   Thyroid
Abdomen   Scars
                                             Masses
                                             Tenderness
                                             Inguinal Glands
                                             Hernia
                                             Bs

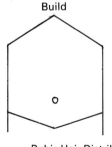

PR   Pubic Hair Distribution

Vaginal Examination
External Urethral Orifice   Vulva
Vagina   Cervix
Uterus   Appendages

B Weight   Urinalysis

Fig. 15.1   a. Gynaecological proforma (History).   b. Gynaecological proforma (Examination).

GENERAL EXAMINATION

Apart from noting the general build of the patient, any pallor of skin or mucous membrane should be looked for, perhaps denoting an anaemia associated with menorrhoagia or malignant disease. Breast examination should whenever possible be included, save in a young unmarried girl (unless pregnancy is suspected) since a breast lesion of some type is found in 1% of all gynaecological patients. Details of breast examination findings should be carefully recorded to avoid this embarrassing examination being repeated unnecessarily frequently.

The procedure for abdominal examination — when this is thought to be necessary — follows that for any suspected intra-abdominal problem. Particular attention however should be paid to the presence or absence of previous laparascopy scars: these can be small and as such easily overlooked. It is useful to remember that an abdominal mass such as an ovarian cyst, will reveal dullness on percussion over the central abdomen, with a tympanitic note in the flanks, whereas with ascites, the converse will be found. Where pregnancy is suspected, the fetal heart will usually be heard with the conventional stethoscope by about 18 weeks gestation, although with a Doptone or Sonicaid machine (using the Doppler effect) the fetal heart can be picked up from the 13th week onwards.

SPECULUM EXAMINATION

Speculum examination of the vagina and cervix assists inspection, and should therefore precede manual examination. Any vaginal discharge present can be seen and removed for examination and culture before it is

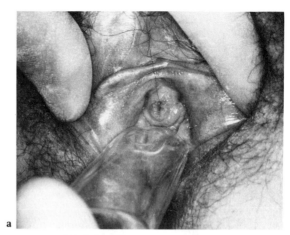
a

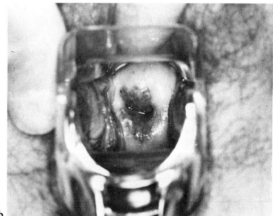
b

Fig. 15.3 Insertion of a Cusco's speculum: a. Introduction. b. Visualisation of the cervix.

contaminated with lubricant. Cellular debris from the cervix, uterus and the vagina to a large extent also should be left undisturbed and can be used for a cervical or vaginal smear, or for cytological study. A bivalve speculum should be used to inspect the vagina and to visualise the cervix (whether the patient is in the dorsal or left lateral position) (Fig. 15.2a, b) while for the assessment of genital prolapse, the Sim's type speculum is preferable (Fig. 15.2c) — with the patient in the left lateral position. The bivalve (Cusco's) type of speculum should be inserted closed (Figs. 15.3a & b) in keeping with the cross section of the vagina. There should be a choice of at least three sizes of speculum available (small, medium or large) and the appropriate size should be selected. Once fixed in position by means of the ratchet the examiner's hand is free to take a high vaginal swab, a cervical smear, or to insert an intra-uterine device (described elsewhere).

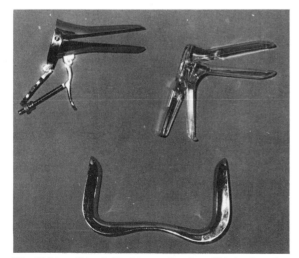

Fig. 15.2 a. Cusco's bivalve speculum (metallic); b. Cusco's bivalve speculum (disposable); c. Sim's double-ended speculum

CERVICAL SMEARS

Figure 15.4 shows the basic equipment necessary for

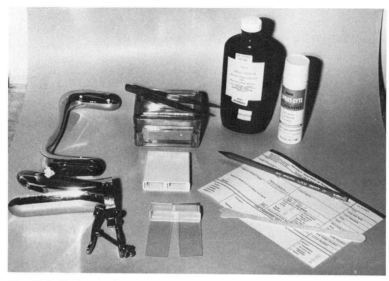

Fig. 15.4   Equipment for taking a cervical smear

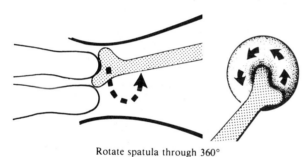

Rotate spatula through 360°

Fig. 15.5   Taking a uterine cervical smear (By courtesy of British Society for Clinical Cytology)

taking a cervical smear. The glass slide (with a ground glass end) should be named in pencil (which does not wash off during fixation) before taking the smear. With the patient in the dorsal or left lateral position and with well adjusted lighting, the clinical appearance of the cervix is noted on visualisation by means of the speculum. The Ayre spatula is then inserted into the cervical os, and rotated through 360° (Fig. 15.5). A florid cervical erosion or an inflammatory cervix may bleed slightly though readily. On withdrawal of the spatula the smear is spread evenly and thinly in one firm stroke along the named glass slide which is then immersed in and covered by fixative for at least 10 minutes. A cervical smear should be taken prior to a bimanual vaginal examination and at the time of routine speculum examination. Lubricant jelly should not be used when taking the smear.

PELVIC EXAMINATION

As in the history-taking, the examination shoould be

conducted systematically, otherwise important information may be missed. A good external light source, such as an anglepoise lamp, is esssential. The examining hand must be gloved; the gloves must be clean though not necessarily surgically sterile. For a gynaecological examination, it is usual to have the patient in the dorsal position (Fig. 15.6) although some gynaecologists prefer the left lateral position (Fig. 15.7). Inspection of the introitus and testing for prolapse is easier with the patient in the left lateral position as is visualising the cervix when vaginal laxity is marked or if the patient is very obese. It should be remembered that from the left lateral position the patient can turn to the dorsal position with the vagin-

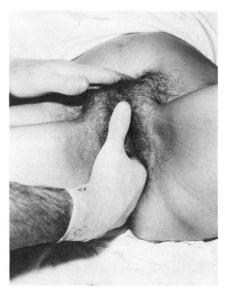

Fig. 15.6   Examination in dorsal position

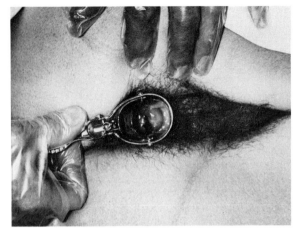

Fig. 15.7 Examination in 'left lateral' position. The upper buttock can obscure the view unless lifted with a hand.

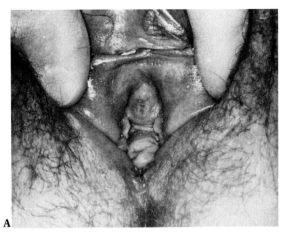

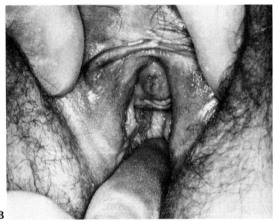

Fig. 15.8 Vaginal examination: A. First stage. B. Later stage.

al hand in situ, and bimanual examination can then be completed. Inspection of the vulva, labia (for redness, excoriation and pigmentation), the perineum and perianal regions (for evidence of previous scars, haemorrhoids, and fissures) is essential. The contour of the vaginal introitus should be noted — gaping and lax in cases of prolapse, while in nullipara it will be virtually closed. With two fingers of the left hand, the labia are gently parted, care being taken to avoid pulling on the pubic hair as this will cause pain and produce spasm (Fig. 15.8a). With the labia still parted, the patient should be asked to cough or bear down, to demonstrate a cystocele or rectocoele; if there is, for example, a second degree uterine prolapse, the cervix will appear at the vulva. A cough will also demonstrate the presence of stress incontinence (so long as the bladder is not completely empty).

With the labia separated by the fingers of the left hand, the first and second fingers of the right hand are now introduced into the vagina. A simple, bland lubricant such as KY jelly is suitable for this procedure, being odourless, colourless, non-irritant and water soluble. To avoid the sensitive clitoris and urethra, the index finger can be carefully invaginated first (Fig. 15.8b), gently pulling down the posterior margin of the vulva towards the anus. The introitus is thus stretched sufficiently and painlessly to allow the introduction of the middle finger. Having done this, the thumb of the right hand should be kept extended, and the elbow pointed well down towards the table (Fig. 15.6).

Systematically, this examination assesses the rugosity of the vaginal mucosa, and any bulging in front or behind is noted. The cervix is then located, and the contour of the external cervical os noted — varying from a small rounded, usually smooth depression in the nulliparous patient, to an irregular transverse slit in the parous pa-

tient. The direction of the cervix should then be noted; where the uterus is retroverted, the cervix will point anteriorly — or even up towards the ceiling. Bimanual examination is essential to bring the uterus and the ovaries within reach. The *abdominal* hand (which is the more important) should be placed initially just below the umbilicus, and moved lower gradually, until the fundus is felt, and presses towards the fingers of the vaginal hand in the anterior fornix. If the uterus is not felt at this stage, it is lying above and behind the abdominal hand. Particular points concerning the cervix and uterus to be noted are the size, shape, position and consistency, mobility, and tenderness on pressure or on movement. The normal uterus and the ovaries are tender when squeezed between the two hands.

It should be borne in mind that rectal examination is a useful adjunct — particularly when vaginal examination is impossible, and it has a special place in the pelvic investigation of babies and children.

Examination under anaesthesia may be necessary where pelvic examination is otherwise difficult or impossible. It cannot be substituted for a gentle unhurried assessment without anaesthesia, as the important sign of tenderness is lost.

HIGH VAGINAL, CERVICAL OR URETHRAL SWABS

With the aid of a speculum, a vaginal swab can be taken by mopping the posterior and lateral fornices with a simple cotton wool bud, and depositing the 'bud' in Stewart's medium, from which trichomonads can be isolated after 48 hours. If there is a microscope in the practice, trichomonads (when deposited on a drop of saline on a slide and covered with a coverslip) can be confirmed in the active state — free flagellae with a rapid whip-like motion; the flagellating membrane can sometimes be seen rippling against the cell wall. The interval between taking the swab and microscopic examination should be as short as possible if accurate results are to be obtained. For the isolation of gonococci swabs specifically from the cervical os, the urethral orifice and the rectum are necessary in view of the predisposition of the organism for this epithelium.

VAGINAL DISCHARGE

At the outset, it should be remembered from physiological principles that a vaginal discharge is normal, and consists of desquamated epithelial cells from the vagina, together with a vaginal transudate, and cervical secretion. This fluid or 'discharge' changes in quantity and quality with the stage of the menstrual cycle, being increased in the premenstrual phase and when the 'ovulation cascade' from the cervix occurs. In pregnancy also there is an increase in both vaginal and cervical discharges. A discharge becomes pathological when an excess of pus cells and infecting organisms are demonstrable along with the desquamated epithelial cells.

Various organisms normally inhabit the vagina, but the Gram-positive anaerobic Doderlein's bacillus is usually predominant. With its production of lactic acid, other organisms are kept in check. The defence mechanism of the vagina is thus directly proportional to the number of Doderlein's bacilli present, although it is further aided by the functional closure of the cervix by mucus — especially if there is a cervical erosion or a significant degree of ectropion. However, during menstruation the cervical plug is absent, and the alkaline menstrual discharge reduces the vaginal acidity. Trichomonal or gonococcal infections, therefore, are more acute during menstruation. The defence mechanism of the genital tract varies also in certain situations:

1. In *childhood* the vaginal epithelium is thin and vulnerable while the endometrium is as yet poorly developed. Susceptibility to ascending infection is therefore obvious.

2. In the *elderly*, the vaginal epithelium becomes thin and pale, while the endometrium has atrophied, so that vaginitis and endometritis become common, and the possibility of pyometra should be borne in mind.

3. In the *puerperium*, when several factors predispose to genital infection:

a. A raw placental site.
b. Minor abrasions or lacerations cause breaks in the epithelial linings of the vagina and cervix.
c. The tissues may be bruised or devitalised.
d. The discharge of liquor and lochia (both alkaline) reduce vaginal acidity.
e. Degenerating blood clots or remnants of decidua or membranes are an ideal medium for incubating invading organisms.
f. The strain of pregnancy and fatigue of confinement, possibly with a degree of anaemia, lower the general resistance of the patient.

Excessive 'discharge' may be due to a cervical erosion (when exposure to the acid vaginal desquamate stimulates the cervix to produce an excess of mucus), ectropion of the cervix (commonly after childbirth and occasionally from surgical injury), the presence of an intra-uterine device (where the tail can irritate the glandular epithelium) and, lastly, patients on oral contraceptives or who are pregnant, have an increased degree of vaginal desquamate.

VAGINITIS

Since numerous organisms normally inhabit the vagina, an acute infection could be attributed to any of these — streptococcus (anaerobic and aerobic, haemolytic and non-haemolytic), staphylococcus, *Escherichia coli*, gonococcus, pneumococcus, *Mycobacterium tuberculosis*, *Cl. welchii*, or the treponema pallidum, as well as the well known parasites *Trichomonas vaginalis*, *Candida albicans*, *Pediculus pubis*, and tinea. Some of these organisms (even *Cl. welchii*) can be found in the vagina without being pathogenic, and their presence can represent either a normal or a carrier state. The commonest infections met with in general practice are trichomonal vaginitis, monilial vaginitis and senile vaginitis. An offensive discharge due to a foreign body, such as a forgotten tampon, or condom, must always be borne in mind.

SENILE VAGINITIS

This condition is associated with a loss of resistance of the vaginal tissues. Apart from a mottled red vagina, attributed to normal climacteric change, there may well also be a purulent discharge — usuaally yellowish, sometimes bloodstained — causing soreness of the vulva with some excoriation in the more severe cases. Multiple reddened areas may be seen in the vault and around the urethral orifice. Patchy ulceration can result in adhesions forming between the anterior and posterior walls to produce stenosing or partial closure of the vagina. Any patient of post-menopausal age who presents with bleeding or blood staining requires an examination under anaesthesia and diagnostic curretage, and cervical cytology or biopsy are essential, since even if vaginitis is present, the patient could additionally have a carcinoma of the body of the uterus.

The principle of treatment is to restore the viability of the vaginal epithelium by the local application of an oestrogen containing cream, such as dienoestrol for 2 to 3 weeks. Alternatively, oestrogens can be given in pessary form, combined with lactic acid (0.5% to 1%) to be inserted into the vagina each night. After the course of hormone therapy, atrophy of the vaginal mucosa will recur, if at all, very gradually.

TRICHOMONAL VAGINITIS

This is a protozoal infection caused by *Trichomonas vaginalis*, and is found in approximately 50% of women complaining of discharge. Being a sexually transmitted disease, it is most common in the younger adult population. The trichomonas group of organisms is a large one and some members can be found in the bladder and the large bowel. The *Trichomonas vaginalis* (morphologically different from the the other forms) is approximately the size of a polymorphonuclear leucocyte, although usually ovoid or pear-shaped, with five flagellae, one of which is bound to the cell wall by a thin membrane.

Clinically, the most severe form of trichomonal vaginitis is usually seen in women who have recently been infected for the first time. Such a patient will complain of a profuse offensive vagnal discharge, with soreness of the skin over the vulva, groins and peri-anal area, and often extending over quite a large area on the inner aspect of the thighs. There is also usually some irritation of the vulva and the vagina. Bright red erythematous areas can extend on to the thighs, and encircle the anus. The inexperienced eye may readily confuse the appearance with that of a fungal skin infection. The vulva and introitus are also bright red, while a purulent discharge (greeny-yellow in colour, characteristically with a slightly frothy appearance, and with a pathognomonic musty odour) is evident. Internal examination reveals obvious vaginitis, with prominent rugae due to swelling of the mucous membrane which is bright red in colour.

Milder forms are much more common and the patient complains of an offensive discharge with, perhaps, some vulval irritation. External examination may well reveal no abnormality, but on insertion of a speculum, some purulent discharge will be evident in the vaginal vault, often with a few bubbles suggesting a 'frothy' tendency and there will be evidence of vaginitis.

Even when the diagnosis seems obvious from the history and clinical findings, the possibility of co-existing infection must always be borne in mind — particularly with gonorrhoea, and especially when the trichomonal infestation has been recently acquired. Likewise it is prudent to look for infection by *Candida albicans* since, if this is present, a severe fungal vaginitis may develop when the trichomoniasis has been controlled.

The standard treatment is the oral administration of metronidazole (Flagyl) in a dose of 200 mg three times daily or nimorazole (Naxogin) for 7 days although it is claimed that short intensive courses are just as effective. Alcohol should be avoided during treatment with this drug, as it sometimes causes vomiting. Better results are obtained if a second course is given after an interval of 1 week, but in any case, an observation period of 3 months, with repetition of treatment if vaginal swabs again become positive, is desirable. Since as many as 60% of husbands of women suffering from trichomonal vaginitis can be shown to harbour the parasite in the urethra and its associated glands, or under the prepuce, it is wise to treat the male partner of every woman suffering from trichomonal vaginitis, giving him the equivalent dosage of metronidazole simultaneously. Trichomonal infections which prove difficult to eradicate may have a reservoir of infection in the bladder or the urethra. Repeated courses of treatment will then be required. Where it is thought that candidiasis is also present, a course of fungicidal pessaries (such as nystatin pessaries BPC) should be used during the course of treatment with metronidazole.

MONILIAL VAGINITIS (THRUSH)

Vaginitis due to *Candida albicans* is less intense than in acute trichomonal vaginitis. The discharge is thin and 'cheesy' and the classical appearance of white adherent plaques on the vaginal wall is frequently seen. This fungal infection thrives in an acid medium (pH 5.0–6.5) and symptoms are thus temporarily relieved during menstruation, when the vagina is more alkaline, or by bathing or douching with a solution of 1% sodium bicarbonate. The exudate is not offensive, but does cause severe pruritus. In its most severe forms, the vaginitis can produce bleeding which may cause anxiety — especially during pregnancy. A number of conditions other than pregnancy predispose to a monilial vaginitis: the use of an oral contraceptive, diabetes mellitus, and in association with or following a course of antibiotic treatment eliminating cohabiting organisms. Vaginal infection is sometimes associated with candidiasis elsewhere in the same individual and can be contracted from a lesion on the hands or the genitalia of the husband. A combination of candidal and trichomonal infection is not uncommon, but the concomitant infection is not always evident until the dominant organism (the trichomonas) has been eliminated. The persistence of symptoms after treatment therefore calls for repeated cultures.

Candidal infection is generally easy to cure, except during pregnancy when it may linger or relapse. A number of patients outwith pregnancy do appear to have persistent recurrences and it should be remembered that there is a distribution of *C. albicans* in the body, being demonstrable in the mouths of 25% of all women, on the peri-anal skins of 8% and in the vaginas of 20–25% (Jeffcoate 1975). Nystatin pessaries at night for 2 weeks is probably still the drug of first choice, but other useful preparations are clotrimazole (Canesten), miconazole nitrate (Monistat or Gyno-daktarin), or econazole nitrate (Gyno-Pevaryl). These preparations can be used for a shorter time, with success, in courses of from 1 to 6 days. In resistant cases (probably due to reinfection from the alimentary canal) further courses of fungicidal pessaries can be combined with oral nystatin tablets 2 gm daily in divided doses for 2 weeks, while the search for any underlying causes of recurrence is pursued. The sexual partners of women with thrush sometimes complain of penile irritation especially in uncircumcised individuals, and the male partner can be treated with the same cream preparation, applying this daily after bathing. Even when the male partner is apparently symptom-free it is worth treating both partners if the patient has recurrent monilial vaginitis.

HERPES GENITALIS

This is caused by the herpes simplex virus, and can be sexually transmitted. It produces severe ulceration and a discharge arises from secondary infection. Considerable vulvo-vaginal discomfort ensues and the characterstic small ulcers are extremely tender. Treatment is seldom satisfactory and is mainly symptomatic, relying on saline packs. In the early stages of the lesions, painting with idoxuridine may abort them.

NON-SPECIFIC GENITAL INFECTION

Since there is epidemiological evidence that non-specific urethritis is sexually transmissible, some female contacts must have a comparable non-specific genital infection. While knowledge of the causes of the condition in the male remains unclear, identification of female contacts who should be treated is difficult. Many authorities recommend a course of tetracycline on epidemiological grounds to exclude associated infections. Signs of cervical inflammation or inflammatory changes on a cervical smear are not in themselves a certain indication for antibiotic therapy.

In a survey of the Well Woman Clinic in the author's group practice, vaginal infections (demonstrated by culture) were, as might be expected, more common in the sexually active age groups with an incidence of 13% in the 20–29 age group, reducing to 7.2% in the 40–49 age group, and 5.6% in the post-menopausal group (unpublished data). Among patients who consulted on account of gynaecological symptoms over an 8-year period, 25% presented with vaginal discharge as one of their problems if not the major issue. Such patients present usually because there has been a noticeable change in the leucorrhoea, and the great majority are able to control this normal desquamation with sensible personal hygiene.

VAGINAL DISCHARGE IN THE CHILD

There are two common times when vaginal discharge may present in childhood:

1. At birth — new born babies may have a mucoid vaginal discharge for the first 7 to 10 days of life; this is thought to be due to stimulation of the uterus and vagina by placental oestrogens. No treatment is required and the discharge will disappear within a week or two.

2. Around puberty — usually 2 or 3 years before or after the menarche. This can become offensive when secondary infection occurs — due to the thin vulnerable vaginal epithelium. Treatment will depend on the organisms detected from vaginal swabs, but this examination must be very gently completed — with the child's mother present in the consulting room — with the minimum of effort required to obtain a satisfactory vaginal swab.

DISORDERS OF MENSTRUATION

DYSMENORRHOEA

It is accepted that more than 50% of women experience some degree of discomfort around the time of menstruation. The criteria for a formal diagnosis of dysmenorrhoea depends on whether the pain is sufficient to interfere with normal day-to-day activities. With this definition it is estimated that some 10% of schoolgirls experience menstrual pain sufficient to keep them away from school. Fewer girls and young women seem to consult nowadays with a complaint of dysmenorrhoea — reflecting, perhaps, either a more sensible outlook on parents' part, or the increasing use of the oral contraceptive in younger age groups.

An accurate history is essential to define the nature of the pain, its site and relation to the onset of menstruation and whether or not it occurs at times other than during a period. Symptoms of premenstrual tension, such as breast tenderness, abdominal discomfort, a 'bloated' sensation, headache, irritability, backache and even depression may be associated with considerable dysmenorrhoea, and treatment of these symptoms can frequently reduce the dysmenorrhoea to a considerable degree, provided there is no associated pelvic disease.

It is useful to think of patients with dysmenorrhoea in two groups:

1. Those *without* associated pelvic disease (primary dysmenorrhoea).
2. Those *with* associated pelvic disease (secondary dysmenorrhoea)

Primary dysmenorrhoea

The pain is present from the start of menstruation and lasts for a few hours, or up to 24 hours. The pain is sharp and colicky, situated centrally in the lower abdomen and in the upper anterior part of the thighs. Sometimes it is associated with nausea, vomiting, headache, and occasionally with bowel or urinary problems. Characteristically, many girls are pain-free for many months or even some years after the menarche; later, often quite suddenly, in the 17–24 year old group, the pain of menstruation begins and worsens.

A vaginal (or rectal) examination is necessary if some pelvic abnormality is suspected. Only in older patients is one likely to find a pelvic abnormality such as a cervical polyp, or a uterine fibroid. Discreet enquiry should be made regarding the possible presence of an intra-uterine contraceptive device and background factors such as the home environment (an over-protective mother), stress factors either at home, in school, or socially, should be probed, and alleviated where possible.

Treatment

If the patient is under the age of 16 years she and her mother should be reassured that these period pains are simply signs of maturing feminine function and fertility. Both mother and daughter may have a blinkered view of menstruation and sex, and time taken to explain the physiology of menstruation and the mechanism of the pain, is time well spent. A distinct note of optimism for improvement in the future is also important. General advice regarding hygiene, rest and simple analgesia, such as soluble aspirin, should be all that is necessary. Since primary dysmenorrhoea is associated with an increased production of prostaglandin synthetase, specific inhibitors such as mefenamic acid, indomethacin, or ketoprofen have proved to be valuable analgesic assets.

If these methods prove of no avail, the most certain treatment is with the contraceptive pill. Anovulatory cycles should be obtained by the use of a 'combined' oral contraceptve for a limited period of between four and six cycles. Alternatively, where contraceptive cover is not necessary a progestogen such as dydrogesterone (10 mg twice daily) can be given up 3 week cycles from the fifth day after period flow begins. A full gynaecological investigation becomes necessary if relief is not obtained after six cycles of such therapy. Congenital uterine abnormality, such as a bicornuate uterus, or endometriosis, would then have to be excluded.

Secondary dysmenorrhoea

In this group, the dysmenorrhoea is secondary to some pelvic pathology, such as a uterine fibroid, pelvic inflammatory disease or endometriosis. The pelvic or lower abdominal pain usually precedes menstruation by a few days and except when associated with endometriosis, is relieved with the onset of the flow. Pain is less commonly a feature of uterine fibroids, unless they are submucous in situation, when they tend to become pedunculated with repeated expulsive attempts by the uterus. Endometriosis can be extremely painful — starting premenstrually and increasing in severity through the period without remission, until cessation of menstruation. Secondary dysmenorrhoea is usually only one of a number of symptoms and these may be associated with menorrhagia, metrorrhagia or dyspareunia.

Pelvic examination usually reveals the nature of the condition but further investigation such as a laparoscopy to confirm a diagnosis of endometriosis may be necessary.

Treatment varies with the underlying cause and is frequently surgical — where further childbearing is planned, fibroids should be enucleated and the uterus reconstituted to allow it to support a pregnancy at a later date. Figure 15.9 shows a sizeable myoma removed from a nulliparous patient who had been on an oral contraceptive for a number of years, but who latterly had consider-

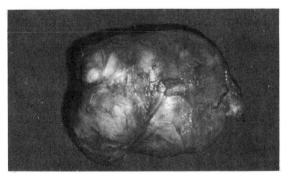

Fig. 15.9   A myoma (uterine fibroid) following enucleation (10 cm long). The patient (on oral contraceptive) presented latterly with secondary dysmenorrhoea.

able secondary dysmenorrhoea. After myomectomy oral contraception was resumed for 18 months and her first pregnancy had a satisfactory outcome. When endometriosis is the problem, its management depends on the extent of the disease. When it is limited in its severity menstruation should be suppressed for at least 6 months by means of continuous progestogen therapy or by a prolonged course of danazol. Pregnancy usually causes a marked remission in symptoms. More severe or persistent cases, though not normally associated with infertility, require local surgical treatment, or in cases of widespread disease, by pelvic clearance.

Dysmenorrhoea remains a symptom which, in the young patient, is almost invariably physiological and requires no elaborate investigation before treatment. In the older patient, it is usually secondary in type, whether from a puerperal or post-abortal infection, or other pathological lesion, the cause of which must be found, prior to appropriate treatment.

THE PREMENSTRUAL SYNDROME

Although for most women menstruation is merely a physiological phenomenon asssociated with some abdominal discomfort or pain, between 30 and 40% are affected with a number of other symptoms which begin about a week or so premenstrually, and which wane after the start of the menstrual flow. This syndrome can be troublesome in any age group but is more often a problem to women in the 35–45 year age group and more so in women with irregular menstruation. The incidence appears unrelated to past childbearing. Variable headache, irritability, tension and a tendency to depression are often present together with vague symptoms such as a bloated feeling in the abdomen, palpitations, dizziness and swelling of the fingers and legs. Retention of salt and water associated with a high circulating level of oestrogen was thought to be the precipitating factor, but it is now believed that in view of the complex hypothalamic/pituitary/ovarian interplay, a two-level aetiology (hypothalamus–ovary) is more likely. The role of prostaglandins in this context is being investigated, since peak levels of prostaglandin production in the menstrual cycle appear to correspond well with the timing of symptoms of the premenstrual syndrome.

Treatment

The tolerance of women to the premenstrual syndrome varies, just as with other conditions. Many of the symptoms are difficult to quantify and it is an advantage to know the patient and her family background and such factors as unemployment within the household, and stresses with teenage children. Many women with the syndrome feel troubled and anxious about the effects of

their feelings on the rest of the family. Some of the resultant family upset or even disruption may cause feelings of guilt. At the same time these women are more liable to an increasing incidence of migraine, asthma, absence from work, failure of examinations, petty crimes, liability to accident, and even attempted suicide. With such a wide range of symptoms and their implications, precise treatment is not easy, and the high rate of placebo response in controlled trials is well known.

Sympathetic understanding and a good listening ear are first priorities in therapy. Always leave the door open for the worried patient to return and discuss the problem again, and to consider further treatment.

Particular symptoms in individual patients appear to remain fairly constant. Many more women have a sensation of fullness in the abdomen or general fluid retention than can be shown to gain weight before menstruation. Bearing in mind a physiological tendency to premenstrual fluid retention — or at least fluid adjustment, a small dose of a diuretic, such as 2.5 mg bendrofluazide daily for 10 days premenstrually often brings considerable relief. Symptoms such as irritability or anxiety will usually benefit from small doses of diazepam (2 mg twice daily for, say, 7 days) in the second half of each menstrual cycle. Other drugs suggested are combinations of a tranquilliser and a diuretic, such as Tenavoid (bendrofluazide 3 mg and meprobamate 200 mg) but polypharmacy in general terms is to be deprecated as the dose proportions cannot be adjusted.

Prostaglandin inhibitors such as mefenamic acid have been shown to significantly improve premenstrual symptoms, while at the same time also reducing associated dysmenorrhoea or menorrhagia. Where breast symptoms (swelling and pain) predominate, danazol is useful (increasing from 200 mg towards 800 mg daily) but side effects such as nausea, dizzines and sickness may be intolerable to some patients. It is as yet doubtful whether symptoms such as generalised fluid retention or mood swings are helped by bromocriptine, but where mastodynia is the predominant symptom, 1.25 mg bromocriptine daily increasing gradually to 2.5 mg bd by the end of 2 weeks from day 10 until the start of menstruation is of value. The motto should be short courses of treatment for specific symptoms, tailored to the individual patient, with repeated courses only if strictly necessary.

ABNORMAL BLEEDING FROM THE GENITAL TRACT

The temptation to perpetuate titles such as epimenorrhoea, polymenorrhoea and epimenorrhagia should be resisted. Only three labels merit description here:

1. Menorrhagia (heavy and prolonged, but regular periods).

2. Metrorrhagia (heavy but irregular periods).
3. Intermenstrual bleeding (bleeding between periods).

Causes can be considered under two broad groups:

a. With a local pelvic cause.
b. With no abnormal physical findings — dysfunctional uterine bleeding.

The essential defect in the syndrome of 'dysfunctional uterine bleeding' is an imbalance in the secretion of oestrogen and progesterone by the ovary. Thus it can be caused by ovarian disease (Stein-Leventhal syndrome with, classically, polycystic ovaries) or may be secondary to disorders in the pituitary or hypothalamus.

LOCAL PELVIC CAUSES

1. Conditions related to pregnancy or the prevention of pregnancy:
   a. Abortion (threatened or incomplete)
   b. Ectopic pregnancy
   c. Hydatidiform mole
   d. Choriocarcinoma
   e. Antepartum or postpartum haemorrhage
   f. Intra-uterine contraceptive device or the oral contraceptive pill.
2. Malignant disease in the pelvis:
   Carcinoma of cervix or body of the uterus, vulva, vagina, ovary or fallopian tube.
3. Cervical erosion.
4. Polypi (cervical or endometrial).
5. Uterine fibroids.
6. Inflammatory conditions:
   a. Salpingitis (post-abortal, or gonococcal)
   b. Endometritis.
7. Uterine displacements:
   a. Retroversion (acute).
   b. Prolapse with decubitus ulceration.
8. Trauma:
   a. Coital injury, particularly ruptured hymen
   b. Injury from an accident
   c. Malposition or translocation of an intra-uterine device.
9. Urethral caruncle (a scarlet polyp arising from the posterior margin of the urethral meatus).

DYSFUNCTIONAL UTERINE BLEEDING

General causes

1. Emotional disorders and anxiety states. Women vary quite markedly in their criteria for abnormal bleeding. Patients who have had 'severe haemorrhage with their periods' for many months are frequently found to have a haemoglobin level of at least 13 g. A background knowledge of the patient and of her family background is of considerable help in assessing the situation. Below the age of 20 years, the disturbance is more likely to be a functional one with a tendency to spontaneous cure. Over the age of 40 years, functional disorders again become common, but the possibility of neoplasm (benign or malignant) must first be excluded.

Emotional and nervous disorders can cause excessive uterine bleeding as well as amenorrhoea. Family or marital crises, change of environment (move of house or change of employment), nervous tension, sexual frustrations, or overwork can all be associated with excessive menstrual loss.

2. Blood disorders. Although anaemia is generally an effect of menorrhagia, it is also said to cause heavy periods. Blood disorders due to coagulation defects, or to capillary fragility can also cause excessive menstrual loss. Thrombocytopenia and leukaemia can possibly present as menorrhagia, or metrorrhagia.

Endocrine causes

1. Iatrogenic — by exogenous hormone therapy — from oestrogens either given as hormone replacement therapy in the perimenopausal era, or in the form of a 'combined' oral contraceptive pill.

2. At puberty. Menorrhagia may occur from puberty to around the age of 20 years. Early periods can sometimes be prolonged, heavy and irregular, and anaemia can result. These early periods are invariably anovular in type, and even in extreme, sometimes alarming, cases, no basis other than a psychogenic one can be suggested. Presumably irregular ovarian activity with variable hormone production is responsible for the heavy bleeding.

3. Perimenopausal bleeding is quite common, and any such bleeding which is irregular, heavy and of longer duration than formerly, requires urgent investigation. Again, it may well be an anovular type of meorrhagia, with a picture of metropathic haemorrhagica.

4. Post-menopausal bleeding is by definition bleeding from the genital tract occurring 12 months or more after the last menstrual period. This always requires urgent investigation — detailed examination under anaesthesia, and diagnostic curettage of the uterus, is obligatory — with malignancy always in mind — whether the patient has been on hormone replacement therapy or not, and even if cervical and vaginal smears are normal.

5. Metropathia haemorrhagica. Characteristically the picture is one of acyclical endometrial bleeding with a heavy painless loss lasting up to several weeks, sometimes preceded by an interval of amenorrhoea of some 6 to 8 weeks. The picture is the result of excessive oestrogen production by the ovary, without the usual luteal activity. This continued high level of endogenous oestrogen gives rise to cystic glandular hyperplasia of the endometrium — the classical Swiss cheese pattern of

endometrium (Fig. 15.10). The uterus may well be bulky and the ovaries a little enlarged. Curettage, with demonstration of cystic hyperplasia of the endometrium histologically, confirms the diagnosis.

6. Thyroid (particularly hypothyroidism) or adrenal disorder.

INVESTIGATION OF ABNORMAL BLEEDING

History
The importance of the history again cannot be overstressed — the time of onset and description of the bleeding, its relationship to puberty or to the menopause, whether a recent pregnancy has occurred, or whether the patient has been prescribed any form of hormone therapy recently by another doctor. If the picture is obscure, and there is no urgency, the patient can be asked to keep a 'menstrual calendar' which can be helpful in outlining any pattern to the bleeding — or alternatively can be reassuring that there is nothing significantly amiss.

Examination
Examination will note any obesity, hypertension, peripheral oedema, hirsutism, thyroid enlargement, glycosuria or haematuria. A local pelvic cause of the bleeding should be excluded by bimanual and speculum ex-amination but the scope of this examination will depend on the age and marital status of the patient. Where it proves difficult to complete a pelvic examination, examination under anaesthesia is in the patient's best interests, since an endometrial biopsy can be done as well as a biopsy of cervix if any doubtful lesion is noted on initial inspection. The more irregular the bleeding the greater is the indication for curettage. All cases of inter-menstrual bleeding should be regarded as abnormal until proved otherwise (Dewhurst 1972)

Blood should be taken for haemoglobin estimation, and film and platelet count, white cell count and erythrocyte sedimentation rate should be included. Thyroid function tests will be indicated in appropriated cases. Ultrasonography can prove invaluable if a pelvic mass or an early pregnancy is suspected. An immunological pregnancy tests (in dilution) is helpful when significant bleeding complicates an early pregnancy. Laparoscopy is indicated when continuing doubt about the aetiology of the abnormal uterine bleeding exists.

TREATMENT OF ABNORMAL BLEEDING

The treatment of those with an organic cause is determined by the cause found. When bleeding has been due to an injury or to a foreign body, the proper examination

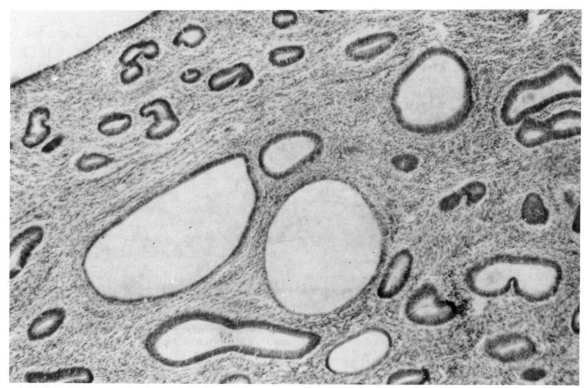

Fig. 15.10 Cystic glandular hyperplasia of the endometrium ('Swiss cheese pattern')

and exploration is only feasible in a gynaecological theatre, under general anaesthesia.

In those with dysfunctional type bleeding two governing principles should be remembered:

1. The young patient should be reviewed at intervals since in many cases the situation will resolve spontaneously. Curettage can be delayed in women in the early reproductive years provided there is no particular cause for concern; in women over 35 years this procedure is mandatory since treatment should be prompt and complete (Gold 1975).

2. The aim of treatment in true functional disturbance is to control symptoms since spontaneous cure usually results. Sometimes a combination of organic and functional causes may exist:

> a 36-year-old teacher, presented with a history of increasing menorrhagia, together with a long history of severe dysmenorrhoea with associated migrainous headaches. The patient, nulliparous and unmarried, had for some time been unable to work for 2 or 3 days during every period. With this brief history there seemed obviously to a large functional factor, but a pelvic swelling was noted on abdominal examination, and gentle bimanual examination confirmed an irregularly enlarged firm uterus which was the seat of multiple fibroids.

It would be unreasonable to procrastinate in such circumstances and a detailed examination under anaesthesia together with curettage of the uterus is obligatory. If suspicions of numerous sizeable fibroids are confirmed hysterectomy would be the likeliest course of action in view of the history, that the patient had no plans of marriage and, in particular, no wish to bear children. The cyclical migraine could then be tackled separately.

There are three possible approaches to the treatment of dysfunctional bleeding:

Hormone therapy

1. Progestogens — for example, Primolut N (norethisterone 5 mg) 15–20 mg daily for 10 days each cycle from the 15th day, with an interval of 1 week between cycles.

2. Combined oestrogen-progesterone preparations — norethisterone 1–4 mg with ethinyl oestradiol 0.5 mg (Minovlar, Gynovlar, or Anovlar) in 3-week cycles starting on the fifth day, as for contraceptive purposes.

3. Androgens — these will usually control most types of functional bleeding (10 mg Ultandren (fluoxymesterone) daily for 56 days) but they should be avoided in younger patients or in patients with a tendency to hirsutism, due to its virilising effects.

Surgery

In general, surgery should be the last resort in the young woman, but the first procedure in those over 40 years. In the older woman the need for conservation is unlikely to be pressing, and there is a much greater likelihood of an organic cause for the bleeding, whereas in the young woman, a conservative outlook with a probable spontaneous recovery is enhanced by the need to preserve reproductive function.

1. Curettage. This is primarily a diagnostic procedure, but it often has the effect of reducing excessive uterine bleeding.

2. Hysterectomy. In patients of 40 years or over who have failed to respond to hormone therapy, hysterectomy is probable the treatment of choice. The ovaries may be cystic in which case removal is indicated, but as a general rule, healthy looking ovaries in patients under 40 years would be preserved.

3. Radiotherapy is not now suggested as an alternative form of inducing an artificial menopause unless hysterectomy is refused, or contraindicated on medical grounds.

Other forms of treatment

1. Epsilon-aminocaproic acid (an antifibrinolysin) is of use on an emergency basis as for the treatment of excessive bleeding caused by an intra-uterine device. The dose is 3 g four times daily. Alternatively, the device should be removed.

2. When the bleeding is associated with pregnancy, oxytocics such as ergometrine, syntometrine (ergometrine malleate 500 μg and oxytocin 5 units) by intramuscular injection, or syntocinon (oxytocin 5 units per mol) by intravenous infusion are valuable forms of treatment.

AMENORRHOEA

Amenorrhoea can be primary (menstruation has never occurred), or secondary (where menstruation has been absent for 6 or more months, having previously been normally cyclical). Physiological causes of amenorrhoea such as pregnancy, lactation and the normal menopause must be excluded as the first priority. For menstruation to take place a normal uterus and patent vagina must be present, and the hypothalamus, pituitary and ovaries must be functioning normally. Causes of primary amenorrhoea may be subdivided into:

1. Congenital:

a. Absence, or gross hyperplasia, of uterus or ovaries.

b. Turner's syndrome (gonadal dysgenesis) which is due to dysfunction of the sex chromosome pairs, resulting in 45 instead of 46 chromosomes.

2. Endocrinological: tumours of pituitary and hypothalamus. Conditions such as the Stein-Leventhal syndrome (amenorrhoea, hirsutism and infertility in

association with polycystic ovaries) or Sheehan's syndrome (amenorrhoea with atrophy of genitalia and evidence of hypothyroidism following atrophy of the anterior lobe of the pituitary gland due to ischaemic necrosis) are examples in this group. Cushing's disease, and Addison's disease are similarly due to variations in function of the adrenal cortex.

3. General:

a. Malabsorptive states such as Crohn's disease, or coeliac disease, or debilitating diseases such as pulmonary tuberculosis, chronic nephritis or carcinoma can cause amenorrhoea. Conversely, gross obesity can cause increasing oligomenorrhoea until amenorrhoea occurs.

b. Psychological trauma due to a family crisis, moving house or travel with associated change in climate, or stress related, for instance, to examinations.

c. Anorexia nervosa. This condition, involving self-starving with, usually, signs of quite severe weight loss, is found in 10–15% of patients who complain of amenorrhoea. The figure-conscious teenager losing as little as 10% of her weight can produce amenorrhoea. Treatment is difficult, and involves a psychotherapeutic approach. With a return to normal weight, menstruation usually returns spontaneously.

d. Chronic poisoning (e.g. from lead), chronic alcholism, and drug addiction may all lead to amenorrhoea.

e. 'Post pill amenorrhoea' is not a recognised entity as such but full investigation is required when this symptom continues for longer than 6 months. About 2.2 per 1000 of women taking the pill will be affected to this extent (Golditch 1972). Specialist investigation of these patients is necessary, to exclude such causes as pituitary tumours, adrenal tumours, and the Stein-Leventhal syndrome.

INVESTIGATION

In any case of amenorrhoea, the question of pregnancy must always be kept in mind and excluded with certainty. Investigation of primary amenorrhoea should not be intensive before 18 years of age. Before this time, examination should be merely a general assessment with regard to endocrinological status, and a pelvic examination to exclude cryptomenorrhoea or a major congenital defect. An accurate history is important to pinpoint the mode of onset, and any association with stress, environmental factors, previous illness and weight changes should be noted.

General examination should concentrate particularly on the presence of secondary sex characteristics, the height of the patient and the state of the breasts. Evidence of hirsutism or other endocrine abnormality should be sought, any obesity or malnutrition noted, and anaemia excluded. Pelvic examination will exclude any

congenital abnormality while the size and development of the pelvic organs are assessed, and pregnancy is confirmed or refuted.

Particular investigations include:

1. A pregnancy test, and hormonal assessment by cervical and vaginal cytology, and plasma hormonal profiles including prolactin levels.

2. Radiological examination of chest (for chronic disease) and of the pituitary fossa (to exclude a pituitary tumour).

3. Blood picture and ESR to demonstrate anaemia, leukaemia or a chronic debilitating disease.

4. Urine analysis to exclude glycosuria and chronic renal disease, together with assays of 17-ketosteroids, 17-hydroxycorticoids, and total oestrogens.

5. Sonar may help to define local pelvic disease.

6. Examination under anaesthesia and endometrial biopsy may be coupled with laparoscopy and ovarian biopsy.

TREATMENT

Specific treatment will be that which is applicable to certain conditions — such as a significant endocrine upset, underlying depression or anxiety. Normal menstruation will recur spontaneously in about 20% of patients and the correction of minor defects such as anaemia or weight problems may be all that is required to restore a normal menstrual pattern.

Should there be no improvement, a test of the response of the endometrium to stimulation can be done by prescribing the contraceptive pill for, say, 3 months. Once it is established that the endometrium will respond with hormone therapy, there is no need to continue treatment merely for the sake of having a period. Treatment with clomiphene citrate or pituitary gonadotrophins should be given when a pregnancy is planned — this requires close and continual supervision within a gynaecological clinic with hormone assay back-up.

What is the place of contraception in the amenorrhoeic woman? Where there is failure of the hypothalamus, pituitary or ovary, there is no need for contraception. Occasionally a woman with hyperprolactinaemia can conceive, so that contraception will be necessary. Of choice, exogenous hormones should be avoided so that a barrier method is to be recommended although a 'progestogen only' pill would be reasonable. However, when amenorrhoea or menstrual irregularity has not been caused by hyperprolactinaemia, there is no contraindication to the combined oral contraceptive. If hyperprolactinaemia is present, then oral contraception, like pregnancy, may stimulate an occult pituitary tumour. 'Post pill amenorrhoea' although not a distinct entity, requires full investigation when it continues beyond 6 months (see ch. 5).

THE MENOPAUSE

The normal menopause, which occurs at about the age of 50 years in the UK (Frommer 1964), is the time when menstruation ceases and is therefore a well defined era in the natural process of ageing. Periods may cease abruptly, or after a time of scanty or infrequent menstruation. The menopause is not related to the age of menarche, though the effect of puberty is less certain. Fertility naturally declines with advancing age, with the proportion of anovulatory cycles increasing to 25% in the 40–45 year age group. Throughout this period of gradual failure of ovarian function (known as the climacteric), oestrogen production falls, while follicle stimulating and luteinising hormone production rises. This fall in oestrogen production results in atrophy of the genitalia, especially noticeable in the vaginal mucosa, and, together with the rising gonadotrophin levels, causes vasomotor instability resulting in hot flushes and sweats. The uterus and pelvic ligaments involute during this time. A little oestrogen is still produced after the menopause (thought to be from the adrenal gland, and extra glandular conversion of plasma androstenedione) (Rader et al 1973).

The symptoms of vasomotor instability are obviously most marked after abrupt surgical or radiation ablation and can be debilitating. Many women after a natural menopause, may experience similar symptoms which may persist over a period of months to a number of years. It is generally felt that the only symptoms related to the deficiency of oestrogen are hot flushes, sweats, and dryness of the vagina, and that consequently only these symptoms are relieved by oestrogen therapy. A minority view is that associated insomnia, fatigue, loss of concentration, depression and diminished sexual responsiveness may also be symptoms of oestrogen deficiency.

Although it has been shown that there is no increased incidence of endogenous depression at this time (Winokur 1973), minor problems such as insomnia, fatigue and loss of concentration are not uncommon. At this stage of life, also, it should be remembered that a woman is often confronted by situations which are changing more rapidly than is her hormonal status. Her children may be leaving home; there may be increasing responsibilities with elderly relatives, and death or serious illness comes to close relatives and friends. Her husband may be preoccupied with his work, with decreasing sexual interests, while at the same time, grandchildren and strange in-laws enter the scene.

In the pre-menopausal woman with symptoms of oestrogen deficiency the diagnosis may be missed unless characteristic sweats and flushes are present. A good case can be made for the use of a low dose oral contraceptive in this age group in that it gives complete contraceptive protection at a time when pregnancy could be a catastrophe and associated with a high incidence of chromo-

somal defects. On the other hand, cyclical oestrogen therapy (with conjugated oestrogens), although improving menstrual irregularity as well as alleviating symptoms, has no certain contraceptive effect. Some preparations are available with an androgen combined with oestrogen but there appears to be little to commend this. A safer and more logical combination is oestrogen with a progestogen: this avoids over-stimulation of the endometrium and produces regular cyclical bleeding. There is now good evidence that well supervised combined hormone therapy for the climacteric syndrome should not produce an increased risk of endometrial pathology (Thom & Studd 1980).

After the menopause, oestrogen therapy should always be given cyclically for 3 weeks out of 4, with regular withdrawal bleeding. Longer-term treatment with a reduced dosage after symptoms are controlled will diminish withdrawal bleeding if not stop it altogether. This area of concern is obviously greatly simplified in women who have had a hysterectomy, and treatment need not be cyclical.

WHICH PATIENTS SHOULD HAVE HORMONE REPLACEMENT THERAPY?

Most women adjust well to the menopause, and may not notice features of oestrogen deficiency. About 25% of women have some significant symptomatology, and probably another 25% seem to give no hint of oestrogen deprivation. If symptoms are persistently troublesome the patient should be well supervised and treatment continued for up to 2 years.

With a life expectancy of nearly 80 years, a great many women are living through more post-menopausal years. The health of some of these women will be affected by oestrogen deficiency, and may be helped considerably by oestrogen replacement therapy without the risk of serious side effcts. The selection of these women so far is initially on a symptomatic basis: without further evidence, it is not justifiable to recommend routine oestrogen replacement therapy in every post-menopausal women. It is worthy of note that recent evidence (Bungay et al 1980) has shown that mental symptoms (such as difficulty with decisions and concentration, anxiety, loss of confidence or insomnia) are related to chronological age rather than clustered at the menopause itself. There is therefore little to be said in favour of tranquillisers or mild sedation in the perimenopausal patient. It requires the courage of one's convictions to withhold therapy when it is not needed. Explanation, support and reassurance can do much to help such patients.

DYSPAREUNIA

Dyspareunia means that coitus is either painful or difficult, and is probably the commonest of all coital problems to confront the doctor. Frigidity implies loss of libido, whereas dyspareunia may be used by a woman to cover up her real problem of frigidity. Usually, it is the woman who consults her doctor; if, at the first consultation, the problem appears to be one involving both partners, then the man should be strongly urged to consult with his partner. This may be difficult since the male partner may not be registered in the same practice and to allow effective management both partners should be urged to register with the same doctor. In assessing a woman presenting with dyspareunia, background knowledge of the patient is very helpful in anticipating possible factors behind her complaint and in being aware that the symptoms presented may mask the true problem. A sympathetic, unhurried approach is important since the patient has obviously been sufficiently concerned about her problem to pluck up courage to come and discuss it. From the numerous 'questions and answers' in women's magazines, and enquiries on phone-in radio programmes there appears to be a large number of women who are apparently unwilling or unable to consult their doctor about relatively simple sexual problems. Perhaps the old adage 'He's always so busy, I don't like to bother him' is a considerable deterrent since such problems will be time-consuming, and there is much to be said for putting aside an extended consultation time for discussion. This gives an opportunity for the partner to be present as well.

MANAGEMENT

The probable site or cause of the problem should be elicited by a careful and tactful history — including the duration of the problem, the frequency of attempted intercourse, the site of the discomfort and whether or not it occurred following childbirth or vaginal surgery. Inspection of the vulva, urethral meatus and introitus (noting any perineal scars or vaginal skin tags) should precede a gentle one-finger examination. If this is achieved satisfactorily, then a speculum examination of the vagina, cervix and posterior fornix can be carried out using a small speculum, and appropriate swabs and a cervical smear taken. Bimanual examination then follows and any uterine displacement or enlargement or adnexal mass is noted, while movement of the uterus is tested to elicit any tenderness or fixation. Where endometriosis is suspected from the history, laparoscopy may be indicated despite negative examination findings, to confirm or refute the diagnosis.

Many of the causes of superficial dyspareunia can be elicited by a careful history and examination, and treated in the primary care setting. Some causes, however, do require a surgical approach; urethral caruncle (diathermy excision), intact hymen (surgical excision), introital narrowing (periniotomy) or congenital absence of vagina (vaginal reconstruction).

In deep dyspareunia, the discomfort or pain is encountered after penetration has occurred. It may not occur until after intercourse and often presents as low abdominal pain, or backache which may persist for hours or even days afterwards. Common causes are chronic pelvic inflammatory disease, retroversion of the uterus (with prolapse of the ovaries into the Pouch of Douglas), endometriosis, ovarian cysts or uterine fibroids (mechanical obstruction) or, occasionally, vault discomfort following a repair operation, or extended hysterectomy. Management of women with deep dyspareunia depends on the established diagnosis, and may involve fairly radical surgery ((such as hysterectomy, or excision of chocolate cysts of the ovary). Patients with vault discomfort after vaginal repair operations should have the cause of the pain explained to them, and alternative positions in coitus suggested. Follow-up must be arranged after any treatment, whether surgical, chemotherapeutic or through counselling, to ensure that the symptom has cleared.

A psychogenic cause must be considered when examination has satisfactorily excluded an organic lesion, or when examination has proved impossible due to vaginismus. Ignorance regarding the technique of intercourse can be surprising; elaborate but misleading folklore can be passed on to the younger generation, while a sexual assault or an unfortunate crude sexual experience can radically affect a woman's future approach to intercourse. Inadequate or erratic contraception with its associated fear of pregnancy is a common aetiological factor. Inhibitions can develop to the extent of producing dyspareunia, or even vaginismus.

A very gentle and patient approach, with much tact and understanding of the background problem is required. The co-operation of both partners is fundamental, and several interviews may be necessary to encourage free discussion. Motivation of the couple remains an essential requirement and this applies as much to the older patient.

THE INFERTILE PATIENT

Childlessness is one of the commonest gynaecological problems which present to the general practitioner. Approximately 10% of all marriages are associated with infertility, with both partners being involved. It is important therefore that both husband and wife should be considered from the outset. The likely multidisciplinary approach (general practitioner, gynaecologist, urologist, and psychosexual counsellor or psychiatrist) emphasises the need for continued and adequate communication.

The basic approach involves a careful history and

physical examination of the female so that obvious causes of infertility such as an absence of vital organs or non-consummation may be revealed. The concept of a 'fertility profile' is to be commended and is useful in systematically attempting to identify the site of the cause so that appropriate investigation and treatment can be carried out. Five levels of tests are used to identify, in ascending order, the possible causes for infertility:

1. Seminal analysis.
2. The cervix — mucus tests and post-coital test.
3. The uterus — hysterogram and endometrial biopsy.
4. Fallopian tubes — laparosopy and hydrotubation or salpingography.
5. The ovary — basal body temperature and hormonal profile.

SEMINAL ANALYSIS

Almost invariably it is the female who presents first for investigation, but it is recognised that the male is responsible in about a third of instances. Seminal analysis should always be carried out by an expert, so that a full profile is made available and further more elaborate investigations and treatments undertaken without delay. A testicular biopsy is indicated (demonstrating, perhaps, marked maturation arrest) when examination of two seminal samples shows evidence of impaired fertility. It should not be forgotten however that in half of the cases where the male is implicated, some element of dysfunction also exists in the female (Buxton & Southern, 1958), so that her investigation should continue in parallel. In the absence of obvious physical abnormality, the sperm count can sometimes be improved by large doses of vitamin C (200 mg daily for 6 months) or fluoxymesterone (Ultandren) 20 mg daily for 3 months.

THE CERVIX

Despite being such a localised region, it is perhaps surprising that abnormalities of the cervix and cervical secretions are considered to be a responsible factor in 5–15% of cases of infertility (Elstein 1974). Tests are aimed at determining whether the spermatozoa are being deposited with receptive and transport-facilitated conditions at the appropriate site. Cervical secretions tend to act as a barrier to sperms in all but the periovular phase of the menstrual cycle (when the mucus is thin and translucent). The traditional post-coital test has largely fallen out of favour since up to 80% of couple may show poor post-coital findings. A true 'cervical infertility factor' is accepted only after an in-vitro invasion test, in which samples of semen and cervical mucus are juxta-

posed and the penetration of the spermatozoa into the mucus observed. Alternatively the distance which spermatozoa pass up a capillary tube filled with cervical mucus in a given time can be assessed.

'Priming' of the cervix by giving the female 0.01 mg of ethinyl oestradiol daily for 7 days pre-ovulation improves the quality of cervical mucus. Sperm penetration may thereby be indirectly aided, thus acting as an effective form of therapy.

Where cervical mucus hostility is a distinct possibility, an immunological reaction must be considered. In the patient with cervical hostility, the sperms appear to lose their mobility and clump together or die when they come in contact with the cervical mucus. The true role of the spermatozoal antibody in female fertility has as yet to be elucidated, and the value of immuno-suppressive drugs or steroids has yet to be proved. The success rate (in terms of pregnancies) of any treatment has not been found greater than that achieved by the mere placebo effect that infertility investigation and treatment has on all infertile couples.

THE UTERUS

Uterine anomalies with distortion of the uterine cavity can be responsible for infertility, but faults in the endometrium are generally responsible. A hysterosalpingogram gives the basic profile with radio-opaque dye injected through the cervix during the proliferation phase of the menstrual cycle. X-ray films show well the contours of the uterine cavity, demonstrating some forms of uterine anomaly, or a deformity of outline by structures such as fibroids, or endometrial polypi. Information about the fallopian tubes (see later) can also be obtained. At the same procedure, endometrial biopsy is carried out, and a simple histological classification of proliferative/secretory endometrium is made. The stage of maturation of the endometrial specimen can be accurately dated to within 1 or 2 days, and from this, the time of ovulation can be estimated. The endometrium should also be sent for culture to exclude tuberculosis.

Corrective surgery (such as myomectomy or separation of adhesions or a septum) is usually necessary when distortion of the uterine cavity is thought to be preventing successful pregnancy. Such treatment involving the uterine region is likely to be more successful when surgery did not involve disruption of the endometrial surface.

THE FALLOPIAN TUBES

Tubal damage is implicated in at least 20% of infertile patients, and this figure is thought to be rising due to the increasing incidence of venereal disease and because of terminations of pregnancy with the increased risk of pelvic infection.

A salpingogram (in conjunction with the hysterogram) is the basic profile, preferably if carried out under direct screening with image intensification. This should demonstrate patency of the tubes, while it can be deduced from the distribution of peritoneal spill and loculation whether any adhesions are present. This procedure has largely replaced tubal insufflation. In fact many gynaecologists are moving towards laparoscopy with hydrotubation (observing the passage of dye such as 1% methylene blue) as their first line of investigation of tubal function — originally advocated by Steptoe (1967). At this investigation it is possible to take an ovarian biopsy, to diathermy patches of endometriosis, or to separate minor adhesions, as well as to correct a markedly retroverted uterus by a suspension procedure.

Reconstructive surgery is the mainstay of treatment for the patient with tubal damage. Re-anastomosis, or re-implantation for a proximal blockage, salpingostomy for a fimbrial end blockage (with or without hydrosalpinx) or salpingolysis (division of peritubal adhesions) can be attempted. It is unusual for endometriosis to be the cause of infertility, but where small areas are noted they should be treated by removal and diathermy.

Results of operative repair of the fallopian tubes following inflammatory disease are not good. In most reported series patency does not guarantee a pregnancy rate above 10% (Speroff et al 1974). Post-operative hydrotubation with solutions containing hydrocortisone, or chymotripsin may help to delay the onset of adhesions. A frank discussion with the couple is therefore essential

before any attempts at tubal surgery are initiated. The breakthrough by Steptoe and Edwards in the field of extra-corporeal fertilisation may well provide the ultimate answer in cases of extensive tubal damage and blockage.

THE OVARY

In the fertile patient, the two basic functions of the ovary (the production of ova, and of oestrogen and progesterone) are of equal concern. It must be remembered from physiological principles that variants of normal in the cervix, uterus or the fallopian tubes may be indicators of ovarian dysfunction. The functions and interplay of the hypothalamus–pituitary axis hormones, the thyroid, uterus and ovaries are extremely complex, but a working knowledge is necessary before relevant investigations can be carried out, results interpreted and appropriate treatment commenced.

Basal body temperature: careful and assiduous recording of basal body temperature over a number of months can often demonstrate the regular occurrence of ovulation. Temperatures are normally lower in the first part of the cycle; a slight dip may occur at ovulation, and more usually a distinct rise will be noted in the second half of the cycle (a reflection of the production of progesterone from the corpus luteum). Figure 15.11 illustrates the type of pattern one can expect in the normal cycle. Where conception occurs, during maintenance of a temperature chart by a patient, the slight elevation of temperature in the luteal phase is continued beyond the

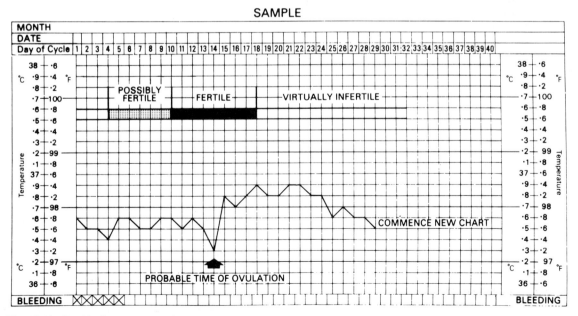

Fig. 15.11 Basal body temperature chart

'missed period' (see Fig. 5.3, p. 53). The chorionic gonadotrophin produced by the trophoblast maintains progesterone production by the corpus luteum. Much more reliable temperature charts can be assured if the clinic nurse or practice nurse teaches the patient how to take her temperature correctly and how to read the thermometer accurately. This investigation may detect intermittent cyclical abnormalities such as a defective proliferative phase, or a poor luteal phase.

The introduction of direct assay for a female hormone profile has now overshadowed vaginal cytoendocrinology (the examination and interpretation of serial vaginal smears throughout the menstrual cycle). Oestrogen assays in the secretory phase are useful in assessing ovarian function, while the FSH and LH levels in plasma are also helpful. Adequately raised plasma progesterone levels in the mid-secretory phase of the menstrual cycle (greater than 30 nmol/l between 5 and 10 days before the next period) is now an accepted criterion for ovulation and avoids the necessity of frequent endometrial biopsy or basal temperature charts.

More detailed hormonal profiles require specialist assessment and monitoring as does the treatment of ovarian dysfunction. This may be secondary to a systemic organic disease, such as a pituitary tumour, and the cause must be treated before attempting the induction of ovulation. Thus full investigation is essential before commencing treatment. Treatment of established disorders of ovarian steroid release should be within a specialist clinic with readily available immunoassay facilities to monitor therapy with clomiphene citrate, for example, in order to stimulate ovulation, or with gonadotrophins when daily hormone assays are required. Careful assessment and selection of patients is thus essential, as well as subsequent monitoring of response, to ensure the best chance of a successful outcome.

In general terms, a couple beginning to have doubts about their ability to conceive may only require simple reassurance. Some straightforward tests however such as a full blood count, X-ray of chest, and a basal temperature chart in the first instance can be coupled with seminal analysis of the husband to help pinpoint the cause of the apparent subfertility. Specialist referral is to be recommended whenever the history or examination indicates this approach, or when a year or more has passed without conception being achieved. A systematic approach, as outlined, helps to pinpoint accurately the source of the problem. This enables a fairly accurate prognosis in many instances, as well as enabling a rational guide to the selection of further investigations and treatment.

GYNAECOLOGICAL EMERGENCIES

From the viewpoint of general practice, gynaecological emergencies can be associated with the uterus (abortion), with the tubes (ectopic pregnancy and salpingitis) and with the ovaries (torsion of a tumour or rupture of a cyst).

ABORTION

Firstly it is essential to establish the likelihood of pregnancy. Bleeding can be a sign of imminent abortion or of an ectopic pregnancy. In abortion, the order of events is always characteristically *pregnancy*, *bleeding* and *pain*. The bleeding is due to separation of the chorion from the decidua associated sooner or later with active contractions of the uterine muscle. The pain which follows is due to the uterus expelling the products (or part thereof) of conception. The pain is therefore felt mostly in the lower abdomen, and, when contractions are powerful, also in the lower back.

While abortion is 'threatened' and there is no pain, bleeding will be slight. This situation is not an emergency. Should the abortion become inevitable, uterine bleeding may be profuse. Pain may well be severe, and a vaginal examination, which should always be done, shows the cervix to be dilated to some extent. Blood clots may be noted in the vagina, and sometimes products of conception (as blood clots) may be felt within the cervical canal; they should be removed digitally. The general condition of the patient must also be assessed, with particular note being made of signs of shock. In the home, the foot of the bed should be elevated, morphine can be given for pain and anxiety, and 1 ml of Syntometrine (which contains 5 units of syntocinon and 0.5 mg ergometrine) given intravenously to ensure contraction of the uterine muscle to stop further bleeding. (The syntocinon causes a rapid contraction of the uterus, while the ergometrine maintains a sustained contraction.) When the abortion has become inevitable, or incomplete, Syntometrine should be given once before the patient is transferred to avoid the risk of prolonged bleeding (albeit slight) and of sepsis. In most pregnancies that abort spontaneously before the 14th week, developmental arrest of the fetus has occurred at an early stage and usually an interval of weeks has elapsed between developmental arrest and abortion. The experienced ultrasonographer can predict the outcome with such certainty, that patients with threatened abortion can be managed at home and periods of unnecessary hospitalisation avoided.

The two major complications of abortion are haemorrhage and infection. Infection is more common where abortion has been self-induced or attempted by someone else. In these cases, a few days may have elapsed since the interference. Such patients can be very ill and toxic, with a high fever (around 39°C) and a tachycardia. The vagina feels tender and 'hot' and a mixture of blood, blood clots and products of conception can be seen. Admission to hospital is essential to ensure adequate and immediate antibiotic cover prior to evacuation of the uterus — the contents of which remain an expanding reservoir of bacterial infection. The possibility of infection with the organisms of gas gangrene should be borne in mind when there has been an interval of several days since the abortion (spontaneous, 'therapeutic', or criminal) occurred. In the older patient, it is possible to confuse metropathia haemorrhagica (variable amenorrhoea followed by brisk bleeding, but *without* pain) with abortion. Metropathia is due to an endocrine imbalance, usually in the perimenopausal era, which requires hormone therapy rather than ergometrine and syntometrine. Curettage of the uterus is obligatory in order to establish the diagnosis and in particular, to exclude malignancy.

SALPINGITIS

Acute salpingitis is usually caused by an ascending infection from the lower genital tract — commonly postpartum, or post-abortion, when resistance to infection is much reduced, or when a virulent gonococcus overwhelms the defences. A tuberculous infection of the fallopian tubes is blood borne, and rarely presents in an acute form. An acute form of salpingitis can arise as a flare up of a chronically or subacutely inflamed tube; this variant presents at the time of a period, or towards the end of it, probably due to the increased vascularity of the genital tract at this time.

There is, invariably, acute lower abdominal tenderness, with some guarding, and on bimanual examination the vagina is strikingly hot, while the exquisite pelvic tenderness precludes the definition of any mass. As with a septic abortion a pyrexia in the region of 40°C can be found; the tongue is usually clean, and fetor oris is absent, thus virtually excluding appendicitis. Such a high pyrexia is common to very few surgical causes, but includes acute cholecystitis, pyelonephritis, and basal pneumonia. Antibiotic therapy should be withheld, as with septic abortion, until at least all appropriate bacteriological swabs have been taken. It should be remembered that where gonorrhoea is suspected, serological tests for both syphilis and gonorrhoea are necessary.

The treatment is essentially conservative, with antibiotics, including metronidazole. Where ectopic pregnancy or appendicitis is suspected, laparoscopy or indeed laparotomy is required. If laparotomy demonstrates an acute salpingitis (usually bilteral) bacteriological swabs are taken from both tubes, and any surgical interference with the tubes is avoided. The major consideration is the preservation of fertility by energetic treatment of the acute condition in order to maintain normal function of the tubes. Salpingitis is closely associated with sexual activity and reproduction, so that its maximum incidence is in the 18–30 year age group.

ECTOPIC PREGNANCY

By definition, an ectopic pregnancy is one in which the fertilised ovum becomes implanted in a site other than the uterine cavity. It occurs most commonly in the fallopian tube, when strictly speaking, it is a tubal pregnancy. The incidence of ectopic pregnancy varies in different parts of the country, and in different parts of the world, reflecting the varying incidence of pelvic inflammatory diseases. Possible sites of ectopic pregnancy are:

— the fallopian tube
— the ovary
— on the peritoneum of the abdominal cacity
— the broad ligament
— the uterine horn
— a rudimentary uterine horn
— the cervix.

The fallopian tube is by far the most common site of inflammation, so it will be considered in greater detail.

The whole process of fertilisation and cell division through the morula to the blastocyst stage (by which time differentiation into the amniotic cavity, the yolk sac, and the embryonic sac surrounded by trophoblast has occurred) is finely timed, with little acceptable margin of error. Normally the blastocyst is embedded in the uterus about the 22nd day of a 28-day cycle — propelled along the fallopian tube by the action of the ciliated epithelium, and by the peristaltic action of the muscular coats.

Any undue delay in transport of the fertilised egg will precipitate its development and embedding in the fallopian tube. Delay can occur through either:

1. Developmental errors of the tube (hypoplasia or undue tortuosity).

2. Distortion of the tube (by uterine fibroids, or broad ligament cysts).

3. Previous inflammatory disease which may be peritubal, due for example to a previous appendicitis, or intra-tubal from infection with gonorrhoea or tuberculosis. This inflammation has usually been mild, since an acute form would block the tubes.

The clinical picture, therefore, may not include a clear-cut history of salpingitis, but the possibility of infection of the tubes following any pregnancy, abortion, or gonococcal infection, must be remembered.

4. Over-development of the ovum — either through excessive trophoblastic activity or by transmigration of the fertilised ovum. This phenomenon of external migration of the ovum to the contralateral tube is not altogether rare — as evidenced by the finding of the

corpus luteum in the ovary on the side opposite to that of the tubal pregnancy.

Classically, the patient is about 2 weeks overdue with her period, so there may be symptoms and signs of early pregnancy. Initially there is pain in the lower abdomen, usually towards one iliac fossa since the pain is caused by the vigorous peristaltic action of the affected tube. The pain is often transient or fleeting but can be so acute at times as to cause dizziness or faintness. Whenever such symptoms are associated with delayed menses, the patient should be admitted to hospital. The burrowing characteristic of the trophoblast causes it to eat into the tubal wall, and if it erodes a larger blood vessel, massive intraperitoneal bleeding can occur, causing shock and circulatory collapse with associated tachycardia, a thready pulse and low blood pressure. This situation is a true emergency and the patient must have a laparotomy as quickly as possible to stop the bleeding. Attempted resuscitation prior to the patient being in theatre is of no avail.

This classical acute form of ectopic pregnancy is fairly uncommon, occurring in only about 20% of cases. The picture may be much more obscure, with an ill-defined disturbance of menstrual regularity and some vague lower abdominal pain which the patient may attribute to dysmenorrhoea as the only symptom. The triad of amenorrhoea (of very variable duration), of pain (often with giddiness), and slight vaginal bleeding *in that order* should be sought. With abortion (the commonest differential diagnosis) the sequence is amenorrhoea, bleeding (due to separation of the chorion from the uterine wall) and pain (due to uterine contractions).

Bleeding at the site of embedding can be slow and the tube may thus be able to expand and accommodate it. Intermittent lower abdominal pain can then be the only clue. Constant slight bleeding at this time associated with some vague abdominal pain (due to the contraction of the tube) is thus very significant.

Tubal abortion is another variant. Variable amenorrhoea occurs with an associated intermittent lower abdominal pain which precedes the possible detachment of the conceptus from the tubal wall. The conceptus is shed into the abdominal cavity with slight, if slow, intraabdominal bleeding which gives rise to recurrent lower abdominal pain. If there is sufficient blood to track up the paracolic gutter, some shoulder tip pain occurs following irritation of the phrenic nerve. If blood collects in the Pouch of Douglas with haematocele formation, palpation may reveal a boggy mass behind the uterus. While clinical anaemia is quite possible from this cause, the bleeding from the embedding site usually stops, and the whole episode is over. Very exceptionally, the expelled ovum can remain viable, and progresses to an intraabdominal pregnancy.

Considering the spectrum of variation in presentation, the diagnosis of ectopic pregnancy can be either straightforward or very difficult. The history, accurately interpreted in the light of disturbed physiology, is the major factor in diagnosis, while a continuing high index of suspicion on the part of the doctor is as important. Emphasis must be laid on amenorrhoea, pain, slight vaginal bleeding, dizziness or faintness, and continual slight vaginal bleeding. Laparoscopy as a diagnostic tool has proved extremely useful in doubtful cases. Exclusion of an ectopic gestation by this means can save a patient many long days in hospital — this is particularly valuable where there are young children in the household.

THE OVARY

Lower abdominal pain at the time of ovulation (Mittelschmerz) is not uncommon, and is usually mild. It can recur on the same side, or may move from side to side with successive ovulations. Occasionally it can be severe, and may be sporadic. Appendicitis has to be excluded when it occurs on the right side. Simple analgesia and explanation are all that is usually required.

Three emergency situations can arise with an ovarian cyst:

Torsion
Torsion is heralded by sudden severe abdominal pain, often on getting out of bed or after some sharp movement. Vomiting frequently occurs at the time of torsion. The presence of a large tender tense abdominal swelling can be confirmed on bimanual examination. By and large, only benign tumours undergo torsion of their pedicles: malignant, inflammatory and endometriotic tumours become fixed to the pelvic wall early in their development, and thus cannot twist.

Haemorrhage
Severe abdominal pain associated with a mass arising from the pelvis is found when there is bleeding within a cyst. Such tumours may be endometriotic but, more commonly, are malignant.

Rupture
Acute pain is invariably the presenting symptom, with perhaps a feeling that something has given way. The picture is that of an 'acute abdomen' for which surgery cannot be avoided.

Benign ovarian tumours are much more common and are slow-growing. Women will put up with a gradually increasing abdominal girth, attributing it to middle-aged spread, and the larger tumours are predominantly benign. Most ovarian tumours are felt in the posterior fornix, where the Pouch of Douglas is in close relationship with the vaginal mucosa.

All pelvic masses should be assessed by a gynaecologist, since the large majority require surgical treatment. The ultimate diagnosis may only be made after laparotomy (a double pathology is always a possibility) with appropriate classification of the tumour dependent on histological examination.

GENITAL CANCER

CARCINOMA OF THE VULVA

Pre-malignancy

Considerable confusion and difference of opinion exists regarding the group of conditions known as the chronic epithelial vulval dystrophies. The significant type of 'white vulva' in this context is leukoplakia, where fissures appear in the white patches on the vulvar skin, which looks thickened and macerated. The label leukoplakia is usually reserved for cases in which the changes are regarded by the histo-pathologist as 'pre-malignant'. The basal layer of the epithelium becomes irregular with loss of nuclear polarity and increased mitotic activity, some of which may be aberrant. The possibility of transition to carcinoma is real, and such patients should be reviewed regularly, with repeat biopsies every 6 to 12 months. Vulvectomy is nowadays considered only following histological reports of changes amounting to pre-invasive carcinoma, or as a last resort, when the intractible itch cannot be satisfactorily relieved.

Carcinoma

Carcinoma of the vulva comprises only 3 to 4% of all genital cancers. It is primarily a disease of the elderly, with most patients well beyond the menopause. It is thought that 15–20% of patients with leukoplakia will eventually develop carcinoma.

There is often a long history of pruritus with eventually an offensive discharge, or post-menopausal bleeding. An ulcer of variable size is apparent, without there being necessarily palpable enlargement of the inguinal or femoral glands on either side. Spread can be by direct invasion to surrounding tissues, by contact producing a 'kissing' ulcer on the opposite labium, or by lymphatic spread, which occurs in at least 50% of patients. The sequence of glandular involvement is superficial inguinal, femoral, external iliac, common iliac, and aortic groups.

A biopsy is essential to confirm the malignancy of the lesion. The treatment of choice is surgical, involving radical vulvectomy which involves the excision of the superficial and deep inguinal glands, and the gland of Cloquet in the femoral canal. Formerly only partial closure of the wound was carried out, and the central area is left to granulate over the ensuing 4 to 6 weeks; primary closure is usually possible now. Palliative treatment by means of radium needles which can sometimes effect a cure is possible where there are contraindications to major surgery.

VAGINAL CARCINOMA

Vaginal carcinoma is usually a metastasis from a malignant growth elsewhere in the pelvis. The primary form is very uncommon, but its possibility in young girls whose mothers were on oestrogen during that pregnancy must be borne in bind. A carcinoma in-situ can have a localised or patchy distribution in the vagina, and may be associated with similar lesions on the vulva or cervix. The epithelium may appear to be no more than a little reddened so that the lesion is often discovered by means of vaginal cytology.

The growth in the vagina usually occurs high on the posterior vaginal wall opposite to the external os. A history of exposure to a pessary (not necessarily a neglected one) is obtained in 25% of cases. Carcinoma of the vagina spreads quickly through its thin mucosa to involve the bladder, the rectum, the uterosacral ligaments, the cervix and the vulva. Patients are usually aged between 60 and 80 years and present with symptoms of irregular or contact bleeding, and an offensive discharge which is often blood-stained. The lesion is usually an ulcer with a hard base, and rolled edges, which become fixed to deeper tissues at an early stage: it bleeds readily on touching, having a friable surface.

'In-situ' lesions, provided they are symptom free, are treated conservatively, with regular medical review. Radiotherapy is felt to be the best form of treatment for invasive carcinoma, despite the close proximity of the bladder and rectum. Alternatively, radical surgery which includes either the excision of the whole vagina and uterus may be indicated.

Secondary malignant lesions of the vagina occur either directly from the local sites or indirectly through the bloodstream or by lymphatic spread. They usually appear in the form of isolated nodules that are found low in the anterior vaginal wall. Metastases can arise from any organ but are often from a renal primary, and, more particularly, from a choriocarcinoma or adenocarcinoma of the body of the uterus.

CARCINOMA OF THE UTERINE CERVIX

Pre-malignant disease of the cervix

Cervical cytology is recognised as a successful technique for diagnosing atypia, and is the only practical method of detecting cervical cancer in its preclinical stages (Wachtel 1973). Although the relationship of an 'in situ' lesion to an invasive one has been questioned, the temporal relationship of the lesion supports the idea of a sequence — the earlier lesions occurring in the younger patients (Langley 1974). In recent years, there has been a general trend in Western nations for increasing numbers of younger women (under 35 years) to develop invasive squamous carcinoma of the cervix (Worth 1974).

If one compares the age distribution of cases of *in-situ* lesions for West Lothian for the periods 1970–75 and 1976–80 then both the numbers of cases (and their relative proportion) in women aged less than 30 shows a striking increase. In 1970–75, there were nine cases aged less than 30 years in this population which represented 13% of all positive smears; by 1967–80, this number had increased to 27 which was 30% of all identified cases. In the new town of Livingston, 53% of all new cases in 1967–80 were aged 20–29. There are difficulties in the epidemiological interpretation of these trends but the numbers just quoted should be sufficient to emphasise the importance of this preventive technique in these age groups.

Ideally, all patients with abnormal cervical cytology, whether suspicious (Grade II) or positive (Grade III) should be subjected to colposcopic assessment of the cervix (Jordan 1980a). The nature and extent of the disease can thereby be accurately assessed, and treatment can be tailored to the needs of the individual patient. If the lesion is pre-malignant, the principle of treatment is to define the extent of the lesion, and to eradicate it by removal or destruction. The timing of this treatment depends on the severity of the lesion, and the circumstancs of the individual patient. If the lesion is carcinoma in-situ, it will be treated within a short period of time (weeks rather than months), whereas in a young patient with a suspicious smear and a known degree of dysplasia, treatment can justifiably be delayed until such time as her family is complete (Fig. 15.12a, b, c). Two reasons have been suggested to support this conservative regime:

1. Some known dysplasias will undergo spontaneous regression.

2. It is accepted physiologically that the cervix of the adolescent, and even the young adult, undergoes metaplasia (normal columnar epithelium being transformed into squamous epithelium) and active metaplasia can be mistaken both cytologically, colposcopically and histologically for epithelial abnormality.

It is therefore important that younger patients with abnormal cytological and colposcopic findings should be assessed carefully before being subjected to any treatment which could possibly adversely affect subsequent childbearing. Where inflammatory changes are noted, any suggestion of underlying malignancy can be double-checked by treating the infection before repeating the smear. Likewise, smears taken at a post-natal examination may demonstrate some features of dysplasia, related to the hormonal imbalance and unstable epithelium at the squamo-columnar junction following childbirth. At the time of the menopause, some smears may well show atypical cells, for which follow-up with repeat smears are required, possibly for a number of years.

Surgical treatment of premalignant disease of the cervix has tended to swing from conization (cone biopsy) of the cervix to the more recent development of cryosurgery or laser treatment. The use of the laser is a most exciting development in this field, since under direct vision by means of the colposcope the premalignant tissue can be destroyed; the energy output of the laser is directed and focused on the affected areas of cervix allowing precise destruction of any epithelial abnormality. Provided the criteria for surgical destruction are met, about 70% of epithelial abnormalities can be treated in the outpatient department without any form of anaesthesia (Jordan 1980b). As far as can be estimated, there is no effect on subsequent fertility or performance during pregnancy or labour. Surgical conization is not without its complications of post-operative haemorrhage, pelvic infection and cervical stenosis; this complication rate has been quantified as 6.6% by Jordan (1980c). No similar long-term follow-up of laser therapy is as yet available, but with the accepted criteria for the technique and tissue destruction to a depth of 5–7 mm, a cure rate of 94% can be expected with a single vaporisation.

It is now accepted (particularly by colposcopists) that hysterectomy is over-treatment for the majority of these lesions and the increasing use of destructive techniques under colposcopic control have proved that conization can also be avoided in most instances. The crux of selection of treatment is the colposcopic assessment and provided the facility is available in the area, no treatment should be undertaken without prior colposcopic assessment, together with an appraisal of individual factors such as age, parity, prolapse, and other uterine pathology.

Invasive carcinoma

Micro-invasive carcinoma occurs when, as the name suggests, there are tiny zones of penetration of abnormal cells through the basement membrane of the cervical epithelium. Although the evolution of the condition from premalignant to micro-invasive changes is still somewhat obscure, most of these lesions are likely to become truly invasive. Punch biopsy at colposcopy will confirm the precise type of lesion and its extent. Hysterectomy is not now recommended without prior colposcopic assessment and biopsy. Where the lesion is thought to be more extensive, reaching near to the vagina, then hysterectomy with a generous cuff of vagina would still be the treatment of choice.

Invasive carcinoma of the cervix is the commonest form of genital cancer and accounts for 6% of deaths from malignant diseases in women. In the past, there has

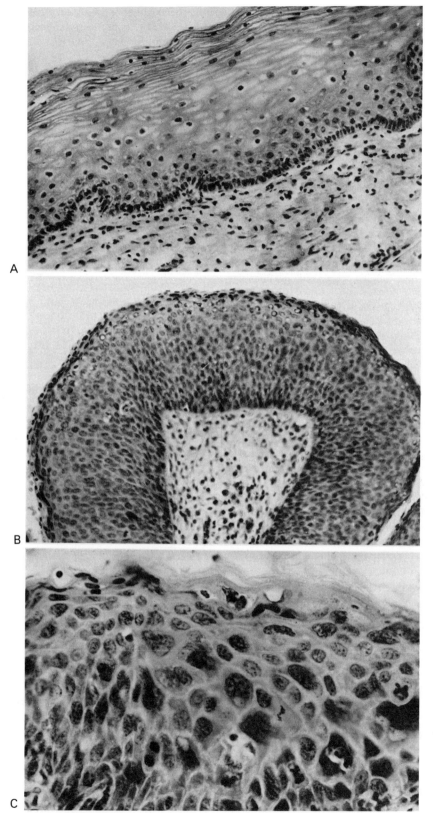

Fig. 15.12   A. Normal (stratified squamous) cervical epithelium. B. Dysplasia of cervical epithelium. C. Carcinoma-in-situ of cervix.

been much controversy concerning the value of cervical screening as a way of reducing the incidence of invasive carcinoma but a significant reduction in mortality has now been demonstrated where continuing screening by cervical cytology is carried out (Dickinson et al 1972, McGregor 1973). Canadian experience has shown a clear relationship between the intensity of screening programmes and the reduction in the mortality rate (British Medical Journal 1976). As one would expect, invasive carcinoma of the cervix is more prevalent in later age groups than the *in-situ* lesion; one difficulty in interpreting the effects of screening programmes concerns the 'natural' interval in which the in-situ lesion might progress to an invasive carcinoma and variations in this interval in different groups of women. Data from West Lothian and from Livingston New Town, however, suggest that the age of onset of invasive carcinoma may also be shifting towards earlier ages. In 1970–75, only 13 of the 50 cases in West Lothian were aged less than 50 compared to 20 out of 42 cases in the period 1976–80; 13 of these 20 cases were aged between 30 and 39.

Important aetiological factors include previous childbearing (it is rare in childless women), low socioeconomic status, and an association with coitus (the earlier in life that coitus starts, and the greater number of coital partners, the greater is the risk). There is thus a group of women in the community who are 'at risk' and who are least likely to use the screening facilities open to them. It should be emphasised that the educational process is a continuing one. A letter of invitation to take part in cervical screeninng is not enough; time and effort in the one-to-one situation between doctor and patient (for example when mother is attending with some of the family) or between nurse and patient (either in the treatment room or with the community nurse or health visitor in home) is necessary if the cervical screening is to reach this at risk group of patients.

In the following order, the clinical picture consists of:

Bleeding — often post-coital or after digital examination, or presenting as a prolongation of a normal period. In the post-menopausal patient, the onset is usually gradual, with intermittent slight spotting. The pattern of bleeding thereafter may be quite haphazard, and may in fact reach alarming proportions if a sizeable vessel is eroded.

Discharge — inevitably, the surface of the tumour becomes infected as it ulcerates, causing an offensive discharge which is thin, and serosanguineous. A cervical smear at this stage is of no consequence, and may, if it can be interpreted, show no alarming evidence.

Pain — extension of the growth to involve the pelvic nerves produces a deep persistent pain in the lower abdomen, lower back, the groins and, later, in the legs.

Anaemia, weakness and weight loss develop in the course of the disease, while in the later stages, faecal or urinary incontinence occurs due to fistula formation, and swelling of one or both legs can occur due to lymphatic obstruction.

Examination almost invariably shows blood on the examining finger, but outlining a cauliflower-type growth, with friable edges or an ulcer crater with indurated edges, confirms the suspicion. Speculum examination will demonstrate one of these lesions, probably with some contact bleeding or with the appearance of one or two crumbs of friable tissue which have broken off in the course of visualisation of the cervix. Apart from some fixation of the cervix, spread of the lesion to the parametrium or uterosacral ligaments is best demonstrated on rectal examination.

Urgent referral of such patients to a consultative gynaecological clinic is mandatory, since detailed examination and assessment under anaesthetic is required to stage the disease as well as to obtain a biopsy specimen to confirm the diagnosis by histological examination.

Surgical treatment in the form of Wertheim's hysterectomy is the preferred treatment for the earlier stages of invasive carcinoma of cervix. The more advanced cervical lesions are initially treated with irradiation therapy and secondary operative treatment is reserved for those in whom irradiation fails (Mattingly 1980). It is believed that it is the initial treatment — whether by surgery or irradiation — that provides the best chance for long-term cure of this disease. This implies that treatment should be in the most experienced hands, since secondary treatment for recurrent disease offers only limited long-term cure.

Studies of deaths from cancer of the cervix have shown that 90% occur in the unscreened population. Comparing patients with invasive carcinoma with controls matched for age, parity and social class, McGregor (1973) discovered a far lower screening rate in those with carcinoma. The incidence of carcinoma of cervix has increased in England in the last decade, while in Scotland it remains static. However, if data for Grampian and Tayside, two areas where screening is actively pursued, are excluded the incidence in the remaining areas of Scotland is increasing in the same way as in England. There is thus a responsibility for the general practitioner to pursue cervical screening, preferably on an organised basis, but to be prepared to attempt to obtain cervical smears from a high-risk patient who attends the surgery for any reason, since she is one who would be most unlikely to attend a special clinic.

CARCINOMA OF THE UTERUS

Carcinoma of the body of the uterus has now reached an incidence slightly greater than carcinoma of the cervix and there has not been an appropriate fall in carcinoma of the cervix to account for this increase. The condition commonly affects post-menopausal women, and unlike carcinoma of the cervix, at least 40% of the women so affected are multiparous. The clinical features are similar to those of cervical carcinoma:

Bleeding — either post-menopausal, or very irregular bleeding in the perimenopausal era.

Discharge — usually thin, watery but offensive.

Pain — again this is a late symptom, after the lesion has spread to the parametrium or via the peritoneum to the tubes and ovaries.

Clinically, there may be little if any evidence of the disease. The uterus may be small and atrophic (in keeping with the greater incidence after the menopause), but eventually the inguinal lymph glands are involved, becoming enlarged and palpable. Diagnosis must involve endometrial biopsy for histological confirmation of the disease.

Treatment includes a combination of surgery and radiotherapy, recent opinion favouring a radical hysterectomy followed by radiotherapy. There is unfortunately no reliable method of detecting the lesion in its earliest stages. Out-patient or 'office' techniques give a reasonable cytology sample but their greatest limitation is in giving a clear idea of what is happening, and where. It is believed in gynaecological circles that both post-menopausal and peri-menopausal bleeding are not taken seriously enough by busy general practitioners. Too often, perhaps, a variety of hormones are prescribed to control irregular menstruation, and patients may be prescribed progestogens, oestrogen replacement therapy, or a 'combined' pill preparation as a primary form of treatment without an attempt being made to establish a specific diagnosis — and in particular to exclude malignancy.

Carcinoma of the body of the uterus may be heading for epidemic proportions in the middle-aged and older woman. Epidemiological studies (particularly in the United States of America) leave little doubt that oestrogen therapy is a cause of endometrial cancer. The cancers induced by oestrogens seem mostly to be detected at an early age (perhaps a reflection of the surveillance of these women while on treatment) and the mortality associated with such tumours is said to be low. Some workers (Sturder et al 1978) are convinced that the addition of a progestogen to the oestrogen will eliminate the cancer risk, and that it is the duration rather than the daily dose of progestogen (13 days instead of seven) which is important. In view of some recent concern about the role of progestogens in the aetiology of arterial disease (Kay 1980), any approach to the use of oestrogen–progestogen mixtures in post-menopausal women should be cautious.

OVARIAN CARCINOMA

Ovarian cancer is the fifth mosst common cause of deaths among cancer sites for women, and causes the same number of deaths as cancer of the uterine cervix and cancer of the body of the uterus combined. Because of the insidious growth of ovarian cancer, 80% of patients will have advanced disease at the time of diagnosis. The overall mortality rate from ovarian cancer has increased by nearly 50% in England and Wales in the last 40 years, particularly amongst older women. Risk factors have been found for cancers of the cervix and endometrium, but singularly few have been identified for ovarian cancer. It is becoming apparent that voluntary limitation of family size, with or without infertility, may increase the risk of ovarian cancer. As far as prevention is concerned, it is encouraging to note that a possible association between the use of oral contraceptives and a decreased risk of ovarian cancer has been suggested. Proof of this assertion is awaited with interest.

Ovarian cysts and their possible complications have already been discussed. There is much to be said for the maxim 'lump, cut: no lump, no cut' in dealing with gynaecological tumours, since the differentiation of ovarian tumours is confirmed only on histological examination of the specimen. Many simple tumours are symptomless (Fig. 15.13), and occur mostly within the childbearing ages. Cysts can attain considerable proportions before a patient (or perhaps a friend) realises the changing waistline. Although the possibility of prevention and/ or earlier diagnosis seems remote, screening by ultrasound of the ovaries in women over, say 45 years of age might prove to be as justifiable as in cervical cytology. The 'false positive' rate of such screening, as yet, mitigates against this idea.

When examining the abdomen for a suspected ovarian cyst, the patient's bladder should be empty. Ultrasonography has proved a very useful adjunct to confirm or

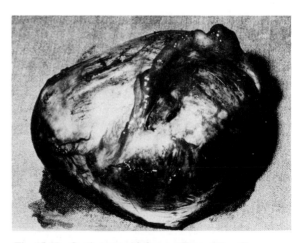

Fig. 15.13   Cystic teratoma of ovary ('Dermoid cyst'). Discovered at screening examination in the Well Woman/Family Planning Clinic. The patient was nulliparous and has since had a successful pregnancy.

refute the presence of an ovarian cyst and can show the presence of loculations. Ascites can also be demonstrated by this means, adding further evidence to suspicions of a malignant ovarian tumour.

Benign ovarian tumours are usually removed easily on laparotomy. At present, no one is satisfied with the current management of ovarian carcinoma — whatever the stage of the disease at the time the diagnosis is confirmed. A confident cure of ovarian carcinoma is not presently possible, but much work is being done on reappraisal of methods of management. Surgery, with or without postoperative radiotherapy, provides both the diagnosis and an attempt at total eradication of the disease. Experts in this field now have a choice of chemotherapy in their hands, and only these experienced colleagues can expect the best results from both the initial and any secondary surgery deemed necessary. Treatment schedules in a number of large centres are being revised and the place of surgery, chemotherapy and radiotherapy reassessed in the management of ovarian cancer.

URINARY PROBLEMS IN GYNAECOLOGY

CYSTITIS

The term 'cystitis' suggests that there is inflammation of the bladder. Commonly, however, it is used to described dysuria and frequency regardless of whether there is any evidence of bladder inflammation. The urethral syndrome is usually reserved for these symptoms presenting without evidence of bacterial infection. Cystitis is extremely common in adult women: in one study 22% of women described symptoms within the previous year, and 10% had consulted their doctor because of them (Waters 1969).

In a recent survey in the Well Woman Clinic in the author's practice, 10% of all patients checked had a demonstrable bacteriuria. Previous evidence suggested that about 4% of non-pregnant women have asymptomatic bacteriuria (Journal of the Royal College of General Practitioners 1977, Graymans et al 1976). Only one-third of the surveyed patients were noted to have *recurrent* infection whereas Graymans (1976) found that bacteriuria occurred more commonly in women with a past history of urinary infection.

The incidence of demonstrable bacteriuria in the clinic survey (Table 15.1) was found to escalate with advancing age, being highest in the post-menopausal group. It did not relate to the childbearing age groups which are accepted as being more sexually active. The incidence of bacteriuria however increased steadily with increasing parity although a high incidence was also found in the group of nulliparous women. Four patients were found to have hypertension associated with bacteriuria.

Table 15.1   Urinary tract infections in a Well Woman Clinic

Related to age	
Under 20	Nil
20–29 years	5.7%
30–39 years	5.3%
40–49 years	21.4%
50+	22.4%
Related to parity	
0	11.7%
1	6.3%
2	8.8%
3	11.9%
4+	15.5%

Investigation should include microscopic examination of the urine and, in older women, the presence of tubercle bacilli and neoplastic cells should be excluded. Bacterial counts can be made from urine held in a domestic refrigerator for up to 72 hours, although leucocytes often degenerate within hours (Triger et al 1966). Intravenous pyelograms are recommended for older women with cystitis of recent onset, and for patients with persistent pyuria or who require cystoscopy for haematuria. Abnormal pyelograms were discovered in 4% of women presenting in general practice with recurrent bacterial cystitis (Manners et al 1973).

Symptoms of uncomplicated cystitis often resolve spontaneously, while increasing fluid intake helps to rid the bladder of more bacteria. Urine should be cultured, particularly if symptoms persist, and an antibacterial prescribed. As short, sharp course of treatment is thought to be acceptable if the infection involves only the lower urinary tract, but since there is no simple way of locating the site of infection, the general rule is to prescribe a 10-day course of therapy. It is worthy of note that for adult women treated in general practice — a 3-day course of treatment was as effective as a course for 10 days (Charlton et al 1976).

What can be done about prevention? A high fluid intake, post-coital micturition, avoidance of excessive intercourse and adequate lubrication during intercourse are desirable and advised, but their actual effectiveness is doubtful. Symptoms induced by coitus are frequently prevented by a single dose of antibiotic (such as cotrimoxazole, or nitrofurantoin). Where attacks are frequent, nightly low dose treatment for 6 to 12 months has been recommended. Wherever possible, antibiotics should be avoided in the first trimester of pregnancy, although teratogenicity is unlikely. In this context, since the fetal mass is increased by two and a half million times between the time of fertilisation and 13 weeks gestation, a very conservative approach with any drug at this finely balanced stage of development is imperative. Prevention and treatment are likely to be particularly difficult in women with large residual volumes of urine, since it is difficult to eradicate bacteria from the urine, resulting in the development of resistant organisms.

STRESS INCONTINENCE

The term 'stress incontinence' is understood to mean the symptom or sign of loss of urine upon physical effort, such as coughing or movement. Stress incontinence is a fairly common problem — affecting patients in all age groups, but more frequently in the elderly. It is regarded as a most embarrassing problem by most patients, who find difficulty in discussing the details. Probably only a small proportion of patients affected by it actually seek medical advice. A number of studies have shown that as many as 50% of young healthy multiparous women are incontinent from time to time, although only about 5% of them find it troublesome. In a general practice survey, there was little increase in the incidence of mild urinary incontinence between the age groups of 15–34 years and 35–65 years, but the incidence of severe incontinence more than doubled in the older group (Thomas et al 1980).

Continence relies on the fact that urethral pressure is always higher than bladder pressure, except during micturition; there is a positive pressure gradient from the urethra to the bladder. Intra-abdominal pressure also affects the bladder pressure, and any coughing or straining, inevitably increasing intra-abdominal pressure, is transmitted to the bladder. With normal anatomy, the bladder neck and proximal urethra lie close to the pelvic floor, so that an increase in intra-abdominal pressure will in fact increase the closing force. However, in some women with anterior vaginal wall prolapse, and resultant cystocele formation, the bladder neck and proximal urethra are below the level of the pelvic floor, so that increasing intra-abdominal pressure is not equally transmitted (below the pelvic floor) resulting in urinary incontinence.

CAUSES OF URINARY INCONTINENCE

Genuine stress incontinence

In most cases, stress incontinence of urine may be the only symptom relating to micturition, there may be no history of pregnancy, urgency, or urge incontinence. Genuine stress incontinence, with its weakened urethral sphincter mechanisms may be associated with multiparity, genital prolapse, or with the genital atrophy of the menopause.

Detrusor instability

This is the second commonest cause of incontinence in women. It occurs by uninhibited detrusor contractions which allow the bladder pressure to exceed the urethral pressure, with consequent incontinence. The actual cause of the detrusor instability is unknown, although in many cases emotional factors are thought to play a part. It can sometimes be secondary to an upper motor neurone lesion, such as in multiple sclerosis. Usually, patients with an unstable bladder have a variety of symptoms, including urgency, urge incontinence, stress incontinence, enuresis and nocturia. Patients with genuine stress incontinence (with weakness of the urethral sphincter mechanism) may, by habit, have diurnal frequency, but no nocturia, unless an infection is present.

Overflow incontinence

This is uncommon, since chronic retention of urine in women is uncommon, and often no cause can be found. A pelvic mass, or inflammation of the urethra, vagina or vulva or a lower motor neurone lesion may be responsible. Drugs such as ganglion blockers, anticholinergic agents, ß-adrenergic stimulants or tricyclic antidepressants can also cause retention of urine. Although patients may present in a number of ways — with dribbling or stress incontinence, or passing small amounts of urine at frequent intervals — diagnosis is confirmed on finding an enlarged bladder at examination.

Functional

This group, in which no organic cause can be found for incontinence, frequently have an associated anxiety state, which responds to psychotherapy.

Congenital abnormalities

Conditions such as epispadias and ectopic ureters are rare, and should have been evaluated at birth.

The importance of an accurate and detailed history must be emphasised. Basically, stress incontinence is associated with urethral sphincter weakness (genuine stress incontinence). While urge incontinence is related to detrusor instability, stress incontinence, however, can be a symptom of any of these conditions, while urgency or urge incontinence may be sensory rather than motor — inflammation of the mucosa such as cystitis, a calculus, or a bladder tumour may be the cause. Frequency of micturition is a symptom commonly associated with urinary incontinence, but this commonly results from the patient's habit of emptying her bladder frequently — before any heavy housework or before going out shopping. In such cases, the bladder capacity is never 'stretched' and therefore persistent frequency and even urgency is the almost inevitabble sequel. Nocturia is not usually associated with detrusor instability, and drinking habits have to be checked, as well as sleep patterns, apart from intercurrent or recurrent urinary infections.

Clinical examination is much less helpful than an accurate history. Demonstrating the presence of stress incontinence (e.g. on coughing) does not elucidate the cause of the incontinence. In long-standing cases, excoriation of the vulva verifies the chronicity of the problem. Vaginal examination will exclude any pelvic pathology, and might reveal scarring from previous surgery or trauma. Genital prolapse and cystourethrocele may also be found, but again this does not indicate the cause of the incontinence.

Where the history is complicated, or the problem recurrent, more elaborate investigations are necessary including a micturating cystography, and cystometry. Urine culture is essential in every case, since an infection may be responsible for the symptomatology. Catheterisation itself can precipiate urinary infection, which in turn can invalidate more elaborate investigations. For detrusor instability, drug treatment is worthy of trial in the first instance, since it is not so amenable to surgical treatment: this is not surprising considering the varied procedures suggested — denervation of the bladder, cystoplasty, or sacral neurectomy. Emepronium bromide (Cetiprin) or flavoxate hydrochloride (Urispas) are probably first choice drugs. Temporary relief of symptoms is achieved in about a third of patients. Where nocturia and enuresis are predominant, imipramine has proved helpful. Bladder drill is an important adjuvant to treatment of idiopathic detrusor instability, but it requires continual motivation and exhortation of the patient. The theory of failure of cortical inhibition is gaining popularity and recently interest in bladder drill has grown (Cardozo 1981).

Pelvic floor exercises are of use in the post-partum patient or where levator muscle tone is poor, for example after surgery. Obese patients and patients with a chronic cough require appropriate measures which indirectly will help to reduce intra-abdominal pressure. Sometimes obesity may be the result rather than the cause of the urinary incontinence, since some women so afflicted have an increasing reluctance to leave the house, where they probably eat compulsively, and become overweight. Patients who tend to have a high fluid intake should be advised to restrict their drinking, particularly if frequency of micturition is a predominant symptom.

Incontinence is an important problem in the elderly patient, particularly if chair or bed bound. The sequelae of pressure sores, established chronic renal infection and the strain on caring relatives can be of greater consequence than is the incontinence. Regular visits from the district nurse will help to avoid the first complication while the use of an appropriate sheath or other urine collection garment — or long-term catheterisation — can limit both pressure sores and the social consequences of being incontinent. Soiled clothes and bedclothes can prove a problem and in many areas a laundry service — organised by the Social Work Department — can be of great assistance.

Stress incontinence is a not uncommon symptom in pregnancy, when it is noted by up to 50% of primigravidae. It is liable to recur in subsequent pregnancies, probably to a greater degree, and if it persists following postnatal examination, despite apparently responsive levator ani muscle tone, it may become a permanent complaint requiring surgical treatment. This sequence of events is not directly related to the number of pregnancies, since the complaint can be admitted by as many as 30% of young normal nulliparous women, albeit more or less as an occasional, relatively trivial accident.

REFERENCES

Bungay G T, Vessey M P, McPherson C K 1980 British Medical Journal 28: 181–183

Cardozo L 1981 Detrusor instability. In: Jordan J A, Stanton S L (eds) Proceedings of a scientific meeting of the Royal College of Gynaecologists. p 45

Charlton C A C et al 1976 Three-day and ten-day chemotherapy for urinary tract infections in general practice. British Medical Journal 00: 124–126

Dewhurst C T D (ed) 1972 Integrated obstetrics and gynaecology for post-graduates. Blackwell Scientific, Oxford, p 606

Dickinson et al 1972 Proceedings of staff meeting. Mayo Clinic Proceedings 47: 534

Elstein M 1974 Clinics in obstetrics and gynaecology 1:2. In: Cooke I D (ed) Management of infertility, Saunders, London, p 345

Frommer D J 1964 British Medical Journal II: 349

Gaymans, Walkenburg et al 1976 Lancet II: 674

Gold J J 1975 Gynaecologic endocrinology. Harper and Row, Hagerstown, p 242

Golditch I M 1972 Post-contraceptive amenorrhoea. Obstetrics and Gynaecology 39: 903

Jeffcoate T N A 1975a Principles of gynaecology. Butterworth & Co. London, ch 1, p 3

Jeffcoate T N A 1975b Principles of gynaecology. Butterworth & Co, London, ch 20, p 312

Jordan J A 1977 Colposcopy in gynaecological practice. Proceedings of the first world congress on colposcopy and cervical pathology. p 131

Jordan J A 1980a The modern treatment of pre-malignant disease of the cervix. In: Jordan J A, Singer A (eds) Proceedings of a scientific meetinng of the Royal College of Gynaecologists, p 25

Jordan J A 1980b Ibid p 32

Jordan J A 1980c Ibid p 28

Journal of the Royal College of General Practitioners 1977 27: 131 Editorial

Kay C R 1980 The happiness pill. Journal of the Royal College of General Practitioners 30: 8

Langley F A 1974 Pre-malignancy in gynaecology. British Journal of Hospital Medicine 12: 79

Leading article 1976 British Medical Journal 2: 569

Lloyd G 1976 Case for the treatment of minor gynaecological conditions in general practice. Update 12: 1279–1283

Manners B T B, Grob P R, Dulake C, Grieve N W T 1973 Urinary tract infection. Oxford University Press, London, p 186

Mattingley R F 1980 The surgical treatment of cervical cancer — factors influencing cure. In: Jordan J A, Singer A (eds) Proceedings of a scientific meeting of the Royal College of Gynaecologists, p 41

McGregor J E 1973 Paper presented to the World Association for Gynaecological Cancer Prevention, Saltzburg

Monaghan J M 1980 Treatment of carcinoma of the endometrium. In: Jordan J A, Singer A (eds) Proceedings of a scientific meeting of the Royal College of Gynaecologists, p 111

Neilson J P, Hood V D, Whitfield C R 1982 British Journal of Hospital Medicine 27: 236

Rader M D, Flickinger G L, de Villa G D, Mikuta J J, Mikhail G 1973 American Journal of Obstetrics and Gynecology 116: 1069

Speroff L, Glass R H, Kase N 1974 Clinical gynaecologic endocrinology and infertility. Williams and Wilkins, Baltimore, ch 13

Steptoe P C 1967 Laparoscopy in gynaecology. Churchill Livingstone, Edinburgh

Sturder D W, Wade-Evans T, Paterson M EL, Thom M H, Studd J W W 1978 Relations between bleeding pattern, endometrial histology and oestrogen treatment in menopausal women. British Medical Journal I: 1575

Thom M H, Studd J W W 1980 Oestrogens and endometrial hyperplasia. British Journal of Hospital Medicine 23:512

Thomas T N, Plymat K R, Blannin J, Meade T W 1980 Prevalence of urinary incontinence. British Medical Journal 281: 1243

Triger D R, Smith J W G 1966 Journal of Clinical Pathology 19: 443

Wachtel E 1973 The Practitioner 211: 137

Waters W E 1969 British Journal of Preventive and Social Medicine 23: 263

Winokur G 1973 American Journal of Psychiatry 130: 92

Worth A J 1974 Canadian Medical Journal 110: 131

SUGGESTED READING

Barr W 1971 Clinical Gynaecology. Churchill Livingstone, Edinburgh.

Uro-genital problems in the male

INTRODUCTION

The male patient who consults his general practitioner with a symptom referable to the genito-urinary system is likely to be understandably embarrassed and may have delayed some time before deciding to see the doctor. It seems reasonable to take this into account when dealing with the patient and make allowances as appropriate.

Problems such as haematuria and prostatic hypertrophy are common whereas others such as testicular tumour though infrequently seen must be dealt with promptly and correctly.

This chapter attempts to outline the more common and important uro-genital problems in men (Table 16.1) and to give guidance regarding their management.

THE PATIENT WITH HAEMATURIA

Haematuria is a fairly common reason for the male patient to seek his doctor's advice, often urgently. The patient is understandably worried about a possible sinister explanation for this symptom and it would be wrong for the doctor to prematurely over-reassure the patient at an early stage. After taking a clear history it is necessary to confirm the actual presence of blood in the urine by visual examination of the urine or by the use of reagent strips. Microscopy is, however, the only foolproof test for blood in urine. Physical examination in such a case is much less rewarding than time spent on history-taking. A decision must be taken at this stage whether direct referral to a urologist is appropriate or whether some initial investigations should be ordered. Some urologists prefer to see the patient at an early stage as they carry out a routine package of investigations which include cystoscopy. All general practitioners should now be able to have an IVP carried out without too much delay and an MSSU at this stage is also desirable. It should be borne in mind that repeated injections of contrast medium may increase the risk of the patient developing a sensitivity reaction.

Table 16.1 Male uro-genital problems in general practice

The patient with haematuria
The patient who has difficulty with micturition
   Acute retention
   Non-acute difficulty with micturition
The patient with a scrotal swelling
   Testicular tumours
   Epididymo-orchitis
   Hydrocoele
   Cyst of epididymis
   Haematoma
   Torsion of the testis
   Inguinal hernia
Renal and ureteric colic
Renal disease and renal failure
Other male urological problems
   Phimosis
   Paraphimosis
   Balanitis (balano-posthitis)
   Penile warts
Traumatic conditions
   Renal trauma
   Tears of the frenulum of the prepuce
   Testicular haematomas
Vasectomy
Male sub-fertility and infertility
Psychosexual problems

Urinary infection should not be accepted as the explanation for haematuria in the male and lest a bladder tumour go undiagnosed, cystoscopy should always be arranged in addition to the IVP. One infection which should not be forgotten however is tuberculosis of the kidney, bladder or prostate.

The explanation for the bleeding will usually turn out to be one of the following:

Bladder papilloma
Bladder carcinoma
Renal, ureteric or bladder calculus
Renal cyst or renal injury

Table 16.2 also gives some of the less common causes of haematuria.

Table 16.2 Causes of haematuria including less commonly experienced conditions

Haemopoetic	Bleeding diatheses
	Anticoagulant drugs
	Thrombocytopenia
	Haemoglobinuria
Kidney	Polycystic disease
	Infarction
	Tuberculosis
	Trauma
	Tumour
Ureter	Stone
Bladder	Trauma
	Infection
	Tumour
Prostate	Varices
Urethra	Trauma
	Calculus
	Tumour
Non-blood 'haematuria'	Beetroot
	Rhubarb
	Phenolphthalein
	Senna
	Dyes in food

THE PATIENT WHO HAS DIFFICULTY WITH MICTURITION

The patient who has difficulty with micturition will present to the general practitioner either in an acute emergency situation or following gradual deterioration in bladder function.

ACUTE RETENTION

Acute urinary retention is usually the result of prostatic hypertropy. There is often a history of increasingly significant prostatic symptoms and no obvious single factor can be implicated for the complete cessation of urinary flow. Prescribing an anticholinergic drug, such as a tricyclic antidepressant, in a middle-aged or elderly man may precipitate acute retention in a previously apparently asymptomatic patient and the use of such common drugs should be preceded by consideration of their potential side-effects. Consumption of alcohol is all too often a trigger factor in acute retention not only on account of the brisk diuresis which it causes but as a result of congestion of the venous plexus of the prostate, especially if voiding is delayed for social reasons, such as football match or bus run.

Constipation is another common condition of elderly patients and a bowel loaded with hard faeces may be the underlying reason for an episode of acute retention.

The use of 'loop' diuretics with rapid onset of action may precipitate acute retention.

Management of acute retention

Although underlying problems should certainly be dealt with — stopping anticholinergic medication or preventing or treating constipation — bladder catheterisation will almost always be necessary and most general practitioners would at this stage request hospital admission except in outlying or isolated areas. Some hospitals admit such patients directly into the Urology Department but in others the General Surgical Receiving Unit deals with the initial management. Following catheterisation the patient may be discharged back to the general practitioner's care to await elective surgery — often prostatectomy — or may have trans-urethral resection of the prostate or open prostatectomy carried out during this initial hospitalisation.

NON-ACUTE DIFFICULTY WITH MICTURITION

Many patients coming into this category have prostatic hypertrophy and report increasing problems with hesitancy, poor flow, frequency, and terminal dribbling. Rectal examination usually reveals benign hypertrophy of the prostate although in some men the irregular craggy character of a prostatic tumour can be easily identified. If the latter is suspected, estimation of serum prostatic acid phosphatase may be helpful although this can not, of course, be carried out immediately after a rectal examination. Patients with either of these conditions should be referred to the urologist, possibly for surgical treatment at some stage. In the case of the latter condition oral stilboestrol is generally recommended and is often successful in slowing the disease process. The patient may have to be warned and reassured that gynaecomastia can develop while on stilboestrol therapy, and he may, of course, sooner or later present with bony metastases. Care in the later stages of the illness can usually be effectively managed by the general practitioner, consulting his urology, oncology or radiotherapy colleagues when necessary.

From time to time a patient will require long-term catheter drainage at home and the continuous presence of an indwelling catheter may give rise to several problems. Figure 16.1 shows a helpful information sheet prepared by a Urology Department for district nurses and general practitioners involved in the long-term management of such patients.

Prostatitis is usually bacterial and only occasionally tuberculous and may cause symptoms of prostatism or even acute retention. There may be a pyrexia and a leucocytosis and antibiotics are helpful if an early diagnosis is made.

Much less commonly the underlying cause of the patient's difficulties with micturition is a urethral stricture. Urethral strictures are either post-traumatic (following

LONG-TERM CATHETER DRAINAGE

1. Patient's Name _____

   Unit No. _____

   Address: _____

   _____

2. Catheter:　Size:
   　　　　　　Type:
   　　　　　　Volume in balloon:

3. *Date of return appointment for catheter drainage at Southern General Hospital.

4. *Arrangements have been made for change of catheter at home by Community Nurse.

5. *Discharge letter follows.

*Delete if not applicable

Catheter should be irrigated twice weekly if possible. Water is suitable.

Intermittent drainage is best for daytime unless by-passing is a problem. Two to three hourly release is adequate, and prevents erosion of bladder mucosa by the catheter.

By-passing results from bladder irritation or uninhibited bladder contraction. Bladder irritation is made worse by:

1. Large catheters
2. Excessive volume in the catheter balloon. A catheter with 5–10 ml balloon capacity is preferable.
3. Debris in bladder: prevented by irrigation.
4. Concentrated urine: increased fluid intake helps.

In patients with neurological disease, the bladder may be hypersensitive and hyperactive, producing uninhibited contractions and therefore by-passing. Probanthine reduces bladder activity in most patients. If needed, starting dose should be 1 tablet (15 mg) t.i.d., increasing to as much as 2 tablets q.i.d. if necessary provided there are no side effects. Probanthine is contraindicated in the presence of glaucoma.

Continuous drainage overnight is usually preferred since the spigot may come out if the patient is restless. Urine culture will always be positive for patients with indwelling catheters. Antibiotics are only indicated when there is evidence of systemic infection.

More detailed advice is available from the Urology Department, Southern General Hospital. The Department holds a weekly meeting on Fridays at 11.15 a.m. in the Walton Urological Teaching and Research Centre. Community nurses regularly attend and family doctors are welcome to discuss problems of a urological nature then.

Fig. 16.1　Instruction sheet for catheter patients, issued by one Urology Department on discharge (reproduced by kind permission of Mr E.S. Glen Consultant Urologist, Walton Urological Teaching and Research Centre, Southern General Hospital, Glasgow)

injury or instrumentation) or post-gonococcal. Such a patient complains again of poor flow but finds that he can empty his bladder only with increased effort. Treatment usually involves bouginage or urethrotomy or, very rarely, surgical repair or reconstruction. In outlying or rural areas suprapubic cannulation carried out by the general practitioner may be required to relieve retention.

Neurological or pharmacological causes of difficulty with micturition should not be forgotten. Multiple scler-osis will usually be diagnosed on other features of the disease as will spinal injuries or tumours. Anticholinergic drugs causing retention of urine have already been mentioned and a check on what drugs the patient has been taking should be part of the initial assessment of the problem.

Bladder calculus may present with difficulty in mic-turition as it acts like a ball-valve producing a 'stop-start' effect to voiding. Pan is usually a feature.

Urinary tract obstruction at any level may lead to hydronephrosis and occasionally symptoms referable to the dilatation of renal pelvis and calyces may be the initial presentation. Loin pain is the primary symptom but infection may lead to fever and pyuria. The kidney may be palpable in such cases and is likely to be tender.

THE PATIENT WITH A SCROTAL SWELLING

Scrotal swellings are usually the result of one of the following:

Testicular tumour
Epididymo-orchitis
Hydrocoele
Cyst of epididymis
Varicocoele
Haematoma
Torsion of the testis
Inguinal hernia

TESTICULAR TUMOURS

About 60% of tumours of the testis are seminomas which are relatively slow growing and usually occur between 30 and 40 years of age. The remaining 40% are teratomas which occur more commonly in the 20–30 age group and spread more rapidly, particularly to lungs and liver. Early diagnosis is essential and the urologist will usually proceed quickly to orchidectomy followed by radiotherapy of the para-aortic nodes. Chemotherapy is also being used in certain specialist units.

EPIDIDYMO-ORCHITIS

Mumps orchitis is usually diagnosed from the accompanying parotid swelling and fertility may be impaired by residual damage. Bacterial infection is best treated by bed rest, antibiotics and a scrotal support.

HYDROCOELE

Hydrocoeles may be primary or secondary to tumour or inflammation of the underlying testis or epididymis. It is important to remember this latter group and not to delay in early referral to the urologist for further investigation.

CYSTS OF EPIDIDYMIS

These need only be removed surgically if giving rise to symptoms. They are not uncommon and tend to be recurrent.

VARICOCOELES

Commoner on the left than the right, a varicocoele may be of relevance as a cause of defective spermatogenesis. Surgical treatment may be warranted on these grounds or if the condition is causing some degree of discomfort.

HAEMATOMA

Scrotal haematomas are the result of direct trauma or are occasionally post-operative such as following vasectomy. The prescription of a scrotal support can afford considerable symptomatic relief.

TORSION OF THE TESTIS

Occurring usually in children or adolescents torsion of the testis is a surgical emergency which presents as an acutely swollen and painful testis associated with pain in the lower abdomen. If untreated, irreversible, infarction of the testis will occur within a few hours. Surgical exploration is carried out forthwith and fixation in the scrotum performed unless infarction is advanced and orchidectomy is thus indicated.

INGUINAL HERNIA

Inguinal hernia should be included in a list of causes of scrotal swelling but its management is of course more related to the surgical condition in general than to a urological problem.

RENAL AND URETERIC COLIC

The drugs of choice for acute renal or ureteric colic are pethidine (100 mg) or morphine (15 mg). They should be given by intramuscular injection and repeated as required. Atropine (0.6–1.2 mg) subcutaneously should also be given to counteract smooth muscle spasm. Coupled with a high fluid intake this may be all the treatment that is required and the smaller stone may pass spontaneously. In the case of larger stones surgical removal may be necessary and urological help is again required.

Some thought should be given to the possibility of an underlying disorder of calcium and phosphate metabolism: occasionally calculi are the result of a parathyroid tumour.

Any patient who has formed a urinary tract calculus should be advised strongly regarding the importance of a high fluid intake in addition to any other measures designed to prevent recurrence, such as the lowering of an elevated serum uric acid with allopurinol.

RENAL DISEASE AND RENAL FAILURE

The general practitioner will be called upon to deal with glomerulonephritis, polycystic disease or other parenchymal kidney disease only rarely. The cases of renal failure which he sees will more usually be in elderly patients in whom impairment of cerebral function and poor excretion of drugs may be a major problem.

For younger patients with renal failure kidney transplantation is the only alternative to long-term dialysis at home or in hospital. As part of his increasing role in health education the general practitioner can assist the transplantation programme by making donor cards easily available and being ready and willing to answer any questions which a potential donor card carrier or even a distressed relative might have (Fig. 16.2).

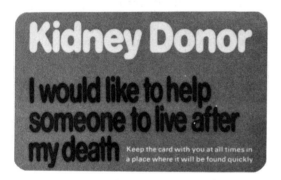

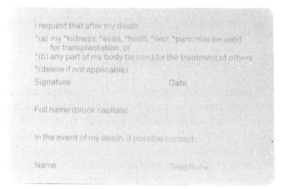

Fig. 16.2 Kidney donor card

Patients on home dialysis generally keep in close contact with their hospital dialysis unit who are likely to welcome increased contact and liaison with the general practitioner.

The social and psychological problems that can result from such an abnormal and dependent lifestyle should be remembered and every step possible taken to minimise them.

OTHER MALE UROLOGICAL PROBLEMS

PHIMOSIS

True congenital narrowing of the preputial orifice is not frequently seen and most cases brought to the general practitioner are of non-retractile prepuce which may be present normally until 3–4 years of age. Forcible retraction of the prepuce should be discouraged and any action such as referral to a paediatric surgeon deferred until the age of 4 unless the case is one of true congenital narrowing.

PARAPHIMOSIS

This condition may present as something of an emergency. If initial attempts at reducing the prepuce (which has become retracted around the corona) fail then surgical referral will be necessary. In most cases circumcision is subsequently advised.

BALANITIS (BALANO-POSTHITIS)

This condition involves simple redness and irritation of the glans and prepuce more often than an acute inflammation of established bacterial infection. The underlying infective agent is often fungal and can be associated with a female partner's vaginal candidiasis. Treatment with a topical antifungal such as nystatin, miconazole or clotrimazole is usually effective but continuation of treatment beyond symptomatic relief must be emphasised as recurrence, as with all fungal infections, is a potential problem.

PENILE WARTS

Although topically applied treatment can be carried out without referral, most cases of penile warts probably warrant referral to the urologist or dermatologist and early, efficient treatment should make the presentation of advanced, widespread collections of genital warts relatively uncommon.

TRAUMATIC CONDITIONS

RENAL TRAUMA

Blunt injury to the kidneys is not uncommon and can result from a kick or a fall such as those sustained while climbing, mountaineering or horse-riding. The presence of microscopic haematuria should be excluded and an IVP arranged if the injury is at all severe. The general practitioner should not hesitate to seek help from the urologist in such cases.

TEARS OF THE FRENULUM OF THE PREPUCE

The presentation of a tear usually involves an embarrassed young man who experiences brisk bleeding from the inferior aspect of the glans following sexual intercourse, often for the first time. The blood loss from the vessel in the frenulum may appear quite considerable before haemostasis is established either spontaneously or by suturing. Treatment of any kind is however rarely necessary and firm reassurance is usually all that is required. The condition may occasionally be recurrent.

TESTICULAR HAEMATOMA

This has already been described in the section on scrotal swelling.

VASECTOMY

Male sterilisation has become an increasingly popular method of contraception and this minor procedure is now performed by many general practitioners. Referral may also be made to the local urology outpatient department or to a urologist privately.

The Family Planning Association also arrange vasectomy if a couple request this at one of the Family Planning clinics.

The procedure is safe and simple but several points are worth emphasising. Pre-vasectomy counselling can be carried out satisfactorily by the general practitioner with his personal knowledge of the family circumstances, both socially and as regards health. The irreversibility of the procedure must be emphasised to the couple and consideration given to the stability of the marriage and the health of existing children.

MALE SUB-FERTILITY OR INFERTILITY

The problem of infertility is one of the most sensitive with which a patient may approach his doctor. Before referring his patient the general practitioner should carry out a brief examination in order to avoid missing an obvious testicular or penile abnormality. Investigations should be carried out simultaneously by urologist and gynaecologist although often disappointingly little close liaison seems to take place. The general practitioner should act as a co-ordinator in such cases if he is indeed responsible for both partners. The treatment of male infertility may involve androgen therapy or correction of a varicocoele but little effective therapy is available for many patients.

PSYCHOSEXUAL PROBLEMS

Problems of this nature may be relatively straightforward or may involve repeated counselling sessions which can be very time-consuming. If the general practitioner feels in any way unhappy about dealing personally with such a patient he should seek the help of a colleague either within the practice or at a psychosexual clinic, which are run by the Family Planning Association and by some psychiatrists and psychologists.

Impotence is a common example of such a problem and undiagnosed alcoholism should be high on the list of possible causes. Diabetes should not be forgotten as a cause of sexual problems and depressive illness may also present in this way. Side-effects of any drug therapy should also be considered as the older antihypertensive agents such as methyldopa were frequently responsible for causing impotence. Drug therapy should also be borne in mind when investigating patients who complain of a failure to maintain erection which, along with premature ejaculation, constitutes a large proportion of the remaining male psychosexual problems.

Sexually transmitted diseases

INTRODUCTION

According to returns made to the World Health Organization approximately 200 million new cases of gonorrhoea and 40 million new cases of syphilis are notified each year. This is thought to be an underestimate (Adler 1982). In the United Kingdom consultants in charge of clinics for sexually transmitted disease (STD) are required to make quarterly returns to the Chief Medical Officers of the respective counties. This requirement is made in Veneral Disease Regulations of 1916 which also provided for the establishment of a free and confidential service for the treatment of venereal disease in clinics under the auspices of local authorities. Currently the total number of cases seen at the 230 clinics throughout the United Kingdom is just over half a million per annum. About a quarter of these cases are of non-specific genital infection. A further quarter are conditions requiring no treatment but include patients asking for reassurance, check-ups or advice. Syphilis, gonorrhoea and chancroid, the diseases originally designated as Venereal in the Regulations of 1916, account for only 15% of the total seen in clinics today.

The figures provided by the returns from the clinics are subject to some controversy, but there is no doubt that the incidence of sexually transmitted diseases in the United Kingdom is increasing. A large majority of patients who suspect that they might be suffering from these diseases do not consult their own general practitioner, but attend a clinic, consult a doctor other than their own or just wait for spontaneous recovery.

Probably the commonest reason for patients not consulting their own doctor is shame and fear that their family or spouse could somehow hear about their problem. Women are more likely to consult their general practitioner with symptoms that could be due to a sexually transmitted disease, but seldom admit suspicion about their cause. The general practitioner's knowledge of the patient, the family and the marital relationship can be helpful in deciding what investigations to pursue, but often such knowledge can lull the doctor into a sense of false security. The place of the general practitioner in the management of these diseases is in some respects controversial and can only be considered alongside the services provided by the hospital clinics specialising in these diseases.

HOSPITAL CLINICS FOR SEXUALLY TRANSMITTED DISEASES

In 1948 the National Health Service took over the responsibility for the clinics established under the Venereal Disease Regulations of 1916. This continuity of service has produced a national, efficient and comprehensive service, totally free of any charges to the patient. The clinics are open and no referral letters are necessary. Communication from clinic to clinic is efficient so that a patient moving from place to place can be provided with continuity of care.

The aims of the clinics are not only to investigate patients suspected of having a sexually transmitted disease and treat them if necessary, but to make contact with the sexual partners of those found to be infected. Most clinics have on their staff professional contact tracers. Patients who are anxious but not suffering from infection can be reassured, thus preventing much deep mental suffering and anxiety.

THE ROLE OF THE GENERAL PRACTITIONER

In many situations in general practice, the establishment of a firm diagnosis is often not of fundamental importance because many of the problems encountered can be solved without making one. In the management of sexually transmitted diseases a firm diagnosis is of prime importance and it should be established before treatment is started. The high incidence of sexually transmitted disease in the community and the relatively few cases that present themselves to their doctor create a problem. How often is the possibility of gonorrhoea considered in the case of a happily married woman who complains of a vaginal discharge? If in fact she is suffering from gonorrhoea and a firm diagnosis is made, should the disease be treated in general practice or the patient referred to the clinic?

The good management of sexually transmitted disease depends upon early diagnosis by microscopy, access to an expert bacteriological service, adequate treatment and the ability to follow up contacts. Many general practitioners are prepared to use a microscope, can perform a Gram stain and the majority have access to a bacteriological laboratory. All can learn the appropriate treatment. However, to take an example, a search for intracellular Gram negative diplococci on an occasional basis presents problems and an even greater difficulty arises when the doctor is faced with making contact with the sexual partners of the infected patient: frequently they are the patients of other doctors.

The conclusion must be that in the majority of cases it is preferable to refer the patient to the hospital clinic. Some patients will of course refuse this advice leaving the doctor with the responsibility of managing the case himself or risk that the patient shall have no treatment at all. It is primarily for this situation that this chapter is written.

THE PRESENTATION AND DIAGNOSIS OF SEXUALLY TRANSMITTED DISEASES

MEDICAL HISTORY

The general practitioner in taking a history from a patient whom he suspects as having a sexually transmitted disease requires considerable tact and discretion. The doctor at the hospital clinic can often be more direct. The nature and duration of the symptoms should be determined as must the details of sexual contacts. Methods of contraception are important as are any symptoms or illness in sexual partners. It is possible that the partner is already attending another doctor or a hospital and it is important to make enquiries concerning the diagnosis made and the treatment prescribed. Very frequently answers to these enquiries are vague, unhelpful and often misleading.

Presentation and diagnosis in the male

The commonest presenting symptoms are penile discharge, dysuria and frequency, urethral or penile irritation, sores or lumps on the penis, or a rash involving the penis or, more rarely, the abdomen. Men presenting with symptoms that could be those of sexually transmitted disease should be subjected to a careful physical and bacteriological routine. The absence of physical signs does not exclude the presence of disease.

Examination

The external genitalia should be inspected, the inguinal lumph nodes, testes, epididymes and spermatic cords palpated. The uncircumcised prepuce should be retracted and any inflammation or lesions of the glans or foreskin noted. Phimosis may make a complete retraction of the prepuce impossible. Frequently a bead of pus may be seen issuing from the urethral meatus, but if this is not apparent then the penile urethra should be massaged gently when a bead of pus can sometimes be extruded through the meatus in cases of urethritis. This is an important sign in making a distinction between a balano-posthitis or urethritis in the patient with a phimosis.

The anal region and perineum should be inspected as should the thighs, buttocks and abdomen. In homosexuals a proctoscopic examination should be performed so that a swab can be taken from the rectal mucosa.

Bacteriology

Swabs should be taken for microscopy and culture. The bacteriological swab should be inserted into the urethral meatus and then spread on to a slide for subsequent Gram staining. Another swab should be inoculated into a transport medium. The sooner that the specimens can be delivered to the hospital the more likely it is that a diagnosis can be made. If there is a balano-posthitis swabs should be inoculated into transport medium for Candida and the herpes simplex virus. If a primary chancre is suspected the patient should be referred for a specialist opinion. The absence of physical signs should not inhibit the taking of a urethral swab for culture; 10% of men suffering from gonorrhoea are symptom-free and have no apparent discharge. It is preferable to make these tests on patients who have not passed urine for at least 1 hour or more before the examination.

The two glass urine test

This is a simple test to detect the presence of urethritis but it is of little value if the patient has passed urine within 1 hour of the examination and should only be performed after taking a bacteriological swab as detailed above. The patient should pass 2 inches (5 cm) of urine into the first glass and the remainder into the second. A solution of 20% acetic acid is poured into both glasses. The presence of threads in the first and clarity in the second indicates anterior urethritis. Threads in the second glass suggests a posterior urethritis or prostatitis. The urine should always be tested for protein and glucose.

Presentation and diagnosis in the female

The commonest presenting symptoms are vaginal discharge, vulval soreness or irritation, dysuria and frequency, rashes or lumps around the vulva or anus and dyspareunia. Less frequently there may be a rash or lumps on the thighs or abdomen or in regions remote from the genitals. Hardly a surgery session passes without at least one woman presenting with at least one of these symptoms and the possibility of sexually transmitted disease must be considered in all potentially sexually active women.

A large number of women suffering from sexually transmitted disease are symptom-free. The majority of women attending hospital clinics do so because their sexual partners have asked them to do so, because he himself has a sexually transmitted disease, because the woman herself suspects that her partner is being promiscuous, or because she has been asked to do so by the clinic contact tracer. 60% of women infected with gonorrhoea and over 9% of women suffering from non-specific genital infection are symptom-free. If a sexually transmitted disease is suspected for any reason a careful physical and bacteriological routine must be followed.

Examination

The pubic, vulval, perineal and anal regions should be inspected and the inguinal glands palpated. The abdomen and thighs should be inspected for rashes or lumps. A speculum should be used to inspect the vagina and cervix and any abnormality noted. A high vaginal swab should be obtained from the posterior fornix. If microscopy is available the swab should be mixed with a drop of normal saline on a slide using a cover slip and examined for *Trichomonas vaginalis*. A second swab should be taken for inoculation into a transport medium. The cervix should be cleaned with a cotton wool swab on the end of a pair of forceps and, having inspected the cervix for any abnormality, a bacteriological swab should be rotated just inside the os and then smeared onto a clean slide which should be Gram stained. Another bacteriological swab should be inoculated into the transport medium. A smear should be taken for cervical cytology.

The speculum should be withdrawn with gentle anterior pressure which has the effect of milking the urethra. A further specimen should be taken from the urethral orifice and smeared onto a slide for Gram staining, and another inoculated into the transport medium.

A bimanual pelvic examination should be performed in all cases and urine should be tested for protein and glucose. If the history suggests a urinary tract infection a mid stream specimen should be sent for examination in the laboratory. In all cases blood should be taken for serological tests for syphilis.

VAGINAL DISCHARGE

In all cases an abdominal, bimanual pelvic examination and a speculum examination should be performed. In most cases, unless for example an obvious neoplasm is suspected or a foreign body found, bacteriological swabs should be taken for examination in the laboratory. It is wrong to assume that there is a Candidal or Trichomonal infection on clinical evidence only. *Candida albicans* is responsible for many cases of vaginal discharge and *Trichomonas vaginalis* is also frequently the causative agent, but a high vaginal swab will confirm or deny their presence. If negative cultures are reported and the symptoms and signs persist then other more serious causes must be looked for.

Not to perform a vaginal examination in a case of vaginal discharge and for a colleague later to retrieve a tampon from high up in the vagina can be the source of acute embarrassment.

GONORRHOEA

The causal agent is *Neisseria gonorrhoeae*, a delicate organism which does not survive long outside the body. Under the microscope it is a Gram negative intracellular diplococcus. Its identification depends upon taking specimens from the sites likely to harbour it. It has an affinity for columnar epithelium and therefore in the male it is most likely to be found in the anterior urethra but can also be found in the pharynx and, in homosexuals, in the rectum. In females the most likely site to find it is the cervical canal. It can also be found in the urethra, rectum and in the pharynx if there is a history of orogenital sex. A significant number of cases will be missed unless specimens from the less likely sites of infection are examined. The gonococcus does not thrive in vaginal secretions and many laboratories do not even attempt to culture the organism from vaginal swabs. A high vaginal swab is of no use if a diagnosis of gonorrhoea is suspected.

CLINICAL GONORRHOEA IN THE MALE

The incubation period is 2 to 7 days but can be from 2 to 10 days. The initial infection in the genital tract is an anterior urethritis presenting with dysuria and irritation quickly followed by a purulent urethral discharge. Complications are posterior urethritis, prostatitis, trigonitis and epididymitis, usually unilateral, and much less frequently, arthritis. A patient who suspects that he might have been exposed to the disease must always be investigated. About 10% of cases of men with gonorrhoea are symptom-free.

CLINICAL GONORRHOEA IN THE FEMALE

In women the incubation period is difficult to determine. 60% of women suffering from gonorrhoea are symptom-free and attend only because they think that they might have been exposed to infection. Initially the infection in the genital tract is usually a cervicitis but frequently there is also a urethritis. In the 40% of women who do have symptoms the commonest are an increased vaginal discharge and dysuria and frequency. Often the patient will say that she has 'cystitis'. The most serious complication is salpingitis.

On examination clinical signs may be scanty or absent. An excess of vaginal secretion may be noted, there may be a cervicitis with pus issuing from the os, and the urethra may be inflamed with a bead of pus issuing from the meatus.

TREATMENT OF GONORRHOEA

The drug of choice is a penicillin. Ampicillin 3.0 g should be given orally in a single dose preceded by probenecid 1.0 g in order to enhance absorption. Patients allergic to penicillin should be given tetracycline 500 mg q.i.d. for 7 days. Certain strains of the gonococcus have developed resistance to penicillin. This is uncommon in the United Kingdom but is increasingly frequent abroad, especially in South East Asia. The bacteriological laboratories in the United Kingdom will alert the practitioner if resistance is present and such cases should be referred for specialist treatment.

Complications can be serious in the untreated case. In women the infection may become established as a chronic cervicitis and therefore a reservoir of infection for sexual partners. It can track up the genital tract causing acute salpingitis with the subsequent risk of permanent sterility. A bimanual examination is therefore essential.

NON-GENITAL GONORRHOEA

Gonorrhoeal infection remote from the genital tract is becoming more common. The practice of oro-genital sex has increased the frequency of gonococcal pharyngitis. Rectal infection is common in male homosexuals and also is remarkably frequent in women and indeed it is estimated that if a rectal swab is not taken as a routine some 6% of cases of female gonorrhoea could be missed altogether.

Follow-up for cure is essential. Men should be re-examined microscopically and bacteriologically 7 and 10–14 days after treatment. The two glass urine test should be performed on both these occasions because, in the absence of persistent gonorrhoeal infection, the patient might be suffering from non-specific urethritis which is frequently concurrent with gonorrhoea. Women require three investigations at weekly intervals after treatment before cure can be confirmed. The persistence of pus in the cervical canal indicates non-specific genital infection which requires treatment.

NON-SPECIFIC GENITAL INFECTION

It is estimated that approximately 25% of all cases attending clinics in the United Kingdom are diagnosed as non-specific genital infection. Non-specific urethritis (NSU) is the most common diagnosis made in male patients.

No agent can be isolated and the diagnosis is made by the exclusion of other known causes of urethritis.

NON-SPECIFIC URETHRITIS

The incubation period varies from 5 days to 1 month. The commonest symptoms are dysuria and frequency, meatal irritation and a urethral discharge which can be mucoid but is frequently purulent and is *indistinguishable* from gonorrhoea. A diagnosis is made on the presence of pus cells only on a Gram stain smear and in some clinics, the presence of threads in the first glass of the two glass urine test. Frequently the infection is concurrent with gonorrhoea. Complications are trigonitis, epididymitis and Reiters syndrome.

NON-SPECIFIC GENITAL INFECTION IN WOMEN

The majority of women are *symptom-free* and usually they attend as contacts of men suffering from NSU. Those with symptoms have an increase in vaginal discharge, dysuria and frequency.

REITERS SYNDROME

Classically this is a triple syndrome of non-specific urethritis, conjunctivitis and arthritis. Often the ophthalmic element is missing. It occurs most frequently in young men. The ophthalmic and urethral elements usually disappear within a week or two but the arthritis persists for a longer period and may recur at intervals and can give rise to a chronic arthritis with joint deformities.

Treatment of non specific genital infection

Tetracyclines are the drugs of choice. Men suffering from NSU should be given tetracycline 250 mg q.i.d. for 3 weeks. Abstinence from sexual intercourse and alcohol should be advised to reduce the incidence of relapse which otherwise is high. Dairy foods should be avoided when taking tetracyclines. At the end of treatment a two glass urine test is performed and if threads are still present in the first glass metronidazole (Flagyl) 400 mg b.d. for 5 days should be prescribed and thereafter the two glass urine test repeated. Because relapse after treatment is common in NSU the disease is the cause of much anxiety and distress. Much patience and reassurance is required in a relapsing case.

Women suffering from non-specific genital infection and those who are contacts of NSU should be given tetracycline 250 mg q.i.d. for 14 days and required to abstain from sexual intercourse, alcohol and dairy products. A follow-up bacteriological examination should be performed at the end of treatment.

TRICHOMONIASIS

Trichomonas vaginalis, a flagellate protozoon, is a frequent cause of infection in the genital tract. In women it causes vaginitis and vaginal discharge, classically copious, frothy and creamy green but not always so. Symptoms are a heavy discharge, soreness and itching, dysuria and frequency. A diagnosis is made by inoculating a high vaginal swab into a transport medium for examination at the laboratory. If microscopy is available an immediate diagnosis is possible. Men are usually asymptomatic but occasionally trichomonas can cause a urethritis.

The treatment is metronidazole 400 mg b.d. orally for 5 days. The sexual partner must be given concurrent treatment. It is imperative to follow-up all cases of trichomoniasis in women because there is sometimes an association with gonorrhoea which it frequently masks on the first examination. After treatment the culture tests should be repeated and it is especially important to repeat the cervical culture to exclude gonorrhoea.

CANDIDIASIS

Candida albicans, a yeast- like fungus, is a common cause of vaginitis. It can be spread by sexual intercourse but it is not necessarily sexually transmitted. Infection of the genital tract can occur by spread from the bowel.

The increase in the incidence of Candidiasis could be due to the use of the contraceptive pill and also to the use of antibiotics. Symptoms in women are itching, dysuria and soreness. On examination there can be vulval reddening sometimes with considerable oedema. Frequently there is a white lumpy discharge but in many cases the discharge may be absent despite acute symptoms and speculum examination can be very painful. In all cases the urine must be tested for glucose.

Men frequently are symptom-free but they may complain of irritation of the glans and on examination there may be a patchy erythema.

The treatment in women is anticandidal pessaries such as clotrimazole (Canesten) 200 mg at night for 3 nights. The sexual partner should use an anti-candidal cream on the penis for 3 nights even if he is symptom-free. In women some cases are very resistant to treatment and may require oral agents such as ketoconazole (Nizoral) and consideration must be given to other measures such as stopping the oral contraceptive pill, the avoidance of tight jeans and the excessive use of antibiotics. In all cases prone to recurrent attacks of Candidiasis the prescription of an antibiotic should be accompanied by prophylactic use of anti-candidal pessaries. The recurrent case of candidal infection is a fairly common and difficult problem requiring much patience in its management.

SYPHILIS

Syphilis is caused by the *Treponema pallidum*, a corkscrew organism which can only remain alive for a short time outside the human body but, within, it spreads and thrives. Almost from the moment of the initial infection the disease becomes systemic and can involve any organ or structure. It is spread usually by sexual intercourse but it can be acquired congenitally.

DIAGNOSIS

The diagnosis of syphilis has such serious consequences that to rely upon a clinical assessment alone can lead to disaster and laboratory tests are essential.

Serological tests
Several serological tests are in current use in the United Kingdom for the screening of syphilis and in making an evaluation of the response to treatment. The disease requires specialist management and therefore the general practitioner is only concerned with screening for the disease. In many centres the two serological tests most commonly used for screening purposes are:

1. The Venereal Disease Research Laboratory (VDRL) Test
This test detects non-specific antibodies and can become positive 10–14 days after the appearance of the primary lesion, but it may not do so for 5 or 6 weeks. In primary syphilis it is positive in 76% of cases.

2. The Treponema pallidum Haemaglutination (TPHA) Test
This test detects antibodies for pathogenic treponemes and is more effective in the diagnosis of late and latent syphilis. It is positive only in 50% of cases of primary syphilis, but in secondary latent and late syphilis it is positive in 100% of cases.

The VDRL and TPHA in combination provide a highly efficient screen for the detection of syphilis and they are used on a national scale for screening ante-natal cases in the United Kingdom and also by the National Blood Transfusion Service. A positive result warrants referral for specialist opinion so that a firm diagnosis can be made. Positive serological tests do not necessarily mean that patients have syphilis. An administrative error is always possible and therefore the tests must be repeated.

Other treponemal diseases such as Yaws give positive results to serological tests for syphilis and this fact is especially important when dealing with members of the immigrant population.

Microscopy

The identification of the *Treponema pallidum* from specimens obtained from lesions in the primary and secondary stages of the disease require dark ground illumination techniques not usually available to the general practitioner.

CLINICAL SYPHILIS

Syphilis is the supreme mimic and can be mistaken for many other diseases because of the variety of its symptoms and signs. In the United Kingdom it is relatively uncommon except in male homosexuals. Abroad, especially outside Europe, it is more common in heterosexuals and it is important to remember this in someone recently returned from elsewhere.

For the purposes of description the disease can be divided into three stages, but such divisions are arbitrary and the stages may overlap.

Primary syphilis

The incubation period varies from 10 to 90 days, usually about 3 weeks. The primary lesion, the chancre, occurs at the site where the organism has entered the body but even before its development dissemination of the organism throughout the body has occurred.

The chancre appears as a painless, indolent ulcer surrounded by a dull red halo which feels hard on palpation. Even without treatment the lesion will heal spontaneously over several weeks. Within a day or two of the appearance of the chancre there is a painless enlargement of the regional lumph nodes and, if the genitals are involved this sign is easily elicited. Secondary infection of the chancre changes the clinical picture so that the chancre itself is painful and there is a painful and tender lymphadenitis.

In women and heterosexual men, 90% of chancres are genital, but the anal region is a frequent site in homosexual men as is the mouth and throat.

The differential diagnosis is from genital herpes, candidiasis and balanitis, but any ulcerative lesion of the genitals should be considered to be syphilitic unless proved otherwise.

Secondary syphilis

The lesions of the secondary stages of the disease are the result of the widespread dissemination of the organism throughout the body and usually occur 4 to 8 weeks after the appearance of the chancre which in many cases has not been noticed by the patient. In 30% of patients showing the signs of secondary syphilis a healing primary chancre can be identified.

There may be a general malaise with fever, rashes and lesions of the mucous membranes, aching in bones and joints, painful swollen glands, and a patchy alopecia is not uncommon. At this stage of the disease lesions of mucous membranes are especially infectious. Serological tests for syphilis are positive in 100% of cases.

Latent and late syphilis

The latent period between the initial infection and the late manifestations of the disease usually lasts many years. Late syphilis is characterised by the gumma and other destructive lesions which can occur in any organ or any system in the body. The possibility of syphilis in its later stages should be kept in mind particularly when dealing with a patient who is a male homosexual.

The treatment of syphilis

The general practitioner does not have a place in the treatment of this disease. The drug of choice is penicillin and it is remarkable that the *Treponema pallidum* has yet not developed any resistance to this drug. The interpretation of serological tests during treatment is one that requires expertise and specialisation and should not be undertaken by those who are not experienced.

HERPES GENITALIS

Herpes genitalis is a common viral disease characterised by groups of vesicles on the genitals and a tendency to recurrence. In men the lesions occur on the glans and penile shaft and in women most commonly on the vulva, but also in the anal region, vagina and cervix. In both sexes the lesions can be very painful and are liable to secondary infection. There is no specific treatment for this disease but saline baths are soothing. Herpetic lesions in the pregnant woman are dangerous to the infant at delivery.

A firm diagnosis can be made by inoculating a swab into a viral culture medium. Herpetic lesions must be differentiated from the primary chancre of syphilis and in all cases serological tests for syphilis are essential. In women cervical cytology is important and should be repeated at yearly intervals.

GENITAL WARTS

Genital warts are common in both sexes, are often symptomless, but just as frequently cosmetically unaccept-able. They are caused by a virus and are infectious either from a sexual partner or by self-inoculation, for example from a hand. They are more likely to occur in moist situations especially under the prepuce in the male and on the vulva in the female. Treatment is the application of an alcoholic solution of 25% Podophyllin at weekly intervals. In order to avoid a painful reaction the area infected should be bathed about 6 hours after treatment. In severe infections it is sometimes necessary to repeat the treatment for several weeks.

PEDICULOSIS PUBIS

The crab louse *Phthirus pubis*, is usually spread sexually and most frequently it is confined to the hairs of the pubic and peri-anal regions but rarely it spreads onto other hirsute areas below the scalp. The main symptom is irritation. It is difficult to identify because usually it is immobile but can be seen as greyish dots the size of a pinhead at the roots of hairs. Treatment with gamma benzene hydrochloride BP in a detergent base (Quellada) or with malathion applied as a shampoo (Prioderm Cream Shampoo).

THE INVESTIGATION OF A SUSPECTED CASE OF STD — A SUMMARY

Medical history   Symptomatology, nature and duration
Details of sexual contact

— any symptoms, diagnosis or treat-ment given

In men   Physical examination
— penile discharge, rashes, sores, lumps
Bacteriology
— urethral swab in transport medium to laboratory
— Gram staining if microscopy avail-able
Two glass urine test

In women   Physical examination
— vaginal discharge, rashes, lumps or sores on genitals or elsewhere
Bacteriology
— vaginal, cervical and urethral swabs in transport medium to laboratory
— Gram staining and search for tricho-monas if microscopy avaiable

REFERENCE

Adler M W 1982 Journal of the Royal Society of Medicine: 75:4–6

FURTHER READING

Caterall R D 1974 A short textbook of venereology. English Universities Press, London
Robertson D H H, McMillan A, Young H 1980 Clinical practice in sexually transmissable diseases. Pitman Medical, London

Locomotor disorders

INTRODUCTION

Before many months have elapsed, the new entrant to general practice begins to realise how common are disorders of the locomotor system among the patients he sees in his surgery and in their homes. Sometimes, because of the many dialect words used by patients in different parts of the country to describe their symptoms, the doctor may have difficulty in deciding initially what system is affected. The doctor may then become more puzzled as he realises how few of these conditions appear to fit in with the familiar clinical entities of the medical school and hospital training. Indeed often the patient's view of the problem — 'It's my back again,' or 'Just another touch of my rheumatism' is as precise as is the doctor's diagnosis.

Puzzlement may turn to despair when the next discovery is made — that the patient's expectations of the doctor are lower in this area of medicine than any other — 'I don't suppose you'll be able to do anything for it' is an oft-repeated refrain. The general practitioner is usually consulted after advice has been sought from lay persons, and perhaps the local pharmacist, but before the patient consults an osteopath. Morell & Wale (1976) observed that only one symptom in 37 noted by a sample of patients led to a medical consultation. The commonest locomotor symptom, backache, was the third most common of all symptoms appreciated by the patients, but was only the sixth most common symptom for which medical advice was sought. The inference is that a greater proportion of backache sufferers decide against medical attention than do sufferers from other symptoms, such as sore throat or cough. The doctor, indeed, seems merely the tip of the iceberg of disease. While we cannot ignore the massive bulk of the iceberg, we have to direct our efforts at what is visible. What is the visible tip of the iceberg?

MORBIDITY PATTERNS OF LOCOMOTOR DISORDERS

The most complete record of morbidity patterns is 'Morbidity Statistics from General Practice, Second National Study 1970–71' published in 1974. This study shows that the consultation rate per 1000 population per annum for all diseases and conditions is 3009, and for diseases of the musculo-skeletal system and connective tissue 206, that is nearly 7% of the total. The commonest condition seen is back pain — adding together the various rubrics containing different back pain diagnoses gives a consultation rate of 65 per 1000 population. This is followed by osteoarthritis and allied conditions with a consultation rate of 43, and rheumatoid arthritis and allied conditions with 19. All other conditions are relatively uncommon (Table 18.1).

This pattern of morbidity is likely to be very different from that which the trainee has experienced in hospital work, where there is a much higher incidence of rheumatoid arthritis, and other forms of inflammatory joint disease. One or two further points need to be made about morbidity patterns. Many people assume that the vast majority of locomotor disorders are due to the wear and tear of the ageing process, and that, therefore, their incidence increases with age. This is generally correct with regard to osteoarthritis, but is not true of low back pain, for which the maximum incidence is in the age range 34–45, and falls to low levels in the elderly.

BACK PAIN

EPIDEMIOLOGY

As previously noted, back pain is the commonest symptom of locomotor system disorder presented to the general practitioner. Approximately 20–22 persons per 1000 will consult each year because of low back pain, and although some studies have shown a slight excess of males consulting, this may be due to the needs of National Insurance Certification, as community studies have shown that more females than males are bothered with back pain (Nagi et al 1973). The age group most commonly afflicted is 30–60.

Occupational factors can be important: miners, dockers, workers in heavy industry, and those who have to lift

Table 18.1 Diseases of locomotor system — consultation rates per 1000 population (Adapted from the 2nd National Morbidity Study 1974)

Disease	Consultation rate per 1000 population
Back pain	65
Osteoarthritis	43
Rheumatoid arthritis	19
Non-articular rheumatism	14
Other forms of arthritis and rheumatism	9
Tenosynovitis	6
Bursitis	4
Other forms of internal derangement of knee	4
Torn meniscus of knee	3
Synovitis	3
Flat foot	1
Hallux valgus and corns	1
Other diseases of locomotor system	18

or stoop a lot at work have a high incidence of back pain. Having a sedentary occupation, and driving a motor vehicle have also been implicated as occupational risk factors. The low back is the commonest site, followed by the cervical and then the thoracic regions.

DIAGNOSTIC MODELS

At this point, the different models of the diagnostic process used by specialists on the one hand and general practitioners on the other should be considered (see also ch. 2). The hospital model, as taught to medical students, is to list all signs and symptoms and detail all possible causes of the condition, then try to match up the two lists to produce the best fit. Most general practice consultations do not follow this scheme, and can perhaps be best represented by the following diagram (Fig. 18.1). At each step in the diagnostic process the doctor forms a hypothesis which he then proceeds to test. If the test of the hypothesis proves it to be wrong he can form a new hypothesis. If the test proves it right he can decide to stay at that level, or may take the next step to a higher level of diagnosis. Each hypothesis can be tested by history, examination, investigation or by management and by the passage of time. This concept is alien to the medical school model based on 'no treatment before diagnosis' but the theory is borne out by direct observation of general practitioners at work.

Consider an example. A patient comes in with a painful expression on his face, and a slight stoop. He sits down carefully and slowly and says 'I've got a pain in my back'. At this stage the first hypothesis is formed: 'This patient has pain arising from his spine. It is severe enough to cause him to consult, yet not so severe that it prevents him from coming.' This initial hypothesis is

tested by inquiring into the history: sudden onset when lifting, worse when bending, helped by rest. If the initial hypothesis is not confirmed, then it may be rejected and a further hypothesis formed, such as 'This is kidney pain' and enquiry directed towards the urinary tract. If the initial hypothesis is confirmed by the history, the doctor may wish to refine it further by examination, for example by eliciting tenderness and noting restricted spinal movements. At this step all the doctor can fairly say is that the hypothesis of (spinal) back pain is confirmed. He may wish to try to achieve a higher level of diagnosis — the patient has a prolapsed intervertebral disc — or he may decide to stay at the level attained. The doctor may attempt to reach a higher diagnostic level in the expectation that this further hypothesis will be refuted: he may look for sign of a prolapsed disc and find none. It is just as important for some hypotheses to be rejected as it is for them to be confirmed. After all, failure to find evidence of a prolapsed disc is just as important in management as is positive evidence. Thus many diagnostic encounters stop at this relatively low level — there is little point in trying to step up higher. The general practitioner is recognising that there appears to be no worthwhile gain in attempting to refine his diagnosis, but stating implicitly that there is no serious condition that requires further investigation and treatment.

ACUTE LOW BACK PAIN

This often seems to arise from overloading spinal structures, as most people are aware of from personal experience. There seem to be two common modes of onset: (a) instantaneous, during a lifting, bending, or twisting movement, and (b) a gradually increasing pain beginning usually some hours after some strenuous or unaccus-

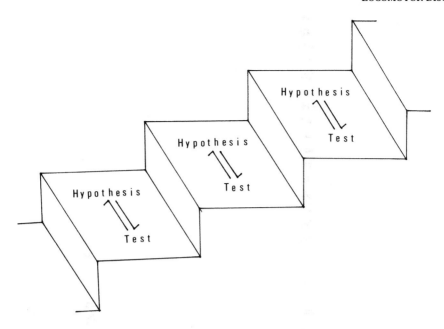

Fig. 18.1 The diagnostic ladder

tomed exercise, such as digging. In the second type, the patient may have gone to bed symptom-free and awakened the following morning to find that he cannot easily get out of bed due to pain.

Examination
It is frequently only too obvious that the patient is in pain and unable to move his back. When undressed, there is usually marked spasm of the paravertebral muscles and often a scoliosis. One or more movements of the spine are usually restricted, and straight leg raising may also be slightly diminished. Although there is often referral of pain to buttock or thigh, it does not extend below the knee and neurological signs are absent.

Treatment
Acute back pain is usually self-limiting and the aim of treatment is to relieve symptoms. The main methods of doing this are by the prescription of analgesics, rest in the most comfortable position, usually lying flat on a firm surface, and local heat. Some people advocate spinal manipulation, especially if pain persists after a few days of complete rest, on the assumption that most cases are due to a 'stuck joint' (intervertebral or facet joint derangement). There is some evidence that although in some cases there is relief from pain in the first day or so this advantage disappears after about 2 weeks.

This situation gives a good opportunity for the general practitioner to use health education in an attempt to minimise the chance of recurrence. Patients are never more receptive to advice about posture, lifting, exercis-ing, or to the importance of a firm mattress, than when they are actually afflicted with back pain. Various drug companies and the Back Pain Association (address at end of chapter) produce booklets which can be given to patients to reinforce this advice.

Management is often part of the diagnostic process of general practitioners, and a good example of this is acute low back pain. In the initial phases it is often impossible to exclude more serious conditions such as prolapsed intervertebral disc or spondylolisthesis. The initial treatment of these conditions is much the same as any acute low back pain, but if symptomatic management fails to produce the expected improvement within 7 to 14 days then a further level of diagnosis should be attempted.

PROLAPSED INTERVERTEBRAL DISC

This condition may occur with or without nerve root involvement. The diagnosis is usually not so obvious if there is no nerve root involvement, and may be based on no more than a hunch when an acute low back pain resolves more slowly than usual. Prolapsed intervertebral disc is by far the commonest diagnosis if signs of nerve root involvement are found, but it is as well to remember that a few cases of sciatica are due to other causes. It remains a presumptive diagnosis in most cases, as very few patients have radiculograms and even fewer have surgery to confirm the diagnosis.

Examination
The features mentioned under 'acute low back pain' are

present. In addition, there are often signs and symptoms of nerve root compression, although these may not be present initially, and sometimes never appear. Symptoms of nerve root compression include pain, numbness and paraesthesiae in the distribution of the affected nerve, and the signs are muscle weakness, diminished reflexes and hypoaesthesia of the affected area. There are charts of dermatomes in most neurology and rheumatology textbooks which can help to establish which is the nerve root affected.

There is often considerable muscle spasm which limits spinal movements. Straight leg raising on the side of the disc protrusion is restricted by a variable amount, often to 30° or less. Straight leg raising on the opposite side often provokes pain on the affected side. Lasègue's test is also a useful adjunct to diagnosis — the leg is lowered slightly from the position in which pain was initially provoked, then the foot is dorsiflexed, thus stretching the sciatic nerve, the test being positive if the pain returns with this manoeuvre.

Treatment
There is one situation that requires immediate referral for hospital management — the very rare condition of cauda equine involvement, which usually presents with bilateral leg pain and weakness, disordered bladder function or acute retention of urine. The majority of these patients require urgent surgical treatment to relieve the pressure on the nerve roots before permanent damage results. Most other patients can be managed entirely by the general practitioner, by advising rest and ensuring adequate analgesia. Bed rest may need to be continued for 1 or 2 weeks, or occasionally longer, and the patient should be visited regularly at home to assess progress. Sometimes parenteral opiates are required initially for analgesia, but in most cases oral medication, using dihydrocodeine or a similar relatively powerful analgesic is sufficient. There is usually a slow improvement and recovery can take up to 4 to 6 weeks. If patient and doctor are happy with this progress, then little else need be done. During the recovery stage an X-ray of the lumbar spine is often obtained but this is usually more useful in reassuring the patient that his doctor is helping him in every way he can than it is of practical value in management. During the recovery stage the doctor should again reinforce the message that prevention is better than cure.

Referral
Some back pain patients are referred to specialists — usually orthopaedic surgeons or rheumatologists. There are no hard and fast rules that can be laid down about referral as each patient presents an individual problem that should be dealt with on an individual basis. The decision about referral can be initiated by either the doctor or the patient (or his relatives) but in most cases it is best to come to a joint decision.

The doctor usually wishes to refer if he is unsure of the diagnosis, is unhappy about the rate of progress, or because he thinks the patient requires some specialised skill he cannot offer. The patient can sometimes doubt the doctor's diagnosis and may occasionally feel happier to have some specific skilled procedure carried out. The most usual reason is that the patient wishes to be referred because he is dissatisfied with his rate of progress.

Some further aspects of prolapsed intervertebral discs will be discussed in the section on chronic back pain.

CHRONIC LOW BACK PAIN

Chronic low back pain may be the result of an acute low back pain which does not resolve, or the patient may complain of persistent discomfort with recurrent more painful episodes. It is difficult to be dogmatic about when back pain becomes chronic but as a general rule, most attacks of acute pain will resolve in 4 to 6 weeks.

The first problem of chronic low back pain to be considered is one of diagnosis, and it may be as well to consider the two types of chronic back pain separately. In the patient with an unresolved acute attack, the first step is to take stock and review the presumptive diagnosis and the management prescribed. Further steps should be taken up the stairway of diagnosis and in most instances there is a need for further information, unless on reviewing the evidence he has already gathered, the doctor realises he has made a mistake which can be rectified without any further action. Additional information can be obtained by radiology and laboratory tests or from specialist referral.

Radiology
X-rays of the spine may show evidence of fracture, infection, degenerative changes or congenital abnormalities, or may suggest osteoporosis, ankylosing spondylitis, or secondary neoplasm. X-rays are sometimes reported as showing disc space narrowing. This may imply localised spondylosis — wear and tear of this disc — or indicate an old disc lesion, perhaps resulting from previous trauma. It is important to realise that a narrowed disc space does not necessarily indicate a recent prolapsed disc.

Laboratory tests
The most useful tests are the ESR and full blood count and these should be performed on all patients with chronic back pain. Occasionally other tests are indicated by aspects of the history or X-ray appearances, such as serum calcium, phosphorus and alkaline phosphatase in suspected metabolic bone disease or secondary cancer.

Specialist opinion

If the general practitioner still cannot provide a confident diagnosis and is therefore unable to formulate a plan of management then he should refer the problem to a specialist colleague.

These diagnostic steps may also be necessary in the patient who presents with a long-standing history of back pain though in such cases the diagnosis is often suggested by the history. In many instances the problem may be linked to poor posture or working conditions in factory, shop or home, or poor vehicle seating.

There is often surprisingly little to find on examination and consequently the detailed history of the complaint including exacerbating and relieving factors is of great importance. Occasionally the back pain can be abolished by a simple change in the patient's environment such as replacement of a worn-out mattress with a firm one, or the provision of a lumbar cushion for a car or lorry seat.

Management

Some specific abnormalities such as metabolic bone disease, may have specific remedies. There are, however, some general principles of management that are common to all patients with chronic low back pain.

Whereas rest is one of the most important therapeutic measures in acute back pain, it can be side effects just as severe as any drug. Prolonged bed-rest can lead to demineralisation of bones and muscle weakness which in turn can themselves lead to back pain. More serious, however, is the attitude of mind that can be engendered by excessive rest. The patient may become lethargic and dispirited and unwilling to undertake any activity for fear of provoking further pain. The doctor should guard against the infectious pessimism of the patient and instead should discover what activities he is capable of doing, then encourage him to build upon these activities rather than to bemoan what he cannot do.

In the recovery period, patients are usually taught back exercises which they should continue afterwards — even when the pain has largely subsided. As well as this, many patients can be encouraged to take up more general exercise, such as swimming, which can have long-term beneficial effects, especially if it leads to a change of life-style: walking or cycling rather than always driving.

A few patients continue to suffer such severe pain and disability that they cannot return to their former occupation. In these cases, the Disablement Resettlement Officer at the local Department of Employment may be able to help in placing the patient in a more suitable job, possibly after a course of rehabilitation and training.

THORACIC SPINAL PAIN

The thoracic spine is often not recognised as the source of pain, which is often referred to the anterior or posterior chest, upper abdomen, or upper limb, and it may cause confusion with pain from other sites. This may be a cause of anxiety to the patient who imagines that he has heart or lung disease, as well as a diagnostic pitfall for the doctor. The pain may indeed mimic cardiac infarction or pleurisy. However, the general wellbeing of the patient will direct the doctor to look to the thoracic spine for the cause of a pain which is brought on, or made worse, by certain spinal movements, such as a sudden twist, as when a driver looks over his shoulder when reversing his car.

Examination

It is important to be able to reassure the patient that his heart and lungs are sound, so the chest should be carefully examined and the blood pressure checked as a matter of routine. When the thoracic spine is examined, there may be little to find, but careful inspection and palpation often reveals local tenderness and some muscle spasm around the affected area. A tender spot around one of the costo-vertebral junctions may be found giving rise to speculation that derangement of one of these joints is the source of pain.

Management

As already mentioned, the patient may need reassurance about the origin and nature of the pain. This together with the knowledge that the pain is usually self-limiting is sufficient in many cases. Treatment of such patients by spinal manipulation — in the hands of a trained professional — may shorten the duration of the symptoms, or indeed, may instantly abolish the pain.

Although the vast majority of cases of thoracic pain are self-limiting, they are, however, often recurrent. Patient education is therefore an important part of the management, and all that may be required is for the doctor to elicit a history of exacerbating factors and give advice about their avoidance. In many cases the patient's posture is poor, and he should be shown how it can be improved. Leaflets obtainable from the Back Pain Association are a useful adjunct. Simple rotation exercises of the spine can be helpful, and can be demonstrated in the surgery.

Before leaving the problem of thoracic spinal pain, mention should be made of epiphysitis in teenagers (osteochondritis or Scheuermann's disease). The pain is often not severe, but persists for months or even a year or so. The diagnosis can often be confirmed by X-ray which shows Schmorl's nodes, but it may be difficult to persuade the patient and parents that no treatment is necessary, and that the symptoms will eventually subside. Occasionally in severe cases bed-rest is required to avoid future deformity.

WRY NECK

This is not an unusual problem, particularly in children and young adults. The diagnosis is usually evident as the patient walks through the door, the head being held to one side by spasm of the sternomastoid muscle. The usual history is 'I don't know how it happened. It was like it when I awoke.' Further examination shows the restricted movement brought about my muscle spasm and confirms the absence of any cervical adenitis that might be irritating the sternomastoid and provoking secondary spasm.

Management

Muscle spasm can be relieved by heat from a scarf or padded hot water bottle or by cold from an icepack or an ethyl chloride spray. Manipulation may be successful. However, in young children, it is probably best to do nothing except advise rest and aspirin and explain that, although the cause is not known, the symptoms will disappear within a few days.

CERVICAL SPONDYLOSIS

This is the result of a series of complicated degenerative changes affecting many of the structures of the cervical spine. The same processes can also involve the thoracic and lumbar areas and much of what is written here is applicable also to these other areas of the spine. Typically there is intervertebral disc degeneration leading to disc space narrowing with subsequent osteophytosis and arthritis of the intervertebral facet joints. Cervical spondylosis can have many manifestations ranging from limb paraesthesiae to drop attacks. The symptoms can be divided into local and distal, which in turn can be further subdivided into vascular and neurological.

Local symptoms

These include pain which is referred to the shoulders and upper arms, and limitation of movement.

Distal symptoms

Vascular

The patient may feel giddy or faint, especially when looking and reaching upwards, due to compression of the vertebral arteries by osteophytes, leading to hypoxia of the brain stem. In severe cases, this can cause drop attacks.

Neurological

Osteophyte formation may lead to nerve root compression in the intervertebral foramina, the distribution of pain or paraesthesiae depending upon the level of compression. Very occasionally there is spinal cord compression causing weakness of the legs. With regard to pain and paraesthesiae in the arms, it is sometimes difficult to be sure that cervical spondylosis is the cause of the symptoms. An X-ray is not often useful — there seldom seems any correlation between the site and severity of the symptoms and the location and degree of radiological change. The patient may need referral to a specialist for further investigations such as nerve conduction tests, to exclude carpal tunnel or ulnar nerve entrapment syndromes.

Management

Cervical spondylosis is a chronic condition running a fluctuating course. The general practitioner therefore may need to deal only with his patient's exacerbations, and may not see him for long periods. Here again, the avoidance of exacerbating factors should be stressed. Many patients are worse at night due to the neck being overflexed by too high a pillow. Conversely pain can sometimes be aggravated by too low a pillow, allowing the neck to go into side flexion when the patient lies on his side. A careful history helps in solving this paradox. Analgesic and muscle relaxant drugs are often prescribed but it is doubtful whether the non-steroidal anti-inflammatory drugs are of any value in cervical spondylosis.

If these measures fail, the patient may be helped by physiotherapy, (neck traction or mobilising exercises) or by the provision of a soft collar. Under the NHS, many patients will have to be sent to a hospital out-patient consultative clinic before physiotherapy or an aid such as a collar can be provided, although some physiotherapy departments provide open access for general practitioners. This can mean a wait of many months before treatment can begin, and the doctor may come under increasing pressure to 'do something'. While it is possible to obtain immediate treatment for acute cases by referral to an emergency clinic, or by asking the consultant to see the patient urgently, it is obvious that not all patients can be regarded as justifying immediate action. Delay in referral is one reason why the patient may enquire about a private referral to specialist or physiotherapist, or may go off to an osteopath. However, the patient can gain some relief from a partial immobilisation of the neck. A temporary collar for night use can be made from some folded newspapers inserted into a length of stockinette bandage, and some patients fashion their own collars from a length of felt.

THE ACUTELY INFLAMED JOINT

Reference to Table 18.1 earlier in this chapter will show that rheumatoid arthritis is the commonest cause of inflammatory joint disease, but this is of little help to the general practitioner confronted by a patient with an acutely inflamed joint. Rheumatoid arthritis may be at the back of the doctor's mind (and at the front of the patient's) but there are many other possibilities to be considered. The features of the history and examination that should be considered depend on circumstances. If a middle-aged man limps in and says he has a red, throbbing swelling at the base of his big toe, the initial hypothesis is that he has gout, which can be confirmed by measuring his serum uric acid. The same man coming in with pain in several joints of several weeks duration together with general malaise is likely to be initially diagnosed as 'possible rheumatoid arthritis' and confirmation sought by requesting and ESR and test for rheumatoid factor. As every patient, and every consultation, is different it is difficult to lay down exact guidelines about what aspects of history and examination should be noted. Common to every consultation, however, is the background knowledge of the patient and his family, and their reaction to previous ill-health.

The doctor's assessment starts as soon as he sees the patient. Although this may be formed from impressions, or 'clinical hunches', it is often of value.

RHEUMATOID ARTHRITIS

With this, the commonest inflammatory joint disease, psoriatic arthropathy and other types of sero-negative arthritis will be included along with other conditions which in some way mimic rheumatoid arthritis. The precise clinicopathological diagnosis is of importance, but more so to the rheumatologist than the general practitioner, who is going to manage the patient in much the same way, whatever the precise diagnosis. The first step is to make a diagnosis, often not an easy task as rheumatoid arthritis may present with one, or many affected joints, in varying degrees of severity, in virtually any age group and with a very variable clinical course. Once the diagnosis has been considered, it can often be confirmed by finding a raised ESR, a positive test for rheumatoid factor, such as the latext test, or by certain distinctive X-ray or clinical features as in the case of psoriatic arthropathy. Sometimes the patient may need referral to a specialist or help in diagnosis, especially if there seems to be significant clinical evidence of arthritis with negative or equivocal test results, or if the general practitioner wishes to advance the diagnostic process to a higher level: in differentiating between possible causes of sero-negative arthritis. While the diagnostic process is going on, the doctor should be aware of his patient's anxieties about the diagnosis and prognosis and attempt to allay any unnecessary fears.

Having arrived at a diagnosis, the steps in management depend vey much on individual circumstances and va-

rious factors need to be taken into account. The question 'How are these symptoms affecting this patient at the present time?' is a useful first step in formulating a management plan. The therapeutic aspects of management will have been suggested by the rheumatologist if the patient has been referred. The specialist is most likely to be useful in providing specific treatments, such as steroid injections into affected joints, physiotherapy, the provision of splints, and the supervision of therapies rare in the general practitioner's experience, such as gold injections, chloroquine and penicillamine. The general practitioner is most likely to help the patient with day-by-day management, with the supervision of the drug regime, with discussion on prognosis and possible future problems and with advice about where to seek help with the provision of aids and adaptations to the home. As many of these points are common to other locomotor disorders they are discussed later in this chapter in the section on general principles of treatment.

GOUT

This cause of an acutely inflamed joint should not be forgotten. The diagnosis is often fairly obvious when the classical site, the first metatarsophalangeal joint, is affected, but it is as well to remember that other joints can be involved and gout should be considered in every case of acute joint inflammation. It should be remembered that clinical gout can be the result of long-term therapy with a thiazide diuretic. It must also be borne in mind that the first metatarsophalangeal joint can become inflamed from other causes, such as infection and trauma. The clinical hypothesis of acute gout therefore needs to be tested by the result of the serum uric acid estimation.

The traditional therapy for acute gout is colchicine, which is still used although a non-steroidal anti-inflammatory drug such as indomethacin (Indocid) 25–50 mg three times a day is also of help. The acute attack lasts only a few days, for which the patient is usually very grateful, and often apprehensive about the possibility of recurrence. Serum uric acid-lowering drugs, such as allupurinol (Zyloric) and probenecid (Benemid) are available for the secondary prevention of gout, and their use should be discussed with the patient. Many patients do not wish to take regular prophylactic treatment since acute attacks may occur very infrequently, and because the acute condition responds quickly to treatment. This can leave a dilemma — to what extent should the doctor attempt to coerce the patient by warning him of the possibility of increasing attacks and the long-term effects of a raised serum uric acid, and to what extent should he encourage his patient to make his own decisions about his health and his medical treatment. It is as well to remember that any decision made by doctor or patient can be modified in the light of experience: the patient may be only too willing to change his mind and start prophylactic therapy if he does have repeated painful attacks of gout. A more common occurrence is that the patient stops treatment because he has not had any further attacks. The doctor may know nothing of this until the patient re-presents with a new attack.

DEGENERATIVE JOINT DISEASE

OSTEOARTHRITIS

In all its forms, osteoarthritis is the commonest locomotor disorder in general practice. The prevalence of osteoarthritis increases with age until it is almost universal in the elderly. Osteoarthritis is a general term, and is applied to the condition which affects small finger joints, as well as the destruction of a solitary large joint such as the hip. While it is unimportant to consider the precise aetiology of the different forms of osteoarthritis, it is of more importance when management is considered. Although no pathological changes of osteoarthritis may be found on X-ray there is often a variable degree of disability and pain. The management strategy therefore needs to keep in mind the severity and site of the patient's symptoms, and their effects in terms of disability. The main symptoms of osteoarthritis are pain, restricted movement or stiffness, and joint instability, especially of the large weight-bearing joints.

Pain

Pain is usually the symptom which brings the patient to the doctor and for which self-medication has almost invariably been tried beforehand. Most patients will have tried a variety of analgesic tablets and most also will have purchased creams or liniments for rubbing into the painful area. Some will also have tried various forms of heat, such as infra-red lamps, or heat pads. The patient should be encouraged to persist with any remedy that has been found helpful, even although there may be no scientific proof of its efficacy. He may have come because of inadequate pain relief from the remedies he has tried, and is thus seeking stronger and more effective drugs.

Rest is a good pain reliever, and may be necessary in some cases, especially during an acute exacerbation. Because of the long-term nature of the disorder, however, complete rest is rarely possible or advisable, and a balance needs to be struck between advising beneficial rest in the acute phase, and sufficient activity to prevent secondary stiffness and to promote mental activity and wellbeing.

Stiffness

This symptom is occasionally more prominent than is

pain — the patient may notice difficulty in performing a habitual task, such as climbing stairs, or getting into a car. However, it is more often noted during the examination of a patient who has presented with a painful joint, and to some extent may be due to secondary muscle spasm in an attempt to protect the joint. In this case, it may be abolished by adequate analgesia. Stiffness is, however, frequently due to changes within the joint, and is thus not helped by analgesics. There may be some value in advising regular passive exercises to maintain as much range of movement as possible, with active exercise to maintain muscle strength. It is sometimes necessary to refer a patient for physiotherapy but in many cases giving advice on exercises is all that is necessary.

Instability of joints

Patients may complain of the joint 'giving way'. This is especially true of the weight-bearing joints, the knees in particular. It can be difficult in some instances to differentiate between a joint giving way and other forms of drop attack in the elderly, such as vertebrobasilar insufficiency, or Adams-Stokes' attacks, as the patient sometimes gives only a hazy history, especially if concussion follows the fall.

The provision of some kind of external prop often helps. The choice of walking stick, walking tripod, crutch or Zimmer frame depends on the degree of disability and what the patient will accept — there is little point in the patient being given a Zimmer if it will remain unused, as the patient doesn't like using it, or doesn't have room to manoeuvre it in a small or overcrowded room. Occasionally a leg caliper or other aid may be prescribed, though more usually in instability of neurological origin. In some cases, different aids may be provided for different times, such as a walking stick for use indoors and a walking frame for outdoors.

SOFT TISSUE RHEUMATISM

Although many conditions included under this heading are common in general practice, they are seen less frequently in hospital practice, thus presenting the new entrant to general practice with problems in recognition and management. There are a number of syndromes which the general practitioner should be able to recognise and treat effectively, usually without recourse to hospital facilities.

TENNIS ELBOW

This is usually due to a chronic strain of the attachment of the forearm extensor muscles to the lateral humeral epicondyle although it sometimes is the result of an acute injury which partially tears the musculotendinous attachment. There may be a history of occupational use of the forearms, such as in lathe operators, or unaccustomed overusage in weekend do-it-yourself enthusiasts: it rarely occurs from playing tennis. There is pain and tenderness around the lateral epicondyle with possible radiation down the forearm and restricted ability to lift objects, especially if heavy, such as a teapot or saucepan full of potatoes. The condition is often recurrent over several years.

Treatment

Treatment consists of rest in mild cases, if necessary with a sling, and with analgesics as required. The amount of rest required is variable — avoidance of lifting may be sufficient, but if the condition is of occupational origin, time off work may be necessary. Some benefit can be obtained by applying elastoplast strapping or an elasticated stockinette (Tubigrip) bandage around the upper forearms. If this fails, or in severe cases from the outset, long-acting local corticosteroids should be considered. There are a number of products available, and there is no clear evidence that any product is better than its competitors; methylprednisolone (Depo-Medrone) or triamcinalone (Kenalog) are of value. 0.5–1 ml is injected along with 0.5 ml lignocaine into and around the site of maximum tenderness (not pain), and the patient should be warned that there may be increased pain for a day or two before any benefit is noticed. For this reason it is wise not to treat both elbows simultaneously in a patient who has both affected. Improvement usually continues for about 3 weeks and the need for a further injection can be assessed at that time. Very rarely a third injection is indicated, but any sign of steroid-induced skin atrophy overlying the site of the previous injection is a contraindication to further therapy of this kind. Treatment failures at this stage will probably require referral to a rheumatologist. The same considerations apply if the medial epicondyle is affected (golfer's elbow).

PLANTAR FASCIITIS

Like tennis elbow, plantar fasciitis is the result of strain or injury, usually at the site of the tendoperiosteal junction between the plantar fascia and calcaneum. The diagnosis is usually made on the history of pain in the heel felt when walking, and tenderness is found over the anterior–inferior edge of the calcaneum. The diagnosis does not depend on the X-ray appearance of a calcaneal spur, which may appear late due to periosteal reaction. Treatment with injected corticosteroids is usually successful and careful padding to protect the painful area may also be necessary.

THE PAINFUL SHOULDER

The painful shoulder is a common problem found more usually in middle aged and elderly patients. There is continuing controversy regarding the aetiology and pathology of shoulder pain and indeed whether the various clinical syndromes — pericapsulitis of the shoulder, frozen shoulder, painful arc syndrome, rotator cuff lesions — are different stages of the same process. It is generally assumed that the process is initiated by minor, repeated trauma which tears the shoulder capsule. This causes pain around the shoulder, often extending down the arm. The patient may complain that he cannot lie on the affected side when in bed. Examination may reveal a tender area in the shoulder region and limited movement of the joint. If the limitation is not too severe, a *painful arc* is sometimes found during abduction of the shoulder joint, indicating a supraspinatus lesion. If more severe, there is often no movement at the shoulder itself (frozen shoulder) and the patient may have learned to partially compensate for this lack of movement by rotation of the scapula.

Treatment

A mixture of local steroid and local anaesthetic should be injected, either into the joint itself, using an anterior or posterior approach, or into the subacromial bursa using a lateral approach. A steroid injection can completely cure a rotator cuff lesion such as supraspinatus tendinitis; in a frozen shoulder it will relieve pain, while movements will remain restricted. Local heat sometimes helps to relieve pain, and can easily be applied at home by the patient using a heat pad or hot water bottle. Supported movements of the shoulder can be allowed but active use, especially lifting or carrying heavy objects, should be discouraged.

BURSITIS

There are many different forms of bursitis known, but relatively few are commonly seen in general practice. Over-use and trauma are the aetiological factors that seem common to all forms of bursitis. The sites that are commonly affected include the following:

Bunions over the first metatarsal head, aggravated by hallux valgus, or tight shoes; there is a probable hereditary element in many cases.

Calcaneal bursae which appear between the skin and the achilles tendon, caused by friction from footwear.

Housemaid's knee never seen in housemaids (owing to the demise of this occupation), but sometimes seen in joiners or electricians who spend a lot of time on hands and knees at work.

Olecranon bursitis (sometimes called student's elbow) is common in anyone wh sits with the elbow pressed against a firm surface.

Treatment

Often an explanation to the patient of the cause and benign nature of the condition is sufficient, especially if the patient can avoid aggravating the inflamed bursa. If the swelling is large and is interfering with function — specially likely to occur with bursae at the elbows and knees — fluid should be aspirated and a tight crepe or tubular stockinette bandage applied. Rarely this causes the formation of a chronic sinus, which may also develop if the bursa discharges spontaneously. If a sinus does occur, or if the bursa does not disappear with appropriate rest and support, referral to an orthopaedic surgeon for excision may be necessary.

POLYMYALGIA RHEUMATICA

This diagnosis should be considered in any elderly person who complains of muscle pain and stiffness of sudden onset. The muscles of the shoulder region are most commonly affected but the pelvic muscles are sometimes involved. The ESR is always high (>70 mm/hr) but care should be taken that there is no other reason for this before diagnosing polymyalgia rheumatica.

Treatment

There is usually a swift resolution of symptoms with a moderate dose of steroids — 15–20 mg prednisolone daily. The dosage is then reduced to the minimum compatible with relief of symptoms, and may need to be continued for several years. Where there is an associated temporal arteritis, the inital dosage of steroids needs to be higher (30–40 mg daily). Since this condition may develop later, patients should be asked to report any episodes of temporal headache or visual disturbance.

'NON-SPECIFIC RHEUMATISM'

Rheumatism, fibrositis and similar terms appear more commonly in old medical records than they do today. Diagnostic fashions change but this change is most likely indicative of greater precision in diagnosis. However, despite greater diagnostic awareness there are some patients in whom an accurate diagnosis seems impossible, and a 'low-level' diagnosis, such as 'non-specific rheumatism', has to be made. In a few cases a more accurate diagnosis may be possible as time passes, and more specific management can then be planned.

PSYCHOLOGICAL ASPECTS OF DISORDERS OF THE LOCOMOTOR SYSTEM

General practitioners should be aware of the multifactorial aetiology of disease and in particular the medical, psychological and social aspects. The complications of disease, not only in medical but also psychological and social terms, also need to be considered.

LIFE EVENTS

Stress factors often lead to the onset of disease and earlier mortality, as shown most dramatically in the work of Parkes et al (1969) who demonstrated that there was an increased likelihood of death in the 10 months following a close bereavement. There is evidence that this also occurs in a non-lethal form. Rose (1975) found that there were more 'life events', such as travel, family changes, in patients with pain in the back and neck than in a control group of patients.

ANXIETY

It has been shown elsewhere (Gilchrist 1976) that patients presenting with back pain are more likely to have had a diagnosis made of anxiety in the preceding few years than patients who did not have low back pain. The physiological expression of anxiety — muscle tension — may be an important aetiological factor in some locomotor disorders, and tense muscles by themselves can provoke pain. It was first shown many years ago by Holmes & Wolff (1950) that back pain patients had pain and generalised overactivity of trunk muscles in anxiety-provoking situations. This implies that management of the patient's anxiety may have a large part to play in the alleviation of pain. Indeed some authors, including Sarno (1974), have suggested that one group of patients with back pain may be suffering from 'tension myositis', where anxiety causes pain in the absence of any physical lesion.

DEPRESSION

There is evidence that patients who have chronic pain also suffer from depression (Sternbach et al 1973, Lloyd et al 1979). The most probable explanation is that depression develops as a consequence of chronic pain, although it is possible that having a depression-prone personality may make a patient more susceptible to any condition causing chronic pain. Depression does not occur solely as a result of pain in the locomotor system, but it does often occur in patients with chronic low back pain or rheumatoid arthritis; as well as the destruction of bones and joints, there is often destruction of the patient's personality and social functioning. Because of pain and disability, he cannot follow his usual job or social activities. He becomes unemployed, impoverished and consequently decreases his social activities, reinforcing his lowered self-esteem and social isolation, thus deepening the depression.

Treatment

Treating such a depressed patient is a difficult task. Pursuing ever more elusive physical 'causes' of the pain is unlikely to be of much benefit. The patient may well require investigation and treatment of, say, a prolapsed intervertebral disc, but there is usually little benefit to be gained from referral to a variety of specialists who successively prove unable to 'cure' the pain. As well as treating the pain by whatever method seems appropriate, the doctor will also have to tackle the problems of his patient's psychological and social malfunction. How can his depression be treated? How can his social activities be renewed? Measures may include pharmacological treatment of depression; referral to the Disablement Resettlement Officer of the Department of Employment to help find suitable work; encouragement to join patient groups or self-help schemes to widen the patient's restricted social horizons. The general practitioner usually has to act not only as personal doctor to the patient but also as family doctor to the other members of the family who may be affected by the illness of the patient, and discussion with the spouse or other members of the family may help resolve family conflicts which are affecting the situation.

Many patients will feel angry and resentful that they have a long-term disabling illness which cannot be cured as an appendicectomy cures appendicitis. This anger may be directed inwardly, aggravating the pain and disability, or outwardly, disturbing relationships with family, friends and doctor. The patient may need counselling to help him see how his anger can be adversely affecting him.

SEXUAL PROBLEMS

Patients with disorders of the locomotor system may have sexual problems of either a mechanical or psychological nature. For example, intercourse may become difficult in a patient with arthritis of the hip because of an inadequate range of abduction or rotation. Discussion of the problem with the patient may lead to a solution such as advice on alternative positions of intercourse, surgery to improve the mobility of the hip, or discussion about methods of expressing affection without intercourse. The problem may be psychological — possibly mediated through the libido-lessening effect of depression. Even in the absence of overt depression, there may be diminished libido, possibly due to fear of provoking pain or causing further damage to inflamed tissues. The general practitioner should be prepared to explore these matters with the patient and his spouse. In many cases simple reassurance that intercourse will not cause further physical harm is adequate, but in some cases the psychosexual problem is another facet of the entire life problem of the patient and cannot be treated in isolation.

GENERAL PRINCIPLES OF TREATMENT OF LOCOMOTOR DISORDERS

Often, the aim of treatment is to allow the maximum opportunity for the body to heal itself, there being little that medicine can offer to alter the course of the condition. Much of treatment is directed towards the alleviation of symptoms which to a greater or lesser extent can be adapted to most disorders of the locomotor system.

REST

Rest is an important therapeutic measure and should never be forgotten. A painful or acutely inflamed joint settles more quickly if adequate rest is advised. In the case of the spine or lower limb joints bed-rest is often required but in the case of upper limb joints avoidance of use is usually sufficient. The amount of rest required often cannot be predicted accurately in advance, and medical practice is often the result of a series of compromises — against the beneficial effects of prolonged rest one must set the adverse effects such as osteoporosis, muscle weakness or the development of an 'invalid' lifestyle.

SUPPORT

There are many forms of support that can be applied in general practice without referral to hospital services for specialised collars, corsets or splints.

The most adequate support for the spine is a good, firm bed, and if the patient with back pain is seen at home a check should be made on the bed as well as the patient's back. If it is so soft that the patient sinks into it so that there is clearly no support, a board under the mattress may help, or alternatively resting on a mattress on the floor may be easier.

Peripheral joints can be supported in a variety of ways. If the patient is confined to bed — during an acute exacerbation of rheumatoid arthritis — a painful limb joint can be supported by a pillow. If the patient is remaining mobile there are a variety of supporting bandages which can be used, examples include Elastoplast strapping, Viscopaste, crepe bandage, and Tubigrip. The advantages of the first two are good support and the ability to remain in place for a week or more with no interference from the patient. Their disadvantages are their relative rigidity, so that if applied over a swollen joint they may loosen as the swelling goes down, and they can be difficult to apply and remove. Crepe bandages are easy to remove but difficult to apply properly, and as they have to be reapplied frequently, the patient or a relative needs to be shown how to reapply them properly. Elasticated surgical tubular stockinette (Tubigrip) offers a good compromise — it is firm, comes in different sizes for different areas of the body, can be easily applied and removed and does not require any great skill in application. Elastic hosiery kneecaps and anklets can also be very useful for patients with recurrent problems of these joints.

PHYSICAL METHODS OF TREATMENT

Heat, cold, ultrasound and short-wave diathermy are among the physical methods of treating locomotor disorders, but only the use of heat and cold is likely to be possible in general practice. Heat has long been used as a method of relieving pain and muscle spasm in locomotor disorders, and can be applied in a variety of ways, including infra-red lamp, heat pad, hot water bottle and massaging-in embrocations. The benefit, if any, is usually short-lived, but even so can often be a psychological comfort to the patient.

Cold, in the form of ice-packs or aerosol sprays, may have a wider use. Ice is of value in the immediate treatment of muscle and ligament injuries where its vasoconstrictive effect minimises bruising and exudative swelling. It is worth trying the application of ice-packs at frequent intervals for the first day or so after any traumatic lesion of the locomotor system.

DRUG THERAPY

Apart from a few instances where drugs have disease-modifying properties such as penicillamine, gold and chloroquine in rheumatoid arthritis, and allopurinol in gout, most drugs are prescribed for symptomatic reasons, of which pain relief is by far the commonest. As well as analgesics with no anti-inflammatory action, the doctor can choose from a wide variety of drugs whose analgesic effect depends on their anti-inflammatory properties — the non-steroidal anti-inflammatory drugs (NSAIs). The British National Formulary lists 21 such

agents and more are being introduced at frequent intervals. The BNF can be used to select an NSAI, but the doctor should ask himself — should one be chosen at all in a given case, rather than a simple analgesic? It is now widely held that in many cases of, say, osteoarthritis during an acute exacerbation, some inflammation occurs in the joints due to synovitis and crystal deposition, and NSAIs appear to produce better results than simplle analgesics. Whichever drug or drugs the general practitioner chooses from the wide range available, it is wise to become familiar with only a few. It should always be remembered that drugs are very rarely the only form of treatment required despite the enthusiasm with which they are promoted by the pharmaceutical industry.

Corticosteroids
Except in a few exceptional conditions, such as polymyalgia rheumatica and the systemic connective tissue diseases, systemic corticosteroids should not be used routinely in rheumatic disorders. Experience has shown that although they often have initial beneficial effects in rheumatoid arthritis, there is no lasting benefit as judged after 2 years or so. The possible complications of steroid treatment far outweigh any possible short-term benefits. Locally injected steroids, however, largely avoid the systemic side-effects of oral steroids, and have an important part to play in the management of joint and soft-tissue conditions. While many techniques should properly remain in the province of the specialist it should not be beyond the competence of the general practitioner to learn the indications for and techniques of injecting tennis elbows, painful shoulders and similar conditions as outlined earlier. It is far better to learn these techniques under personal supervision than from the pages of a book, and the doctor would be wise to seek such help before treating his own patients.

MOVEMENT

The same principles of learning by practical experience under supervision apply to the techniques of manipulation which are practised by some general practitioners and which are outside the scope of this book. However, all general practitioners should be able to recommend some simple exercises to help mobilise joints and build up weakened muscles. Perhaps the most common advice about exercise and movement given by general practitioners to their patients relates to back disorders. The patient should be advised and shown proper methods of lifting and bending to avoid undue strain on the spine. There is evidence that by using the abdominal muscles to increase intra-abdominal pressure during lifting, the spine can be stabilised to some extent. It would therefore seem reasonable to advise exercises to strengthen the abdominal muscles as an aid to prevent recurrences in back pain patients who cannot avoid lifting. The Back Pain Association publish a number of booklets which give useful information on exercises and methods of lifting. Many patients benefit physically and psychologically from exercise, and swimming and cycling can be recommended.

Specialist referral

Patients may need to be referred to a specialist, either for help in diagnosis or in management. The number of patients referred will depend to some extent on the facilities available to the general practitioner. In the NHS all general practitioners should have open access to hospital laboratories and to X-ray departments, at least for plain radiographs. Laboratory or X-ray facilities will probably be required in less than 10% of cases involving the locomotor system, and a smaller percentage will need to be referred for specialist advice.

AIDS FOR THE DISABLED

There are a number of sources of aids for disabled people, and there is often an overlap between such agencies.

HOSPITALS

Patients may be supplied with crutches or walking frames through the hospital if they are in-patients or out-patients. In most cases articles are supplied for short-term loan, although this is variable. Items such as lumbar supports and footwear are specially made by trained fitters, and can only be obtained through the hospital service, unless the patient wishes to purchase them privately.

ARTIFICIAL LIMB AND APPLIANCE CENTRES

These are special centres of the DHSS which deal with artificial limbs, and major appliances such as wheelchairs. Most of the work with limbless patients is of course initiated by hospital specialists, and the general practitioner may have very infrequent contact with his local centre, except for referral back of patients if and when problems arise. The general practitioner is much more likely to use these centres to provide wheelchairs. The DHSS provides a booklet detailing the types of wheelchairs available and their modifications. A suitable wheelchair can be ordered directly by sending in a form, AOF 5G, or the centre can be asked to assess the patient and provide a suitable model.

SOCIAL SERVICES DEPARTMENT OF LOCAL AUTHORITY

The local social services department is a major source of aids and appliances for the disabled. Services range from the provision of walking sticks and frames, through bath seats and grab-rails, to adaptation of the house by arranging for the construction of ramps for wheelchair access, widening doors and sometimes installation of a home lift. In straightforward cases, the doctor should be able to request the provision of the necessary article, but in complicated problems the Adviser to the Disabled should be consulted, who can visit the patient and make recommendations about appliances and any adaptations to the home that may be required.

Social services departments can also help with holiday arrangements for the disabled, either in a local authority or voluntary holiday home. A social worker may need to be involved to help with the social problems faced by many disabled people — the problems of acceptance of their disability, anger and frustration, isolation and loneliness.

Lastly, social services departments can provide Home Helps and Meals on Wheels for disabled people where required.

DEPARTMENT OF HEALTH AND SOCIAL SECURITY

Many patients with locomotor disorders will be in receipt of benefits from the DHSS — either sickness or invalidity benefit, retirement pension or supplementary benefit. Patients with disorders of mobility may also be eligible for a range of extra benefits such as a heating allowance, if the person is housebound and cannot move around freely, or an attendance allowance, if the person requires close supervision or care.

VOLUNTARY ORGANISATIONS

There are many organisations involved with the care of the disabled in general and some are principally concerned with people with particular diseases. Both the Arthritis and Rheumatism Council* and the Back Pain Association† have local branches to help sufferers, as well as raise money for research and educational activities. Other charities may provide holidays, outings or grants for particular groups such as ex-servicemen and retired

* Headquarters address: Arthritis and Rheumatism Council, 41 Eagle Street, LONDON, WC1R 4AR
† Headquarters address: Back Pain Association, Grundy House, 31–33 Park Road Teddington, Middlesex, TW11 OAB

Post Office employees, and these activities can often lighten the load that a disabled person and his relatives have to bear.

COMMUNITY NURSING SERVICE

Many disabled persons may require the services of a community nurse, for bathing or general nursing care. The community nurse may request special equipment such as a ripple bed, sheepskins or hoist from the health authority or the social services department. The general practitioner should have a close working relationship with the community nurse to ensure that all patients who might benefit from nursing services receive them, that the patient's management can be jointly planned and that the nurse can report on progress or any problems which may arise. As the needs of the disabled are often multiple, varied and unique to the patient, the general practitioner may have to work closely with many others also contributing to the care of the patient.

ACKNOWLEDGEMENT

I wish to thank Dr Douglas Golding for his criticism and advice in the preparation of this chapter.

REFERENCES

British National Formulary 1982 3rd edn. British Medical Association and the Pharmaceutical Society of Great Britain, London

Gilchrist I C 1976 Psychiatric and social factors related to low back pain in general practice. Rheumatology and Rehabilitation 15:101–107

Holmes T H, Wolff H G 1950 Life situations, emotions and backache. In: Life stress and bodily disease. Research Publications, Association for Research in Nervous and Mental Disease 29:750–772

Lloyd G G, Wolkind S N, Greenwood R, Harris O J 1979 A psychiatric study of patients with persistent low back pain. Rheumatology and Rehabilitation 18:30–34

Morrell D C, Wale C J 1976 Symptoms perceived and recorded by patients. Journal of the Royal College of General Practitioners 26:398–403

Nagi S Z, Riley L E, Newby L G 1973 A social epidemiology of back pain in a general population. Journal of Chronic Disease 26:769–779

Office of Population Censuses and Surveys 1974 Morbidity statistics from general practice. Second National Study 1970–71. HMSO, London

Parkes C M, Benjamin B, Fitzgerald R G 1969 Broken heart: a statistical study of increased mortality among widowers. British Medical Journal 1:740–743

Rose H S 1975 The lives of patients before presentation with pain in the neck or back. Journal of the Royal College of General Practitioners 25:771–772

Sarno J E 1974 Psychogenic backache: the missing dimension. Journal of Family Practice 5:353–357

Sternbach R A, Wolf S R, Murphy R W, Akeson W H 1973 Aspects of chronic low back pain. Psychosomatics 18:52–56

RECOMMENDED READING
Golding D N 1982 A synopsis of rheumatic diseases, 4th edn. Wright, Bristol

Central nervous system disorders

INTRODUCTION

It is difficult for the general practitioner to achieve and maintain competence in the field of neurological disorders; the knowledge and skills acquired in undergraduate and postgraduate education, even if supplemented by reading textbooks of neurology, seem inadequate and even fade in an area of work where although there are many presenting symptoms which are referable to the central nervous system there are nevertheless few central nervous system disorders or diseases, apart from migraine, epilepsy, cerebro-vascular disorders and Parkinson's disease. Even these can give rise to difficulties. In addition, the anxiety not to miss a rare but potentially disastrous diagnosis such as brain tumour, vascular abnormalities or early evidence of multiple sclerosis, strongly influences practice and especially referral to and dependence upon specialists.

THE FIELD OF WORK

PATIENT CONSULTATION RATES

Consultation rates are available from general practice morbidity recording (RCGP OPCS 1974). Table 19.1 shows the main groups of central nervous system diseases

Table 19.1 Annual patient consulting rates for diseases of central nervous system

Disease	Patients consulting		
	per 1000	per 2500	% of total
Cerebrovascular disorders	6	15	20
Migraine	7	18	24 ⎫
Headaches	4	10	13 ⎬ 37
Vertigo	8	20	26 ⎭
Epilepsy	3	7	10 ⎫
Paralysis agitans	1	3	4 ⎬ 17
Multiple sclerosis	1	2	3 ⎭
New growths	0.1	0.25	1
		(1 in 4 yrs)	
Total	30	75	100

seen in general practice in a year both per 1000 of population and in a list of 2500 patients. The total of 75 includes new patients as well as those with established conditions and combine annual incidence and prevalence.

The disorders vary in how common they are and also in how commonly they are seen by the doctor, consultation rates relate to severity, patient expectations and doctor concern.

One new patient with multiple sclerosis will be seen once in 15 years, and there will be one or two new cases of epilepsy each year. Almost all patients with stroke will be seen in the course of a year, rather more than half the patients with epilepsy and only one-tenth of those with migraine.

There is a balance of care between patient, practitioner and hospital; acute situations of severe stroke, status epilepticus and perhaps exacerbation of multiple sclerosis require hospital in-patient care; the hospital specialist service may be essential in establishing the diagnosis and looked to for guidance about treatment. The hospital may attempt to provide continuity of supervision for a proportion of patients with chronic disease but cannot for all and certainly not all patients with epilepsy. Continuing medical care is the responsibility of the general practitioner and how he faces up to this determines its quality.

EVALUATION OF CARE

GENERAL PRACTICE VIEWED FROM HOSPITAL

The perspective of hospital doctors (Harwood 1982) gives some insight into the general practitioner's contribution. The following are common criticisms:

1. *Failure to obtain an adequate history* which provides the diagnosis in 80% of cases; and allied to this referrals requesting tests, especially scans and EEGs in the mistaken belief that these have greater diagnostic validity than basic clinical evaluation, associated with the myth that an EEG is needed to make a diagnosis of epilepsy.

2. *Failure to cope with commonly occurring problems:*

a. Not recognising adolescent faints, which are referred as possible epilepsy.

b. Not appreciating that ill-defined transitory and migratory sensations of numbness are unimportant.

c. Failure to evaluate common causes of headache.

3. Reluctance to manage chronic disorders and their medication, such as epilepsy and Parkinson's disease.

4. Failure to recognise that patients and pathology change and that this has implications for management, and also lessons for hospital doctors.

GOALS FOR CARE

Acceptable goals include:

Prevention; early accurate diagnosis; treatment to cure, relieve and limit disability. Failure to achieve these goals appears to be due to:

1. Lack of basic clinical knowledge and skill.
2. Poor communication with patient and colleagues.
3. Failure to keep abreast of developments in medicine, therapeutics and support services and failure to exploit them.
4. Lack of resources or organisation to put into practice what is possible.
5. Attitudes about the job, restricting what is done.

These barriers are both philosophical and practical. Each general practitioner must decide how much time and effort is justified for screening, reviewing patients and keeping up-to-date. The author's philosophy gives priority to early diagnosis and more effective management of known patients, over screening; towards enabling patients and relatives to cope with their disorder by teaching them about it and providing support and supervision which includes doctor-initiated follow-up for at-risk patients.

Clinical knowledge

It is essential to have good accounts of neurological diseases and the treatment available as 'bench books' in the consulting room. Reading, combined with good clinical descriptions from one's own patients is the best way to acquire expertise in recognising patterns. W.B. Matthews' (1975) textbook *Practical Neurology* and *Medicine* Third Series 31–34, the monthly add-on journal, are especially helpful. Therapeutics, except in very recent publications, is liable to be so out of date as to be unhelpful and with reference to anticonvulsants and recent advances even harmful. The British National Formulary (1983) is invaluable and should be referred to when unfamiliar drugs are encountered, the appendices on drug interaction should always be scrutinised. Reactions are very common amongst drugs effective in central nervous system disorders.

Clinical skills

History

Each generation, it seems, has to learn that a good history is fundamental to sound practice; unhurried history-taking, especially with patients handicapped by being unaware of what has happened to them or unable to communicate adequately demonstrably leads to mistakes. To take time, if necessary to see witnesses, is difficult, but it pays.

Examination

Although it is neither realistic nor necessary for a general practitioner to be able to carry out a detailed neurological examination and pinpoint lesions with anatomical precision, and examination matters less than history, it is nevertheless important. Valuable and obvious information is missed by failure to carry out a simple examination especially regarding function, e.g. walking, dressing, writing.

Telling the patient

Patient understanding is vital in chronic diseases especially if how they live or take their pills is crucial to optimum benefit. Remembering to teach the patient and providing or advising booklets like *Epilepsy Explained*, (Laidlaw 1980), *Migraine and other Headaches*, (Wilkinson 1980) and *Parkinson's Disease*, (Godwin-Austen 1979) are of great importance.

Organising the practice

Disease registers even for a limited number of chronic diseases enable the review of patients for individual care, audit and recall.

Using outside resources

In addition to specialist neurological services it is important to establish relationships with other sources of help particularly for those with disabling illness, in particular the remedial professions and Social Services. Where resources such as physiotherapy, are not available they should be argued for. Where they are theoretically available but not readily forthcoming, e.g. aids and alterations by the Social Services, then the general practitioner must pressure on the patient's behalf. The various sorts of financial help available need to be borne in mind and check lists help; it is not uncommon, for example, to forget that patients on anticonvulsants are entitled to free prescriptions.

CEREBRO-VASCULAR DISORDERS — STROKE

The annual incidence of stroke is between one and two

per 1000; it increases with age, with a mean age for men of 67 years, and of women 71 years. The average general practitioner will thus see five new cases each year. Most cases (80%) will be due to cerebral infarction, about 10% to intra-cerebral haemorrhage and 10% to subarachnoid haemorrhage; one patient with the latter will present every 2 years. Underlying hypertension will be present in over a third, with about half of these being poorly controlled or undiagnosed.

Outcome of stroke

Accounts vary especially for early mortality (Fry 1979, Waters & Parkin 1982). 30% or more die in the first month, half of these in the first 24 hours; 50% make a good recovery in a month (but 40% of these will have a further stroke); 20% will already be severely handicapped by the end of the first month. In round terms about a third of survivors will be recovered and well, a third moderately handicapped and a third severely handicapped. The overall 5-year survival rate is 30–50% and the average general practitioner will have 20 disabled patients on his list.

STROKE PREVENTION

Of the central nervous system disorders stroke is the only one which so far allows much scope for prevention. Screening for and treating hypertension is known to reduce the incidence of stroke, and arguments for screening and then treating what amounts to 10% of the adult population are well described (Hart 1980, Ramsay 1981). In addition to screening for hypertension better efforts could be made to achieve good control in those already diagnosed; it is salutory to reflect that of cases of hypertension detected only half are treated and only half of these are treated satisfactorily.

A few strokes, or repeat strokes from emboli, may be avoided by attention to such causes as mitral stenosis and atrial fibrillation.

STROKE MANAGEMENT — HOME OR HOSPITAL

The arguments for admission of all strokes to hospital focus on the reduced risk of complications such as bronchopneumonia, deep venous thrombosis, bedsores, and better functional recovery. In practical terms however not all patients can go into hospital and not all want or need to. Severity, age and social conditions decide. It appears (Waters & Parkin 1982) that patients kept at home are less likely to benefit from remedial therapy such as physiotherapy and speech therapy; this should be remedied. All stroke patients managed at home with any

significant handicap should be assessed by a physiotherapist and speech therapist, and be visited at home by an occupational therapist or experienced social worker to give advice about aids and structural alteration (Table 19.2).

The long-term management of the patient who has survived a stroke concerns several members of the practice team. The patient is likely to be elderly and to have several co-existing medical problems which will require treatment regimes that may change with age and the progress of each condition. Hypertension may have provoked the stroke and will require even more rigid control if a further vascular accident is to be avoided. The patient will need to be encouraged to optimise any functional recovery, and the relatives to continue to include the patient in normal family life: the patient with speech problems resulting from a right-sided hemiplegia is frequently ignored by relatives who may regard the speech impediment as indicating loss of intellect. Some degree of emotional lability or frank depression is common following major strokes: the former due to cerebral damage with the latter, to an extent, a reflection of the patient's distress at loss of independence. Both manifestations may require drug therapy, and both can be minimised if relations understand and show a constructive sympathy.

Again, depending on the degree of resulting disability, regular visits by the district nurse may be needed for duties that include personal bathing and care of pressure areas. A home help and meals-on-wheels may be necessary if independent existence is to continue and, most importantly, the physical and mental health of the caring relative or relatives requires attention to allow this support to be continuing.

Regular admission of the patient to hospital for 'holiday care' is one means by which the health of the caring relatives can be maintained and their support of the patient extended.

MIGRAINE AND HEADACHE

Figures derived from population surveys vary considerably because of the problem of definition and the commoness of headaches. Up to 19% of men and 29% of women have been estimated to have had migraine at some time in their lives. It is generally held that between 5 and 7% of the population suffer in any year, but only

Table 19.2

1. Practice organisation. List and review known hypertensives. Pursue adequate control.
2. Plan of management for strokes at home to include remedial professionals and provision of aids and alterations
3. District criteria for stroke management

one in 10 consult their general practitioner. Although most patients with migraine or recurrent headahces have infrequent attacks of variable severity, a significant minority have major disability.

As a profession we have been limited in what we can do by a lack of understanding of the causes of headache and of the value of different therapies. Useful lessons have been learned from the expertise developed in the 'Migraine Clinics' set up in city centres, to carry out research, provide emergency treatment and give advice to patients referred by general practitioners. Results have included a methodical approach to management, a critical evaluation of different therapies, but the most useful is the simple discovery that metoclopramide (10 mg) given early in an attack followed 10 or 15 minutes later by an analgesic is effective in most cases.

CAUSES OF HEADACHE

In most patients presenting with headache there is little difficulty in diagnosing the cause quickly and treatment is equally straightforward. The list of possibilities is endless but Table 19.3 shows the commonest.

Headaches due to intracranial causes are very much less common but important because of their serious nature.

SERIOUS CAUSES OF HEADACHE

The important, serious or life-threatening causes are:

— Meningitis
— Subarachnoid haemorrhage
— Temporal arteritis
— Intracranial tumour

Early diagnosis is desirable in all but crucial in the first three where delay may lead to a potentially avoidable disaster. Common reasons for delay include a failure to see the patient early (either patient or doctor delay) and failure to act quickly when the diagnosis is suspected. The doctor may miss the diagnosis because the patient is

Table 19.3 Commonest causes of headache

1. Headache associated with fever or infection
2. Referred pain from:
   Eye   Sinuses   Cervical spine
   Teeth or Temporo-mandibular joint
3. Tension headache
4. Migraine
5. Neuritis and neuralgia:
   Herpetic neuralgia
   Trigeminal (and glossopharyngeal) neuralgia
6. Temporal arteritis

known to have had headaches previously, or has more than one possible cause for the symptoms, or because the presentation is atypical, perhaps with the patient omitting to complain of headache.

Meningitis
Most patients with meningitis complain of a prodromal respiratory tract illness, and severe headache and are found to have marked nuchal rigidity. It should be remembered however that the clinical signs of meningitis may not become apparent until some hours after the onset of the headache: the severity of the headache is the clue and the patient should be repeatedly examined if the diagnosis is not to be missed. Extremes of age also tend to be associated with atypical presentation and altered symptomatology. The commonest causative organism in meningitis is a virus: meningococcal meningitis is rare but like other types of pyogenic meningitis carries a worse prognosis unless diagnosed at an early stage. Pyogenic meningitis is characterised by sudden onset, high fever, irritability, severe headache, vomiting and frequently convulsions. In infants neck rigidity is less common but increased intra-cranial pressure can be detected by feeling the anterior fontanelle. Nuchal rigidity is a more consistent sign in the older child and adults. The purpuric rash, often associated with meningococcal meningitis is a valuable diagnostic sign. The much less common, but important, tuberculous meningitis generally shows a slow progressive course with headache, stupor, vomiting and irritability as the usual presenting features. Whatever the infecting organism all patients with meningitis — suspected or proven — should be admitted to hospital for definitive investigation and treatment.

Subarachnoid haemorrhage
Early diagnosis and urgent, normally operative, treatment is essential if a high mortality is to be avoided. The typical presentation of a very sudden severe occipital headache in an adolescent or young adult is the most useful. Diagnostic problems can occur if the symptomatology is atypical or if the patient also suffers from severe headache such as migraine. Again this is a diagnosis to be remembered and admission of the patient is the correct approach if it is suspected.

Temporal arteritis
This is an uncommon complaint and full of pitfalls if not classical. The pain may be atypical, pulsation may be present and tenderness slight. One well-remembered elderly patient lost the vision in one eye as we awaited the result of a further ESR, the first having been only slightly raised. In conclusion, all patients complaining of severe headache should be seen urgently. If in doubt, especially about neck stiffness, admit to hospital; if temporal arteritis is at all a possibility, don't wait! Treat with steroids.

Intra-cranial tumours

Doctors as well as patients associate headache with a brain tumour; parents especially so with severe headaches in children. The commonest cause of severe headache, however, is migraine although the features of periodicity, nausea and vomiting are common to both migraine and space-occupying lesions. The general practitioner is likely to see one patient with an intra-cranial neoplasm every 8 years. In adults the cause is likely to be secondary metastases from bronchus, breast or kidney. In children cerebral tumour is the second commonest cancer and is invariably invasive and progressive.

Signs and symptoms

There are three sources of the signs and symptoms: increasing cranial pressure, infiltration of structures causing loss of function and focal irritation producing epilepsy. The increasing pressure has three consequences: headache, vomiting and visual disturbance.

Where headache is a symptom other neurological or ocular signs or symptoms are commonly present or will develop within a few weeks; in children it has been observed (Honig & Charney 1982) that of 72 children with cerebral tumour with headache, 68 had neurological or ocular signs, or both, at the time of diagnosis, 49 had ataxia, 18 had head tilt and 63 had papilloedema. Abnormal signs developed within 2 weeks of the headaches in 33 children, within 8 weeks in 51 and by 24 weeks in the remainder of the 68.

Headaches may be similar to those with a benign cause but the following features are emphasised and are similar in adults:

1. Recurrent morning headache.
2. Headaches awakening from sleep.
3. Intense, prolonged incapacitating headache.
4. Changes in the quality, frequency and pattern of headaches.
5. Vomiting associated with headaches. (Vomiting may be projectile and not preceded by nausea.)

THE COMMONER CAUSES OF HEADACHE

Tension headache

Tension headache is said to be the commonest cause of headache, possibly because the label tends to be applied to most headaches that worry the patient and which cannot be attributed to some other condition such as migraine. It is also referred to as the 'muscle contraction headache' because of its association with tension of the scalp and neck muscles. Textbook accounts vary in descriptions but the following are common features:

— Band-like sensation around head
— Bi-frontal or occipital
— Usually bilateral
— Sometimes a constant ache with sharp jabs
— Doesn't usually affect sleep
— Not associated with vomiting

Neurologists are pessimistic about the outcome of explanation or treatment, but they do see the worst and the most chronic. In general practice there are many headaches associated with muscle tension, often due to stress or fatigue and prolonged concentration, sometimes associated with depression, and they usually respond to commonsense advice and simple analgesics. The chronic and persistent varieties exist but fortunately do not dominate the scene; in common with some severe migraine sufferers, such patients may not be helped by the doctor, but may improve when important aspects of their lives change, for example an end to an unsatisfactory marriage, a change of job or a change of inner attitude from religious or spiritual experience. The cornerstone of treatment for tension headache is the identification — and acceptance by the patient — of the likely stressful cause. The tendency to tension headaches will only improve when the patient understands and accepts the explanation for her symptoms and as a consequence takes some steps to remove the source of stress. This can seldom be achieved quickly or easily and several careful explanatory consultations may be needed. Once the patient has understood the problem supportive counselling from the doctor is more effective than analgesics or anxiolytic drugs.

It is important to remember that tension headache may co-exist with migraine; the latter may be unsuspected but may cause much of the incapacity. Although the diagnosis is usually established by the history, examination is important (especially fundi and blood pressure) to exclude other causes and to strengthen the doctor's explanation and make it more acceptable.

Hypertension is not normally a cause of headache but it is generally thought to be so by lay people and fears about this may be the reason for the consultation.

MIGRAINE

Definition and diagnosis

The simplest definition is 'recurrent headache, accompanied by a visual or gastro-intestinal disturbance or both with freedom between attacks'.

Attacks may be preceded by or associated with marked sensory, motor or mood disturbances; these may be dramatic and especially alarming in a first attack if hemianopia, unilateral paraesthesiae or transitory hemiplegia are present. Features other than headache may be variable, mild and sometimes absent and although some authorities regard the presence of either vomiting or visual disturbances as necessary for diagnosis, epidemiological studies do not support this view. Much episodic headache, even if not unilateral and without other symptoms, is probably common migraine.

Types of migraine

The diagnosis rests on pattern recognition and there is little difficulty with classical migraine. It is not the authors' purpose to provide extensive descriptions but the following aspects are emphasised: there is a wide variety of presentation; although there may be an underlying structural cause in rarer presentations such as familial hemiplegic migraine or ophthalmoplegic migraine, this is unlikely to be so in classical migraine even in severe and highly dramatic presentations. Migrainous neuralgia, although relatively uncommon and perhaps not true migraine, merits particular mention since it is not always recognised and yet is very responsive to treatment.

Migrainous neuralgia — 'cluster headache'

Episodes of pain, usually very severe, occur in and around one eye. The pain may radiate to the forehead, cheek and temple. It tends to recur daily for several weeks often awakening the patient in the early hours, and may last from between 15 minutes to 2 hours and recur several times in a 24-hour period. The eye may become red and run and the nostril on the same side may also run or become blocked. Partial ptosis and oedema of the eyelids may be present; occasionally Horner's Syndrome is seen. It is commoner in men than in women and attacks are frequently provoked by excess alcohol.

Treatment is very effective and traditionally involved an injection of ergotamine tartrate each night until the cluster is thought to be over. The injectable form is not currently available but suppositories or inhalation by aerosol work just as well. Failing that, methysergide 1 mg increasing to 2 mg t.d.s. is effective and although there are reservations about its safety, it is needed only for a few weeks at a time.

Management of migraine

The aim is to have the patient manage his own migraine. He will do this better if he knows what it is, what might cause it in his case, what is happening during an attack and how an attack may be cut short or modified.

The diagnosis and pattern of events or possible precipitating causes may not be immediately clear, and to involve the patient as a detective by keeping a diary of symptoms and associated circumstances may make a dubious diagnosis clear and teach the patient about the things which have triggered his attacks (Table 19.4).

It is worthwhile writing descriptions of the individual's attacks in his case notes: this will demonstrate the variety of presentation and avoids the predicament of not knowing what the patient means when he consults at a later date.

Table 19.4 Trigger factors in migraine

1. Dietary factors:	cheese
	chocolate
	alcohol
	citrus fruits
2. Allergy:	wheat
	milk
	eggs
	fish
	tea
3. Sleep:	too much or too little
4. Hormonal:	premenstrually
	contraceptive pill
5. Environment:	heat
	noise
	light
6. Psychological:	anxiety
	depression
	frustration

It is useful in explanation to say 'that the aura is caused by blood vessels in the brain constricting and the headache by blood vessels expanding again, the particular neurological symptoms present in each case depending upon which bit of brain is affected'. If this is done the value of taking ergotamine early enough to influence events is more likely to be appreciated. The failure of drugs to work because of poor absorption when nausea and vomiting are present is readily grasped as is the value of taking a drug such as metoclopramide together with or followed later by an analgesic.

The value of sleep in resolving attacks may need stressing and that it is worthwhile to give in sometimes and lie down in order to have a shorter attack.

Drug treatment

The reader is advised to refer to up-to-date accounts of current drug therapy.

Acute attack:

1. Lie down in a darkened room.

2. Try a simple analgesic first, if necessary with metoclopramide, 10 mg at the time or 10–15 minutes earlier.

3. The place of ergotamine tartrate is well established but it should be remembered that it itself may cause nausea and vomiting. Repeated use may lead to habituation and attempts at withdrawal may precipitate headaches. Ergotamine should never be given together with methysergide because of the risk of arterial occlusion; it should not be prescribed for hemiplegic migraine.

Prevention of attacks

Very few patients require interval treatment and patients with frequent severe attacks frequently have an underlying psychological problem. Beta adrenergic blockers help some patients, propanolol being the most commonly used in a dose of 20 mg b.d. to 80 mg t.d.s. Clonidine in a dose of 25 μg b.d. to 50 μg t.d.s. is effective in some patients as is pizotifen in a dose of 0.5 to 2 mg t.d.s. Methysergide, already mentioned, is often effective but the rare, though serious, side-effect of retroperitoneal fibrosis discourages its use, especially long-term. Mild sedatives, tranquillisers and tricyclic antidepressants also have their place.

EPILEPSY

The prevalence of epilepsy varies between seven per 1000 in children to half that in adults. It varies considerably between practices but the average general practitioner will have 12 patients with epilepsy, one-third of them children. He will see one or two new cases each year.

Two-thirds of the children will become seizure-free in adult life; three-quarters of the adults will have had their first seizure in childhood or adolescence. Of the adults who develop epilepsy, 10% will have an underlying intracranial tumour.

There can be few conditions in which the potential for improved care so far exceeds the reality than in epilepsy; both the evidence about shortcomings and about advances which make improvement possible are well-documented (Table 19.5).

Misdiagnoses

None would argue that accurate diagnosis should be the basis of treatment, and yet surveys (Jeavons 1975) found that up to 20% of patients attending epilepsy clinics are wrongly diagnosed. Misdiagnosis appears to stem from the following:

— Inadequate history-making
— The occurence of clonic movements or incontinence
— The existence of a family history of epilepsy
— Previous febrile convulsions, or
— An abnormal EEG
    and most fundamentally:
— Insufficient knowledge of the nature of epilepsy

Shortcomings identified by patients include: failure to explain the purpose of anti-epileptic drugs, polypharmacy in response to repeat seizures and ignorance of blood-level monitoring.

One survey of adults with epilepsy in general practice (Hopkins & Scambler 1977) identified the following problems:

— Inadequate communication of the diagnosis
— Inadequate medication and follow-up supervision related to the patient's needs

The authors considered that anticonvulsant treatment was conservative both in choice and quantity of drug and

half of those having generalised seizures monthly or more frequently were probably under-treated. Continuing medical supervision seemed random and half of the few still attending hospital clinics had rare seizures while some of those with very frequent seizures did not even see their general practitioner for months at a time.

Effective anticonvulsants have been available for many years and the traditional regimens, based on multiple drug therapy, evolved partly because of the belief that the effects of anti-epileptics were additive or as a further response to repeat seizures in a patient who was already on one or more drugs. Advances in the past few years, the ability to monitor serum levels and the improved understanding of pharmacokinetics of anticonvulsant drugs have called into question the time-honoured practice.

Shorvon and his colleagues (1978) having already ascertained that where two drugs were being taken improvement in control was usually associated with optimum levels of at least one drug, then demonstrated that 76 to 88% of new patients could be controlled with a single drug. Later they demonstrated (Shorvon & Reynolds 1979) that polypharmacy could be reduced in chronic epilepsy with reduction to a single drug in 72% of patients with improvement in seizure control in 55% and a striking improvement in mental functioning in 55%.

Audits in general practice, although varying in their conclusions, mainly support the view that the management of epilepsy is unsatisfactory and that there is a possibility of producing marked improvement.

In the practice of one of the authors (Taylor 1980) (6500 patients) of 35 patients diagnosed with epilepsy, three were considered misdiagnosed; careful adjustment of anticonvulsants led to improvement in seizure control in 27%, and polypharmacy was reduced in 24%. Some patients were tolerating chronic drug toxicity, and frequent seizures both generalised and partial which were unknown to the family doctor. Out of five who were handicapped by the condition, improvement in control and reduction of side-effects made it possible for one to return to work and for another to contemplate it. Overall improvements were considered to be due not simply to more effective prescribing but also to a better understanding of the nature of epilepsy and the purpose of medication by patients and relatives. From the foregoing, the shortcomings in care and therefore the oppor-

Table 19.5

1. Up to 20% of patients labelled 'epileptic' misdiagnosed
2. Doctors fail to explain about epilepsy and about drugs
3. Follow-up supervision is often unrelated to need
4. Most new patients controlled with a single drug
5. Reducing polypharmacy in chronic patients improves seizure control and wellbeing in up to 55% of patients

tunity to transform it lie in the initial diagnosis, the use of drugs and supervision and doctor–patient communication.

Diagnosis

Mis-diagnosis of grand mal is common usually because of the presence of jerking movements or incontinence of micturition, symptoms which can also occur in syncope *after* loss of consciousness unlike a true epileptic seizure in which the abnormal movements *coincide* with loss of consciousness. There are other differences; after syncope the patient will come round and be perfectly well in a short period of time whereas the tonic clonic seizure patient is likely to be confused, sleepy and have a headache. The complex partial seizures of psychomotor epilepsy are often missed because of the lack of a good description or the failure of the doctor to recognise it. Absence associated with this group of seizures may be confused with petit mal which is quite different, has a different prognosis and responds to different therapy. A clear description of events must be sought from a witness.

Type of epilepsy

A review of patients with seizures in a single general practice will reveal almost as many different types of seizure as patients, and show that many individuals have more than one type of seizure. Making sense of this is difficult and a simple classification (Table 19.6) is helpful as a basis for action.

For practical purposes in determining treatment the majority of seizures may be divided into two kinds, generalised seizures and partial (focal) seizures. Many of the latter may become generalised as seizure activity spreads leading to a tonic clonic fit. Very full descriptions

Table 19.6 Classification of seizures

Generalised seizures
1. Grand mal:
   Tonic clonic seizures
   Without aura or evidence of a focal onset
2. Petit mal:
   Absence

Partial seizures
1. Simple
   No impairment of consciousness:
   Symptom relates to focus of origin, e.g. motor, sensory, affective, cognitive, olfactory, psyche
2. Complex partial:
   With impairment of consciousness:
   a. Simple onset
      or
   b. Impaired consciousness from onset.
3. Generalised tonic-clonic seizures:
   a. Evolved from a partial focal seizure
   b. Spontaneous but EEG evidence of focus

are available (Laidlaw & Richens 1982) and are a valuable reference. A clear and simple account is available in a booklet written for patients and relatives and therefore easy for doctors to understand (Laidlaw & Laidlaw 1980). Since there are obvious misunderstandings the simpler classification is here described in detail. Less common forms of epilepsy, especially of childhood, are not included (see Robinson 1980).

Generalised seizures

These fall into two groups:

1. *Grand mal* tonic clonic seizures in which there is *no* evidence of focal onset, for example an aura, motor activity as in Jacksonian epilepsy, or bizarre behaviour from a psychomotor focus.

2. *Petit mal* absence which is almost totally a problem of childhood. This is a brief absence often associated with movement (which has a typical rhythm at three beats per second) usually localised to the eyelids but sometimes involving the arms. In most patients an attack may be provoked by a 3-minute period of hyperventilation. This is one condition in which the EEG pattern is especially helpful in showing a regular synchrous generalised three cycles per second spike wave pattern. The combination of grand mal with petit mal is termed *primary generalised epilepsy*; this is important from a therapeutic point of view since sodium valproate is effective against both these types of seizure and will be the drug of choice when they occur together.

Partial seizures (including those evolving to generalised tonic clonic seizures)

Grand mal tonic clonic seizures with an underlying focal source are commoner than primary generalised grand mal and many patients have more than one type of seizure. Not uncommonly a patient who one day has an olfactory aura succeeded by a tonic clonic seizure may on other days experience a brief aura only or the process may be so rapid that the focal symptom or aura is not perceived.

Implications of seizure type for treatment

Drugs are more effective in controlling generalised seizures than partial seizures and some drugs are more effective than others. When treatment is started with an anticonvulsant fewer tonic clonic seizures may result but partial attacks may persist, not always progressing to secondary generalisation. Although the aim is to abolish seizures, this is not always desirable and an occasional aura or absence or even a complex partial seizure may be preferable to drug side-effects.

The diagnosis of epilepsy is essentially clinical; EEG and other investigations do not *prove* epilepsy but help to define what sort it might be. One seizure does not comprise epilepsy (Table 19.7).

Table 19.7

1. A witnessed account is mandatory
2. Diagnosis is clinical
3. EEG does not mean epilepsy but helps to define it
4. Epilepsy is more than one seizure

Choice of anticonvulsant

The choice of most anticonvulsants has been established over many years by their empirical use mainly in combinations and although the improved therapy of single drug therapy has been established there is still uncertainty about the relative merits of individual drugs for particular seizures.

Table 19.8 provides a list of first line anticonvulsants with optimum serum levels (Reynolds 1978). Phenytoin and carbamazepine have generally been regarded as equally effective against grand mal and partial seizures but there is increased support for the use of the latter as the drug of choice for partial seizures, and especially complex partial psychomotor seizures (synonym temporal lobe epilepsy).

Primidone and phenobarbitone are effective, the former due to its metabolism to phenobarbitone. These two drugs and clonazepam (Rivotril) are generally too sedating and are too prone to cause behavioural disturbance to encourage first choice for chronic use. Sodium valproate (Epilim) although effective against tonic clonic seizures is probably not so effective against partial seizures.

Since two-thirds of adults with epilepsy have a partial seizure with grand mal or other evidence of focal onset, either carbamazepine or phenytoin is now likely to be prescribed singly as first choice, depending on the preference of the clinician. Both drugs have toxic side-effects but phenytoin gives most problems in this respect and its optimal use in more severe and intractable epilepsy requires meticulous dose adjustment to give control while avoiding toxicity.

Starting anticonvulsant therapy

Only one or two new patients on a general practitioner's list will develop epilepsy each year and although he may not initiate treatment he will be involved in supervising medication, and may need to change it. The current best choice for grand mal seizures with or without evidence of partial onset is carbamazepine followed by phenytoin, sodium valproate and phenobarbitone in that order. Whichever drug is selected a low dose should be started, increasing until seizures are controlled or side-effects appear. Although the patient should be seen frequently, drug dosage should not be increased at too short intervals. Since the aim is to produce stable serum levels a knowledge of the half life of the drug helps to judge the intervals at which the dose should be increased. As a basic guide four to five half-lives are needed before a steady serum level is achieved.

Most anticonvulsants may be given in daily or twice-daily doses, even those drugs with a short half-life such as sodium valproate or carbamazepine (Table 19.9). It is probably better to work out with the patient what suits him best.

Individual anticonvulsants

The current BNF gives the dose range for different ages but does not help in advising how to build up the dose and the following may be helpful for the common individual anticonvulsants.

Carbamazepine: dizziness, drowsiness and gastro-intestinal disturbance may be a problem, especially early in treatment. For this reason it is best started in adults at a dose of 100 mg b.d. increased by 200 mg daily at a minimum of fortnightly intervals. Serum levels are very variable between individuals and the average daily dose is 600 mg, maximum 1200 mg.

Phenytoin: for adults start with 200 mg daily either in a single or a divided dose, and adjust no more than once a month. If serum levels are not available and seizures persist increase to 300 mg daily and thereafter, increase the daily dose by 50 mg each month until seizures stop or signs of toxicity develop, in which case stop treatment for 2 days and restart on a lower dose, e.g. 25 mg less per day.

If serum levels are available (having started on 200 mg daily) and serum concentration is less than 8 μg/mol (32

Table 19.8   First line anticonvulsants and optimum serum levels

Type of epilepsy	Drug	Optimum serum levels (μg/ml)	(μmol)
Tonic clonic (grand mal) or partial (focal) $\pm$ tonic clonic	Phenobarbitone	15–40	45–105
	Phenytoin	10–20	40–80
	Primidone	as for phenobarbitone	
	Carbamazepine	4–10	15–42
	Clonazepam	?	?
	Sodium valproate	50–100	300–650
Petit mal	Ethosuccimide	40–80	280–710
	Clonazepam	?	?
	Sodium valproate	50–100	300–650

Table 19.9 Pharmacokinetic data for anticonvulsants

Drug		Serum half-life	Minimum daily dosage intervals	Suggested interval dose adjustment
Phenytoin		1–4 days	Daily	3–4 weeks
Carbamazepine	New	24–46 h	b.d.	2–3 weeks
	Chronic	8–19 h		
Phenobarbitone		2–5 days	Daily	4 weeks
Primidone			t.d.s.	4 weeks
Sodium valproate		6–10 h	b.d. or daily	2–3 weeks
Clonazepam		20–40 h	b.d.	2–3 weeks
Ethosuccimide		2½–4 days	Daily	4 weeks

* True half life in chronic therapy not available
† Despite short half-life a daily dose may be adequate

μmol/l) increase by 100 mg daily; if 8–12 μg/mol (32–48 μmol/l) increase by 50 mg daily; above 12 μg/mol (48 μmol/l) increase by 25 mg daily. Average adult dose is 350 mg, maximum 600 mg.

Phenobarbitone: (also *primidone*): is started in a dose of 30 mg daily. Increase to 60 mg after 1 week if drowsiness is not a problem and then increase by 30 mg/day every 4 weeks. As much as 150 mg daily may be required. Upper limits are determined by individual tolerance to side-effects.

Sodium valproate: this is effective against grand mal but probably not against partial seizures. It is the drug of choice for petit mal with grand mal; despite its short half-life twice-daily dosage is usually effective. The dose range is 400 mg daily to 2.5 g. Although regarded as a safe drug, sodium valproate may cause hair-thinning, weight gain, behavioural problems in children and rarely encephalopathy with increased frequency of seizures. Thrombocytopenia, impaired liver function and pancreatitis may also occur.

Ethosuccamide: (*Zarontin*) is the drug of choice for petit mal alone, at a dose of approximately 20 mg/kg in 24 hours. Once daily administration is satisfactory but this may cause gastro-intestinal side-effects and make it necessary to take in a divided dose. It is usual in practice to start with a dose of 500 mg daily in adults and older children, 250 mg in children under six, increasing at intervals of 7 days.

Reviewing long-term therapy

In providing continuity of care for the dozen or so patients on his list the practitioner has to cope with the good and bad consequences of past prescribing, face the challenge of reviewing his patients on long-term therapy, and identify those suffering from side-effects, polypharmacy or poor control, before attempting the perhaps hazardous course of simplifying or changing

treatment. The current edition of the improved British National Formulary will prove a help as will *The Adult Epileptic* (Taylor 1982) in *Long-term Prescribing* (Wilkes 0000). (It is important to refer to the Tables on drug interaction at the rear of the BNF.)

If after reviewing established patients on multiple therapy they are found to be well, seizure-free and free from appreciable side-effects they should be left alone unless they specifically wish to consider withdrawal of medication. If side-effects and/or seizures are present, consideration should be given to simplifying therapy but it must be borne in mind that there is a small risk of withdrawal seizures and for a smaller number, a danger of worsening their epilepsy. For the majority there is the likelihood of better control and reduced drug toxicity.

Confidence should be placed in the drug likely to be most effective ensuring that its dosage is such that its serum levels are in the optimum range before any other drugs are withdrawn. Reduction in dosage should involve one drug at a time and it is safer to take many weeks between individual dose changes and 2 to 3 months to withdraw a single drug.

Changing therapy

Where seizures are not controlled on one drug (85% are likely to be) the choice lies between adding a second drug and then either accepting polypharmacy or transferring to the second. Since there is evidence that having a second drug makes little if any difference there can be no objection to changing over completely. It is essential however that the first drug should not be withdrawn suddenly but gradually over many weeks and not until the new drug is providing serum levels in the optimum range. Stopping the first drug may lead to withdrawal seizures and the temptation to abandon withdrawal may be difficult to resist. Phenobarbitone is especially prone to cause these problems.

Whether starting or changing therapy, some understanding of pharmacology is required.

Essential basic pharmacological facts

Drug therapy is aimed at achieving and maintaining an effective concentration of the appropriate anticonvulsant in brain tissue whilst avoiding adverse effects. The concept of maintaining an effective concentration is most important since continuing seizures may be due to 'withdrawal seizures' associated with a sudden drop in drug levels, this is not the same as loss of control.

Anticonvulsant serum levels

Monitoring serum levels provides a useful check on compliance, unexpected toxicity on a small dose may be demonstrated to be due to a low rate of metabolism and poor control to be associated with low serum level despite standard dosage in high metabolisers, (this is especially true of phenytoin). There is nevertheless real danger that serum levels rather than the patient may be treated.

The so-called optimum serum levels are in fact merely a guide. In less severe epilepsy, 30% will be seizure-free on low dosage and low serum levels and in these circumstances it is not necessary to take a larger dose. Occasionally it is worthwhile pressing above the optimum range, as long as intolerable side-effects do not appear.

It is possible to have toxic levels in brain tissue with normal or low serum levels if serum levels are reduced by displacement of anticonvulsant from protein binding. This has important consequences when other drugs are taken with phenytoin which is 80% protein bound. The combination of sodium valproate with phenytoin, which is becoming increasingly common, may lead to a situation with low phenytoin serum levels but dangerously high brain levels, since valproate displaces phenytoin from protein binding. A way out is to do anticonvulsant assay of saliva.

Table 19.10 shows the main factors influencing blood serum levels.

Table 19.10 Factors determining serum anticonvulsant levels

Absorption
Distribution   — protein binding
Metabolism   — hepatic enzymes
Renal elimination

These all influence the plasma half-life and form a necessary guide to:
   Frequency of dosage
   Time to steady serum level
   Minimum intervals for dose adjustment
These factors may be influenced by:
   Age
   Disease
   or
   Drug interactions

Absorption

Abnormal drug absorption is not the source of many problems with preparations in use in the United Kingdom. Suspensions should be well shaken to ensure that the dose does not vary. Most important and not widely appreciated is the fact that intramuscular injections are *slowly* absorbed and therefore phenytoin, diazepam and phenobarbitone given *intamuscularly* are useless in *status epilepticus* which requires intravenous or rectal diazepam or intramuscular paraldehyde.

Metabolism

Anticonvulsants are removed from the plasma by liver metabolism to yield metabolites excreted by the kidneys; this varies considerably between individuals and shows up in the wide variation of dosage needed to produce comparable drug serum levels. This is especially true with phenytoin. A small increase in phenytoin dose within the 'therapeutic range' may lead to toxic serum levels; conversely, an equally dramatic fall in serum levels as a consequence of missed doses may lead to withdrawal seizures. The practical importance of this is that the dose of all anticonvulsant drugs should be gradually increased to gain seizure control but in the case of phenytoin the extra daily doses should be very small once near or within the so-called therapeutic range, 25 mg if within it (see above).

Drug interaction

Hepatic metabolism of drugs may be increased or inhibited and either may cause problems. Many of the anticonvulsants are powerful enzyme inducers capable of increasing the metabolism of other drugs and of each other. Phenytoin, primidone, phenobarbitone and carbamazepine are all enzyme inducers. On the other hand pheneturide (Benuride) and sulthiame (Ospolot) inhibit phenytoin metabolism and raise its serum levels.

Other drugs also interfere with anticonvulsants: isoniazid, prescribed for tuberculosis, and viloxazine, for depression, inhibit phenytoin as does the now commonly prescribed anti-ulcer drug cimetidine (Tagamet). Prescribing cimetidine may therefore lead to phenytoin toxicity. Therapeutic failures in the use of griseofulvin for fungal infections, tricyclic antidepressants and the oral contraceptive pill may be due to the effects of anticonvulsants on the liver.

The patient with epilepsy

Advice, guidance and drug treatment must be relevant to the patient's particular seizure disorder, life and circumstances, and may have to be adjusted as life moves on and circumstances change.

Compliance whether conforming to general advice about activities such as driving, swimming or continuing to take medication must be based on an understanding by the patient of the nature of the illness, the purpose of the medication, how it works, and what can cause it to fail and what problems this might create. It is helpful for the doctor to have a list of points which should be covered over a number of consultations depending upon their relevance at the time (Table 19.11).

Explaining about epilepsy and treatment
The helpful booklet by Laidlaw (1980) has already been referred to; in addition the British Epilepsy Association provides useful literature. Apart from the obvious points on the list it is helpful to explain epilepsy in terms of electrical activity. The localised burst causing partial attacks such as auras or more complicated partial seizures and funny behaviour which either occasionally, or for some people frequently, lead on to a generalised spread of activity which causes the major tonic clonic seizure.

It seems to be particularly helpful if the individual can be assisted to understand the nature of their own particular fits and by discussion to identify what might set them off: loss of sleep, tiredness, boredom, tension, menstruation, alcohol, TV or missed tablets. It is useful also to point out that the opposite may ward off seizures: activity, involvement, and regular rest.

Dealing with a fit
Although it is important that close relatives are told what to do by the doctor the patient needs to be able to explain to a wider circle of acquaintances. Useful pamphlets are available through the British Epilepsy Association, and support simple sensible advice about dealing with isolated seizures. It is important to emphasise the need to seek medical aid for repeated seizures in status epilepticus which should be regarded as a serious emergency.

Table 19.11   Points to be covered during consultation

Fits
What causes fits?   What happens?
What causes *your* fits?
What sets them off?
Avoiding fits
Dealing with fits
— Single
— Status epilepticus
Rest
Work
Recreation
Alcohol
Driving — the law
Marriage — Oral contraception
Children
— Danger of inheriting
— Teratogenic effects

Drugs
How they work
Your drugs
How to take them so that they work

Marriage and children
Most of the other points in Table 19.11 are self-explanatory, some more important than others and some assume greater importance as life goes on; the choice of oral contraceptive and decisions about having children. With regard to pregnancy two main issues arise, the risk of having children who will develop epilepsy and the risk to the developing fetus of maternal drug treatment. The risk of epilepsy in a child is approximately 1 in 30 if one parent is affected and this risk of course does not apply if the epilepsy is due to acquired disease, such as trauma. If both parents have epilepsy or if there is a strong family history the risks are considerably greater and genetic counselling may be needed to establish the exact risk. The risk of fetal abnormalities is slightly increased in a mother with epilepsy, and drug therapy itself is associated with congenital abnormalities such as hair-lip, cleft palate or heart defects. The risk, however, is small, it is more likely with phenytoin and phenobarbitone but because of polypharmacy there is uncertainty and any drug is suspect.

As a general rule the risk of seizures should guide decisions about therapy and the decision to withdraw anticonvulsants is probably unwise once pregnancy has started.

Treatment of status epileptics
Repeated partial seizures are not such an urgent matter but repeated tonic clonic seizures lasting for *longer than 10 minutes* have a substantial mortality rate and may lead to further neurological damage in survivors. Sometimes this is not clear to relatives, or their doctors, who may have become confident in the capacity of relatives to cope with seizures.

Treatment in adults is by intravenous diazepam in a dose of 5–10 mg or clonazepam 1 mg, given over 2 to 3 minutes and repeated if necessary after 30 to 60 minutes. There is a risk of apnoea, which is greater in children, and ideally means of resuscitation should be available. An alternative is intramuscular paraldehyde 8–10 ml but this takes 30 minutes to act. If it is difficult to get into a vein, particularly in children, rectal diazepam maybe given in a dose of 0.5 mg/kg. The risk of apnoea is said to be less and it is effective; parents may safely be supplied with plastic syringes — not needles — and ampoules of diazepam if they have children prone to febrile convulsions.

Seizures in childhood and convulsions associated with fever
Full descriptions of the many seizure disorders of childhood and their management are well described elsewhere (Laidlaw 1976, Robinson 1980, Hoskin 1981).

The commonest seizures in childhood are those associated with fever. These occur between the age of 6 months and 5 years and since there is evidence that repeated or prolonged febrile convulsions are associated with subsequent development of temporal lobe epilepsy it is important to treat attacks effectively. Parents should be well instructed in measures to reduce body temperature during infections, using paracetamol or aspirin and reduction of body temperature by tepid sponging. It is important to stress that it is necessary to undress the child fully, otherwise the forehead may be dabbed whilst the rest of the child is cocooned. Rectal diazepam or intramuscular paraldehyde may be given by parents at the onset of the attack and it may be preferable to treat attacks in this way as an alternative to prophylaxis with anticonvulsants. Unfortunately the most effective drug in this regard, phenobarbitone, is associated with behaviour problems in many children. If the rectal temperature rises above 36.5°C, sponging, particularly including the head, should continue for half-an-hour, possibly in a tepid bath. (Ice-cold water should not be used as it causes peripheral constriction and the body core retains its heat.)

Psychomotor or temporal lobe attacks and petit mal with or without associated tonic clonic seizures may develop later in childhood. Differentiating them and treating them follows the same lines as for adults and have been described earlier.

Admission to hospital is indicated for an initial seizure with fever because of the risk of undiagnosed meningitis, and also for any subsequent seizure which lasts longer than 10 minutes.

Stopping therapy

After many years seizure-free it may be reasonable to consider withdrawing anticonvulsants. The decision can be difficult and weighing benefits and risks is a matter for individual decision. The following points should be borne in mind: two out of three children with epilepsy in childhood become seizure-free and adults on anticonvulsants who have been seizure-free since childhood may reasonably consider withdrawal. The likelihood of relapse as might be expected is related to the extent and siting of any organic focal lesion. Consequently very abnormal EEG's, a history of very frequent seizures in the past, difficulty in control, evidence of brain damage or a history of non-febrile seizures at an early age are all factors associated with the likelihood of relapse.

It is current practice to attempt withdrawal after 2 to 3 seizure-free years in patients who have had occasional seizures. About 30% of this group will relapse after 2 years. As in changing or simplifying therapy, withdrawal should be very slow over several months with one drug at a time, leaving the most potent until last.

PARKINSON'S DISEASE

The onset is usually in the fifth or sixth decade, with a prevalence of 1 or 2 per 1000 rising to 5 per 1000 in the over 50's. Each general practitioner will have only one or two patients disabled with this condition.

The problems

Diagnostic difficulties
Early symptoms are often unrecognised especially if tremor is not marked.

Treatment difficulties
The advent of levodopa has radically changed management. Although all do not benefit equally, the effects on some in the short term have been dramatic. In the long term complications and varying difficulties occur both from the developing disease and the treatment; not surprisingly general practitioners with few patients are likely to be unaware of the variety of problems and side-effects and possible ways of avoiding or surmounting some of them.

Diagnosis

There is no diagnostic laboratory test and diagnosis rests on clinical judgement. The important signs are tremor, rigidity and bradykinesia.

Early symptoms

Early symptoms include:

— Painful limb and trunk muscles
— Nocturnal spasms and cramps
— Fatigue and difficulty coping with skilled tasks, e.g. writing or cleaning

The fully established clinical picture with mask-like face, poverty of expression, slow response, flexed posture and pill rolling is striking and easily recognised. Early clues include impairment of arm swinging and enhancement of latent rigidity and cog-wheeling by vigorous voluntary movement of the *other* limb. An associated depression is common and well known but hallucinations may also occur in the untreated disease and may be provoked by almost any of the medications used.

The patient needs an adequate explanation of his condition and simple concepts about the cause of the disease, how it progresses and how treatment works are helpful for patients and relatives. Guidelines used by the authors include:

Cause
Cells in parts of the brain (brain stem) concerned with movement control are not working, their job is to produce a chemical messenger (dopamine) which is necessary for messages to pass between special nerve connections. Lack of dopamine causes the symptoms. Similar symptoms may be produced by some drugs: reserpine

produces them by depleting dopamine and phenothiazines by blocking dopamine receptors.

Progress

The disease is progressive and there is no cure, although severity varies: fortunately treatment which makes up for the missing dopamine may relieve many of the symptoms and allow a normal life span. (Prior to modern treatment, two-thirds would deteriorate remorselessly and a quarter would die from a chest infection within 5 years.)

Treatment

The missing dopamine can be made up for in two ways:

1. Reducing the effect of another chemical (acetylcholine) which normally balances the effects of dopamine. These anticholinergic drugs help modestly with tremor, drooling and muscle stiffness but have the well-known side-effects of dry mouth, blurring of vision, increased constipation, and have a danger of precipitating glaucoma or prostatic obstruction. (Confusion and hallucinations which sometimes occur may be reversed by 0.5 mg of physostigmine subcutaneously.)

2. Providing extra dopamine or stimulating dopamine receptors with other drugs. Amantadine possibly works by freeing dopamine but does not often help for more than a few weeks. Bromocriptine stimulates dopaminergic receptors and has similar side-effects to levodopa.

Levodopa is converted into dopamine in the body: the latter has many side-effects especially peripherally but these can be overcome by giving at the same time a peripheral decarboxylase inhibitor; this works by preventing the breakdown of levodopa in the body but not in the brain. The two combinations used in this country are Sinemet and Medopar.

Levodopa side-effects include hallucinations and nausea, which may be limited by slow introduction of the drug or by giving metoclopramide, and postural hypotension.

With prolonged usage increased involuntary movements, associated with a high dose, become more frequent. After 2 to 3 years the effects may wear off after an hour where they previously lasted 4 to 5 hours. Sudden freezing may occur alternating with the involuntary movements.

Some of these problems may be overcome by smaller, more frequent dosage of levodopa combinations, or reduction in dose with the addition of bromocriptine.

Deciding upon treatment

The problems with long-term levodopa therapy despite the early honeymoon period, have led to some opinions favouring withholding levodopa and relying upon anticholinergics as long as possible. Where handicap is not severe and symptoms mainly consist of temor or stiffness

this is reasonable. The authors believe that the patient should be able to choose: honeymoon with possible relapse and problems, or more limited initial improvement but with the likelihood of a longer help from treatment.

A good current resume of therapy is given by Stern G (1982) in *Medical Treatment of Parkinsonism*, Prescribers Journal, February 1982, Vol. 22: No. 1.

MULTIPLE SCLEROSIS

This is the commonest chronic disabling condition of young people in the British Isles. However, the average general practitioner will only have two or three people on his list with this diagnosis. It was first described as a separate disease in 1868 by the great French neurologist Charcot (1872), though what he wrote then could hardly be altered except by speculation if it were written today. Theories about causation, treatment and management are legion and as such illustrate the paucity of hard facts available. The youth of many sufferers brings to mind the large social implications of the problem, i.e. wage earners, mothers, dependent children. It is this aspect which is often the most distressing feature of management.

EPIDEMIOLOGY

The two most commonly used statistics are incidence and prevalence of a disease. The former is the number of new cases in a population in a given time and the latter the number of cases present at a set moment. Where multiple sclerosis is concerned these figures are at best good approximations (Kurtzke 1977); incidence 1–2/100 000 and prevalence 50/100 000. These figures are for the UK and within it there are wide variations, the most striking being dependent on latitude. On the south coast 25/100 000 is usually an accepted figure whereas in the Orkneys and Shetlands quotations in excess of 100/100 000 (the highest in the world) are made. Certainly latitude seems important but there are notable exceptions: Japan although in the same latitude as the British Isles has a very low figure but when it occurs it is apparently a more severe disease. As a general rule the latitude idea holds true, similar levels being found in Western Europe, British Isles and America (Northern hemisphere), while comparable figures are found in Australia and New Zealand (Southern hemisphere). There are in addition some areas of high local levels which have led to speculation that common environmental factors are at work; detailed studies have failed to reveal them.

Presentation

Multiple sclerosis is a disease of the central nervous

system and as a result possible symptoms are many. However, there are some modes of presentation more commonly seen than others (Table 19.12).

The initial symptoms rapidly resolve almost without exception and since they are frequently similar to symptoms which have a 'neurotic' rather than a neurological basis it is encumbent on the good general practitioner to distinguish accurately between them. Failure to do so may lead to excessive and unnecessary anxieties.

Course and prognosis

One of the most striking features of multiple sclerosis is the very wide variation which may be seen in any group of patients, ranging from a rapidly disabling condition leading to the death of a patient in 5 years, to a few symptomless plaques discovered at post mortem in old age following death from a totally unrelated cause. The vast majority of sufferers naturally lie between these two extremes. What will be described is a fairly average pattern and readers should bear in mind that almost any other sequence of events is possible. The initial symptoms usually resolve completely and the true diagnosis may not even be suspected. The patient then remains well for several months or even years — in remission. New symptoms then appear and on this occasion do not entirely resolve — relapse.

This sequence of relapses and remissions continues every 6 to 12 months for 3 to 5 years. A stage is then reached when the patient is partly disabled, with weakness of legs and a poor gait often with frequency and urgency of micturition; but life is tolerable. There then follows about 7 to 10 years of relative stability until a major relapse occurs from which there is little or no recovery. Progress is then steadily downhill leading to death from kidney or respiratory failure or intercurrent infection. The life span for this sequence is 20 to 25 years (McAlpine 1972). Once again it must be emphasised that this is a generalisation. 5% of patients will die inside the first 5 years, conversely, if there is very little disability after 5 years, then the outlook is good. After 10 years, one-third have little or no disability. After 15 years, one-quarter have little or no disability. After 20 years, the figure is one in five.

Table 19.12 The percentage frequencies for types of neurological deficit in the onset bout

Pyramidal	45
Cerebellar	44
Brainstem	47
Sensory	42
Optic signs	24
Bowel/bladder	8
Cerebral — total	9
Cerebral — mentation	2
Other	8

Aetiology

Despite many years of intensive research, no single cause has been demonstrated. There is clearly a genetic factor — 7/1000 in close relatives against 1–2/1000 in the general population. There is a fairly well defined age distribution and also the previously mentioned latitude effect. Individually these are all seen in other diseases, but together they form a unique combination which has to be explained in any final description of the disease.

High on the list of suspects are:

1. Slow viruses (Norrby 1974), especially the measles virus.

2. Autoimmunity (Myers 1975) possibly to myelin, which is inherently abnormal in multiple sclerosis sufferers.

3. Errors in metabolism of fatty acids (Crawford 1979, Miller 1973).

Recently another possibility has been put forward:

4. Chronic fat embolism (James 1982, Neubauer 1980) which is being investigated at the present time.

Causes of relapse are rather less controversial, though any sufferer will tell stories of a relapse which followed an identified event. Viral infections and stress (physical or emotional) are of great importance and ought to be avoided if possible. Unfortunately, it is very easy after a relapse to look back and see something to blame, usually in error.

Role of the general practitioner

There are two areas where the general practitioner has an important role to play. The first is in diagnosis (Field 1977): not so much in making the initial diagnosis, but in identifying relapses for what they are and taking appropriate action. The second role is a supportive one both for the patient and relatives.

Diagnosis

It is important to remember that multiple sclerosis is a disease of relapse and remission, only 10% of patients never have this episodic pattern to their illness, but have a relentlessly progressive disease. In the usual form the neurologist will clearly be required. The one single factor of multiple sclerosis that is regarded by many of paramount importance in order to make a diagnosis is the relapsing nature of the disease. This means that many people do not get an answer to the question 'What have I got, doctor?' until they are in their first relapse, by which time they may have reached a point of less than full recovery. In the initial attack one must exclude other disorders and therefore blood, CSF, radiology and CT scans are important. Unfortunately very few will have any changes in these parameters. Field (1974) has developed a test which shows promise of being specific though it is not yet widely accepted. It depends on the mobility of the RBC's in an electrophoretic field. The changes from normal are small and this limits its usefulness in the general laboratory. Subsequent relapses should be recognised for what they are and treatment with ACTH (Rose 1969) started immediately. If a community physiotherapist is available she should be involved at this early stage. There is no evidence that this aggressive policy has any long-term advantage, but the patient is up and about again a lot faster than if a laissez faire policy is followed. The range of symptoms is great and we are grateful to those neurologists such as McAlpine (1972) who have followed their patients for many years. Table 19.13 gives his analysis of symptoms occurring singly or in combination.

It is clear that medicine has little to offer the average patient. They can however do much for themselves. Patients should be encouraged to join a self help group such as the Multiple Sclerosis Society or ARMS (Action for Research into Multiple Sclerosis). Such groups offer contact with other people with multiple sclerosis together with positive advice and encouragement. There are two books that are useful for the sufferer and also of value to the busy general practitioner, (neither are long and both are easy to read), *Multiple Sclerosis — a self help guide to its management* by Judy Graham (published by Thorsons) and *Multiple Sclerosis — The Facts* by Bryan Matthews (published by Oxford University Press).

DISCUSSIONS WITH PATIENTS

What does one tell the patient, if anything? The authors are very much in favour of the truth. The problem is how to tell it without appearing callous. Another important problem is the lack of any firm diagnosis, especially in the early stage of the illness. Few specialists will say after an initial attack, 'This is multiple sclerosis'. Even of those who do, 25% will change that opinion by the end of 4 years. So again, what does one say? Evidence is increasing to show that early attention to a healthy diet, good general fitness, avoidance of fatigue and a positive approach to the problem can slow down the rate of deterioration. Judy Graham illustrates this well in her book on self-help management.

For a long time it has been said with confidence by textbooks of neurology that multiple sclerosis is a primary de-myelinating disease of the central nervous system. This fails to recognise or attempt any explanaation of the fact that damage to axons in the peripheral nervous system has been described many times. It also makes no effort to explain why most sufferers have problems related to the autonomic nervous system which is non-myelinated — in bladder and bowel control. Cross-sections of the spinal cord show that damage appears to be fairly evenly spread between both grey and white matter, so clearly the story is not as simple as it might appear.

The easiest way of explaining the problem to the patient is to liken a nerve fibre to an electric wire which has to be insulated in order to carry a current without discharging to earth, comparing the myelin sheath to the insulating coat on the wire. Simple diagrams drawn at the desk in front of the patient are very valuable. Explanations of all sorts of illnesses are retained much better by their recipient if there is a visual record that they can refer to later. Studies have also shown that information given in the surgery is better understood and remembered if accompanied by some form of simple documentation.

The established patient is a different prospect. He or she usually knows the diagnosis and fears that every new symptom heralds a relapse; a view that has to be discouraged, but in its place the patient must be helped to recognise a relapse when it does occur. This may be the appearance of new symptoms and signs or sudden worsening of existing ones. It is always good advice to wait a few days because things may improve spontaneously and often do so without active intervention. If the symptom does not, a course of intra-muscular injections of ACTH in a dose of 80 units/day for 5 days should be given, slowly reducing the dose so that the whole course runs 13–14 days. Where the relapse is largely of physical capabilities an experienced physiotherapist can provide great help, keeping in mind that the object is to maintain normal function — not to produce a champion athlete. A slow deterioration rarely improves with this regime and any active treatment has little to offer in this sad situation.

THE LONG SUFFERING NEW PATIENT

New patients appear from time to time with this problem and almost without exception will be taking a whole host of drugs, many of which will not be needed. Some may be suffering from past enthusiasms, such as tenotomies to stop muscle spasm, so they cannot produce that movement now even though they have not had spasms for years. Multiple sclerosis sufferers have many anxieties, and depression is a common problem which requires specific treatment, but many will be on long-term benzo-

Table 19.13   Incidence of initial symptoms

Motor weakness	40%
Optic neuritis	22%
Paraesthesiae	21%
Double vision	12%
Vertigo/vomiting	5%
Disturbance of micturition	5%
Other types (hemiplegia, trigeminal neuralgia, facial palsy, deafness)	below 5%

diazepines without any real justification. Is diazepam really a good muscle relaxant? Certainly not long-term.

In recent years new drugs such as baclofen have appeared which do reduce spasticity; they have a place in the management of multiple sclerosis but great care has to be exercised since for some people the spasticity may be all that keeps them on their feet! A change from spasticity to flaccidity is not recommended.

Another enthusiasm from the past is the monthly injection of vitamin B_{12} — a useless treatment but one to which many older patients cling with great avidity. The message therefore is 'take care' since many people will be happier with your active interest than with your inappropriate prescription.

Help for the disabled

Chronic disability is not confined to multiple sclerosis and many of the problems can be seen in relation to a wide range of pathologies. A recent study of disability gave the breakdown in Table 19.14.

Existing criteria are based largely on patients who are already in care or for whom some type of residential placement is being contemplated. These assessments are often of little value to the patient or his supporters planning an independent lifestyle. People can often be helped a great deal by a sympathetic look at the home and the organisation of any adjustments that may be necessary. The Social Service Department may need to be cajoled into action, helping with ramps, stair lifts, hand rails or bathroom adaptations. In the latter case an imaginative appreciation of the problem can be most helpful; stereotyped alterations are sometimes no better than the original.

It is also important that the problems is not forgotten once the work has been done. Handicaps, particularly of a neurological nature are rarely static and reassessment at, for example, annual intervals could anticipate difficulties before they become problems. It should not be overlooked that handicapped people may be reluctant to discuss their problems and need to be encouraged to make their needs known at an early stage; the wheels of bureaucracy turn slowly, and a kick in the right place at the right time can work wonders.

Table 19.14 Claimants for mobility allowance. Diagnosis by body system (Robertson GM, RCGP July 1982)

System	Cases	Percentage
Central nervous	193	40.6
Locomotor	174	36.6
Cardiovascular	50	10.3
Respiratory	30	6.3
Malignancies	9	1.9
Amputations	6	1.3
Endocrine	8	1.7
Blood and blood forming organs	2	0.4

REFERENCES

British National Formulary 1982 No. 4. British Medical Association and Pharmaceutical Society of Great Britain.

Charcot J M 1872 Maladies du systeme nerveux, 1; de la sclerose en plaques disseminee. Anat. Pathol. Delahaye, Paris

Crawford M A, Budowski P, Hassam A G 1979 Dietary management in multiple sclerosis. Proceedings of the Nutrition Society 38: 373

Field E J 1977 Multiple sclerosis. A critical conspectus. MIP Press Ltd., Lancaster

Field E J, Shenton B K, Joyce G 1974 Specific laboratory test for multiple sclerosis. British Medical Journal 1: 412

Fry J 1979 Common diseases, 2nd edn. MIP Press Ltd, Lancaster

Godwin-Austen R B 1979 Parkinson's Disease, 6th edn. Parkinson's Disease Society, London

Hart J T 1980 Hypotension. Library of General Practice Vol. 1 Churchill Livingstone, Edinburgh

Harwood G 1982 The GP and the specialist neurology. British Medical Journal 1170

Honig P J, Charney E B 1982 Children with brain tumour headaches — distinguishing features. American Journal of Diseases of Children 136: 121–5

Hosking G 1982 Children with neurological disorders. In: Wilkes E (ed) Long-term prescribing. Faber and Faber, London

James P B 1982 Evidence for subacute fat embolism as the cause of multiple sclerosis. Lancet, February

Jeavons P M 1975 The practical management of epilepsy. Update 10: 269–280

Kurtzke J F 1977 Multiple sclerosis from an epidemiological viewpoint. In: Field E J (ed) Multiple sclerosis — a critical conspectus. MTP Press Ltd, Lancaster

Laidlaw M V, Laidlaw J 1980 Epilepsy explained. Churchill Livingstone, Edinburgh

Laidlaw J, Richens A (eds) 1982 A textbook of epilepsy, 2nd edn. Churchill Livingstone, Edinburgh

McAlpine D, Lumsden C E, Acheson E D 1972 Multiple sclerosis — a re-appraisal, 2nd edn. Churchill Livingstone, Edinburgh

Matthews W B 1975 Practical neurology, 3rd edn. Blackwell Scientific Publications, London

Medical Association and Pharmaceutical Society of Great Britain Medicine 3rd Series 1978 pps. 31, 32, 33, 34 Parts 1–4. Medical Education (International) Ltd., Oxford

Millar J H D et al 1973 British Medical Journal 1:765

Myers L W et al 1975 Cell-mediated immunity to isolated oligodendroglia in multiple sclerosis. Archives of Neurology 32: 354

Neubauer R A 1980 Exposure of multiple sclerosis patients to hyperbaric oxygen at 1.5–2 ATA. A preliminary report. Journal of the Florida Medical Association

Norrby E et al 1974 Comparison of antibodies against viruses in CSF and serum samples from patients with multiple sclerosis. Infectious Immunology 10: 688

Ramsey L E 1982 Hypertension. In: Wilkes E (ed) Long-term prescribing. Faber & Faber, London

RCGP/OPCS 1974 Studies on Medical and Population Subjects No. 26 — Morbidity Statistics from General Practice, 2nd National Study 1970–71. HMSO, London

Reynolds E H 1978 Drug treatment of epilepsy. Lancet 2: 721–725

Robinson R 1978 Seizure disorders in childhood. Medicine 3rd Series: 32 pp 1624–1630. Medical Education (International) Ltd, Oxford

Rose S A et al 1969 Co-operative study in the evaluation of therapy in multiple sclerosis. ACTH vs. placebo in acute exacerbations. Transactions of the American Neurological Association 94: 126

Shorvon S D, Chadwick D, Galbraith A W, Reynolds E H 1978 One drug for epilepsy. British Medical Journal 474

Shorvon S D, Reynolds E H 1979 Reduction in polypharmacy for epilepsy. British Medical Journal 2: 1023–1025

Taylor W P 1982 The adult epileptic. In: Wilkes E (ed) Long-term prescribing. Faber & Faber, London, p 65–79

Waters H J, Perlion J M 1982 Study of stroke patients in a single general practice. British Medical Journal 284: 791

Wilkes E (ed) Long-term prescribing. Faber & Faber, London

Wilkinson M 1980 Migraine and other headaches. British Medical Association, London

General practice dermatology

INTRODUCTION

Senior medical students, trainee general practitioners and many general practice principals confess considerable ignorance of the diagnosis and management of skin disorders. The blame for this lies equally with University curriculum committees, which are heavily biased in favour of general medicine and surgery, and with dermatologists whose teaching is usually based on patients at the hospital end of the disease spectrum. A further difficulty is that the hospital environment aids efficacy and compliance, so that treatments used in hospital may be less effective or even inappropriate for patients who are treated in the community. That some general practitioners are competent in the diagnosis and treatment of skin disorders owes as much to learning in their early days by trial and error as it does to reading or postgraduate courses.

This chapter is an introduction to the diagnosis and management of skin disorders in the environment of general practice. It is an attempt to clarify the maze of descriptive terms, to improve on the 'best bet' diagnosis and to suggest a rational approach to the growing number of topical treatments that are available.

CLASSIFICATION OF SKIN DISEASE

Some framework is essential to learning about skin disorders and is helpful in their recognition and management. Traditionally, classification of skin disease has been on a morphological or regional basis: this is a method that is logical for lectures and articles in journals, but does not help one to learn about the overall pattern of skin disorders. In this chapter a pathological classification of skin disorders will be used (Table 20.1). This approach may not satisfy the specialist and it is a less precise system of classification in that some disorders are not due to a single cause, for example atopic patients are more likely to develop allergies, and chemical irritation of the skin predisposes to a true allergic sensitisation.

The three main divisions of skin disorders are congential, constitutional and acquired.

Congenital disorders are due either to defective skin formation or to abnormal collections of cutaneous elements. These are present at birth, but may not manifest themselves immediately.

Constitutional disorders are the result of an inherited predisposition and will manifest themselves at some time in the patient's life.

Acquired disorders do not usually require any predisposition and any patient may develop these diseases.

The word 'eczema' is used when there is no obvious cause, that is, when the condition has a constitutional basis. The term 'dermatitis' is used when the cause is known. This distinction must be explained to the patient since dermatitis can often imply fault or neglect on the part of an employer.

PREVALENCE OF SKIN DISORDERS IN GENERAL PRACTICE

In 1980, the author conducted a 6-month survey of the skin conditions for which he was consulted. In the latter part of this chapter the figure in brackets after the dis-

Table 20.1   Classification of skin disease

Congenital
1. Naevi (birth marks)
2. Ichthyosis
3. Rare conditions

Constitutional
1. Eczemas
2. Psoriasis

Acquired
1. Infections, infestations and insect bites
2. Physical and chemical damage
3. Allergy
4. Endocrine related
5. Vascular
6. Degeneration
7. Neoplastic
8. Autoimmune
9. Unknown

order indicates the frequency of the condition as a percentage of the total number of skin consultations in that survey. It is accepted that the results of surveys of this type cannot always be applied elsewhere because of variations in social class, local types of employment, and racial differences in the frequency of certain disorders together with the doctor's particular interest in certain diseases or age groups. However, it represents the results of fairly accurate diagnoses made in a general practice composed mainly of patients in social classes 3 and 4. One interesting finding was that endocrine related conditions (acne, rosacea and peri-oral dermatitis), skin infections, constitutional eczemas and psoriasis accounted for 73% of the skin disease consultations. A good knowledge of the diagnosis and management of these conditions gives any general practitioner a firm foundation in general practice dermatology.

THE MANAGEMENT OF SKIN DISORDERS IN GENERAL PRACTICE

The first step in management is the recognition of the skin disorder. An adequate history is important in coming to a diagnosis and to elicit causative factors, such as tonsillitis in guttate psoriasis or cleansers in irritant dermatitis. The diagnosis may be based on a judgement of its likelihood — for example, from a family history — or from the expected frequency of various disorders from personal experience or that of others. Most doctors have a good pictorial memory and remembering the appearance of conditions in previous patients in whom the diagnosis was known or visualising coloured photographs from textbooks, journals or lectures can aid the diagnosis. The use of photographs in a well illustrated textbook of dermatology, for example Levene's *A Colour Atlas of Dermatology* or Fry's *Dermatology*, will be helpful when reading the description of skin disorders in this chapter. With experience, 'spot diagnoses' of conditions such as acne, psoriasis and pityriasis rosea become easier. A major difficulty is that the general practitioner may see the very early signs of an eruption at a stage when a firm diagnosis is impossible. In this situation the extended consultation can be of value.

The second step in management is to identify the *cause* of the eruption and, where possible, to explain it to the patient. If a cause can be found then the third step is to give advice on *prevention*. These three steps should be completed before prescribing the appropriate *treatment*, which is the last step.

THE TREATMENT OF SKIN DISORDERS IN GENERAL PRACTICE

Treatment should not be empirical, apart from the use of the traditional lotion on an acute eruption or an ointment on a scaly eruption. As far as possible, the treatment should be specific — topical antibiotics antibiotics for impetigo, systemic antibiotics for severe acne, or topical steroids for eczema. Topical steroids are discussed later in this chapter but care should be taken that their use is appropriate to the site and severity of the eruption and to the age of the patient.

MANAGEMENT OF SPECIFIC SKIN DISORDERS

CONGENITAL CONDITIONS

Naevi or birth marks (0.3%)
These are an important although infrequent reason for a consultation since they persist throughout life and can be a cause of distress and concern to parents.

Strawberry angioma (0.14%)
These appear soon after birth, enlarge for about 1 year and regress slowly over 3 to 5 years. They may bleed readily, but this can be controlled by direct pressure. Trauma from plastic pants may induce the earlier regression of a lesion in the napkin area and the use of a topical fluorinated steroid may speed involution. Redundant tissue may require the attention of a plastic surgeon once involution is complete.

Capillary angioma
May be helped in later life by tattoing or by camouflage make-up.

Warty naevi
A life-long blemish usually having a curious linear, rather than dermatome pattern. Dermabrasion can help, but it may have to be used repeatedly.

Moles (0.14%)
These are so common that patients seldom mention them. However, they can cause considerable distress to young adult females and excision by a plastic surgeon should be considered. Any change in the size or appearance of a mole is a cause for concern, if not for a second opinion.

Ichthyosis
Ichthyosis is seldom present at birth. It presents in childhood as dry skin or as scaling skin in adults. There are different varieties and some clear up at puberty. They are an indication for emollients (such as emulsifying ointment, lanolin and vaseline in equal parts, Oilatum emollient), but not for topical steroids unless there is a secondary eczema from scratching. Ichthyosis should not be confused with follicular plugging which produces a roughness of the extensor surface of the thighs and upper

arms. This responds to firm scrubbing at the end of a bath, possibly after the prior application of 3% salicylic acid in soft paraffin for 12 hours.

Rare conditions

Medical curiosities usually only seen in hospital practice. One 'collodion baby' and one case of epidermolysis bullosa simplex have been countered in 18 years in a practice averaging 10 500 patients.

CONSTITUTIONAL CONDITIONS (30%)

Eczemas (20%)

The word 'eczema' is derived from the Greek and literally means to 'boil out', indicating the resemblance of the typical vesicles of eczema to bubbles rising in boiling water. If present, these bubbles confirm the diagnosis of eczema (dermatitis), but the term is extended to many forms of erythema and slight scaling. An alternative working definition is: 'if it looks like eczema, it is eczema!' This definition commends itself as personal experience grows.

Atopic eczema (5.8%)

This condition is allied to asthma and hay fever and there is often a family history of one or other of these two complaints or of eczema itself. There is some abnormality of the immune mechanism manifesting itself in multiple positive responses on skin prick testing and on RAST testing. Sufferers from this disorder have, on average, a higher level of IgE than the normal population. The condition may start at any age, but most commonly in infancy when it presents on the face or trunk. Exacerbations are commonly associated with teething, but teething proceeds from 6 to 24 months and it is too simple to regard each exacerbation as a manifestation of teething. After teething is completed, exacerbations may well continue and there are no controlled observations to indicate a direct link. After the early manifestation on the face and trunk, the eruption spreads to involve the limbs, especially the wrists, fingers and the posterior hip flexure in toddlers. The eruption waxes and wanes and 75% of these infants will be free of their disorder by the age of 5 years. If the disease continues beyond 2 or 3 years, it may predominate in the antecubital and popliteal fossae while continuing on the face, body and extremities. The typical antecubital and popliteal distribution, without lesions elsewhere, is not usual until the late childhood or teenage period. Those unfortunate to have the disease into adult life are more likely to have lesions on the face and the extensor surfaces of the limbs than on the flexures.

Infants aged between 2 and 6 months are predisposed to eczema on the face, neck and upper chest. Commonly, this only lasts a month or two and *atopic* eczema should not be diagnosed before the infant is 6 months old. It is best to consider these infants as suffering from *infantile* eczema (1.4%) although infants who have eczema for only a short period during infancy may be part of the spectrum of atopic eczema.

Atopic eczema may become secondarily infected by bacteria or rarely, by herpes simplex virus and the practitioner must be alert for this possibility. Exacerbations on the face shortly after respiratory infections usually indicate viral super infection. Toddlers and older children with severe, crusted, flexural exacerbations should be considered to have secondary bacterial infection. Both infections are associated with excessive crusting and herpes simplex infection causes a 'burning' discomfort. Bacterial super-infection should be treated with topical or systemic antibiotics as for impetigo, depending on the location and the degree of constitutional upset (see p. 250); herpes simplex infection responds to topical idoxuridine (see p. 251). If there is no super-infection, atopic eczema should be treated according to the principles outlined in the section of this chapter devoted to the use of topical steroids.

Idiopathic foot eczema of infancy (0.72%)

This appears to be a localised variant of atopic eczema: there seems to be an increased incidence of atopy in close relatives. However, it first appears at a later age, usually between 5 and 8 years, and regresses at puberty. It affects the flexor surface of both feet, usually the distal third including the toes, but may affect the heels. It has a shining, erythematous appearance with scaling and fissuring. A similar eruption may occur at the same time on the thumb and index finger although this eruption on the fingers usually affects young adults in whom the feet are not affected. Normally the eruption is symptomless, becoming 'burning' when there is marked erythema and painful when fissures develop. Tinea infections rarely occur in children and present in the flexures of the lateral toes rather than on the pads of the medial toes. Allergy to shoe materials affects the thinner skin on the extensor surface; maceration of the skin of the sole of the feet presents as a matt, soggy surface on the contact areas of the soles of the feet in teenagers and young adults.

Idiopathic foot eczema waxes and wanes like atopic eczema and is usually worse in winter. Ventilated footwear, such as sandals, should be worn when reasonable and natural-fibre socks sometimes help. Fluorinated steroid ointments are required when the eruption is acute and the following application:

Salicyclic acid ointment	
Starch glycerine	} of each 50 g
Soft paraffin	

should be applied at night when the eruption is milder,

preferably after steeping the feet in water for 15–20 minutes.

Pompholyx (2.5%)

This affects the palms and palmar surface of the fingers and the flexor surface of the insteps of the feet and toes. This is a post-pubertal form of constitutional eczema and the typical vesicles of eczema are usually obvious on the palms or fingers. The vesicles are 1–3 mm in diameter and usually skin coloured, unlike the larger (3–5 mm) yellow pustules of palmar and plantar psoriasis. An older generation of dermatologists equated pompholyx with tinea infection of the palms and soles. In this latter eruption vesicles are absent and fine scaling is the most obvious feature. Examination of scrapings at the Regional Mycology Laboratory will confirm or refute the diagnosis. The affected extremities are 'burning' or intensely itchy and made worse by irritants such as detergents. Irritant or allergic dermatitis affects the thinner skin of the extensor surfaces of the extremities and it is unusual to find definite vesicles. Sweating from excessive heat or nervous tension exacerbates pompholyx.

The management of pompholyx is difficult in general practice. Ideally, the patient should be put to rest and wrapped gently in cotton wool. In practice, the patient should be advised to avoid all irritants and excessive sweating. If protective gloves are worn, for example for housework, these should be removed immediately after wet work is completed. A topical fluorinated steroid is required for this eruption and should be applied night and morning, and after the hands have been in water. Acute or prolonged eruptions require clobetasol propionate. Like the other forms of eczema pompholyx shows relapses and remissions with eventual total remission. It may be accompanied by eczema on the limbs and trunk.

Discoid eczema (0.4%)

This is an uncommon eruption affecting limbs and trunk. As the name implies, it is a discoid area of eczema 1.5–3 cm in diameter. There is not usually as much scaling as is present in psoriasis and the edge is not raised as it is in ringworm infections. The presence of a domestic pet, especially a kitten, will suggest, and laboratory examination of scrapings will confirm, ringworm infection.

The lesions of granuloma annulare are usually solitary and have a characteristic purplish appearance with an annular series of small domes completing the circle. These are symptomless. The 'herald patch' of pityriasis rosea will be followed by the typical eruption within 14 days and fixed drug eruptions, from substances such as phenolphthalein, can be excluded in the routine history.

Like other constitutional eczemas, discoid eczema comes and goes and eventually remission is complete. Its course usually runs in months rather than in years. Dilute topical fluorinated steroids are required to control it.

Seborrhoeic eczema of adults (1.7%)

Seborrhoeic eczema typically occurs on the scalp, behind the ears and centrally on the front and back of the chest. Uncommonly, it appears in the axillae and groins. On the scalp and behind the ears, the striking feature is scaling on an erythematous base, and erythema with some scaling are the features of the other sites. Acne of the face and seborrhoeic eczema of the scalp and chest commonly occur together in adults. Psoriasis of the scalp is usually 'lumpy' and evidence of psoriasis elsewhere should be sought. Seborrhoeic eczema of infancy is a hallowed diagnosis. It is probably a misnomer and psoriasiform napkin eruption or flexural infantile eczema are more appropriate since both these descriptive labels have prognostic significance (Neville & Finn 1975). Seborrhoeic infants do not become seborrhoeic adults. Adult seborrhoeic eczema responds to a 1% hydrocortisone–antiseptic combination on the trunk and behind the ears, but requires a less acceptable treatment for the scalp. A suitable preparation is:

Salicylic acid	2%
Precip. sulphur	2%
Emulsifying ointment to 200 g	

This should be applied daily, removed by shampooing and re-applied until the scaling has cleared. Fluorinated steroid scalp preparations may be partially effective.

'Cradle cap' in infants and young children is so common that it is hardly a skin disease although mothers seek advice for it. The following preparation is useful:

Salicylic acid	½–1%
Precip. sulphur	½–1%
Aqueous cream to 100 g	

This cream is applied every 24 hours after shampooing and will remove the scaling in a few days; it can then be used intermittently until the condition resolves.

Psoriasis (10.4%)

This condition can be the most difficult to treat in general practice. For some patients it is minimal, with infrequent relapses, and easily hidden from the public by clothing; for others, it separates them from the other 98% of the population who are not predisposed to the disease and forces them to live a life restricted by various veils or screens. A few who are severely affected can disregard their appearance and have a normal family and working life, but most have a poor image of themselves. If this leads to undue anxiety, according to the author's local trainers' group, it tends to prolong exacerbations. Otherwise 'stress', apart from catastrophic events, appears to play little part in initiating or maintaining outbreaks of psoriasis. Some doctors, seeing only selected cases, have come to different conclusions and have helped to perpetuate the lay myth that permeates into the medical profession that psoriasis is a 'nervous' disease. This myth should be laid at the earliest opportunity. It has been shown that most patients who develop psoriasis belong to specific antigenic phenotypes and will develop the disease at some time in their lives with the first signs appearing any time between infancy and old age. The spectrum varies from psoriasiform napkin dermatitis in infants to scaling lesions on limbs and trunk, unlike any other skin disease, to isolated typical lesions on limbs, trunk or scalp in children and young adults and to the typical lesions of guttate or formal psoriasis. Always inspect the finger nails for pitting or separation of the distal nail plate from its bed, and examine the elbows, knees and scalp for similar lesions when unusual scaling lesions appear for the first time on the limbs or trunk. Psoriasis is not always 'typical' and once the diagnosis has been made (and entered on the summary card or sheet) all scaling eruptions should be so diagnosed until proved otherwise.

Various triggers may provoke psoriasis. Napkin eruptions in infants, streptococcal sore throats in children and catastrophic nervous upset in adults may be trigger factors in those predisposed. Trauma to the skin may result in Koebner's phenomenon of psoriasis at the site of trauma.

Management of psoriasis

The history should include the past played by trigger factors and any seasonal variations, in particular the response to natural sunlight. The 'hang-up' of psoriasis being a nervous disorder should be removed in the vast majority of patients and an explanation of the tendency to spontaneous remission and its predilection for areas easily covered by garments should be given. When the trigger of streptococcal tonsillitis recurs frequently, tonsillectomy should be considered, and the use of artificial ultraviolet light can be encouraged when the history supports its use.

The treatment of psoriasis depends on the severity and extent of the eruption, or how much the patient is affected psychologically by the condition and on whether the patient has used tar or tar derivatives in previous episodes. A list of prescriptions is given at the end of this section; different preparations are referred to by the prefix P and the number of the prescription in the discussion which follows.

Infants with psoriasiform napkin eruptions should be treated with a 1% hydrocortisone/anticandidal/antiseptic ointment until the eruption settles. This can take from 2 to 6 weeks. These infants thrive normally and show no tendency to scratch. Guttate psoriasis has a natural tendency to remission and tar treatment may exacerbate the eruption. Although the parents or the patient may be presenting for 'cure' mild treatments are indicated (P1, P2). Any episode of sore throat merits treatment with phenoxymethyl penicillin in full dosage. Unfortunately,

in some patients the eruption persists beyond 3 to 4 months and may develop into more typical lesions of psoriasis. The treatment for established psoriasis is indicated at that stage and the use of a tar preparation will not cause exacerbation. Typically, psoriasis presents with scaling plaques on the elbows, knees and sacrum or nummular lesions on the limbs and trunk. If these are localised and not causing problems, mild treatments (P1, P2) are indicated initially. If the patient is sufficiently motivated to use staining treatments, the milder preparations (P3, P4) can be started. If these fail to produce an improvement, or if the patient has previously used tar, the more messy, staining treatments (P5, P6) may be used. The strength of prescription (P6) should be increased at 4- to 7-day intervals depending on the response. If the patient has never used tar preparations before, inspection and changes of strength, if indicated, are appropriate at weekly intervals. Localised plaques may respond best to dithranol (P7). The patient should be advised to smear vaseline around the plaque and to wear rubber gloves when applying dithranol; he should be warned that tar and dithranol leave a permanent stain in contact fabrics.

Scalp psoriasis does not respond well to topical fluorinated scalp preparations, which may keep the condition at bay when more specific treatments cannot be used. Regular shampooing (P8) will help to remove obvious scaling. Dithranol preparations (P4) are helpful in some cases, but may stain the forehead, ears and neck and will give fair hair an orange appearance. Tar preparations (P9) are the most effective and can be used when the patient will be at home for at least 12 hours (preferably 24 hours) and can apply the ointment daily over several days. Most patients maintain reasonable control by using a tar preparation at weekends with steroid preparations and shampoos during the week.

Psoriasis of the palms and soles can be very scaly and uncomfortable and often leads to painful fissuring. Strong salicylic acid (P10) or dithranol preparations (P3, 4 or 7) may help, but sometimes the only treatment likely to help is clobetasol propionate applied night and morning with a salicyclic acid preparation used several times during the day.

Patients with psoriasis on the back of the hands are unwilling to draw attention to it by the use of tar or dithranol and fluorinated steroid ointments are the only effective alternatives. Similarly, although psoriasis rarely appears on the face other than at the hair margin, diluted or full strength fluorinated steroid ointments allow patients to lead a more normal life. Side-effects of fluorinated steroids do not seem to occur as readily when used to treat psoriasis as they do in eczema, and most patients will regard any side-effects as a small price to pay for the freedom it brings to their lifestyle. Flexural and genital psoriasis respond best to 1% hydrocortisone–antiseptic combinations, but can be extremely persistent. Tar and dithranol preparations should never be used on these areas.

There is no successful treatment for the nail changes of psoriasis and psoriatic anthropathy should be treated in the same way as rheumatoid arthritis.

Prescriptions used for psoriasis

P1	Salicylic acid	2–5%
	Soft paraffin to	100%
P2	Resorcin	2%
	Salicylic acid	3%
	Liquor picis carbonis	4%
	Lanolin	20%
	Soft paraffin to	100%
P3	Dithrocream	0.1, 0.25, 0.5%
P4	Psoradrate	0.1–0.2%
P5	Coal tar and salicylic acid ointment BNF	
P6	Crude coal tar	2–4–6–10%
	Zinc oxide	2%
	Starch	25%
	Soft paraffin to	100%
	Crude coal tar	20%
	Zinc oxide	20%
	Lanolin	20%
	Soft paraffin to	100%
P7	Dithranol	0.1–0.2%
	Lassar's paste to	100%
P8	Polytar liquid	
P9	Oil of cade	6–12%
	Salicylic acid	3–6%
	Emulsifying ointment to	100%
P10	Salicylic acid	5–10%
	Soft paraffin to	100 g

ACQUIRED SKIN DISEASES

Infections (21.1%)

Bacterial infections (3.9%)

Impetigo (1.6%). A superficial infection of the skin occurring on any site, most commonly on the face. Crusting is variable and is most marked on the scalp. Occasionally, the blistering (bullous) variety is encountered. It may be superimposed on other skin disorders such as atopic eczema or herpes simplex infections and, when this occurs, the impetigo should be treated first. It responds to most topical antibacterial preparations but systemic antibiotics appropriate to gram positive infections are indicated when there is constitutional illness, when the impetigo is persistent or recurrent, or when it occurs on the scalp.

Abscesses (1.0%). Vary from folliculitis to carbuncles. They are commonly multiple or recurrent and indicate colonisation of the skin by *Staph. aureus*. A three-pronged attack is usually required; a topical anti-bacterial applied to and around the lesions, the appropriate systemic antibiotic and twice daily washing or bathinng with pHiso-MED.

Superficial skin sepsis (0.9%). Usually affects the hands and fingers of those affected by xeroderma or irritant dermatitis. It does not show the same crusting as does impetigo, penetrates deeper into the skin and is more painful and is not localised like an abscess. Topical anti-bacterials and washing with pHiso-MED are usually effective. Systemic antibiotics effective against Gram positive organisms are indicated when these local measures fail.

Acute paronychia (0.3%). Can be regarded either as a surgical or as a dermatological complaint. Chronic paronychia is more definitely a dermatological problem and is discussed under fungal infections. The acute variety initially affects one side of the nail fold and is extremely painful. Pus becomes evident within a few days and the correct treatment is incision when pus is evident. An incision about 0.5 cm in length, made with a 21-gauge needle is adequate. Deeper incision, under ring block may be more satisfying for the inexperienced, but is seldom necessary. Topical antibiotics are ineffective but systemic antibiotics hasten resolution.

Pyogenic granuloma (0.1%). A curious rarity. It is more vascular than a wart, but not usually suggestive of a skin neoplasm. It may respond to the application of copper sulphate crystals, but its suspicious appearance warrants referral for destruction by liquid nitrogen or removal by excision biopsy.

Viral infections (12%)

Warts (9.4%). Account for the majority of viral skin eruptions and appear in four forms in general practice.

1. *Plantar warts* (7.4%) are prevalent where there is a local swimming pool or when schoolchildren have a communal shower after physical education. If there is doubt whether a plantar lesion is a wart or a callosity (corn), paring with a No. 15 blade will reveal the pin-point bleeding points from the capillaries of a wart. Since plantar warts restrict the social and recreational activities of children and young adults, treatment is justified although time-consuming and prolonged. If the warts are painful, parents should be shown how to pare off the necrotic surface material with a No. 15 scalpel blade. Soft paraffin should be smeared around the wart and the affected part steeped in 5% formalin solution for 15 minutes each night. The formalin can be poured back into the container after use. The wart should be pared down, after steeping, every third night. Plantar warts which are not painful may respond to podophyllin. A suitable preparation is Posalfilin and an instruction sheet helps compliance. Again, twice-weeekly paring is essen-

tial. After 6 weeks treatment with formalin solution or podophyllin the patient should be reviewed. If there is obvious improvement after paring off the necrotic surface, the treatment should be continued and reassessed after 6 weeks. If there is no improvement after 6 weeks, or the wart is not cured after 12 weeks, more active treatment is justified. The following keratolytic paste is useful:

Salicylic acid	12 g
Trichloracetic acid	5 g
Glycerine	5 ml

This is applied to the wart after paring, a piece of gauze swab adequate to cover the wart is applied to prevent spread of the paste and the application is kept in place by three turns of Elastoplast 1″ bandage. The patient is instructed to keep the dressing dry and in place until review 1 week later. The dressing may become wet in the weekly bath which should be allowed on the night before the review! After paring off the necrotic debris the treatment is repeated. Usually four or five treatments result in cure, depending on the vigour of the paring of the necrotic debris after treatment. Liquid nitrogen treatment applied at the hospital will help to cure stubborn plantar wards. Multiple warts in clusters (mosaic warts) are much more stubborn and the use of liquid nitrogen earlier in treatment should be considered. It must be pointed out that liquid nitrogen application is very painful and should be avoided in young children. Patience and perseverance with the topical paste is usually painless and successful in such patients.

2. *Common warts* (1.7%) will involute spontaneously in 18–24 months if ignored. However, parents, teachers and, unfortunately, some school nurses may wish treatment for them. Topical treatments combined with abrasion may make them less obvious, but seldom cure. In children and young adult males it is best not to treat them and await spontaneous involution. Peri-ungual warts may be painful and liable to trauma and treatment with podophyllin (Posalfilin) occluded with zinc oxide adhesive tape may be helpful. Failure after 2 months treatment of these warts warrants consideration of treatment with liquid nitrogen. Teenage girls and adults who have attempted to cure their warts with proprietary treatments may be prepared to suffer liquid nitrogen therapy. This form of treatment is painful and motivation is required since treatment may have to be repeated. If possible, warts on the hands, fingers and knees should be regarded as part of normal development and no action should be initiated by the medical or nursing profession.

3. *Filiform warts* (0.14%) occur around the lips and nose. They grow further from the skin surface in these sites since they experience less friction. They are unsightly and do not respond to topical wart treatment. Referral is indicated for destruction with liquid nitrogen or cautery.

4. *Penile* (0.14%) and vulvar warts are smaller and more discrete than the larger venereal warts (condylomata accuminata). If there is doubt, the appropriate VDRL serology should be tested. These warts respond to podophyllin in tincture of compound benzoin. Initially 12.5% podophyllin should be painted on and washed off after 2 hours. The treatment should be repeated at weekly intervals and the duration of application doubled. If after three applications, cure has not been achieved 25% podophyllin should be applied and the time of application doubled at weekly intervals. If this does not produce cure, or if there are extensive vaginal warts, cautery under general anaesthetic is usually required.

Mollusca contagiosa (0.14%). More frequent if there is a local swimming pool and in children with active atopic eczema. They appear as smooth 'warts' with an umbilicated centre. If left untreated they will become inflamed and enlarged after several months and then involute spontaneously. Before this occurs however they may become numerous and unsightly and treatment is usually justified. Treatments recommended include curettage, painting with strong iodine or phenol, piercing with a sharpened orange stick and the application of liquid nitrogen. These remedies are all extremely painful, if not barbaric in children, and a simple alternative method is to squeeze the lesions between the thumb nails and express the white contents. Uusally, three lesions can be treated at a session and the parent should repeat the treatment twice weekly and then scrub the thumb nails! Patients with obvious lesions on the eyelids should be referred to an ophthalmologist for curettage under general anaesthetic.

Herpes simplex (1.7%). Infection usually occurs on the lower third of the face during a febrile illness or after exposure to strong sunlight. It should be remembered that the lesions may occur at any site and can be recurrent. Unusual sites include the fingers, the sole of the foot and the peri-anal region. The history and appearance are typical. For 24 to 48 hours the patient notices a 'burning' feeling after which the typical vesicles appear. The lesions then become crusted and usually heal within a week unless secondary impetigo develops. Recurrent lesions occur at any age after infancy. When the lesions are infrequent, the application of povidone-iodine paint is adequate, but when the condition occurs frequently or causes considerable distress, such as when lesions are on the index finger of the dominant hand or on the face, 5% idoxuridine in dimethyl sulphoxide is justified despite its expense. This treatment should be started as soon as the patient notices the 'burning' feeling and it should be discontinued after 4 days. When extensive herpes simplex infection complicates atopic eczema, 5% idoxuridine in dimethyl sulphoxide should be applied immediately; a consultant opinion may be required to allay the anxiety of patient or doctor.

Herpes simplex stomatitis (0.14%). Causes considerable distress to parents and to the patient, who is usually a toddler. Multiple, superficial lesions are present on the tongue and around the oral cavity. There is fever, local lymphadenopathy and reluctance to feed because of pain. The eruption lasts for approximately 1 week and during this time both the child and his parents are miserable. There is no specific therapy but advice on antipyretics, fluid replacement and mouth washes should be given.

Herpes zoster (0.58%). Infection is easily diagnosed once the eruption has appeared. The prodromal pain can be confusing, but its unilateral and segmental distribution should arouse suspicion. In younger patients, dabbing with some form of alcohol and dusting with talcum powder plus the prescription of an appropriate analgesic is adequate. In patients over 60 years in whom postherpetic pain may become a problem or if the patient is otherwise debilitated, the 4-hourly application of 5% idoxuridine in dimethyl sulphoxide is justified. This treatment must be started immediately the diagnosis is considered and continued for 4 days only. The results of early use can be dramatic. If the diagnosis is not made until the eruption is established, amantadine 100 mg capsules should be prescribed four times daily for 2 weeks. There is some evidence that this antiviral drug may decrease the duration of the eruption and of the post-herpetic neuralgia.

Fungal infections (5.2%)
Fungal infections of the skin respond only to specific antifungal agents and the older remedies are specific only for *Candida albicans*, for ringworm or for *P. versicolour* fungi.

Ringworm infections (1.7%). Affect the feet or rarely the hands, the flexures, or may appear as typical annular lesions when animals are the source of the infection.

Tinea pedis (0.72%). Affects the webs of the toes and their flexor surfaces. The lateral toes are the most likely to be affected. Pompholyx appears as vesicles and scaling rather than maceration and scaling, is more likely to affect the medial toes or instep and is associated with severe itching or burning discomfort. Idiopathic foot eczema affects pre-pubertal children, involves the pads of the toes and the sole of the foot and presents as shining erythema and scaling.

Chronic or recurrent tinea pedis usually involves the toe-nails. The nails become thickened, lose their lustre and become brownish in colour. If the diagnosis is supported by identification of fungi by the mycology laboratory (scrapings or clippings may be sent in a paper packet through the ordinary post) treatment with griseofulvin, 500 mg daily for 1 year, may result in cure in a small proportion of patients. Its use can only be supported if

the affected toe-nails are causing pain. Rarely, tinea may affect the insteps and palms, when erythema and fine scaling are the main features rather than the vesicles of pompholyx. The diagnosis is made by the examination of scrapings by the mycology laboratory.

Tinea cruris (1.0%). Usually affects the inguinal flexures in people who sweat excessively. It presents as a velvety erythema with a fairly distinct margin.

Animal ringworm. With its typical, raised, annular, nodular appearance the condition is infrequent, but should be suspected, when there is close contact with kittens or calves. On the scalp it develops rapidly and may mimic an abscess; however, the scalp lesions are not pustular and should not be incised. The diagnosis can be confirmed by examination under ultraviolet light or by mycological examination of hairs removed from the lesion.

Tinea (or ringworm) infections respond readily to tolnaftate, clotrimazole or miconazole creams. If relapse occurs rapidly, if the lesions are extensive or if there is involvement of the scalp, oral griseofulvin 500 mg daily for 4 to 6 weeks should be combined with topical therapy.

Candida albicans (3.5%). Usually affects the skin in otherwise healthy people unlike systemic candidosis which selects those with serious life-threatening disorders.

Chronic paronychia (1.2%). May complicate atopic eczema or may be the result of prolonged immerson in water. There is swelling and tenderness of the finger just proximal to the nail fold, but the pain is not the extreme pain of acute (bacterial) paronchyia and a pustule at the edge of the nail fold does not appear. A small bead of pus may however be expressed at the nail fold. The disorder is due to *Candida albicans* invasion and the edge of the nail may have a greenish colour. Secondary bacterial infection may cause a painful exacerbation. Treatment is with an antifungal/antiseptic lotion applied every 2 hours during the day and an antibiotic cream such as gentamycin, applied at night. Erythromycin 250 mg q.i.d. should be prescribed during an exacerbation. These treatments are effective if the patient can avoid prolonged immersion of the hands in water for several months. Busy housewifes and kitchen workers may find this impossible.

Cutaneous candidosis (0.14%). May occur in the finger webs if the fingers are constantly apposed by deformity or if they are frequently wet.

Oral candidosis (1.0%). Occurs after antibiotic therapy, especially if prolonged, and in patients who have complete sets of dentures. If the dentures are ill-fitting, angular stomatitis occurs. In the author's experience, angular stomatitis is more commonly associated with oral candidosis or ill-fitting dentures and is seldom associated with iron or vitamin B deficiency. The oral cavity is inflamed, especially under the dentures, and white aggregates of

Candida albicans may be seen on the hard palate, on the buccal mucosa or on the inner surface of the dentures. The tongue usually appears smooth, red and shining (glossitis). The condition responds to amphotericin B lozenges sucked four times daily between meals, for 10 days. Ill-fitting dentures require to be adjusted.

Oral candidosis in infants may cause refusal of feeds and is readily diagnosed since the aggregates of *Candida albicans* on the mucosa are obvious. Treatment with nystatin oral suspension 100 000 units four times daily may be effective, but 0.5% gentian violet always works when painted around the mouth four times daily. Treatment is continued until the mouth appears to be normal.

Candidal napkin eruptions (1.2%). There is good evidence that *Candida albicans* is a major causative factor in symmetrical napkin eruptions which involve the flexures. This condition is distinguished from ammoniacal dermatitis by peripheral 'satellite' lesions beyond the confluent eruption which has fringe scaling surrounding an area of dull erythema. This contrasts sharply with ammoniacal napkin dermatitis when affects the prominent areas — the buttocks, scrotum, vulva and areas where the plastic pants are held in contact at the periphery of the napkin area. Chemical napkin dermatitis has a shining, scaling appearance when mild, causes erosions when severe and *always* spares the flexures within the napkin area. Both eruptions may be partly due to bacterial colonisation of the inflamed areas.

Psoriasiform napkin dermatitis (1.0%). Presents as a candidal napkin eruption with a secondary nummular, scaling eruption on the limbs and trunk. When the face is involved, there is thick scaling of the eyebrows and this is usually associated with thick crusting on the scalp. The mother must be instructed to discard the plastic pants and expose the baby's buttocks as much as possible until the eruption clears. The eruption always responds to a combined anticandidal/antiseptic weak hydrocortisone preparation (1% Nystaform H.C. ointment, Trimovate, Daktacort cream) applied to all affected areas over 2 to 6 weeks. The scalp scaling responds to the prescription for seborrhoea capitis provided on page 248. Some infants develop *symmetrical intertrigo* (0.1%) of the napkin area without any secondary eruption. This should be treated in the same way as psoriasiform napkin dermatitis.

Infestations (2.5%)

Scabies (1.3%)

More likely when personal hygiene is poor. However, nurses who are in close contact with patients who have poor personal hygiene for psychological reasons are prone to this infestation. Those who frequently stay in 'overnight' accommodation are similarly at an increased risk. Even fastidious people on holiday may be unfortunate, especially if sleeping in caravans or in less reputable holiday accommodation. Children who stay overnight with friends or relatives are at increased risk and may quickly spread the infestation around the household. There is a delay of 4 to 6 weeks between exposure and the development of overt infestation and the source may not be obvious at first. A careful history can usually pinpoint the source and persuade the patient and relatives that this is not always a 'dirty' disease. The appropriate treatment is to apply a gamma benzene hexachloride preparation over the whole body surface after bathing on the first night, to repeat the application without a bath on the second night. All contact clothing and bed linen should be changed and well laundered (after the cleansing bath) and replaced by well laundered substitutes. All children and parents should be treated simultaneously, but unmarried, older teenagers and adults do not usually pass on the disease except to their bed-fellows and treatment should be limited to these close contacts.

Normally, the lesions of scabies do not appear on the face, except in young babies who may develop inflamed scabetic papules on the cheeks and feet: these may persist after treatment, although they are not infectious.

Scabies causes profound itching — particularly during the night — and there may be secondary eczematisation. Treatment must first be directed at the infestation and any residual eczema treated afterwards with crotamiton-hydrocortisone (EURAX) cream.

Pediculosis capitis

Mainly affects children with long hair, and parents may have to have their guilt feelings allayed when the school nurse finds the infestation in their child. Live insects are usually found only in children where family hygiene or supervision is poor and the diagnosis is usually made by finding nits (eggs) attached firmly to hair shafts close to the scalp. Unlike dandruff, these cannot be moved except by pulling them up and off the hair shaft. Infestation should always be suspected when impetigo of the scalp is diagnosed.

Pediculosis pubis

Usually results from a sexual encounter with an unhygienic partner and the insects, although small, are usually obvious. Both infestations respond to the application of 0.5% malathion lotion for 12 hours. This treatment should precede topical treatment of scalp impetigo, although systemic antibiotics — if required — can be started immediately.

Insect bites (1.4%)

Such bites present as raised papules of varying size with a central punctum. The grouped, recurrent lesions of flea bites have to be explained to parents who think that these 'heat spots' or 'hives' are due to some ingested allergen. It may defuse the aggression of the parents to state that fleas visit doctors and their children as well as their patients. The patient's sheets, night attire, and underwear require to be dusted daily with an insecticide dusting powder until no fresh lesions have appeared for 10 days. Fleas require a feed of blood every 5 to 7 days and when 10 days have passed without fresh lesions it can be assumed that the unwelcome visitor has perished or has sought fresh pastures. Domestic pets may be the source of the offending insect and will require treatment with an appropriate insecticide dusting powder. Some patients, usually children, appear to be truly allergic to contact with even fragments of dead insects which parasitise domestic pets, and develop a more generalised itching, papular eruption. If dusting the pet with an insecticide powder and regular vacuum-cleaning of every nook and cranny does not result in resolution of the eruption, removal of even the most cherished pet may be necessary. Before this drastic decision is made, support from a specialist may be required. An unusual situation may arise when a family moves into a house where there was previously a domestic pet and the allergen is not obvious. However, the itching papules are typical and a careful history will indicate the cause. Generous dusting with insecticide powder and regular vacuum cleaning will result in resolution of the problem over a few months.

Other insects may cause raised, itching lesions with a central punctum or even blisters, but usually the history will reveal the offender — midges in Scotland, mosquitoes in warmer climes.

Physical and chemical causes (7.5%)

Neurodermatitis (1.4%)

Occurs more frequently in females and is caused by repeated scratching of accessible sites such as the elbow, back of the neck and the medial side of the leg just above the ankle. In some cases an itch may initiate the eruption which is then perpetuated by repeated scratching. Lichenified atopic eczema occurs on the flexor aspects of the joints and, up to a point, is a form of neurodermatitis due to repeated scratching of an itching eruption. Lesions over the extensor aspect of the elbows may mimic psoriasis, but evidence of psoriasis elsewhere is absent. Perfume dermatitis occurs just under the angle of the jaw rather than on the nape of the neck and can be clarified by the history. The nature of the eruption must be explained to the patient and a fluorinated steroid should be applied as often as the patient realises that she is scratching. Gradually, the eruption resolves when application of the steroid should be decreased, but continued, until the skin is smooth and no longer itches.

Lip licking (0.43%)

Due to a combination of licking dry lips and friction from the teeth or finger nails. The eruption is characterised by scaling of the lips spreading on to the adjacent areas

beyond the vermilion border of the lips. In peri-oral dermatitis there is an unaffected area of normal skin between the lips and the eruption. Lip licking is impossible to treat unless the patient ceases to irritate the lips. Dilute hydrocortisone in a water repellent base (Cobadex 0.5% cream) applied every 2 hours can help resolution.

Callosities (0.14%)

Occur where there is considerable, repeated friction or pressure on the palms and soles. On the feet they may mimic plantar warts, but they appear in an older age group and occur on the toes where they are exposed to pressure due to tight fitting shoes, or under the metatarsal heads if the transverse arch has fallen. Advice regarding proper footwear and padding, and treatment by a chiropodist may help if the patient is prepared to co-operate. Rarely the assistance of an orthopaedic surgeon is required to deal with exostoses of the metatarsals or to correct gross abnormalities of the toes.

Infantile sweat rash (0.58%)

Occurs on the cheeks of babies who are covered with excessive layers of clothing in a warm environment. The eruption is due to a combination of warmth and immature sweat glands and is most noticeable on the side of the face on which the child has been sleeping. The papular and erythematous eruption may spread to the limbs and trunk if the baby is heated excessively. The mother should be instructed to count the number of layers of clothing in which she herself feels comfortable at rest and to cover the baby with one more layer. A 1% hydrocortisone cream will be necessary if the eruption is severe or extensive.

Pruritus ani (1.0%)

Due to excessive warmth and moisture, especially if the patient has an above average amount of hair in that region. It is aggravated by scratching and may be complicated by C. albicans infection if the patient has recently received systemic antibiotics.

Pruritus vulvae (0.29%)

Due to the same factors as pruritus ani, but glycosuria should always be excluded, especially in the obese; tight fitting underwear may be a factor in younger women. Both eruptions are more common in anxiety-prone patients and scratching, which is both hurtful yet satisfying, perpetuates the eruptions. A combined antiseptic/anticandidal/1% hydrocortisone cream should be applied, initially as often as the patient finds that she is scratching and eventually twice daily until the itch ceases.

Irritant dermatitis (3.0%)

Most commonly due to excessive immersion of the hands

in detergents and particularly if there is a tendency to eczema. Mothers with young infants and kitchen workers are most commonly affected. Workmen who use harsh cleansers too often or who are in contact with irritant chemicals, such as cement, may be at risk of contracting allergic contact dermatitis due to the increased permeability of the chemically irritated skin. Advice is more important than topical steroids in the management of this condition.

Ultraviolet light will cause erythema or blistering if there is over exposure, but some people are predisposed to an eczematous eruption, especially on the back of the hands and face, without over-exposure. If eruptions occur in moderate sunlight or are extensive, referral for exclusion of errors of porphyrin metabolism is necessary. Some drugs (sulphonamides, chlorpromazine, nalidixic acid, benoxaprofen) are associated with skin eruptions but only when the patient is exposed to strong sunlight.

Ammoniacal napkin dermatitis (0.58%)

This condition is worst at the areas of maximum contact with sodden napkins and is usually in proportion to the duration of contact. Persistence of the eruption, despite good maternal care, suggests a tendency to eczema. The mother should be instructed to expose the napkin area as much as possible, change napkins as soon as they are wet, and discard plastic pants, until the skin has returned to normal. Since bacterial and candidal infection appear to play some part in this eruption, a combined antibacterial/anticandidal/1% hydrocortisone preparation should be applied twice daily until the skin returns to normal.

Allergy (3.5%)

If atopic eczema is excluded, allergy plays a smaller part in the aetiology of skin conditions than most general practitioners believe.

Urticaria (3.5%)

May be cholinergic, being provoked by changes in temperature and appearing as scattered nummular or annular raised, itching areas which recur over a prolonged period. No obvious ingested allergen can be identified in this type of eruption and an antihistamine-decongestant preparation of the kind usually prescribed for rhinitis, offers the best suppression. The more dramatic map-like, extensive urticaria occurs less frequently and a specific allergen can be identified in about 50% of these patients. Drugs, such as penicillin and aspirin, food, such as fish, curry and shellfish and household plants are the most common causes, but almost any chemical present in food or in the atmosphere can be responsible and can only be identified by careful history-taking. Severe urticaria may result if tetanus injections are given too often, or too close together. Antihistamines should be used if there is no obvious allergen, or until the allergen is identified and avoided.

Erythema multiforme (0.29%)

An extensive eruption secondary to another skin eruption which is usually viral or due to a drug allergy. The lesions are extensive and annular or target-shaped. The patient is toxic and can be seriously ill when the mucosae are involved. Extensive cholinergic urticaria or extensive animal ringworm may be considered if there is no primary viral lesion or history of drug ingestion. Treatment is with antihistamines in mild instances, but a consultant opinion is required if the patient is toxic.

Sensitisation eczema (0.14%)

Appears when there is an acute eczema on any site. The sensitisation eczema is a secondary response and treatment should be aimed at the primary eruption with a soothing treatment for the secondary eruption.

Drug eruptions (0.43%)

Due mainly to penicillins and sulphonamides, but may be due to any drug. Penicillin eruptions are urticarial when due to the penicillin radicle and will appear when any penicillin is ingested, and morbilliform when due to amoxicillin and ampicillin. Sulphonamide eruptions are more common in sunny weather on the exposed surfaces and are usually a mixture of urticaria and eczema. Almost any drug can cause a rash, but so too can the disease for which the drug was prescribed and it can be difficult to decide if the disease or the drug is responsible for the eruption. Specific RAST testing may aid accuracy.

Contact dermatitis (2.6%)

Appears initially at the site of contact, but spread may occur to other areas. It is more frequent in women. A good history, plus clinical suspicion aroused by the site of the eruption, will provide a provisional diagnosis. If proof is required, subsequent provocation by the allergen, after the initial eruption has cleared, will result in recurrence.

Nickel dermatitis occurs where 'cheap' metal is in contact with the skin, for example, ear-rings, jean-studs, metal clips on brassieres. Cosmetic dermatitis is seen on the lips or eyelids and perfume dermatitis on the sides of the neck or behind the ears. Men are more likely than women to develop industrial contact dermatitis, mainly because cement is so widely used in the building industry. If the history and presentation do not indicate a definite diagnosis, patch testing with common allergens can be performed by a dermatologist. The management must include advice about avoiding the allergen, or protecting the skin from it; only then is the appropriate steroid prescribed. Many patients, especially in the building industry, do not readily accept advice and require repeated treatment for their dermatitis. Advice should continually be offered, but some patients are unable to adapt to other occupations and continue to accept exposure to the allergen and consequent disability.

Endocrine related disorders (21.6%)

Acne (17.9%)

Acne is so common that it is almost a part of adolescence or young adult life and a description is not required. It is the patient — not the physician — who has the problem and two pustules can be as psychologically devastating to an immature youth as to a beauty queen. The condition may continue, or even not appear, until full adult maturity is achieved. Mild eruptions of comedones and small papules may respond to abrasives: more extensive papular eruptions with a few pustules to peeling agents; whilst pustular and cystic lesions always require long-term systemic antibiotic therapy. All types of acne respond temporarily to ultraviolet light from the sky or a lamp, and its use can enhance other modes of treatment. When systemic antibiotic therapy is required, treatment may need to be continued for years and females should be cautioned to stop treatment if they think they may be pregnant, since tetracyclines can damage fetal tooth and bone formation. A simple drug regime should be prescribed and the patient advised that little response can be expected in the first month and a good result not before 3 months. Thereafter, the dose is adjusted according to the response. Oxytetracycline 250 mg twice daily before meals, avoiding simultaneous large quantities of milk, alkali, or oral iron, produce a good or excellent result in 90% of patients after 3 months. The few patients who do not respond to this regime usually improve with a regime of erythromycin 250 mg b.d. or co-trimoxazole b.d. for 3 months. Co-trimoxazole should be stopped after 6 months when the remission can be maintained with oxytetracycline or erythromycin even when these antibiotics failed previously.

Rosacea (2.6%)

More common in women and affecting mainly those from 35 to 50 years of age. It affects the central third of the face with a varying combination of mild erythema, papules and pustules. The use of topical steroids causes severe erythema with multiple pustules, and an extension on to the sides of the face; the eruption then becomes very difficult to manage and the erythema may be permanent. Rosacea can be a very satisfying condition for a general practitioner to treat, since it almost always responds well to oral oxytetracycline 250 mg b.d. The dose may be reduced after 6 weeks, depending on the response, and the drug may be discontinued after 3 months. Repeated courses are usually required at intervals over many years and some patients require a low dose of oxytetracycline, 250 mg daily or on alternate days, to subdue the eruption. Rarely erythromycin or co-trimoxazole are required. Occasionally, mixed eruptions of acne and rosacea are encountered and these require the treatment appropriate for acne.

Peri-oral dermatitis (0.87%)

Occurs in adolescents and young adults, almost all of whom are female. It starts as a mild erythema with scaling at the sides of the nose and spreads very slowly. Fluorinated steroids, however, cause it to spread rapidly around the mouth and papules and pustules complicate the eruption. A margin around the vermilion border of the lips is always spared. The correct treatment is to give oral oxytetracycline 250 mg b.d. for 6 weeks and 250 mg daily for a further 6 weeks, with subsequent courses for relapses. When strong topical steroids have been used to treat rosacea or peri-oral dermatitis and have caused the inevitable exacerbation, the use of 1% hydrocortisone lotion or cream may be required to prevent a 'rebound' deterioration before oral tetracycline begins to subdue the eruption.

Hirsutism (0.3%)

Hirsutism can be distressing to the adolescent and the young adult female, whereas older women tolerate it, although they may be unhappy about it. Endocrine investigation is required to exclude rare causes, but most patients have normal hormone profiles and require advice on shaving, bleaching the unwanted hair, depilatory creams or electrolysis.

Vascular disorders (2.9%)

Stasis eczema (1.0%)

Affects older patients who have obvious varicosities. The veins require support with below-knee elastic stockings, if surgical intervention is unjustified for other reasons, and the application of a mild topical steroid will give symptomatic relief.

Stasis ulcers (0.9%)

Will not heal if the limb is oedematous. If the oedema does not respond to firm bandaging, the foot of the bed must be elevated by about 15–18 inches. In the absence of oedema, firm bandaging, combined with any topical antiseptic preparation, will result in gradual healing. Firm support with below-knee elastic stockings usually maintains intact skin. If there is surrounding eczema, zinc oxide cream or a 1% hydrocortisone/antibiotic preparation is indicated, but fluorinated steroids usually cause an increase in the size of the ulcer.

Chilblains (0.6%)

Occur in winter on the fingers, toes and heels of adolescent and young adult females who have cyanosed extremities. The lesions are purple, elevated and fairly localised. Advice on warm clothing and the prescription of a peripheral vasodilator allow the lesions to settle. Patients should not 'toast' themselves on returning indoors over the winter months.

'Vasculitis' (0.4%)

Causes pain and tenderness of the lower one-third of the leg. It occurs in middle-aged females and all investigations (apart from biopsy) are usually normal. Vasculitis seems to respond best to non-steroidal anti-inflammatory drugs.

Degenerative skin disorders (0.9%)

Senile pruritus (0.7%)

A diagnosis of senile pruritus is based on the exclusion of other skin, psychiatric or systemic disorders, such as endocrine or hepatic diseases, in the elderly. The skin appears to be normal, yet the itch may be intense. A dilute fluorinated steroid ointment usually suffices, but hydroxyzine hydrochloride 10 mg t.i.d. may also be required.

Seborrhoeic keratoses (0.1%)

Occur usually on the upper half of the body and are so common that they are usually ignored. However, patients with multiple or large lesions and those with lesions on the face may request treatment. The diagnosis is seldom in doubt because of their brown, slightly raised, 'greasy' appearance, but, if there is doubt, a dermatologist's opinion should be sought. One or two applications, 3 to 4 weeks apart, of trichloracetic acid causes the lesions to blanch, and results in a cure after the crust has separated. Gratitude, disproportionate to the work performed, usually results from this treatment!

Primary skin tumours (0.7%)

These are usually benign and may be ignored if the diagnosis is uncertain. If there is any doubt about their benign nature, referral for excision biopsy is the wise course.

Squamous epithelioma (0.1%)

Presents as an ulcer of varying depth with built up edges. Basal cell carcinomas may not show ulceration and the edge is variable. Both occur more commonly on exposed parts of the body and both require referral. Treatment of basal cell lesions may not be necessary in the very old or ill, provided they are kept under regular review.

Melanomas (0.1%)

Occur on any part of the body and are extremely common. Any change in size or the presence of ulceration requires urgent referral.

Fibromas or 'pimples' (0.1%)

These do not require excision, unless there is doubt as to the diagnosis or they are causing embarrassment.

Chondrodermatitis nodularis chronicus helicis (0.1%)

Presents as a small lesion on the rim of the upper pinna of the ear and causes pain at night when the patient turns on the affected side. The pain is disproportionate to its size and destruction of the lesion with cautery or liquid nitrogen results in cure.

Undiagnosed (0.1%)

Undiagnosed lumps in the skin indicate referral.

Autoimmune conditions (0.7%)

Normally, for the diagnosis of an autoimmune disorder, specific antibodies in serum should be demonstrated or complement shown at the site of pathology. The proven autoimmune disorders, such as pemphigus, pemphigoid, dermatomyositis and SLE, were not encountered in the practice survey mentioned above and descriptions of them can be found in the standard textbooks of dermatology. However, diagnostic techniques at present are limited but the presence of cells usually found in proven, systemic autoimmune disorders or several specific autoantibodies in the serum suggest that the following disorders may have an autoimmune basis.

Alopecia areata (0.4%)

Can affect any hairy area in children and young adults. It is easily diagnosed, since the skin of the affected area is entirely normal. If it is not, referral is indicated, since there are other uncommon forms of patchy baldness. A hopeful prognosis can be given in the first episode if the affected areas are small and localised. No treatment has been shown to be effective and regrowth over several months in almost invariable. Recurrent episodes, extensive hair loss, or a strong family history justify a guarded prognosis and, since hair loss at a young age is so distressing, support from a specialist or the prescription of a wig may be required.

Vitiligo (0.1%)

Can affect any part of the body, but early opinion is usually sought when the exposed parts of the body are affected. Sunlight pigmentation of the normal skin accentuates the effected areas which lack pigmentation. The edge of the lesions have a characteristic curved border. The lesions enlarge and coalesce until fairly extensive areas are affected. There is no safe treatment and camouflage techniques are required. Some dermatology departments have experts to advise on suitable preparations if the local pharmacy's beauty expert is unable to help.

Dermatitis herpetiformis (0.1%)

Occurs on the extensor surface of the limbs and sacrum although typical vesicles (if they have not been destroyed by scratching) may appear anywhere. Since the lesions are so like eczema, the diagnosis is usually confirmed by biopsy and some patients will show a pattern of immunofluorescence. These patients require investigation and supervision by a specialist, since some patients have gluten enteropathy and the drugs used in the treatment of the condition require fine control.

Conditions of unknown aetiology (2.0%)

Pityriasis rosea (0.7%)
Frequently occurs in small outbreaks and usually confers life-long immunity, suggesting an infection by some, as yet unidentified, virus. The eruption is preceded for a few days by a solitary lesion ('herald patch') and then the rest of the eruption appears on the trunk and proximal parts of the limbs. Itching is minimal. The lesions follow a segmental pattern with the long axis of the spots in the line of the dermatome. The lesions are oval, slightly brown, level with the normal skin and have a fine fringe scale. A papular or nodular variant may occur, but the distribution and pattern are characteristic of the more common eruption. VDRL testing should be done in the papular variant. No treatment is required and the eruption clears in 4 to 8 weeks.

Follicular plugging (0.4%)
This condition is common and the doctor is seldom consulted for this abnormality. It is discussed in the section on ichthyosis (p. 246).

Milium cysts (0.3%)
Appear on the cheeks and around the eyes in young adult females. The patient can be shown how to open the lesions with a sterile needle and express the white contents.

Nail dystrophy (0.1%)
Can occur in the presence of eczema, psoriasis, tinea infection, chronic paronychia or lichen planus. In some cases there is no other skin disorder and no history of trauma. No treatment can restore normality, but growth of the nail may gradually result in a normal appearance.

Hair fall (0.1%)
Occurs all the time, but can be excessive and worrying 3 to 4 months after a normal pregnancy or after a serious illness. It is due to an excessive number of hair bulbs entering the resting phase when the old hairs are loose in the hair follicles. It always remits over a few months and the patient should be reassured and advised to treat the hair with respect until the excessive hair fall ceases.

Geographic tongue (0.1%)
A term that describes areas where there is a loss of the normal papillae. Its extent and site vary, but the affected areas are always smooth and red. No investigations are indicated since normal results will be found. No treatment is effective and remission usually occurs.

Pruritus (0.1%)
Pruritis without any skin or systemic disorder in a psychologically normal patient occasionally occurs. Treatment is the same as for senile pruritus (see p. 257) but the physician should keep an open mind about the possibility of infestation or some more serious systemic disorder.

Unclassifiable (0.4%)
Despite considerable experience, some skin eruptions cannot be given a diagnosis. The early eruptions of a definite disease will eventually declare their true nature, while the transient, unclassifiable eruptions will remit.

THE USE OF TOPICAL STEROIDS IN GENERAL PRACTICE

Because they are clean and effective, topical steroids are the mainstay of treatment for pruritic and eczematous conditions in general practice. Because they are so useful, the pharmaceutical industry made them stronger and flooded the market with new preparations. Gradually, it became obvious that the stronger preparations had side effects and the worst side effects occur when they are used inappropriately. An over-reaction has occurred and there is confusion regarding the strength of steroid which should be used.

INDICATIONS

The following conditions respond to the application of topical steroids: constitutional eczemas, irritant and allergic dermatitis, stasis eczema, neurodermatitis, pruritus vulvae and ani, eczematised scabies (after treating the infestation) and psoriasis affecting the hands and feet, flexures, face and scalp.

CONTRAINDICATIONS

Topical steroids must never be used alone when there is infection, or the risk of infection, whether bacterial, viral or fungal. The secondary infection of an eczema or dermatitis is best treated with topical or systemic antibiotics before a topical steroid is prescribed. Acne, rosacea and peri-oral dermatitis are much more difficult to treat when fluorinated steroids have been prescribed. The dry skin (xeroderma), which may persist after atopic eczema, remits, and the frankly scaling skin of ichthyosis does not require steroids, unless scratching causes eczema. Psoriasis of limbs and trunk may seem to improve with the use of topical steroids, but recurs promptly when treatment is discontinued. Recurrence can then be extensive and unstable with the possibility of pustular or exfoliative psoriasis developing.

POTENCY

There is considerable variation in potency of the available topical steroids. The British National Formulary and MIMS have tables indicating the potency of each preparation and the practitioner should select one from each group and become familiar with its use. Some bases (10% urea or 'oily' cream) enhance the potency of the steroid, or are effective in their own right and promote speedier resolution of the eruption.

TOPICAL STEROIDS PLUS ADDED AGENTS

The pharmaceutical industry has presented a bewildering array of combinations of topical steroids and antiseptic or antibacterial agents. Most of the antiseptics are faint yellow dyes and the patient should be warned about their effect on clothing. A combination of 1% hydrocortisone with an antiseptic or antibiotic/antifungal combination is appropriate in napkin rash and in the flexures. Some of the more recent additions to this range of products combine 1% hydrocortisone with an all-purpose, non-staining agent which is effective against most infections. These preparations are a welcome addition for use in general practice.

THE QUANTITY REQUIRED FOR ONE WEEK'S TREATMENT

Unlike swallowing a tablet or 10 ml of medicine, it is necessary to explain to patients that topical steroid preparations must be rubbed into the skin slowly and firmly and that an adequate amount should vanish into the skin. The following amounts should be adequate for 1 week's treatment:

Face	15–30 g
Hands	30–60 g
Limbs	30–120 g
Groins	15–30 g
Napkin area	30–60 g
Trunk — Infant	30–200 g
Adult	100–500 g

SIDE-EFFECTS

Side-effects are local at the site of application. The destruction of connective tissue results in thinning of the dermis, and a consequent loss of support for the dermal blood vessels. Systemic side-effects due to absorption of the corticosteroid are more likely to occur when potent steroids are applied to inflamed areas and in infants and children where the surface to mass ratio is reduced.

Local side-effects
1. Due to local destruction of connective tissue:
   a. Striae
   b. Telangiectasia
   c. Bruising
   d. General transparency of the skin.
2. Acneiform eruption.
3. Growth of hair.
4. Extension or exacerbation in severity of rosacea and peri-oral dermatitis.

Systemic side-effects
1. Cushingoid appearance with gross overuse.
2. Stunting of growth in children.
3. Delayed puberty.
4. Impaired ability to cope with physical stress.

THE APPROPRIATE TOPICAL STEROID

The choice of steroid depends on the site of the eruption, since the epidermis is thicker over some areas than others, the age of the patient and the extent of the eruption, and on the severity of the eruption and its cause. Potent remedies may be appropriate to treat acute, non-recurring eruptions, whereas in long-term eruptions their use would be contraindicated except for occasional use in acute exacerbations.

Age

Infancy	1% hydrocortisone
Toddlers	1% hydrocortisone: rarely, dilute fluorinated steroid on limb flexures.
Children	1% hydrocortisone: occasionally dilute fluorinated steroid on limbs and trunk and fluorinated steroid on limb flexures, hands and feet.
Teenagers and adults	1% hydrocortisone: dilute fluorinated, or full-strength steroids on limbs or trunk: clobetasol propionate on hands and feet.

Site

	Normally
Face	1% hydrocortisone possibly
Axillae	with an antiseptic.
Groins	Rarely — if very acute (and in psoriasis).
Perineum	Dilute fluorinated steroid.
Limbs and trunk	Dilute or full strength fluorinated steroid, depending on severity.
Palms and soles	Fluorinated steroid or clobetasol propionate if acute.

GUIDELINES FOR USE OF TOPICAL STEROIDS

1. The patient should be instructed how to apply the treatment: application more frequently than twice daily is appropriate only when the eruption is very acute. The topical steroid is removed by washing and, in neurodermatitis, by scratching.

2. The steroid appropriate to the severity and site of the eruption and age of the patient should be prescribed.

3. Fluorinated steroids should be prescribed for as short a time as possible and their use should be reviewed periodically. Tragic errors can be made when they are prescribed as 'repeat prescriptions' without clinical review.

4. Avoid the use of fluorinated steroids on the central third of the face for more than 2 weeks.

5. Avoid the extensive application of fluorinated steroids in infancy and childhood.

REFERENCES

Fry L 1978 Dermatology, 2nd edn. Update Publications Ltd, London
Fry L 1982 The G.P. and the specialist — dermatology. British Medical Journal 284: 1093–1094
Levine G M, Calnan C D 1974 A colour atlas of dermatology. Wolfe Medical Books, London
Neville E A, Finn O A 1975 Psoriasiform napkin dermatitis — a follow-up study. British Journal of Dermatology 92: 279–285

Allergic conditions

INTRODUCTION

The term allergy has come to be used increasingly loosely and many patients will use this description for any unwanted effect of a drug, for a foodstuff which causes a minor digestive upset or simply for something which they dislike! In this chapter allergic conditions are considered to be those which involve a Type I or anaphylactic reaction where an antigenic substance reacts with antibody(IgE) on the surface of an already sensitised mast cell. The progress triggers the release of histamine and other vasoactive substances from their 'packaged whorls' within the cell. As with other branches of medicine it is not possible to clearly separate this immunological reaction from the ever present and powerful psychological influences of which we are aware in our day-to-day clinical work. Nowhere is this more dramatically demonstrated than in the much publicised cases of 'total allergy syndrome'. With this background of misunderstanding concerning causative mechanisms and possibly strong psychological overtones, allergic conditions pose a real challenge to the general practitioner, both in terms of diagnosis and investigation and also in management and therapy. Such conditions are well suited to management by the general practitioner with his unique knowledge of the patient, his family and his background. The investigation and treatment of most allergic conditions can be carried out entirely within a general practice setting affording considerable satisfaction to the doctor and convenience for the patient.

FAMILY BACKGROUND AND PAST MEDICAL HISTORY

The triad of asthma, eczema and hay fever has long been recognised. The 'atopic' individual may have an increased family history not only of these three conditions but of urticaria, food allergies, drug allergies and severe reactions to stinging insects. Provision of a haptotype which is protective against allergy is confined to only a minority of the population; the majority of people are at risk of allergy throughout their lives. There is no clear familial pattern to these illnesses and what determines who will, or will not, experience allergy is not well understood. In the patient with an obviously allergic condition a family background or past medical history is of interest only — in the patient with an ill-defined illness, such information may provide an essential clue to the correct diagnosis. Breast feeding is thought to be a protective factor in respect of allergic diseases and it would seem reasonable to add this to the already impressive list of good reasons why ante-natal patients should be encouraged away from artificial feeding.

CLINICAL PATTERNS OF ALLERGIC DISEASE
(Table 21.1)
The antigen challenge may take place on the surface of the respiratory tract (hay fever, asthma), on the surface of the gastro-intestinal tract (food allergy) or may be systemic (insect bites).

Asthma is fully dealt with elsewhere in this book (Ch. 11) as are skin problems (Ch. 20), these conditions will not therefore be discussed in depth.

HAY FEVER

The somewhat inaccurate title of 'hay fever' encompasses both seasonal allergic rhinitis and conjunctivitis although 'fever' is not a feature of the condition and 'hay' may not

Table 21.1 Clinical patterns of allergic disease

Asthma
Allergic rhinitis — seasonal
                             perennial
Skin manifestations — eczema
                                      urticaria
Food allergy — milk allergy in infants
                       ?migraine
                       ?depressive illness
Drug allergy — penicillin
Bites and stings

be involved at all in many cases. Wind-borne pollen from grasses is the common allergen and insect-pollinated plants such as roses and flowers which have relatively heavy pollen are not involved. Tree pollen is a source of trouble in spring while moulds and spores tend to cause autumn exacerbations. House dust mite may be involved throughout the year possibly with spring and autumn peaks.

Rhinitis — and its causes — can be thought of in terms of a spectrum in which hay fever, or the response to a specific allergen, is at one end, and vasomotor rhinitis, which may be compared to asthma, at the other. Patients with vasomotor rhinitis will give negative results to sensitivity tests but many, who fall in the middle of the spectrum, may react to some allergens. It is important to emphasise that all these patients share the common characteristic of an unstable nasal mucosa which is sensitive to a wide range of chemical irritants, which will provoke symptoms. These might include cigarette smoke, paint smells, perfumes and are not themselves mediators of an antigen–antibody reaction; it is inaccurate to say 'I am allergic to smoke'. The unstable nasal mucosa is also acutely sensitive to changes in humidity and this alone may precipitate a bout of sneezing.

Clinical features of hay fever

The basic clinical features of allergic rhinitis and allergic conjunctivitis are well known. Sneezing, blocked nose, watery nasal discharge and itchy, red, watering eyes may occur separately or in combination. Itching of the palate and ears may be troublesome. 30% of hay fever sufferers may experience wheezing and breathlessness at some time. The correct diagnosis may not be obvious in some cases and less common presentations should not be forgotten. Persisting coughs, sore throats and even sinus headache may be overlooked as clues to an allergy. Many atypical presentations occur in children when a more accurate early diagnosis could have beneficial effects on the doctor's long-term management of their problems.

FOOD ALLERGY

Food allergy is a relatively new area and many doctors are understandably dismayed by the potential range of allergens and conditions to which they might contribute.

Milk allergy in infants has long been described and has to be considered as an explanation for vomiting of feeds, albeit rare. The management of such cases usually involves avoidance of cow's milk altogether.

Food allergens are now being implicated in atopic eczema, urticaria, migraine, asthma and even depressive and other psychological illnesses. Diagnosis in such cases is exceedingly difficult and, if the doctor is successful in identifying a responsible allergen, dietary modification resulting in its total exclusion is often virtually impossible to ensure. Accurate food diaries are essential in the elucidation of such cases but possibly the most important stage is simply clinical suspicion that such a problem may exist.

A more dramatic presentation of food allergy is exemplified in the acute anaphylactic reaction which may follow ingestion of shellfish.

STINGING INSECT ALLERGY

Wasp and bee stings are a common problem of the summer, and more particularly, the autumn months. Most are simple local reactions to the insect venom and it is important that topical antihistamines and local anaesthetic preparations be avoided as they regularly lead to a skin sensitisation which is much more severe and unpleasant than the reaction with which they were intended to deal. Of much more importance is hypersensitivity to such stings which can lead to potentially fatal anaphylactic reactions. Such severe reactions may be the result of multiple stings in the vicinity of wasps' nests or beehives but may also be the result of an extreme allergy to such insects. The management of severe anaphylactic reactions is dealt with later in this chapter but once such individuals are identified they should as far as possible avoid any potentially dangerous situations. It may be advisable for them to carry emergency medication for use should the need arise. It is now possible to test patients for allergen specific IgE mediated against such stinging insects using the RAST test to be described below.

DRUG ALLERGY

One sometimes has to ponder just how accurate are patients' histories of 'penicillin allergy' which are all too commonly described, but the possible consequences of giving the drug to a truly allergic patient are so great that most doctors prefer to err on the cautious side. It is however unfortunate that once a patient is labelled as 'penicillin allergic' he is then denied not only phenoxymethypenicillin (penicillin V) but all relatives of the molecule including the ampicillin 'family' and all the extremely useful 'anti-staphylococcal' penicillins. An annoying bout of antibiotic diarrhoea is not 'allergy' nor is the oral or vaginal thrush which sometimes follows antibiotic therapy. One should then avoid labelling a patient 'allergic' to a drug such as penicillin unless this does indeed seem to be the case. A very useful variant of the already mentioned RAST test can determine whether a patient is indeed allergic to the two main determinants of penicillin allergy (see below). The management of any allergic reaction to a drug starts by stopping the drug immediately and simple oral antihistamines will often be more than sufficient to deal with the problem. Emergency measures to deal with acute anaphylactic reaction may be needed in extreme cases.

INVESTIGATIONS FOR THE GENERAL PRACTITIONER (Table 21.2)

CLINICAL HISTORY

No apology is necessary for mentioning once again the importance of a good clinical history. The doctor must be prepared to listen patiently to the patient's own description of his problem and his suggested explanation although this may often be somewhat bizarre. The history may or may not give an all important clue to the offending allergen. Commercially produced clinical allergy history sheets are available which may help the doctor to concentrate on the most useful aspects of such an exercise.

Table 21.2 Investigations for the general practitioner

Skin tests
RIST (Measurement of total IgE)
RAST (measurement of allergen specific IgE)
Measurement of nasal airways resistance

SKIN TESTS (PRICK TESTS) (Table 21.3)

A skin testing outfit is a useful item for the general practitioner's surgery and can consist of a basic set of allergens or may be a comprehensive stock of skin testing solutions. The usefulness of such equipment depends to some extent on the doctor's own interest and experience in this field; it has the disadvantages of being time consuming, somewhat unpleasant for young patients in particular and providing results that are often difficult to interpret. It has been suggested that the practice nurse might carry out these procedures but she must be fully trained in the technique and be able to deal with any

Table 21.3 Suggested useful selection of skin testing solutions

D. pteronyssinus (house dust mite)
House dust
Feather mix
Cat
Dog
Tree mix (early blossoming)
Tree mix (mid blossoming)
Grass mix
Flower mix
Weed mix
Fungi mix

untoward reaction. If the nurse is involved in these tests or in desensitisation injections a doctor must be readily available.

RIST AND RAST TESTS (Figs. 21.1 and 21.2)

These extremely useful tests are likely to become more widely used in general practice as they become better known and more widely available from local laboratories. Both tests can be carried out from one single small venous blood sample. They are unfortunately significantly more expensive than skin tests and this has to be borne in mind.

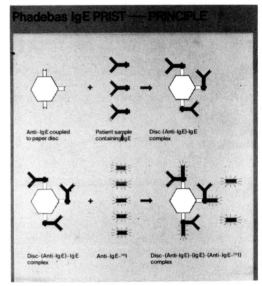

Fig. 21.1 RIST test

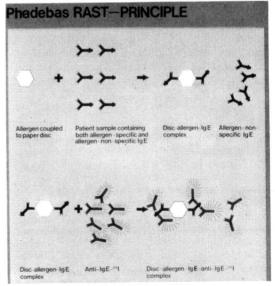

Fig. 21.2 RAST test

The Radio-immunosorbet test (RAST) measures allergen specific IgE and is available for a wide range of allergens including grasses, trees, weeds, moulds and spores, house dust and house dust mite. RAST results are reported in Classes 0–IV as shown in Table 21.4. A small panel of allergens can be tested for initially including the commonly positive substances such as grass, house dust mite and cat epithelium along with a total IgE measurement (using RIST). A negative result in the presence of an elevated total IgE (i.e. more than 100ku/litre) suggests that the responsible allergen or allergens have not been tested for.

Variants of the RAST test are available for stinging insect allergy and for penicillin allergy. It is becoming increasingly obvious with experience that serial measurements of both total IgE and allergen specific IgE are more useful than are isolated tests.

Table 21.4   Classification of RAST results for allergen-specific IgE

Class 0	Undetectable level	
I	Low level	
II	Moderate level	
III	High level	'Positive result'
IV	Very high level	

OTHER INVESTIGATIONS

A method of measuring nasal airways resistance which could be used in the general practitioner's surgery may be available in the forseeable future. Such a measurement could be useful in monitoring the response to treatment in the same way as peak expiratory flow rates are used to monitor lung function. This latter investigation may of course be appropriate in more severe cases of hay fever where there is a degree of pollen asthma.

Other investigations which include nasal provocation tests, blood or nasal eosinophil counts and nasal RIST/RAST tests do not lend themselves to routine use and are more appropriate for research laboratory type investigation.

Table 21.5   Management of allergic conditions

Avoidance measures	
Antihistamines	— oral
	intramuscular
Sodium cromoglycate	— nasal
	inhaled
	oral
	ophthalmic
Corticosteroids	— nasal
	inhaled
	parenteral
	(ophthalmic)
Desensitisation	

MANAGEMENT OF ALLERGIC CONDITIONS
(Table 21.5)

The measures available to deal with allergic conditions can be considered to fall into two broad groups; general or non-specific measures, and specific measures. An example of the former is systemic steroid therapy and of the latter nasal sodium cromoglycate.

AVOIDANCE MEASURES

It seems logical that where a patient has a diagnosed allergy to a substance they should, as far as possible, avoid that allergen. This is, however, often impractical and sometimes almost impossible. Measures designed to reduce exposure to house dust mite may make a considerable difference to a patient's asthma, hay fever or even urticaria but attempts to exclude specific food allergens from the diet are often worthless. Sensible advice should be a balance giving consideration to how seriously unwell the patient is as a result of the allergy and to how disruptive to the patient's normal lifestyle such avoidance measures may be.

ANTIHISTAMINES

The usefulness of antihistamines should not be underestimated when dealing with allergic problems. These drugs are non-specific in their action and act as H_1-receptor blockers so that the prescription of an antihistamine must always be accompanied by a sensibly worded caution in respect of possible drowsiness or alcohol potentiation. The response to these drugs is extremely individual and with some consideration it should often be possible to find a preparation with which sedation is not especially troublesome. Many preparations are available from the pharmacy without prescription and patients can be advised to use such remedies when this is an appropriate decision to take.

SODIUM CROMOGLYCATE

Sodium cromoglycate prevents the release of histamine and other vasoactive substances through the mast cell membrane following sensitisation of the cell. Sodium cromoglycate is topically active and works specifically on the respiratory epithelium, nasal mucosa, conjunctiva or intestine, according to the form of therapy used. This form of treatment is primarily prophylactic and its effect is short-lived. Continuous use five or six times each day is recommended for hay fever and initiation of treatment when symptoms are already established is less effective.

Treatment for any length of time is expensive. Sodium cromoglycate is accepted as an extremely effective drug in allergic asthma.

CORTICOSTEROIDS

Corticosteroids — specifically beclomethasone or betamethasone — by inhalation or nasal spray are useful and widely accepted forms of treatment. This is particularly true of beclomethasone. Continuous medication is important and oro-pharyngeal moniliasis is an occasional complication of inhaled steroids. Oral, and on occasion, intravenous steroids are acceptable in severe asthma unresponsive to other forms of treatment but the use of systemic steroids in hay fever is seldom advisable. Although long-acting triamcinolone injection is used with success repeated requests for such therapy may be a problem.

DESENSITISATION

Desensitisation is specific therapy in the sense that only allergic problems resulting from the allergens in the desensitising vaccine used are being treated. The limitations involved where more than one or a small number of allergens are involved have long been recognised. 'Blind' desensitisation therapy, where proper identification of responsible allergens has not been carried out, should not be performed. This form of treatment is probably more commonly carried out in hay fever where commercial pressures to use a readily available desensitisation course are considerable. Such courses are expensive, often time consuming, and can be potentially hazardous involving as many as 18 injections, and adding a not inconsiderable extra burden to the NHS drugs bill. Experience with a large population of hay fever sufferers raises serious doubts as to the overall usefulness of such therapy. This does not however apply to patients who have had anaphylactic reactions to bee or wasp stings, for whom an effective treatment is now available in the form of graded doses of venom. There is also the suggestion, from work at Great Ormond Street, that injections of dust mite vaccine can now be used effectively in the treatment of asthmatic children with dust-mite sensitivity.

Table 21.6 lists some commonly available desensitisation vaccines. Specific manufacturer's instructions for each product should be followed carefully. Precautions against serious anaphylactic reaction must always be followed. Not only adrenaline injection B.P. but also syringe, needle and tourniquet should be readily available. In the event of such a reaction occurring adrenaline injection 0.5–1.0 ml (0.5–1.0 mg) should be given by the subcutaneous or intramuscular route and repeated if necessary.

EYE PREPARATIONS

Allergic eye connditions (allergic conjunctivitis, vernal conjunctivitis) may or may not occur in conjunction with another system involvement, such as allergic rhinitis. Antihistamine therapy may be of considerable help in this condition but a more specific therapy such as an ophthalmic solution of sodium cromoglycate is also available. Considerable caution must always be exercised before using corticosteroid eye preparations although these may afford considerable relief to a severely inflamed eye that is the result of an allergic reaction.

Table 21.6 Desensitising vaccines

Proprietary name	Type of vaccine	
Alavac-P	Alum precipitated	
Allpyral-G	Alum precipitated	
Norisen grass	Aluminium adsorbed	Grass and Tree Pollens
Pollinex	Tyrosine adsorbed	
Spectralgen 4 Grass Mix	Aqueous solution or Alum precipitated	
Spectralgen 3 Tree Mix	Aqueous solution or Alum precipitated	
Allpyral D. pteronyssinus	Alum precipitated	
Allpyral mite fortified house dust	Alum precipitated	House dust mite
Migen	Tyrosine adsorbed	
Alavac-S	Alum precipitated	
Allpyral specific	Alum precipitated	
Norisen	Aluminium adsorbed	Patient specific
SDV	Aqueous solution	
Spectralgen Single Species	Aqueous solution or Alum precipitated	
Pharmalgen	Freeze dried venom — wasp or bee sting allergy	

ANAPHYLACTIC SHOCK AND ANGIO (NEUROTIC) OEDEMA

Such acute reactions may result from bee or wasp sting, injected vaccine or, occasionally, ingested food allergen. These conditions are of sudden onset and life threatening and the doctor must be prepared to deal with them quickly and efficiently. As mentioned above, adrenaline injection 0.5–1.0 ml, subcutaneously or intramuscularly, should be given. Intravenous corticosteroid such as hydrocortisone hemisuccinate (100 mg) or dexamethasone sodium phosphate (20 mg) can be life-saving.

An injectable antihistamine such as chlorpheniramine (10 mg) can be given by the intramuscular route. Care of the airway and observation of vital signs should be carried out and cardio-respiratory resuscitation performed should this become necessary.

CONCLUSIONS

Allergic conditions offer the general practitioner the opportunity to assess, investigate, and treat the patient often to their mutual satisfaction. There are however many pitfalls in dealing with such conditions which may range from the mildly annoying to the life-threatening.

For the future considerable interest centres on oral mast cell stabilisers and on long-acting antihistamines free from cerebral side-effects.

RECOMMENDED READING

Harland R W 1979 The management of hay fever in general practice. Journal of the Royal College of General Practitioners 29: 265–286

Lessof M H 1982 Allergy, 2nd edn. Update Postgraduate Centre Series, London

Wood S F 1982 Hay fever and its management in general practice. Medicine in Practice 1: 262–265

Diseases of the eye

INTRODUCTION

Diseases of the eye form a small but important part of the family doctor's workload. Pain in the eye or a disturbance of vision can be distressing and worrying to the patient who may fear that permanent damage to his sight will result. Usually patients seek help soon after symptoms develop and this allows a diagnosis to be made and treatment to be started early in the course of the disease. Delay in diagnosis can occur in the elderly who may assume incorrectly that deterioration in vision occurs due to old age, when organic disease is in fact present. Patients may overlook uniocular loss of vision until they happen to cover the good eye when washing.

The eye conditions most commonly seen are bacterial infections which are most prevalent in young children and the elderly. Injuries which are usually superficial occur at all ages, particularly to those working in heavy industry or engaged in home maintenance without safety glasses. Inflammatory disease, such as iritis, is potentially more damaging if early diagnosis is not made and the associated conjunctival inflammation is mistaken for that of bacterial infection. The uncritical use of steroids in eyedrops is particularly hazardous as their administration in keratitis of viral origin can lead to blindness.

An accurate diagnosis must, therefore, always be made in this group of diseases and an early specialist opinion should be sought if the true cause of the patient's symptoms is in doubt.

EQUIPMENT AND EXAMINATION TECHNIQUES

It is most important to obtain a clear and close-up view of the surface of the eye. A good quality magnifying loupe with a focusing torch should be used, and a binocular loupe mounted on a headband will be found valuable as it leaves one hand free to steady the patient's head and the examiner's crouching body.

The visual acuity should be measured using the Snellen test types, or one of its modifications such as the Sheridan Gardner test. The surgery should be arranged to allow the use of this with a reversing mirror if space is short. In the patient's home, rough testing with newspaper print can be used to compare his vision to that of the examiner.

A small supply of drops used in investigation is necessary. Single-dose units such as Minims are ideal and a short-acting mydriatic such as tropicamide 0.5%, pilocarpine 2% as a miotic and 1% amethocaine should be kept ready for use. Dry fluorescein — impregnated strips (e.g. Fluorets) — and chloramphenicol ointment should also be available.

A good ophthalmoscope will have bright even illumination and be reasonably robust. Several makes are available, some combined with an auriscope, and the pocket-sized ones have some advantages for the general practitioner. The best view of the fundus will be obtained in a darkened room where the patient should be instructed to fix his gaze on a picture or something similar.

To examine the right eye the doctor should use his own right eye and hold the instrument in his right hand supporting it also against his own superior orbital margin. By approaching within 2 inches (5 cm) of the patient's eye, the widest possible angle of view of the fundus will be obtained. To examine the left eye, the observer holds the ophthalmoscope in his left hand and uses his left eye.

In old age the pupil becomes smaller and an adequate view can be obtained only after instilling a mydriatic. There is then the risk of inducing angle-closure glaucoma in a susceptible eye and 2% pilocarpine should be used after the examination.

LIMITATIONS OF FUNDUS EXAMINATION

The family doctor will be able to diagnose marked hypertensive vascular changes as well as the haemorrhages and exudates of background diabetic retinopathy. He may see other local changes in the fundus very infrequently and will find their diagnosis difficult. Myopic fundi are difficult to visualise with the direct ophthalmoscope, and the indirect opthalmoscope in the hands of the more experienced will yield a better view. Practising in the use of the direct instrument will pay dividends in obtaining improving results.

CHILDHOOD COMPLAINTS

INFLAMED EYES AND WATERING EYES

In the first few weeks of life, a frequent complaint is of sticky, watery eyes. Examination shows mucus at the inner canthus: the condition is inclusion conjunctivitis caused by chlamydia and it is relieved by tetracycline used as an ointment. More persistent stickiness accompanied by watering indicates congenital blockage of the tear drainage ducts. Pressure with one finger on the skin below the inner canthus may cause the reflux of mucus or pus into the conjunctival sac. By the age of 6 months most cases resolve spontaneously as canalisation of the epithelial cords represnting the ducts occurs. Management consists of temporising with frequent expression of the tear sac followed by antibiotic drops. Syringing and probing the ducts under general anaesthetic can be undertaken after 6 months.

Infants are occasionally seen with gross conjunctival congestion and a copious purulent exudate. This is usually staphylococcal rather than gonococcal in aetiology, but bacteriological swabs should be taken to identify the cause. Energetic treatment is needed as the thin cornea of the neonate can quickly ulcerate and perforate. Topical and systemic antibiotics should produce rapid improvement.

SQUINTS

In the first few months of life the grosser congenital ocular anomalies become apparent. At first, eye movements are random and squint is normal but after a few weeks binocular fixation occurs and the visual axes become aligned. By about 2 months the child fixates moving objects and gazes around the room. Where vision is markedly subnormal, a coarse 'searching' pendular nystagmus develops which may be accompanied by an obvious squint. Weakness of the extraocular muscles shows as asymmetry of the gaze, usually in the horizontal meridian. Suppression of the image in one eye enables the child to avoid troublesome diplopia and a constant squint develops. The aim of treatment is to achieve full visual acuity in each eye with binocular single vision, but unfortunately success is often denied despite early and enthusiastic efforts. Occlusion to force a 'lazy' eye into use will usually be ordered, and an ophthalmic surgeon should be consulted to examine for abnormalities such as cataracts

or congenital scars of the macula, as well as to detect refractive errors which may cause a squint. Examination of the fundus will also exclude the rare but highly malignant retinoblastoma which may interfere with vision and hence cause a squint.

The majority of squints arise when the child becomes more active and interested in detail — between 2 and 4 years. Such squints are apparent in all positions of gaze and there is no extraocular muscle palsy. There may well be a family history of squint, lazy eye or refractive error. Squints may be intermittent initially, being present only when the child is tired, and if convergent, they tend to become constant. Divergent squints are less common and are more frequently intermittent.

DIAGNOSIS OF SQUINT

Some squints are very obvious but in doubtful cases the best simple test is the 'cover test'. The child is encouraged to look at a small attractive object held at normal reading distance — a cartoon character cut out and glued to a tongue depressor is very suitable (a flashlight should be used only if the child will not look at anything else). The examiner then blocks the view from one eye by covering it with a plain card, meanwhile closely watching the uncovered eye. If it was fixing properly it would not move, but if a squint is present the eye moves to take up fixation. The test is then repeated on the other eye and the result noted. There may be no squint present, or a unilateral or bilateral ('alternating') squint.

TREATMENT OF SQUINT

It is important that parents realise that not only is a squint present, but that vision is often impaired, and both aspects require treatment. Occlusion, glasses where indicated, and for some, operation, are the stages to be undertaken. For some, with early treatment a good functional result can be obtained but, for most, some improvement in visual acuity and a cosmetically acceptable appearance are all that can be achieved.

COMMUNITY ASPECTS

A systematic effort is made to detect squints and eye defects by the Health Visitor when visiting an infant at home or during later developmental examinations. Formal vision tests are customary at 5, 7 and 13 years, but there are some advantages in routine tests at 3 or 4 years to replace that at 5. Preschool testing is less likely to cover such a high proportion of the child population however. Where defects are found, the child is referred to an ophthalmologist. Colour vision is also tested at one of the school examinations but there is, of course, no treatment in cases of defect.

THE DIFFERENTIAL DIAGNOSIS OF THE PAINFUL OR RED EYE

This is a worrisome diagnosis for most practitioners. The circumstances may suggest an injury and appropriate action is discussed later in this chapter.

The history is important and can help to establish the diagnosis together with a careful and systematic external examination. The distribution of the vascular congestion often indicates the origin of the disorder. Congestion of the ciliary vessels which surround the cornea suggests corneal or intraocular trouble; conversely congestion deep under the lids suggests conjunctivitis. External examination should include eversion and inspection of the conjunctival surface of the upper lids. Most often, a watering and painful eye is caused by a minor injury or a dendritic ulcer of the cornea.

HERPETIC KERATITIS

Cases of herpetic keratitis presenting *de novo* often give a history of recent coryza. Recurrent ulcers appear for no apparent reason, the eye being irritable and the vision only slightly impaired. There is some ciliary congestion. In established cases, corneal sensation is reduced and touching the cornea with the corner of a tissue fails to elicit a normal blink reflex. However, the only way to make the diagnosis is to visualise the ulcer and this may not be possible without staining the cornea with fluorescein and using the slit-lamp microscope as early lesions produce only a tiny area of epithelial disturbance which cannot otherwise be detected. The branching appearance of a typical ulcer is diagnostic of a herpes simplex infection.

OTHER FORMS OF KERATITIS

Bacterial infection of the small corneal abrasions which follow trauma is common unless topical antibiotics are used early in treatment. The eye is painful and ciliary congestion is marked. There is usually a macroscopic grey patch of corneal infiltrate with a central depression or slough. If severe, there may be a fluid level of pus in the anterior chamber. Peripheral corneal infiltrates also occur in clusters and may be associated with acne rosacea.

CONJUNCTIVITIS

It is easy to recognise bacterial conjunctivitis. The eye is sore with a gritty sensation. There is copious purulent secretion which encrusts the lashes and the eye is uniformly red except in the palpebral aperture. Cases without pus formation are likely to be caused by a virus, frequently Adenovirus type 8. The possibility of herpes simplex infection should be remembered and slit-lamp examination is indicated.

IRIDOCYCLITIS

A sore or aching eye with photophobia and ciliary congestion may have iridocyclitis. The pupil is constricted, the cornea is clear, watering is uncommon and vision is only slightly reduced. Adhesions between iris and lens causing irregularity of the pupil are pathognomonic, but diagnosis usually requires slit-lamp microscopy to see the opalescent aqueous and the inflammatory cells it contains.

ACUTE GLAUCOMA

The diagnosis of established congestive glaucoma is not difficult. Pain in the eye and the supraorbital region is constant, severe and nauseating. Vision is markedly reduced and halos are seen round lights. The pupil is semi-dilated, vertically elongated, non-reactive and the cornea lacks lustre and becomes oedematous. Ciliary congestion and general conjunctival injection are extremely marked.

OPTIC NEURITIS

Optic neuritis also produces pain but only on movement of the eye, especially upwards and sidewards. The eye is white, the pupil is only moderately dilated and is non-reactive or reacts poorly to light. It constricts readily if the fellow eye is illuminated (consensual reflex). Vision is markedly reduced often to 'hand movements' and sometimes there is no light perception.

DIPLOPIA

In adolescents and young adults a complaint of double vision is most commonly due to the breakdown of a pre-existing extraocular muscle imbalance and is thus not of sinister significance.

Cover testing may reveal a squint, but a full evaluation is beyond the scope of general pratice and orthoptic treatment is possible. Trauma to the face and head causing nerve palsy or entrapment of extraocular muscles is another cause of diplopia. Less commonly, double vision in young people is the result of demyelinating disease or myasthenia gravis. Diplopia with facial pain may be due to an intracerebral aneurysm. Older people often complain of double vision when they mean blurring of vision due to uncorrected refractive errors which may occur with early cataract formation. Extraocular muscle palsies quite commonly produce diplopia in elderly people and these are associated with degenerative cerebrovascular disease, hypertension or diabetes. The prognosis for spontaneous recovery is generally good.

INJURIES

MINOR INJURIES

While minor corneal injuries are seen frequently in general practice, conjunctival injuries are relatively uncommon, and symptoms are not severe.

The history may suggest an injury, but it must be remembered that misplaced or loose lashes produce intrinsic trauma. Lashes rubbing the cornea, subtarsal foreign bodies and corneal foreign bodies produce a lot of pain, watering, blepharospasm and photophobia, as well as ciliary congestion. Grit blown into the eye on a windy day may lodge under the upper tarsal plate, scratching the cornea with every blink.

It is often hard to locate a small corneal injury or foreign body, and fluorescein from an impregnated strip of filter paper (Fluoret) dipped in the conjunctival sac will help. The dye stains the epithelial defects bright green, making them more readily visible especially in blue light. A corneal foreign body will look dark against the coloured background of the iris, and should not be confused with an iris freckle. Movement of the observer's head will throw the corneal lesion into apparent relief due to parallax.

TREATMENT OF ULCERS

Unless there is a definite history of injury, all corneal abrasions, ulcers and staining areas should be regarded with the greatest suspicion. If the patient has had a recent cold or 'flu they are probably herpetic lesions. If the eye is but slightly affected, herpes simplex keratitis is the most likely diagnosis. A large ulcer in a really painful injected eye is seldom of viral origin. Steroids should *never* be used when a corneal ulcer is seen or even suspected, but chloramphenicol or another broad spectrum antibiotic in ointment form can be applied safely. If the eye is watering, relief is obtained by closing it and covering it with a gauza pad held by adhesive tape for 12 hours. The pad should be removed as soon as watering stops and this allows frequent topical treatment to be given.

REMOVING FOREIGN BODIES

A good light, and adequate magnification are essential. The cornea is very tough and the chances of puncturing the cornea while removing a particle are very slight. A few drops of amethocaine 0.5% are instilled and the removal accomplished with a sterile disposable large-gauge needle after spreading the lids with the thumb and forefinger of one hand. The conjunctival fornix is filled with antibiotic ointment and the eye padded for 12 hours. If removal has been incomplete, a further attempt may be made in 3 days, using antibiotic ointment in the interval.

MAJOR INJURIES

The signs of a major injury to an eye are not necessarily obvious but all such cases should be immediately referred to an eye unit. Where there is a history of trauma, the following features will suggest a serious eye injury:

1. Reduction of visual acuity. Defective sight preceding the accident should not be assumed without corroboration.
2. Cloudy cornea, hazy aqueous humor or visible blood in the anterior chamber.
3. Immobile, irregular or tremulous pupil.
4. Shallow or absent anterior chamber. This may be combined with a visible corneal wound, a peaked pupil and the iris included in or herniating out of the wound.
5. Visible white lens opacity indicating rupture of the lens capsule.
6. History of sudden brief pain in the eye when using hammer and chisel or high speed drill. Even if the eye appears to be normal there may have been a perforating injury.

SUDDEN LOSS OF VISION

Sudden blindness in one eye is commonly due to either central retinal artery occlusion or to ischaemic optic neuropathy caused by temporal arteritis. The latter diagnosis will be suggested by finding a grossly elevated ESR compatible with systemic collagen disease. Blindness in the fellow eye in this condition can be averted by systemic steroid treatment: an ESR estimation is mandatory in all cases of sudden uniocular blindness in adults.

In patients with sudden gross reduction in vision, the commoner diagnoses are ischaemic neuritis, central retinal vein thrombosis, vitreous haemorrhage and haemorrhage at the macula. These incidents are associated with degenerative vascular disease and are common in diabetics and elderly people. Retinal detachment is another possible diagnosis which tends to be commoner in high myopes and is seen, occasionally, at all ages. The patient can often describe a definite grey blanked-out or curtained area in the visual field of the affected eye.

Rapidly progressive visual loss with severe pain is generally due to acute glaucoma but may accompany a severe exudative iridocyclitis. Retrobulbar neuritis also produces a rapidly progressive visual loss which may be bilateral and is accompanied by a variable amount of pain on eye movement only.

A peculiar type of visual loss which may escape recognition is that of homonymous hemianopia due to cerebrovascular ischaemia. This condition is not uncommon in elderly people and there is often no associated limb or facial weakness. The patient is usually unable to read and often blames his reading glasses or his optician, a he is quite unable to identify his disability. When examined in the consulting room he may be able to read test type well.

It must be especially remembered that the patient may innocently think that his uniocular visual loss is of sudden onsent, simply because he has had ocasion to shut his sound eye and has only then discovered his disability. The late effects of gradual loss of vision may thus become suddenly apparent.

SLOW DETERIORATION IN VISION

This is an encyclopaedic subject. In youth, severe progressive myopia, conical cornea, congenital macular dystrophies, congenital glaucoma, retinitis pigmentosa and neoplastic lesions involving the optic pathways should all be considered. In older people cataract, senile macular degeneration, chronic simple glaucoma, diabetic retinopathy and vitamin B_{12} deficiency (toxic amblyopia) are the common diagnoses. It is often difficult for the practitioner to decide whether some visible cataract is the entire cause of the visual deterioration. Pigmentary changes at the macula may be hard to see and expert evaluation is necessary. Diabetic retinopathy will be suspected in the known diabetic or from testing the urine and making the discovery of diabetes hitherto unsuspected.

Toxic amblyopia is almost always the the result of prolonged heavy pipe smoking in elderly men. Serum B_{12} levels may or may not be reduced and the response to parenteral hydroxycobalamine may be rapid or slow to appear.

Chronic simple glaucoma is not a disease that declares itself: it tends to be discovered at a late stage when vision has already failed in one eye. Disc cupping is often a relatively late sign which may be detected by an alert optician during routine refraction for reading glasses. Tonometry is a technique that requires practice and is not generally performed outside a hospital clinic, and full visual field examination requires time and special skill. Near relatives of glaucoma patients should be screened for the disease using the ophthalmoscope, the applanation tonometer and field-measuring instruments.

SPECTACLES AND REFRACTIVE ERRORS

Children seldom complain of poor eyesight but considerable defects are frequently found and corrected only after routine testing. On the other hand, insecure young adults, especially women, suffer headaches and ill-defined 'eye-strain' which they ascribe to refractive errors. In later years many recall being given spectacles at this time which they later discarded.

Emmetropes will generally need glasses for close work during the later fourth or fifth decade, but those who are slightly hypermetropic will need glasses some years earlier. It should be remembered that premature presbyopia may be a symptom of glaucoma. Bifocals or lenses with a continuously variable focal length (e.g. Varilux) are available for presbyopes who also need a distance correction. The latter are subject to some peripheral spherical aberration, but with perseverance this disadvantage can usually be overcome.

Ordinary refractive errors in adults are fairly stable over a period of years but there tends to be a slow change in the axis of astigmatism so that occasional refraction checks are justified. Lens sclerosis and early cataract alter the situation entirely and frequent changes in correction then become necessary.

After cataract operations, thick heavy convex glass lenses are frequently dispensed which are uncomfortable to wear and tend to make the glasses slip forward on the face. These difficulties can be minimised by choosing a frame with a relatively small diameter of lens, and by using plastic lenticular lenses which, however, add a little to the cost and are more easily scratched.

Microcorneal contact lenses are effective in the correction of many larger refractive errors. Their use in the correction of low myopic errors for cosmetic reasons is less frequently justified. Contact lenses are well tolerated after cataract operations and, except where an intraocular lens implant has been used, provide optimum correction. They made binocular vision possible in uniocular aphakia and give good vision in high myopia and irregular astigmatism. 'Soft' contact lenses are only used where the patient is unable to tolerate a hard lens and they are less durable in use.

BLUNTED SIGHT

Patients with permanently defective sight can be provided with visual aids. Some are helped by reading glasses of increased strength and light-weight magnifying lenses are available through the hospital service or can be purchased comparatively cheaply. Telescopic spectacles are preferred to hand magnifiers by those requiring additional help, and have the advantage that both hands can be used to hold the book or newspaper. Children become adept at the quick scanning movements required by the small field available with the enlarged image. Large print books are very useful and are available from all public libraries.

Persons who are so visually handicapped that they are unable to perform work for which sight is necessary should be registered as blind. The commonly accepted degree of defect is 3/60 in the better eye, but those with field defects may qualify with a better acuity than this. The decision should be made by an eye specialist. Registered blind persons are eligible for a number of welfare benfits including a supplementary pension, an income tax allowance, talking books from the British Talking Book Library and travel concessions on public transport services. White sticks are provided and a blind person may apply for a guide dog, and learn Braille or Moon.

Less severely handicapped patients may be eligible for registration as 'partially sighted'. Their benefits are restricted to talking books and retraining for suitable employment.

Specially trained social workers keep in touch with registered patients and the responsibility for this lies with the Local Authority Social Work Department. Blind children need much attention and care, and should be spoken to much more than usual. It is advisable to keep them at home until school age and then they usually go to residential schools for the blind. Partially-sighted children may be taught in the local school with reading aids and some special teaching methods, but in some cases they may go to a special school for the partially-sighted. Decisions about schooling should be taken after discussions involving people from the education authority and the hospital eye service and a community physician has a useful co-ordinating role.

Persons blinded in adult life can get advice on employment from the social workers for the blind or the disablement resettlement officers of the Department of Employment. Class or individual instruction in Braille or Moon embossed type, typing and handicrafts is available in all areas. Rehabilitation is furthered by residence at centres where retraining in appropriate trades is available. Future employment may be in the community in ordinary occupations or in one of the sheltered workshops for disabled persons.

RECOMMENDED READING

Bedford M A 1971 A colour atlas of ophthalmological diagnosis. Wolfe, London

Chawla H B 1981 Essential ophthalmology. Churchill Livingstone, Edinburgh

Gardiner P A 1979 ABC of ophthalmology. British Medical Association, London

Jackson C R S 1975 The eye in general practice, 7th edn. Churchill Livingstone, Edinburgh

Lim A S M, Constable I J 1979 Colour atlas of ophthalmology. Kimpton, London

Trevor-Roper P D 1980 Lecture notes on ophthalmology, 6th edn. Blackwell, Oxford

Trevor-Roper P D 1981 Pocket consultant of ophthalmology. Grant McIntyre, London

Ear, nose and throat problems

INTRODUCTION

The range of ear nose and throat problems in general practice varies considerably, depending largely on the age of the patient. In the pre-school child most ENT problems are of an infectious origin while disturbances of hearing predominate in the elderly. In all age groups symptoms referable to the ear nose and throat are commonly presented as part of a respiratory tract infection.

TONSILS AND ADENOIDS

FORM AND FUNCTION

The tonsils and adenoids, part of Waldeyer's ring of lymphoid tissue guarding the entry portals to the respiratory and digestive tracts, enlarge in childhood to each a maximum size at about the fifth year, then dwindle to insigificant proportions by the tenth year.

The structure of both tonsils and adenoids provides a large contact surface between epithelium and the contents of the pharyngeal lumen. This is achieved in the adenoids by an arrangement of longitudinal folds, whilst the tonsils bear some 20 branched crypts which greatly increases their surface area.

The functions of the lymphoid tissue include:

1. Manufacture of lymphocytes.
2. Filtration — removal of micro-organisms, bacterial toxins extravascular proteins and foreign articles from lymph.
3. Cellular defence against infection: plasma cells and small round cells, fibroblasts and macrophages are derived from lymphocytes. Lymphocytes themselves probably play only a small phagocytic role, but provide proteolytic enzymes, and are a source of antibodies.
4. Antibody synthesis — in plasma cells.
5. Lymphoid tissue incorporates reticulo-endothelial elements capable of active phagocytosis.

The pharyngeal lymphoid tissue, it seems, collects micro-organisms from the nasal passages and mouth, manufactures antibodies, and absorbs and modifies their toxins, then releases them to the reticulo-endothelial stem throughout the body where they stimulate major antibody production.

In the early years of life, as increasing numbers of 'first time' organisms enter the nose and mouth, the tonsils and adenoids are the site of vigorous and important immunological activity — reflected by the brisk hypertrophy at this age. By the end of childhood their task is complete.

TONSIL AND ADENOID PROBLEMS

Tonsils and adenoids may give rise to difficulties in two principal ways:

Infection

Tonsils and adenoids are sometimes casualties to overwhelming infection. Repeated infections may lead to fibrosis, and micro-abscesses may form, so walled off by fibrous tissue as to be inaccessible to natural immunity processes or to antibodies in the blood stream.

Mucus glands open into the tonsil crypts and their secretion gently flushes the crypts, helping to remove infection and debris. In the lingual tonsils these glands open at the bottom of the crypts, but in the faucial tonsils they open further up the crypts leaving a 'dead space' below. This difference may explain why the faucial tonsils are much more liable to troublesome infection than are the lingual tonsils.

Chronically infected tonsils harbour large numbers of organisms — more than 10^5 per gram of tissue. These are mostly non-pathogenic, a-streptococci and Neisseria predominating (Brook et al 1980). They are associated with complaints of sore throat with fever and malaise more than seven times yearly (Saski & Koss 1978). Adenoids behave similarly (Kueton et al 1982).

Although non-pathogenic organisms are abundant in chronically infected tonsils, pathogens including Group A b-haemolytic streptococci are present in a minority. A distinction must be made between 'surface' and 'core' isolates. In one study (Brooke et al 1980) Group A b-haemolytic streptococci were isolated almost twice as often from the tonsil core after tonsillectomy than from the tonsil surface. Negative throat swabs are therefore an unreliable guide to tonsillar flora. Many of the aerobic and anaerobic organisms isolated from tonsils removed following recurrent tonsillitis are b-lactamase producers, capable of preventing penicillin from eradicating Group A b-haemolytic streptococci. Alternative antibiotics such a lincomycin, clindamycin or oxacillin may be preferable to penicillin since they are effective against b-lactamase producing organisms as well as against streptococci.

Tonsils and adenoids may cause morbidity — even mortality — on account of their size alone.

Better understanding of the threat posed by large tonsils and adenoids began with a report in 1966 (Luke et al) of four children with severe respiratory difficulty resulting from enlarged tonsils and adenoids. All had cardiac enlargement and were cured by adeno-tonsillectomy.

By 1974 Jaffee was able to collect five cases seen within a year of cor pulmonale and congestive cardiac failure, all corrected by removal of tonsils and adenoids. He suggested that less extreme degrees of obstruction must be common. This has been emphasised more recently be Freeland of Oxford (1981) who examined the ECGs of 95 unselected children awaiting tonsillectomy. Three showed right atrial hypertrophy with tall P waves — corrected by operation (Fig. 23.1). Such children with severely enlarged tonsils and adenoids are dull, drowsy, and when asleep breath noisily with periods of apnoea.

POPULARITY OF TONSILLECTOMY

The call for removal of troublesome tonsils is not a modern phenomenon — Cornelius Celsus described a technique for tonsillectomy in the first century AD. Following the advent of anaesthesia tonsillectomy was increasingly performed until by the middle of this century over 200 000 operations were carried out annually in England and Wales. By 1977 this figure had fallen to approximately 100 460, according to estimations based on figures reported by the Office of Population Consensuses and Surveys of the DHSS. Marked regional variations in tonsillectomy operation rates were noted — 242.2 per 100 000 in Yorkshire, for example, against 178.4 per 100 000 in East Anglia. Tonsillectomy is still overall the commonest operation performed.

Tonsillectomy carries a mortality of about 1 per 25 000 — a figure that has remained remarkably constant despite technological advances.

Several reasons may account for the declining popularity of tonsillectomy:

1. Improved living conditions and general health.
2. Increased appreciation that tonsils and adenoids perform a useful role.
3. Increased awareness of the 'natural history' of tonsil and adenoid problems, with a strong tendency to spontaneous resolution.
4. It could also be argued that early administration of antibiotics in tonsillitis has brought about quicker

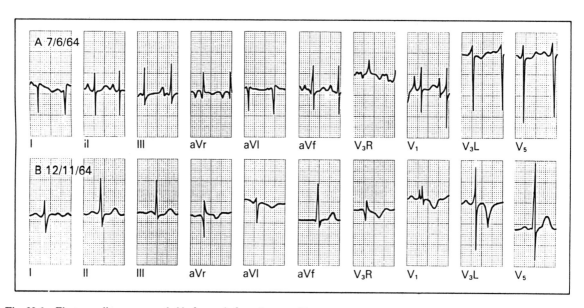

Fig. 23.1 Electrocardiograms recorded before and after adenotonsillectomy

resolution of infection with less permanent damage to tonsillar architecture.

Indications for tonsillectomy

Wood (1973) gives the following indications for tonsillectomy:

1. Repeated attacks of tonsillitis after scrutiny of school record, attack rate, throat swab and serum IgA determination (25% of children suffering recurrent sore throats have a deficiency of IgA and can be expected to continue to have sore throats whether or not their tonsils are removed).
2. Quinsy.
3. Recurrent tonsillitis with otitis media, as in 1.
4. Evidence of chronic streptococcal infection (especially when acute rheumatism has occurred).
5. Gross obstruction of the air passages.

In view of the discrepancies already noted between surface and core bacteriology, throat swabs are an unreliable guide to the presence of chronic infection. Attack rate too can be a misleading yardstick — Paradise (1978) followed up for a year 65 children with at least seven episodes of throat infection in one year, five in each of two consecutive years, or three in each of three years. He found that 43 experienced either no further infections or at the most only one or two infections, mostly mild. Only 11 conformed to the previously reported pattern. The occurrence of quinsy usually implies such a degree of infection, and such damage to tonsillar architecture, as to render further problems almost certain.

Indications for adenoidectomy

Adenoidectomy may be urgently needed where size embarrasses respiration. The value of the operation in the management of middle ear problems is much more controversial. Thus whilst Jordan (1963), discussing the prevention of recurrent otitis media, holds the view 'Adenoidectomy is the first and most important step to be taken in preventing recurrences', Sadé (1979) comments 'Only a large scale, preferably prospective, study could demonstrate conclusively whether adenoidectomy has any minor therapeutic effect or none at all'.

MANAGEMENT OF TONSIL AND ADENOID PROBLEMS IN GENERAL PRACTICE

Protagonists of medical care and of adeno-tonsillectomy in the management of children with recurrent upper respiratory problems have occasionally adopted polarised positions with almost evangelical zeal. The general practitioner is confronted with a confusing array of evidence and opinions, and is obliged to evolve his own policy. Individual circumstances, local facilities, and parental attitudes and expectations influence management.

The author's own approach is to explain to parents the 'natural history' of adeno-tonsillar problems in childhood, emphasising the strong tendency to resolution after the age of 5 to 6 years. Early administration of oral penicillin in more pronounced upper respiratory infections is desirable, in order to minimise structural damage to tonsils from secondary bacterial invasion. Referral for tonsillectomy purely on grounds of infection is seldom necessary. However where enlargement gives rise to airway restriction adeno-tonsillectomy is urgently called for.

OTITIS MEDIA

Otitis media requires prompt treatment with antibiotics to minimise pain and to reduce the risk of perforation of the tympanic membrane and long-term ear damage. The principal pathogenic organisms encountered are *Streptococcus pneumoniae* and *Haemophilus influenzae*. Penicillin V is highly effective for the former, but not for the latter. The consensus reached at a recent international symposium 'Recent Advances in Antimicrobial Therapy for Infection of the Ear, Nose and Throat' (Klein 1981) was that ampicillin, amoxicillin, sulphonamide combined with oral or intramuscular penicillin, erythromycin, cotrimoxazole and cefaclor (Distaclor) are all suitable initial treatments for otitis media. Where significant improvement has not occurred within 48–72 hours a change of antibiotic is indicated.

OTITIS EXTERNA

Otitis externa may lead to conductive hearing loss either by blockage of the external meatus with debris (desquamated epithelial cells, inflammatory exudate, and products of bacterial or fungal overgrowth), or by inflammatory swelling of the meatal walls leading to occlusion of the lumen.

Otitis externa is often part of a generalised eczematous tendency. Excessive exposure to water is a frequent cause. Normally wax secreted by the ceruminous glands (which are confined to the outer third of the meatus) dries and is shed imperceptibly. Frequent entry of water into the external meatus prevents this drying, and encourages accumulation of wax. The normal 'self-cleansing' mechanism furnished by epithelial migration is thus prevented. The resulting warm moist unventilated recess provides an ideal breeding round for bacteria and fungi.

TREATMENT OF OTITIS EXTERNA

This is primarily mechanical. The meatus must be cleaned regularly — every day at first in severe cases. All debris must be removed. This can conveniently be achieved by mopping, using frequently changed pledgets of cotton wool mounted on a Jobson Horne probe. At the beginning of this toilet process it may be helpful to take a swab of the discharge for bacteriological examination. Gentleness is essential, in order to preserve the patient's co-operation. A lamp and head mirror greatly facilitate the procedure.

Where there is much inflammatory swelling of meatal walls insertion of a wick is helpful. Dry gauze should not be used since it tends to stick to the meatus and may be very painful to remove. The gauze may be impregnated with bismuth and iodoform paste, magnesium sulphate and glycerine paste, or an antibiotic/steroid mixture such as Fucidin hydrocortisone ointment.

Once the meatus is clean, suitable topical applications help to combat infection and reduce inflammation. Steroid/antibiotic ointments are commonly used. The risk of development of antibiotic sensitivity, particularly to neomycin, must be borne in mind.

The presence of fungal elements in the debris will usually have been suspected at first inspection — or may come to light with the bacteriology report. Topical antifungal agents such as clotrimazole cream (Canesten) would then be appropriate. Alternatively. nystatin is available as a powder, to be introduced with an insufflator.

For some patients otitis externa is a recurrent problem, and they should be advised to return for toilet of the ear immediately they are aware of discomfort.

GLUE EAR

GENERAL DESCRIPTION

Glue ear is a term first introduced by Jordan of the USA in the 1960's to describe a form of secretory otitis media virtually confined to the age group 6 months to 10 years in which the middle ear beomes filled with sticky thick mucoid material, leading to deafness.

The condition is very common. In a recent study (Tos et al 1982) a type B tympanogram, usually indicating middle ear effusion, was found in 28.6% of apparently healthy 2-year-old children. In a group of healthy four year olds, glue ear or a middle ear pressure of 200 mm H_2O or less making glue ear a likely development was found in 73%. In the light of such figures serous otitis media would appear almost 'normal' at this age. Another feature of glue ear highlighted by this study was the strong tendency to spontaneous recovery — the children were re-examined at 3-monthly intervals and between 78 and 88% were found to have improved. Glue ear fluctuates widely in many children, periods of hearing impairment ending spontaneously to be followed by intervals of good hearing.

Affected children are frequently 'catarrhal'. Their deafness tends to impair emotional, social and academic development. They are often noisy and disobedient (because they cannot hear properly). Misunderstandings with parents and teachers may lead to much unhappiness.

The great majority of affected children make a complete recovery after a period varying from a few months to 2 to 3 years. A small proportion — 0.5% in the above study — do not recover fully, and it is now believed that chronic suppurative otitis media usually arises as a consequence of such permanent tympanic damage.

AETIOLOGY

The aetiology of glue ear remains uncertain. Eustachian obstruction, infection, and allergy have all been incriminated.

Eustachian obstruction

Eustachian obstruction has been known for over two centuries to cause middle ear effusion. In animal experiments obstruction of the Eustachian tube leads to accumulation of serous fluid within a day or so. In patients suffering from Eustachian obstruction progressive negative pressure from air absorption results in transudation from mucosal capillaries of a fluid resembling serum. Anoxia of the epithelium develops, ciliary action is impaired, and metaplasia occurs with an increase in secretory and goblet cells. Subsequently the character of the effusion changes, with an increase in protein and potassium content, accumulation of cells including epithelial cells, lymphocytes and macrophages, and of enzymes (such as dehydrogenases, alkali phosphatase and lysozyme), complement, prostaglandins, and IgA, IgE, IgG and IgM.

Under normal conditions oxygen and nitrogen in the middle ear cavity diffuse into the mucosa creating slight negative pressure. The Eustachian tube is normally closed at rest. During swallowing contraction of the levator palati muscle, attached to the floor of the tube, results in opening of the tube lumen, permitting entry of air to fill the relative vacuum.

Children with cleft palates lack such normal levator palati function — and they almost invariably suffer from glue ear. This observation strongly supports Eustachian obstruction as a cause of glue ear.

INFECTION

Fluid aspirated from the middle ear cavity of patients suffering from glue ear is usually sterile on bacterial culture, and efforts to isolate viruses have generally been unsucessful. In one survey (Klein & Teele 1976) viruses — principally respiratory syncitial virus and influenza virus — were isolated from 29 (4.4%) of 663 middle ear effusions. It is believed by some that infection may frequently play in the initiation, if not the persistence, of glue. However a history of documented acute otitis media is lacking in most glue ear sufferers.

A recent study of middle ear effusions (Juhn 1982) reported positive cultures from fluid aspirated from ears of infants under 1 year. The percentage of positive cultures fell as the age group of the children studied increased. At the same time an increase in IgA and IgG content was noted. The evidence supports infection as an aetiological agent. The increase of immunoglobulins and decrease of percentage of positive cultures suggest that middle ear defence mechanisms develop with age.

Allergy

Allergy was thought by Jordan to play a major role in glue ear. Some investigators (Velt & Sprinkle 1976) have interpreted the immunological features of mucoid effusions as indicating a type II immune complex mechanism. Measurement of specific IgE to house dust mite and grass pollen revealed higher levels in children with glue ear than in a control group (Khan et al 1981). A retrospective study revealed atopy to be twice as common in children with glue ear as in matched controls (Schutte et al 1981).

It is uncertain whether allergy, if it is an important cause of glue ear, makes its contribution mostly by obstructing the Eustachian tube from mucosal swelling, or by causing allergic exudate in the middle ear.

DIAGNOSIS

Diagnosis of glue ear depends primarily upon the index of suspicion and efficiency of the auroscope of the general practitioner.

Children with glue ear may present with recurrent colds, catarrh, earache, noisy behaviour, poor school performance, behaviour disorders — or may be brought because their parents or teachers suspect hearing loss. The condition is often quite unsuspected.

On examination the tympanic membrane is seen to lack normal translucency, the outline of the long process of the incus running parallel, behind, and deep to the handle of the malleous being indiscernible through the drum. The drum itself may take on a variety of hues. Inflation using a rubber bulb attached to the auroscope confirms the immobility of the tympanic membrane. Sometimes the tympanic membrane is grossly retracted — the handle of the malleous may then be pulled up into a more horizontal position and the indrawn tympanic membrane may be seen to be wrapped round the long process of incus and incudo-stapedial joint.

The hearing of children old enough to co-operate may be checked by whispering at 3 feet from the ear — the quietest whisper should normally be audible.

Tuning fork tests reveal a 'negative Rinne' — bone conduction being better than air conduction.

By the age of 4, and sometimes earlier, it may be possible to record a pure tone audiogram.

Acoustic impedence audiometry

Essentially this is a test of the 'stiffness' of the tympanic membrane, and is widely used in hospitals and hearing clinics. It has the advantage of being objective, and therefore available to the youngest age groups. Nowadays the recording is performed automatically by a 'middle ear analyser'.

A plug is placed in the child's external meatus, carrying three tubes. Basically one tube is connected to a sound source, another to a microphone, and the third to a manometer. The analyser varies the pressure in the external meatus progressively from negative to positive, whilst a tone is repeatedly presented and the 'reflected' sound energy measured and recorded automatically.

Examples of normal, negative middle ear pressure and glue ear recordings are shown (Figs. 23.2, 23.3 and 23.4).

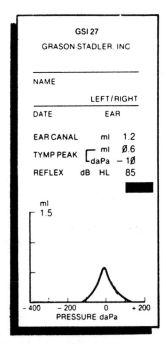

Fig. 23.2 Tympanogram of a normal ear

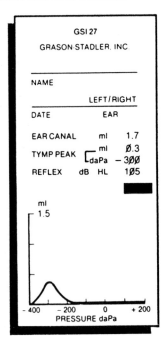

Fig. 23.3   Tympanogram of an ear with negative preessure

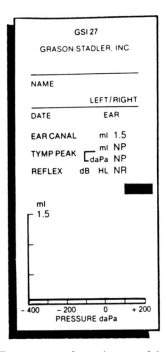

Fig. 23.4   Tympanogram of an ear in a case of glue ear

Screening

Considerable time and expense has been devoted to screening children for glue ear, but practical difficulties have marred the outcome. Too often pure tone audio-

grams have been recorded without prior removal of wax. The middle ear analyser has proved too sensitive — too large a sample of children are picked out by this method, many of whom prove on further investigation to have normal ears. Furthermore, in view of the notoriously fluctuant nature of glue ear, random screening will result in many patients being tested during 'good' intervals and thereby missed. Screening was discussed by eminent international authorities at a Research Conference on Recent Advances in Otitis Media with Effusion in 1977. The Panel noted the continuing uncertainty surrounding aetiology and advantages of treatment of glue ear, and decided that it could not recommend mass screening for the condition.

MANAGEMENT

Since the aetiology of glue ear is uncertain, the condition is liable to resolve spontaneously, and possible long-term harmful effects of treatment are uncertain, firm guidelines for management are difficult to construct.

Treatments advocated include:

1. Steroids, oral or topical.
2. Salicylates or other drugs with anti-prostaglandin effect.
3. Antihistamines.
4. Decongestants.
5. Hyposensitisation (allergy therapy).
6. Mucolytic agents.
7. Politzeration
8. Adenoidectomy.
9. Mastoidectomy.
10. Myringotomy with suction.
11. Tympanostomy tubes (grommets).

Of these measures myringotomy with insertion of grommets produces the most immediate improvement in hearing. However the studies of Sadé (1979) confirm that this benefit is only temporary and that after 6 to 12 months there is no significant difference between the hearing of children who have been left untreated, having merely had a grommet inserted, have had a grommet plus aspiration of glue, or have had aspiration of their glue, a grommet inserted, and adenoidectomy.

It has to be decided therefore whether the benefits of temporary hearing gain outweigh the risks and disadvantages of surgery in each indivdiual case.

One disadvantage of grommet insertion is that swimming has been thought inadvisable. However in a study of 100 children encouraged to swim with their grommets (Jaffee 1981) only three had any subsequent trouble. These developed otorrhoea, which quickly cleared up with ear drops or oral penicillin, and they returned to swimming with no further trouble. All the children had been instructed to put three drops of neomycin/polymyzin/hydrocortisone solution in the ear at bedtime each day that they had been swimming. None had used ear plugs or bathing caps. It would seem unnecessary to prohibit children with grommets from swimming.

In the present state of knowledge a reasonable management plan for glue ear would seem to be:

1. Where hearing loss is not severe — say less than 30 dB at speech frequencies — the upper respiratory tract should be rendered as healthy as possible, with antibiotics, usually penicillin -V where indicated. Regular observation should be made every 1 or 2 months, and a decongestant/antihistamine such as Dimotapp elixir should be prescribed.

2. If hearing loss is over 30 dB and remains so for a few months despite medical treatment the child should be referred for myringotomy and probably insertion of grommets.

The interested general practitioner, with access to audiometry, is the best person to supervise management of children not undergoing surgery. The patient's interests are best served if general practitioner and specialist know one another well enough to co-operate closely.

PERFORATION OF THE TYMPANIC MEMBRANE

When perforation occurs during the course of acute otitis media (a rare happening if treatment is started early), the opportunity to take a swab of the discharge for determination of bacterial sensitivity should be taken. Subsequent antibiotic therapy can then be managed with greater confidence. The possibility also now exists of introducing topical antibiotics into the middle ear cavity. A mixture of chloramphenicol and steroid drops (commercially available as Otopred) is particularly suitable (other antibiotics — especially the aminoglycosides — are potentially ototoxic and better avoided).

Once infection is resolved in acute otitis media, perforations usually heal. Most persisting perforations are in fact long-standing and chronic.

CHRONIC PERFORATIONS OF THE TYMPANIC MEMBRANE

Chronic perforations fall broadly into two groups — central, and marginal.

Central performations are characteristic of tubotympanic chronic suppurative otitis media. Once dry, repair of the perforation by the operation of tympanoplasty should be considered, in order to improve hearing, close a potential route for re-infection, and render swimming a safe pursuit.

Marginal perforations tend to involve the superior and posterior rim of the tympanic membrane. They denote attico-antral disease — a form of chronic suppurative otitis media commonly associated with cholesteatoma formation. Because of this potentially life-threatening complication, such cases should always be referred for full ENT work-up. Surgical exploration of the middle ear or mastoid may be needed.

HEARING PROBLEMS IN ADULTS

Following surveys carried out at Cardiff, Glasgow, Nottingham and Southampton, statistics produced by the Institute of Hearing Research indicate that some 10 million people in this country suffer from some degree of deafness — and over half of these also experience tinnitus.

CAUSES OF DEAFNESS

Chronic suppurative otitis media
This problem has declined dramatically in incidence during the last 20 years, due largely to modern treatment of ear infections with antibiotics.

Noise induced hearing loss
Codes of practice and legislation have been only partially successful in combating noise exposure in industry. Recommendations are not always heeded by management or by workers, and in addition individual susceptibility to noise trauma is considerable, marring the effectiveness of blanket measures. Many older men are hard of hearing as a result of war service, game shooting or target shooting without ear protectors, and frequent attendances at discos produce a toll of hearing loss.

The general public remains surprisingly complacent about the hazard of noise-induced deafness and the general practitioner can play an important educating role. The recording of an audiogram will often bring home to a patient at risk the need to avoid further unnecessary noise trauma.

Otosclerosis
Otosclerosis is the commonest cause of progressive hearing loss in young adults. The incidence is between 3 and 5 per 1000, and the condition often runs in families. Diagnosis is usually easy — any adult with deafness, normal looking tympanic membranes, and negative Rinne responses on tuning fork testing can be referred to an ENT surgeon with a fairly confident diagnosis of otosclerosis. Characteristic audiograms and tympanograms will support the diagnosis (Fig. 23.5). Since 1960 the outlook for sufferers from otosclerosis has dramatically

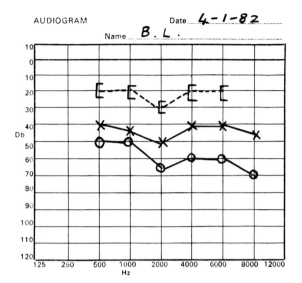

Fig. 23.5 Audiogram in a case of otosclerosis. [--[right ear bone conduction, X---X left ear air conduction, O---O right ear air conduction.

improved with the introduction and development of stapes surgery. For several years many operations were performed whilst the existing 'otosclerosis population' was treated. This is now a mere trickle of new patients presenting. Considerable skill and continuous practice are required for good surgical results to be achieved, and there are now insufficient patients to provide all would-be surgeons with adequate experience. General practitioners may serve their obtosclerosis patients best by referring them to major centres where sufficient clinical material to maintain experience in this shrinking field is available.

Menière's disease
Patients with Menière's disease — a recurring triad of vertigo, deafness and tinnitus described by Prosper Menière of Paris in 1861 — are usually more distressed by the vertigo than by the hearing loss. The doctor however appreciates that the vertigo is self-limiting and amenable to treatment, and tends to be more concerned over hearing loss, which may be progressive and eventually severe. Prolonged administration of betahistine (Serc) appears to benefit some cases and should always be tried. Some authorities, particularly in the USA, believe that a saccus decompression operation should be offered to all patients with continuing symptoms in an endeavour to prevent further hearing loss. Here again the general practitioner may consider referring the patient to a major centre where such surgery is being regularly undertaken. In most patients the disease runs such a mild and short course that medical management alone is adequate.

Deafness may complicate many diseases including de-pression, syphilis, myxoedema, meningitis, Paget's disease and diabetes. Its severity may reflect the standard of care of the disease concerned. Although many drugs are ototxic — especially the aminoglycoside antibiotics, and powerful diuretics given intravenously in high doses — ototoxicity has been more a hospital than a general practice problem.

A substantial but unquantifiable proportion of deafness has a heredity basis. It is common, and in many ways desirable, for two deaf people to marry — they are likely to best understand one another's problems. It would be exceedingly rare for both partners to share the same genetic defect as a cause of their deafness, and surveys have shown no greater incidence of deafness in the offspring of two deaf parents than in those of unions where one parent had normal hearing.

Rubella
Rubella, and in this country to a much lesser extent syphilis, continue to cause congenital deafness. Thanks to the National Health Service system, whereby each doctor has a known list of patients, it is possible to identify all girls of child bearing age, and to ensure, by rubella antibody testing, that they are immune for (or in the case of syphilis, sero-negative). Most girls will have been seen for contraceptive advice when the opportunity should be taken to check rubella antibody status. The age-sex register will serve to ascertain the remainder, who can be summoned for testing. All non-immune patients should be immunised — with 3 months contraceptive cover — and a satisfactory immune response confirmed by a repeat blood test a month later.

Reliance cannot be placed on school pre-pubertal rubella immunisation programmes. Some girls are absent on the injection day, there is no attempt to confirm acquisition of immunity by a subsequent blood test (and faulty 'dud' vaccine batches are not uncommon) and in any cause acquired immunity may have attenuated to ineffective levels by the age of family raising.

Anoxia
Intra-partum anoxia is an important cause of congenital hearing loss (Taylor 1980). The general practitioners preventive role lies in good ante-natal care and the guiding of high risk patients to the best equipped obstetric units.

Presbyacusis
By the sixth decade presbyacusis is emerging as the major cause of hearing loss. It is estimated that one in six of the population over 60, and one in three over 70 need a hearing aid — yet nothing like this number are provided. By the time they require a hearing aid many patients have additional handicaps — arthritis, blindness, general slowness, and faulty co-ordination. Coping with the tiny controls on the hearing aid, flat batteries, fractured leads,

and badly fitting inserts with irritating feed-back may prove daunting. The signals reaching the brain from the degenerated cochlea are liable to be very distorted. It is little wonder that so many patients leave their aids in a drawer. The general practitioner can usually best help by negotiating a fresh visit to the local hearing aid clinic.

Wax

Wax seldom increases hearing loss by more than 20 dB. This is of little significance to a person with normal hearing but to the hearing-impaired this added loss may be crippling. The best drops for softening wax prior to syringing appear to be sodium bicarboanate ear drops BPC. Patients wearing hearing aids seldom accumulate large amounts of wax, but often harbour sufficient wax to block the insert. Removal by mopping with a pledget of cotton wool on a Jobson Horne probe is usually most satisfactory.

CONSEQUENCES OF HEARING LOSS

The handicap of blindness, manifest by dark glasses and a white stick commonly elicits sentiments of sympathy, compassion and the urge to help. Deafness, on the contrary, tends to be either unsuspected — in which case the sufferer may be dismissed as uncommunicative — or else provocative of irritation and even exasperation. It is understandable that many deaf patients become unhappy, depressed, withdrawn and increasingly isolated.

In the family circle they may be unable to participate in the 'cut and thrust' of conversation, and their only hope of communication may be in a 'one to one' conversation with somebody willing to allocate a little time to them.

At work deafness may constitute a severe handicap, especially in tasks involving dealing with the public. It is surprising how successful many patients are in concealing their deafness in a bid to retain their job. Danger exists where heavy machinery is involved, and the deaf are always at risk in traffic.

Recruitment causes added distress to patients with deafness due to cochlear disease — particularly presbyacusis. The phenomenon may be explained in terms of cochlear hair cells. These are arranged in two rows — an outer row with low thresholds responding to sounds of low intensity and happening to be the most vulnerable to degenerative changes, and an inner, more robust row with high thresholds only stimulated by loud signals. In recruitment the outer lay of the hair cells has degenerated. There is no warning of an increasing sound until the threshold for the inner hair cell row is reached, when a loud noise is suddenly heard. Approaching buses are not heard until they appear on top of the victim, with a thunderous roar. Patients do not hear approaching foot-steps and are startled when spoken to — they may physically jump. Recruitment also causes predictable problems with hearing aids.

The general practitioner can often improve the lot of deaf patients by discussing some of these problems with the whole family.

HEARING LOSS AND THE GENERAL PRACTITIONER

In addition to his work in the prevention and management of specific causes of deafness, the general practitioner will encounter deafness incidentally during consultations over other matters. Deaf patients are sometimes either unaware of their handicap, or assume that nothing can be done about it and that it is therefore best ignored. Clues of such unrecognised deafness include unduly loud or quiet speech, mispronounciation of consonants, or close watching of the speaker's face (lip reading).

Directly question about the possibility of deafness, such patients sometimes appear relieved to be able to discuss the matter — it may have caused them uneasiness for some time.

Clinical examination, including whispering tests at 3 feet, will confirm whether there is indeed a problem, and if so, many indicate the diagnosis. Tuning fork testing (Rinne) is invaluable in separating conductive loss — often amenable to surgery — from sensorineural loss in which an aid is usually the only remedy.

The availability of audiometry facilitates further decisions regarding management. If the hearing loss is well below 40 dB at speech frequencies (1000–2000 Hz) the patient will not be seriously handicapped and surgery or hearing aid provision (for conductive or sensorineural losses respectively) are not often required. If the loss is greater than 40 dB, the patient will have a serious social communication handicap and referral to a surgeon or to a hospital furnished with a hearing aid department will be needed.

Modern technology can improve the quality of life out of all recognition for deaf patients. A wide series of hearing aids (available free through the NHS) provides for different types and degrees of deafness. British Telecom are able to supply variable amplication for telephone ear pieces. Front door bells can be modified to flash electric lights. An invaluable piece of equipment is an induction loop lead for television. Plugged into the set, and led to the deaf person's chair, this can be arranged to induce a signal directly into his hearing aid. Much better sound reproduction results, and the set itself can be turned to a volume convenient to others in the room.

Advice and extensive literature is available from the

Royal National Institute for the Deaf, Gower Street, London.

For the last few years the City Litt Institution in London has been training 10 Hearing Therapists annually. It is hoped that this new category of worker will be attached to the ENT departments of district hospitals to help improve the inadequate and haphazard service at present available to the deaf.

Where family relationships are breaking down as a consequence of severe deafness, the Link Centre in Sussex is able to offer accommodation for the patient and spouse or close relative, and such intensive expert rehabilitation has proved invaluable.

REFERENCES

Brook I, Yocum P, Shah K 1980 Surface v. core tonsillar aerobic and anaerobic flora in recurrent tonsillitis. Journal of the American Medical Association 244: 1696–1698

Freeland A 1981 Airway obstruction from adenotonsillar hypertrophy. British Medical Journal 282: 1579–1581

Jaffee I S 1974 Adenotonsillectomy as the treatment of serious medical conditions: five case reports. Laryngoscope 84: 1135

Jaffee B F 1981 Are water and tympanotomy tubes incompatible. Laryngoscope 91: 563

Jordan R E 1963 Secretory otitis media in the etiology of cholesteatoma. Archives of Otolaryngology 78: 261

Juhn S K 1982 Studies on middle ear effusions. Laryngoscope 92: 287–291

Khan J A, Kirkwood E M, Lewis C 1981 Immunological aspects of secretory otitis media in children. IgE and IgA levels in serum and 'glue'. Journal of Laryngology and Otolaryngolory 95: 121–123

Klein J O, Teele D W 1976 Isolation of viruses and mycoplasmas from middle ear effusions. A review. Annals of Otolaryngology 85: Suppl. 25: 140–144

Klein J O 1981 Microbiology and antimicrobial treatment of otitis media. Annals of Otology, Rhinology and Laryngology 90: Suppl. 84

Kveton J F, Pillsbury H C, Saski C T 1982 Nasal obstruction adenoiditis v. adenoid hypertropy. Archives of Otolaryngology 108: 315–318

Luke M J, Mehrizi A, Folger G M, Rowe R D 1966 Chronic nasopharyngeal obstruction as a cause of cardiomegaly, cor pulmonale and pulmonary oedema. Pediatrics 37: 762

Paradise J L 1978 History of recurrent sore throat as an indication for tonsillectomy. Predictive limitations of histories that are undocumented. New England Journal of Medicine 298: 409–412

Report: Annals of Otorhinolaryngology. Supplement 69. Vol. 89 May-June 1980. No. 3 Part 3: 19–21

Sade J 1979 Secretory otitis media and its sequelae. Churchill Livingstone, Edinburgh

Saski C T, Koss N 1978 Chronic bacterial tonsillitis: fact or fiction. Otolaryngologic Clinics of North America 86: 858–864

Schutte P K, Beales D L, Dalton R 1981 Secretory otitis media, a retrospective general practice study. Journal of Laryngology and Otolaryngology 95: 17–22

Taylor I G 1980 The prevention of sensorineural deafness. Journal of Laryngology and Otolaryngology 94: 1327–1343

Tos M, Holm-Jensen S, Soresen CH, Mogensen C 1982 Spontaneous course and frequency of secretory otitis media in 4-year-old children. Archives of Otolaryngology 108: 4–10

Velt R W, Sprinkle P M 1976 Secretory otitis media. An immune complex disease. Otolaryngology, Rhinology, Larynogology 85: Suppl. 25 KP 2: 135

Wood C B S 1973 Tonsillectomy. Practitioner 211: 713

Psychological illness in general practice

The Knowledge which a man can use is the only real knowledge, the only knowledge which has life and growth in it, converts itself into practical power. The rest hangs like dust about the brain or dries like raindrops on the stone — Froude

INTRODUCTION

Formal psychiatric education is now a standard part of the undergraduate experience. However, it still occupies a modest place in most curricula relative to the size of the problem to be faced in general practice. Even with the introduction of compulsory vocational training, a 4 or 6 month period in psychiatry is not a requirement. However it is now possible to do a psychiatric house officer job at pre-registration level as an alternative to medicine or surgery. Regrettably some rotational schemes have recently dropped psychiatry as one of the elements.

It is likely to remain the case for some time that the majority of general practitioners will have acquired skills through experience rather than through training. Those who have had such training will still find that their hospital-based experience provides only a foundation for the development of the appropriate skills and strategies for primary care.

The main purpose of this chapter will be to highlight aspects of mental ill-health which are significant for general practice and particularly areas which are not covered in detail in standard specialist psychiatric texts. However, a sound basic knowledge of psychiatry is an essential beginning. A useful summary is contained in *Notes on Psychiatry* (Ingram et al 1981).

Beginning with a brief appraisal of psychiatry today, alternative models of mental illness will be considered. A syllabus for general practice will be described before going on to epidemiological considerations. This is followed by a review of types of patient care, including an account of the roles of the professional staff involved in this care. Strategies for management will then be looked at, with a more detailed study of a few conditions. The penultimate section deals with the psychological aspects of physical illness, some of which will have been consi-

dered elsewhere in this book. In conclusion, a possible list of books for a personal library in general practice psychiatry is suggested.

The chapter will not cover child and adolescent psychiatry, psychiatry in the senium, alcoholism or forensic psychiatry, nor will the Mental Health Acts be considered.

PSYCHIATRY TODAY

Psychiatry is not, nor will ever be, a science. As Sir William Osler put it:

Our study is man as the subject of accidents or diseases. Were he always, inside and outside, cast in the same mould, instead of differing from his fellow man as much in constitution and his reaction to stimulus as in feature, we should ere this have reached some settled principles in our art.

The Counsels and Ideals of Sir William Osler, 1906

Anthony Clare in his book *Psychiatry in Dissent* suggests that many current diagnostic formulations state little more than recognition that a given set of symptoms and signs resemble a previously recognised pattern. Even in schizophrenic psychosis the debate on a precise definition continues. The result is that many patients, previously diagnosed as suffering from a schizophrenic psychosis, would today be reclassified. This has implications for the continuing management of this small but important area of general practice work (see p. 312).

There is even some debate as to whether mental illness actually exists. Thomas Szasz, Professor of Psychiatry at the State Hospital of New York in Syracuse, New York, seeks to convince us that there is an absolute distinction between bodily and mental dysfunction. There is, in Szasz's view, no clear mental norm from which deviation can easily be measured and, furthermore, any deviation from physical norms found in so-called psychiatric disorders requires the condition to be classified as a physical disease.

Certainly, reaching a diagnosis in psychiatry is rarely easy. Part of the problem is that individually almost all the symptoms found in psychiatry can be experienced by people who are not ill. However, when these symptoms are taken together to form syndromes, psychiatrists have little difficulty in reaching a high measure of diagnostic agreement on psychotic illness. Agreement on diagnosing neuroses, however, falls far short of that high level.

Psychiatric illness is also to some extent cultural. Thus transvestism in some societies is the deviation of a reversed group. A further example may illustrate this. The Royal College of Psychiatrists has been highly critical of the approach of some psychiatrists in Russia who diagnose mental illness in patients whose essential deviation is in their views of the society in which they live. Yet here in the United Kingdom there are organisations who are highly critical of the compulsory detention of some patients and their consequent management, though it is not suggested that this is done for political reasons.

At the present time there is no clear single model of mental illness. Indeed, Clare describes four possible approaches to mental illness:

— Organic
— Psychotherapeutic
— Sociotherapeutic
— Organic and behavioural disorders

Organic

Here the emphasis is on the role of biological factors together with biochemical and physiological dysfunction. Abnormalities are perceived as being best corrected by the use of drugs or other physical treatment. Until recently the ascendency of this model was reflected in the fact that most consultant psychiattrists qualified with a Diploma in Psychological Medicine (DPM) and Membership of the Royal College of Physicians (MRCP) thus emphasising that a sound knowledge of physical medicine was central to any proper psychiatric practice.

Psychotherapeutic

Here the need for any medical qualifications is quite peripheral to the needs of the individual patient or client whose mental health problems can be explained or understood in terms of dysfunction based upon early development. The influence of Freud, Jung, Erikson, Sullivan and Rogers in modern psychiatry is substantial. Their influence, particularly in the middle part of the 20th century, had a profound effect upon the public's perception of mental illness.

Sociotherapeutic

Social dimensions of the individual's life are regarded as of paramount importance in this model. His ability to cope with relationships at various levels, his role in society both in work and leisure, the attitude of society towards him and his response to its demands: these are the areas where work must be carried out to solve the problems of the patient.

Organic and behavioural disorders

Professor Eysenck has proposed this particular division, which allows doctors to continue to deal with organic problems, leaving clinical psychologists to deal with behavioural disorders.

Most general practitioners in the past would have been quite happy either with the first or the fourth model, but it is clear that an overwhelming majority now regard their role as extending well beyond the diagnosis and treatment of formal psychiatric disorders. In a recent survey of experienced general practitioners in the Avon area, 87% regarded the treatment of emotional problems as a major part of general practice and 42% felt they required further training in this field. If the older general practitioners were excluded from the results, this figure would be very much higher (Whitfield & Winter 1980).

ATTITUDES IN GENERAL PRACTICE

Crombie (1972) in proposing a model of the medical care system stated:

> The first thing a general practitioner has to decide is the relative importance of the emotional and physical factors in his patients' problems. Only the general practitioner approaches the matter quite in this way and his ability to do so depends upon his unique previous knowledge of the patient. Where this knowledge is denied to the doctor an assessment has to be made by the more devious and less certain method of evaluating the emotional component by exclusion of the organic. This method of evaluating the emotional component is clumsy and for the 10 to 20% of selected problems which reach the hospital-based doctor it is unsuitable and wasteful of medical resources.

He went on to say that:

> the organic element is less definable in illness encountered in hospital practice. The emotional element, on the other hand, is more important in general practice.

Perhaps today the word 'psychosocial' should be used in place of 'emotional'.

In the the same year the report of a working party entitled *The Future General Practitioner* (Horder et al 1972) outlined the principal educational objectives and goals in the training of a general practitioner. One of the objectives was stated as being the demonstration of self-understanding. There is an Arabian proverb which begins: 'He who knows not and knows not that he knows not is a fool — shun him'. The same proverb goes on to say: 'He that knows not and knows that he knows not is simple — teach him'. However, sometimes teaching alone will prove insufficient and in this case it is more important for a general practitioner to accept his limitations and not endeavour to undertake work in areas to which he finds himself unsuited.

Reference has been made to the importance of self-understanding in doctors. It has been suggested that general practitioners who feel uneasy in certain areas of practice should probably avoid these areas. However, it is also important that the general practitioner should remain inscrutable in the face of, what are for him, embarrassing presentations. Patients will undoubtedly recognise embarassment or a negative response to their psychological problems.

An example of this is in the management of sexual problems. In taking a sexual history it is important that any mutual embarrassment should not get in the way of clearly defining the terms which are being used. Betts and his colleagues at Queen Elizabeth Hospital, Birmingham, have produced a series of educational videotapes on psychosexual interviewing which are excellent. One of these tapes demonstrates with great clarity how both verbal and non-verbal cues betray the attitudes of the doctor. It is important, therefore, to be aware of how much of oneself goes into an interview. Michael Balint reminded us that one of the most potent drugs available in our armamentarium is the doctor himself, but for this to be valuable a proper empathy with the patient must be established.

Mention has been made of the differences between the psychiatry of the psychiatric hospital and its counterpart in the community, and that most general practitioners — established and in training — have to attain the appropriate skills more through experience than from formal instruction. The recognition and management of psychological problems in General Practice is however too important an area of work to be subjected to the imperfect background of experience.

THE LEARNING OF GENERAL PRACTICE PSYCHIATRY

A number of rotating vocational schemes have had a syllabus for psychiatry in general practice published, such as that by Barber & Simpson (1978).

A set of guidelines covering those areas where worthwhile experience should be obtained in a 6 month tenure of a psychiatric hospital post, was drawn up by a joint committee of the Royal College of General Practitioners and Psychiatrists (1980). In summary they were:

1. General psychiatric practice including interview techniques, taking case histories, and making formal diagnoses.
2. Methods of psychiatric treatment, especially the proper use of psychotropic medication and of the more simple psychotherapeutic procedures.

3. Application of the Mental Health Act, with particular reference to the responsibilities of general practitioners.
4. Management of acute psychiatric emergencies.
5. Recognition and management of potential psychiatric emergencies.
6. Liaison with professional workers in the community, especially general practitioners, social workers, and community psychiatric nurses.
7. The long-term care of chronically disabled psychiatric patients.
8. Psychiatric aspects of the aged in the community.
9. Diagnosis and treatment of psychosexual conditions.
10. Counselling, for example in family crises and marital problems.
11. Miscellaneous areas of special experience such as child and family psychiatry, adolescent psychiatry, mental handicap, forensic psychiatry, and dependence on alcohol, tobacco and other drugs.

The trainee needs to identify his own personal training requirements at an early stage to get the best out of both his psychiatric hospital job and his year in general practice. A personal syllabus or check list should be constructed which should recognise the substantial differences between general practice psychiatry and specialist psychiatry. One basis for preparing such a list would be the morbidity prevalence rates in general practice. This would give an initial list comprising in rank order of problems:

1. Depression
2. Anxiety
3. Tension states and psychosomatic disorders
4. Alcoholism and drink problems
5. Heavy smoking problems
6. Marital problems
7. Drug abuse
8. Sleep problems

There are other important areas which cannot be left out, including the psychoses and the dementias, but the top three on the list will account for in excess of half the total workload.

A further important area of knowledge for the general practitioner is in his patient's perception of him as an expert. The following are some of the more unusual questions asked for general practitioners:

1. *From a pregnant woman:* 'I had these terrible dreams that my son and husband are both murdered. Does this mean that the baby has something wrong with it?'

2. *A young mother about her son aged 3:* 'My son is afraid of water, doctor — no, I don't mean swimming, I mean he won't allow me to wash him, he won't drink it, in fact he will have nothing to do with it.

3. A mother on the phone regarding her daughter aged 2½ who had been admitted to the Children's Unit with burns: 'Doctor, I know that you said that we should visit as often as possible and that I should stay with Sheila for as long as possible, but when Tim was in hospital having his tonsils out, the staff advised me not to visit until the next day and then only during visiting hours. Sheila is so upset when we leave her. Don't you think it might be better to visit her less often.'

4. A 60-year-old man: 'I suppose it's inevitable at my age to become impotent, doctor. I find nowadays that I don't always ejaculate when I have intercourse.'

5. A 50-year-old man: 'I have a sleep problem, doctor. I can only sleep for 4 hours every night. My wife says I must do something about it or I will become ill. Is she right?'

6. A son talking about his father aged 76: 'Father's memory is terrible. I told him that he must expect it at his age.'

7. A husband about his wife who had just been diagnosed as having spinal secondaries following a mastectomy 5 years previously: 'The consultant is very nice. He seemed to be quite upset at having to tell me that there was nothing more that they could do for her. He said that he hadn't told her and it was much better not to do so.'

8. A daughter following her father's death: 'My mother sometimes talks to my father. I think that she actually sees or at least feels that he is there. Is she going mad?'

Unless the general practitioner is well acquainted with the normal psychological processes in:

1. Pregnancy and childbirth
2. Child development
3. Hospital admissions for children and adults
4. Sleep
5. Sexuality
6. Aging
7. Terminal illness
8. Bereavement

then he may give wholly inappropriate answers to his patients with considerable damage. Masters & Johnson in their seminal work on *Human Sexual Inadequacy* (1970) reported on a number of sexual problems where the condition had been significantly worsened by the reinforcement given to the condition because of inappropriate counselling by the doctor. The best response that a doctor can make if he does not know the answer is to indicate that he will find out and admit honestly that he does not know rather than make a guess.

The responses to the questions that were given to these patients are listed below:

1. *The pregnant lady* was reassured that such dreams were normal *but* the doctor went on to carry out further investigations despite the absence of any obvious problem. The result was severe anxiety.

2. *The child with water phobia* was referred to a child psychologist. No harm was done, the specific fear disappeared only to be replaced by an equally transient fear of goldfish. Transient phobias are a normal part of child development.

3. *Visiting young children in hospital.* The parents were advised that in view of Sheila's reaction they might be better to curtail their visits. The result was that Sheila became increasingly apathetic and withdrawn. The intervention of a hospital social worker led to a restoration of active and lengthy visiting with beneficial results. Sheila began to object strongly to the parents leaving at the end of visiting — a completely healthy response. The effect of separation, either by parents being in hospital or by children being in hospital, can be severe.

4. *The 60-year-old man with the sexual question.* This patient was referred to a specialist sexual problems clinic and by the time he was seen, he was indeed impotent. His anxiety needed to be managed but he did *not*, in fact, have a sexual problem and was certainly not impotent.

5. *The patient with the sleep problem* was given a barbiturate which did not do much for his sleep pattern but did give rise to a problem of barbiturate dependence with which he presented at a later stage. No treatment should have been necessary unless the patient felt ill as a result of his lack of sleep. Retrospectively he was clear in his own mind that he was perfectly fit and well at the time.

6. *The son's question about the father with the memory problem.* This old man subsequently deteriorated. He was thought to have senile dementia and was admitted to hospital where pseudo dementia of depression was diagnosed. He was treated with antidepressants and had 5 further active and mentally alert years before dying suddenly.

7. *Terminal illness.* The wife's distress was severe and the consultant agreed to move her to a hospice where she was able to confide that she hadn't wanted her husband to know that she was dying because of the distress that it would cause him. The strength of the partnership was restored with the resumption of open communication between them.

8. *Bereavement reaction.* A domiciliary psychiatric visit was arranged. Unfortunately the psychiatrist sat in the husband's chair and interpreted Mrs B's uncommunicative state and lack of movement, when combined with her 'hallucinations', as being a schizophrenic psychosis brought on by the stress of the bereavement. Fortunately the Minister was able to advise that the situation was really quite different and an admission was averted. Mrs B. was having a normal grief reaction.

EPIDEMIOLOGY

The main findings of research into psychiatric morbidity

in the community over the past 30 years have been:

1. That it is substantially different from hospital based studies.
2. That the difference between hospital and community treated psychological illness is not always simply a qualitative one. Not all severe cases are referred and some mild, though usually chronic problems, are referred.
3. That the amount of psychiatric morbidity is hard to quantify. The main difficulty is that of achieving a measure of agreement on what constitutes a 'case'.
4. That much psychiatric morbidity is self-limiting and is hidden either completely or partially from the general practitioner.
5. That more than half the general practitioner's psychiatric workload will be concerned with chronic neurotic patients for whom drug therapy is likely to be of little lasting value and who may require new strategies of management.
6. That there may be a group of vulnerable patients who are more likely to suffer from a number of different physical and psychiatric illnesses at the same time.

PREVALENCE

A number of epidemiological studies undertaken in primary care have produced a wide range of prevalence and incidence rates. Watts in reviewing the Royal College of General Practitioners National Morbidity Survey (1970), found a prevalence of 338.7 per 1000 at risk which constituted almost half of the patients who consulted during the period of the survey. This figure included illnesses classified as psychosomatic or stress disorders. Kessels (1960) in examining the problem in a London setting, looked at various possible levels of 'caseness'. This produced rates varying from 50 per 1000 to 520 per 1000 (Table 24.1). Rates observed in a number of other studies, all of whom endeavoured to achieve a rational level for inclusion of cases, produced prevalence rates varying from 41 to 132 per 1000 at risk and consultation rates of between 8.5% and 65% of all consultations.

These variations in rates of psychological illness have a number of causes. Psychological illness, being so often a

variation of normal behaviour, is exposed to great differences in recognition by both patient and doctor. Again while organic illness frequently has readily identifiable physical characteristics or specific laboratory tests, psychological illness seldom has similar indications of precise diagnosis. Many patients still fear mental illness — when they would not necessarily have the same feelings about a physical complaint — and are thus likely to conceal or not recognise their illness; doctors similarly may be less able or willing to consider a psychological diagnosis, particularly when the patient's presenting complaint is apparently physical. More research, to establish the symptom syndromes of psychological illness, their natural history and response to various management regimes, would allow more precision in diagnosis and thus less variation in rates quoted.

One of the most important epidemiological studies of psychiatric morbidity in the United Kingdom (Shepherd et al 1966) described the characteristics of psychological illness in general practice and the differences between the conditions seen in hospital and the community.

The study covered 50 practices and recognised from the outset that the International Classification of Diseases was too narrow a base. The authors therefore included a second category of what they called Psychiatric Associated Conditions (Table 24.2), in addition to the traditional, formal psychiatric diagnosis.

Table 24.2 Categories of mental illness (from Shepherd & Clare 1981, reproduced by kind permission of the authors and publisher)

Formal psychiatric illness
1. Psychosis (schizophrenia, manic-depressive psychosis, organic psychosis)
2. Mental subnormality
3. Dementia (deterioration of mental powers in excess of normal ageing process)
4. Neurosis (anxiety state, depressive, hysterical, phobic or asthenic reactions; others)
5. Personality disorder

Psychiatric-associated conditions
6. Physical illness   where psychological mechanisms have
7. Physical symptoms   been important in the development of the condition
8. Physical illnesses   which have been elaborated or
9. Physical symptoms   prolonged for psychological reasons
10. Other psychological or social problems

AGE AND SEX

The findings with regard to age and sex in this study have been replicated both in the United Kingdom and abroad. It confirmed the excess of females consulting with a rate of 175 per 1000 persons at risk compared to 97.9 per 1000 for males.

Shepherd also examined the prevalence rates at various ages and found that this was highest for the middle years

Table 24.1 Levels of 'caseness' (from Kessels 1960)

Level	Cumulative rate per 1000 at risk
International Classification of Diseases	50
'Conspicuous' psychiatric morbidity	90
Organic cases lacking detectable cause	380
Psychosomatic disorders	520

for females, whereas for males the rate did not vary significantly from 25 years upwards. This again is at variance with hospital studies where a peak is usually found for both sexes between the 25th and 45th years.

LONGITUDINAL STUDIES

In a 20-year follow-up study of Shepherd's material by Skuse & Dunn (1981) it was found that 75% of the women and over 50% of the men who had remained in the same practice were seen on at least one occasion for a problem regarded as wholly or largely psychiatric by the general practitioner.

CATEGORIES OF PSYCHIATRIC MORBIDITY IN GENERAL PRACTICE

If difficulties in determining overall prevalence rates in general practice seem large, they are as nothing compared to determining individual category rates (Table 24.3).

Shepherd pointed to the substantial differences between patients seen in his study, those seen at Maudsley outpatients and patients admitted to hospital (Table 24.4).

Table 24.3 Patient consulting rates per 1000 at risk for psychiatric morbidity, by sex and diagnostic group (from Shepherd & Clare 1981, reproduced by kind permission of the authors and publisher)

Diagnostic group	Male	Female	Both sexes
Psychoses	2.7	8.6	5.9
Mental subnormality	1.6	2.9	2.3
Dementia	1.2	1.6	1.4
Neuroses	55.7	116.6	88.5
Personality disorder	7.2	4.0	5.5
Formal psychiatric illness★	67.2	131.9	102.1
Psychosomatic conditions	24.5	34.5	29.9
Organic illness with psychiatric overlay	13.1	16.6	15.0
Psychosocial problems	4.6	10.0	7.5
Psychiatric-associated conditions★	38.6	57.2	48.6
Total psychiatric morbidity★	97.9	175.0	139.4
Number of patients at risk	6783	7914	14 697

★These totals cannot be obtained by adding the rates for the relevant diagnostic groups because while a patient may be included in more than one diagnostic group, they will be included only once in the total

Table 24.4 Distribution of the main psychiatric categories: comparison of the present survey with hospital statistics (from Shepherd & Clare 1981, reproduced by kind permission of the authors and publisher)

Category	Community survey %	Maudsley hospital outpatients 1956–1958 %	Mental hospital first admissions England and Wales, 1957 %
Psychoses	4.2	24.5	72.3
Neuroses	63.4	43.6	18.1
Character disorders	3.9	23.2	5.0
Miscellaneous	28.5	8.9	4.6
Total number of cases	2049	6752	48 266

Hodgkin (1978) in his overview of mental illness in general practice produced period prevalence rates for most conditions. His figures, based on 20 years in general practice and a 4-year analysis of his own practice in Canada, have been cross checked against four practices in the North East of England, with a total practice population of 20 000. Table 24.5 gives a compilation of his figures. He himself comments on the uncertainty of the figures for alcoholism and depression.

The problem recognised by Shepherd, and to a lesser extent by Hodgkin, is that the material seen in general practice does not fit into the ICD classification. A more useful approach may prove to be the study of problems as employed by Clarke & Basden in Southampton, or by the author, or by Simpson in Forth Valley.

The prevalence notes in the initial published work of Clarke in 1976 proved remarkably similar to Shepherd's

Table 24.5 Range of diagnostic prevalence (after Hodgkin)

	One year period prevalence, rate per 1000 patients
Anxiety/tension	58.2–132.7
Depression	20 +/−
Manic-depression	20 +/−
Hypochondriasis	3.6–12.2
Insomnia	10–18
Marital problems	9
Hysteria	3.6–12.2
Alcoholism	3.0
Obsessional neurosis	0.8–2.2
Schizophrenia	1.1–1.7
Sexual problems	1.3
Paranoid schizophrenia	0.4
Others	17.5

at 122 per 1000 persons at risk, though a problem list including psychiatric, psychological and psychosocial data shows more of the prolix nature of the problems (Table 24.6).

What is most striking is that all of the studies reviewed showed that anxiety, tension and depression together account for nearly half of all the cases seen. Psychosis, on the other hand, comprises a relatively small part of the general practitioner's workload.

HIDDEN MORBIDITY

In 1963, Last drew attention to the 'iceberg phenomenon' in health care. In 1970, Goldberg & Blackwell used the opportunity afforded them by a psychiatric colleague moving into general practice to study the presentation and identification of psychiatric morbidity. Using the General Health Questionnaire (GHQ) they were able to identify one-third of all significant morbidity which had been missed by this psychiatrically trained general practitioner. This hidden group of patients was not significantly different from the recognised group with respect to either severity or outcome.

Table 24.6 Abbreviated list of problem tallies of psychiatric, psychological and psychosocial morbidity, in rank order, from a total of 170 problems, presented to the primary team (compiled from work done by the author in Bridge of Allan Health Centre and the work of Dr A. Basden (ICI laboratories) using the 'CLINICS' System of data collection at Southampton University Primary Medical Care Centre and reproduced here in this form with his kind permission, from a personal communication, 1982)

	Prevalence
Anxiety	74
Social problems	30
Drinking problems*	26
Acute depression	26
Bereavement	25
Sleep problem	21
Marital problems	20
Over-anxious parent	15
Neurosis	15
Behavioural problems	12
Enuresis	11
Unhappy	10
Social dependency	10
Domestic problem	9
Psychosexual problems	8
Marital breakdown/divorce	7
Speech problems	6
Housing problems	5
Psychosis	4
Relationship problems	4
	338

Total prevalence of all problems 416 per 1000

*This was the Scottish Centre rate — the Southampton rate was less than 10

The study of hidden morbidity patients did show differences in outcome between a treated 'hidden' group and a control 'hidden' group. Both groups showed some initial improvement, particularly in milder cases which would be in keeping with the natural history of mild psychiatric disturbances, although some of the mild cases who were untreated presented later with a more severe episode.

Work in the late 70's has suggested that the GHQ is an insufficiently sensitive tool to identify all the true morbidity, and the Symptom Sign Inventory (SSI) may show earlier work to have underestimated the hidden problem.

Approaching the subject from a different angle, studies in para-suicide, puerperal depression and psychological difficulties following mastectomy, have all shown that, in these areas at least, patients do not always perceive the general practitioner as being the best person to consult. These findings would seem to indicate not only the need for adequate and appropriate psychiatric training if many more patients are not to be missed, but also the need for general practitioners to encourage the development of alternative access to psychiatric services, thus allowing patients to seek help in a variety of ways.

CHRONIC NEUROTIC CASES

In Shepherd's study, the overall proportion of chronic cases was 59% of males and 52.2% of females. Many subsequent studies have confirmed that much psychiatric morbidity is either chronic or recurrent and interrupted by short periods of remission. Fry (1956) reviewing a cohort of patients first presenting with neurotic illness found that 27% of males and 43% of females required further treatment in the follow-up year. A further study found only slightly lower figures for 3, 4, and 5 years follow-up.

Fry's work suggests that there are two discernible groups of patients presenting with neurotic illness. The first, comprising two-fifths of all males and one-fifth of all females, have a single episode. These may be regarded as situational reactions in an otherwise stable personality. The second, a small but significant group who presented at least in 4 out of 5 years with a psychiatric diagnosis, may be a constitutionally vulnerable group. There is considerable evidence that after a number of years in practice, the general practitioner will find that over half the consultations for psychological problems in any given year will fall into the chronic neurotic group. Furthermore he will find that traditional treatments with drugs have little lasting benefit in this group.

Unfortunately, referral to a psychiatrist is unlikely to produce significant benefit in more than a few of the patients. The burden upon the general practitioner created by these patients far exceeds their number or their frequency of consultation. It may be helpful, therefore, at an early stage, to identify these patients and to establish alternative strategies for their management.

Work by Howie (1980), Bain (1981) and Jerrom (1981) has demonstrated in three different settings the effects upon the family of chronic neurosis. The children will have antibiotics prescribed more often, will be referred more often and the spouse and children will consult more often. More studies are needed before the full implications are clarified, but the suggestion is that having identified the chronic neurotic patient the general practitioner will need to be aware of this in consultations with other members of the family.

PSYCHIATRIC AND PHYSICAL MORBIDITY

In studies such as that of Eastwood & Trevelyan (1972) it has been shown that a greater proportion of patients suffering from psychiatric morbidity will also have significant physical illness and that this relationship will occur more frequently than in a control group. Furthermore, it appears that despite the increasing amount of physical illness associated with ageing, the observed excess of major and minor physical problems in the psychiatric group will remain significant. This finding is particularly true for females. The evidence for a 'cluster' effect whereby a number of different physical illnesses can be found in one patient is also more evident in the psychiatric group and the older group of patients. These studies have led some writers to propose the hypothesis that there is a group of patients who are inherently vulnerable both to physical and psychiatric dysfunction.

However, it is also hypothesised that patients with a chronic physical illness are more likely to develop, as a consequence, significant psychological problems. Some of these reactions are discussed on pages 320–323. Whichever of these hypotheses proves to be valid, it lends weight to the need for the general practitioner to assess the mental state of patients with chronic or recurrent physical illness.

REFERRAL TO SPECIALIST SERVICES

As with other areas of illness found in general practice, referral rates vary from practice to practice. An overall average rate would appear to be about one patient in 20, with a range of from one to 10 to one in 40.

General practitioners' referral rates depend upon a number of factors, which includes their own attitude and aptitude as well as the attitude of the patient and his family. There is considerable evidence that the stigma of psychiatric referral can be reduced if the psychiatrist

consults in the primary care setting. There is also evidence that there is less stigma attached to referral to a psychologist or other specialist psychiatric worker than to a psychiatrist. Again, the problem is less if workers are based within the primary care setting.

THE PSYCHIATRIC NETWORK

MODELS OF PATIENT CARE

In developing suitable strategies for actively managing the psychological problems presenting in general practice, no single model of care is universally applicable. In the United Kingdom the usual pattern of access to psychiatric care has been for patients to go to the general practitioner who acts as the main gateway to all other services. The pattern will remain the prime route for the majority of patients, but other modes of access are becoming available (Table 24.7).

Table 24.7 Points of access to the psychiatric network

Health Centre or Surgery
Social Work Area Office
Accident and Emergency Department
Psychiatric Hospital
Police Station
Self Help Groups (See Table 24.14, p. 299)
Walk-in Centre

The general practitioner, in recognising these alternative routes, should ascertain how appropriate or how helpful they are for the community which he serves. Unfortunately communication with the general practitioner by those staff who are working from centres other than primary care centres tends to be rather poor. Yet without adequate information personal care is rendered more difficult.

Table 24.8 is a list of all those who are currently involved at various levels in psychiatric care, and Figures 24.1, 24.2 and 24.3 show alternative models of care, all of which could contain the personnel and facilities which the Health Board and Local Authorities are required to provide in fulfilment of their obligation under the Mental Health Acts.

The team
The team is the main model currently approved for all primary care, but a more appropriate construction may be that of the Network (Fig. 24.3). However, each general practitioner must take from these models what is applicable to the particular circumstances of his own practice.

The ideal team model which has evolved has the merit

Table 24.8 Members of the psychiatric network

Primary team (Direct access)	Specialist team (Indirect or Referred access)	Other groups
General practitioner and secretarial staff	Psychiatrist	Counsellors
Health visitor	Social worker (Specialist)	DRO (Disablement Resettlement Officer)
District nurse	Psychologist	Local Authority Housing Officer
Social Worker	Community psychiatric nurse	Voluntary organisation personnel
Counsellors	Counsellors	

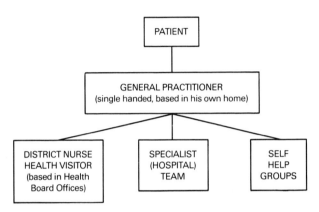

Fig. 24.2 The team model

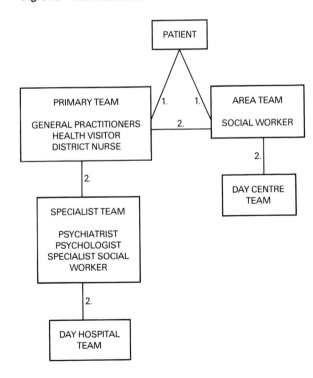

1. Access/Primary level
2. Referal/Secondary level

Fig. 24.1 Early model of patient care

that the primary group shares a defined population. In the author's own practice the situation in 1970 was that the district nurse had her own house and treatment room attached, the health visitor had a base in the nearest town and they both covered an area which included some but not all of the patients from the practice. Because of its catchment area the practice had to work with five different district nurses and five health visitors.

Changes initiated by the Local Authority and subsequently the Health Board have allowed the development of a team serving 5500 patients which consists of three general practitioners, four district nurses, two health visitors, a social worker and a marriage guidance counsellor based in the Health Centre, with specialists consulting in the Health Centre as a back-up.

Whilst the team is an improvement on model 1 (Fig. 24.1), there remain problems with this approach. Firstly, it cannot readily be applied to rural areas; referrals to specialist services are markedly less from rural communities. A recent reminder of this was given in the development of a new district psychology service based in the community covered by the Stirling District of the Forth Valley Health Board, an area of 800 square miles. Reporting the findings after 36 months of operation Jerrom et al (1981) found that 79% of practices in the district had referred patients and out of the remaining 21% who had not referred patients half were rural practices.

Secondly, there is no single model for the team. Health visitors and district nurses, although generally attached to a single practice, may still be attached to a multiplicity of practices, or indeed may still cover a geographical area. Indeed, some urban areas are reverting to this earlier form because of a failure by general practitioners to rationalise their catchment area.

Thirdly, there is an assumption by the general practitioner that he is the undisputed leader in every situation and this may no longer be appropriate or acceptable. For example, a schizophrenic patient returns home from hospital after a first acute episode of illness. He is well maintained on depot medication. What are his problems? Who will be primarily responsible? In a task-orientated team the general practitioner has to keep prime responsibility if he is to remain the leader. If he has no great interest in psychiatry, or in the interpersonal and social

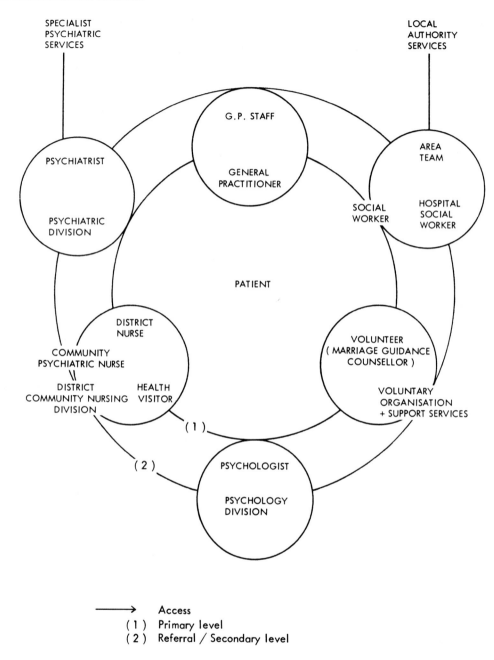

Fig. 24.3   The network model of care

difficulties which predominate in his patient's life, should be still remain the leader? Can he apply himself with efficiency to all the problems which are facing his patient?

Fourthly, the team concept also fails to allow for the realities of line management. Doctors are unique in this respect since all the other professionals in the team have some form of line management. The social worker, the district nurse and the health visitor are all responsible to a manager and are part of their own specialist team.

Fifthly, there is the further problem of confidentiality. Does the team in fact share common records on an open basis? Does the practitioner have open access to social work, health visitor or nursing files, and equally do these members of the team have open access to the general practitioner's records?

Networks and the key worker concept

As Rowbotton & Hey (1978) and Simpson (1981) have argued, the concept of a network is more appropriate in that it allows for great flexibility in the roles played by the individuals and groups that make it up. The general practitioner who reviews his network and identifies gaps in care need not always try to fill them himself. It allows also for the development of the 'key worker' concept. This is a system of care whereby a specified individual is identified to carry prime responsibility for the patient. The key professional has responsibility to liaise with all the others involved at each level and to share information necessary for effective management.

The alternatives to a sophisticated and sometimes complex network with a designated key worker are either a system where many workers pass in and out of the patient's life with no overall co-ordination and a diminution in the quality of care, or an extension by the specialist psychiatric services further into primary care.

MEMBERS OF THE NETWORK AND THEIR ROLES

It is perhaps necessary to say that whatever the traditional role of each profession, these roles need to be adjusted to take full account of the individual's personal skills. The general practitioner who is embarrassed by any discussion of sexual matters is not going to take on sexual counselling. But what then happens to the patient with a sexual problem? Another of the primary or secondary teams may have to take over this area of work. If the skills are not in fact available within the existing network then identification of a gap could result in a decision to bring in a counsellor with marriage guidance experience to advise patients with sexual problems.

THE GENERAL PRACTITIONER

The central function of the general practitioner remains the assessment and diagnosis of the presenting problem. His awareness as a generalist of *all* possible treatment and management options is one of the mainstays of the unique contribution which the doctor makes to the primary network. He need have no fears with regard to his continuing role and status within the network unless he fails to recognise the professionalism, ethical values and independence of his colleagues.

Every general practitioner can benefit from an examination of his own skills and aptitudes and should thereafter attempt to define clearly the role which he feels happy to play. He will then be able to seek complementary skills in his colleagues.

An illustration of the need for complementary skills is to be found in those doctors who find it impossible to cope wtih the psychological management of terminal illness. There are still some doctors who state categorically that they have never told a patient that he is dying. This is often said with some pride. Such doctors fail to accept the variations in response to dying found in patients. By seeking to impose a single psychological state, namely denial of impending death, these doctors seek to avoid what they regard as possible unpleasantness. However, since 80% of their patients will wish to talk about their fears of the process of dying, the doctor will have condemned the majority to an unpleasant death, full of fear, in some cases with great pain or confusion through massive sedation. Far better for such doctors to recognise the problem they themselves have in facing up to the reality of death. They should hand over the psychological care of the patient to a colleague.

HEALTH VISITORS

The training syllabus for health visitors now contains a very substantial element of psychology and psychiatry. There are three main areas where the health visitor already plays an important part, and extension into a number of other areas should be readily achieved with little further training.

Ante-natal mothers

It is evident that pregnant women need more support in the absence of the mothers, fathers, aunts and uncles previously available in the extended family. There is already a ground swell of resentment about the highly technological and scientific manner in which ante-natal and delivery care are managed. Helping parents and sometimes hospital staff to a position of mutual respect and understanding will be an increasing role for the health visitor.

Children

In her work with children a clear understanding of child development and management will allow many psychological problems to be identified at an early stage. Equally important, she may prevent normal features being misinterpreted as 'illness'.

The elderly

Health surveillance can be useful in the elderly not only in picking up early dementia but also in detecting risk factors such as deafness or other sensory deficits, dietary problems, physical illness or increasing isolation. These are often found to be present in depression and paranoid states of the elderly.

Behaviour therapy

A new role for the health visitor which could equally apply to the nurse is in behaviour therapy. Training by clinical psychologists and supervision by them of a programme of therapy agreed between the patient, psychologist and health visitor is one way of coping with the very limited availability of clinical psychologists.

Self-help groups

A further new role is in support of self-help groups. Here the health visitor will need to work in close liaison with the social worker and possibly the psychologist and community psychiatric nurse. The initial process may be aided by a patient participation group.

SOCIAL WORKER

The removal of psychiatric social workers from Health Service employment and their incorporation into Local Authority Social Work Departments has been bitterly resented by many psychiatrists. Doctors have also felt that the parallel introduction of the generalist or generic social worker has done little to enhance the contribution which social workers can make to the care of the mentally ill patient and his family. However, there is already evidence that psychiatric social work as a specialty is once again developing. Moreover, as Whitefield & Winter (1980) reported in a study of general practitioner attitudes, almost three-quarters of those asked indicated a desire to have social work attachment. The development of a strong generic social work presence in primary care, linked to specialist psychiatric social workers, will play an increasing role in patient management over the next decade.

The independence of the social work profession has allowed them to free themselves from a purely medical model, thus enabling them to bring a distinctive approach as a significant contribution to the network. This provides other members of the network with fresh perspectives on the social and interpersonal functioning of the patients.

Although there is some overlap between the roles of health visitor and social worker, general practitioners do perceive some differences. Williams & Clare (1979) analysed those areas where there was a significant negative correlation between the perceived roles of social worker and health visitor. As can be seen from Table 24.9, the practical elements of care are still regarded as being very important in social work. The value of casework was also highly regarded. The study confirmed the advantages laid out in the Mitchell Report (1976) on close and effective liaison between social work and health services through one of the alternative types of linkage to the primary care team suggested by the Report.

Table 24.9 Perceived differences between Health Visitor and Social work roles (after Williams & Clare)

Social work role	Predominantly Health Visitor role
Financial problems	Educational difficulties
Criminal problem in the family	Bereavement
Difficulties in wider family relationships	Mental handicap in the family
Difficulty in other social relationships	Physical disability and handicap
Employment	Psychological and social
Housing	problems in reproduction or pregnancy
	Child care

Models of social work attachment to general practice

Link A

The social worker is based at the practice and is personally responsible for accepting and carrying referrals from members of the practice team. This should not in any way separate her from the area social work team of which she is essentially also a member, with the resources of the social work department directly available.

Link B

The social worker may or may not be based at the practice but is responsible for accepting its referrals initially. She may then either see the patient herself or may ask another member of the social work team to do so as appropriate.

Link C

The social worker is based in the social work department and is named as the person to accept referrals from perhaps several practices. She either sees the patient herself or, in this case more likely, refers him on to an appropriate colleague — for example where the family is already known to another member of the staff!

General practitioners found that they had much greater confidence referring to a social worker colleague whom they knew rather than making referrals to the anonymous 'intake' social worker in an area team. The social workers for their part, felt that they saw clients who would not be likely to come to the area office. They also felt that they were able to do much more preventive work.

Although a number of studies have shown that two-thirds or more of the problems referred continued to be of a practical nature, one-third were what Shepherd has described as 'quasi psychotherapeutic'. Shepherd also stressed the concept of 'social brokerage', the role of liaison and advocacy on behalf of the client with and to other groups.

There is some evidence again that a sub-group of the chronic neurotic patients who are poorly organised and have a high level of social dysfunction, can derive particular benefit from social work intervention.

Apart from the effect upon the patient and his family, the intervention of the social worker can change the doctor/patient relationship. This is particularly true if the doctor, adhering to the organic model, is flexible enough to perceive the importance of information couched in terms of the sociotherapeutic model. Thus the doctor may become more aware of social factors in the illness or the behavioural response of his patient to illness. He may come to accept both the social causes and consequences of the disease and be prepared to help as an advocate in social welfare problems. If he does so he will have incorporated at least part of the socio-psycho-therapeutic model into his approach.

In conclusion, it should perhaps be pointed out that none of the studies reviewed showed any reductions in the time spent by doctors on patients' problems after a social worker joined the group. Indeed, the opposite was often the case. However, the benefits to the patient appeared to be quite significant.

DISTRICT NURSE

Lithium monitoring clinics and depot injection clinics are often run by hospital staff. This is in part because it is believed that hospital based care is more likely to ensure the proper after-care that maintenance therapy of manic-depressive and schizophrenic patients requires. Non-attenders will be assiduously followed up, early signs of deterioration will be spotted and psychiatrists will be on hand for consultation.

A case can be made for these clinics as part of primary care. The main advantage seems to be in a reduction in the 'illness' role of the patient. Continuing attendance at the hospital has a profound influence upon the attitudes of patients. Additionally, greater consistency in the personnel giving care may be achieved in a primary setting. One acceptable middle course is to bring the community psychiatric nurse into the primary centre, working alongside the district nurse and health visitor.

The nurse may also be involved in the supervision of the patient with marked suicidal ideation. Hitherto most psychiatrists would recommend referral or admission of those at risk. However, the threshold for admission can safely be raised provided that close supervision is maintained. The nurse can be involved both in a supportive role and in dispensing medication on the basis of a previously agreed schedule.

The district nurse is often the key worker in terminal cases. It is therefore valuable that she should have experience of hospice work or should receive additional train-

ing in the psychological management of the terminally ill. The nurse may be the most appropriate member of the network to monitor the grief reaction following terminal illness, and to provide counselling in such a situation.

COUNSELLOR

Counselling will be considered as a strategy under management (see p. 303). Again it is necessary to consider whether there is a role for a counsellor in the primary care setting, where he or she may be more effective and more acceptable to patients. The endorsement of referral from the general practitioner appears to be helpful. Furthermore, it is clear that patients are less likely to feel that such a referral is a rejection by the doctor when it is to a named counsellor within the same primary setting. The problems which may usefully be referred to a counsellor are listed in Table 24.10.

Waydenfield (1980) examined the work of nine counsellors over a 2-year period in nine practices involving 35 general practitioners and 79 500 patients. The results suggest that there is significant benefit as determined by five different measurements:

1. There is improvement in the referred problem as assessed by the general practitioner and counsellor independently.
2. There is a beneficial effect by way of reduced consultations with the general practitioner on comparison of a 6 months consultation rate before and after counselling.
3. In a particular group where marital therapy was predominant, there was an improvement in the consultation rates of both the spouse and of the children, as well as for the index group of 99 patients.
4. The use of prescribed medicines dropped.
5. The referral rate to other agencies declined.

It should not be thought that such counsellors are without training. Indeed, the Marriage Guidance Council, in an analysis of applicants, found that only 40% of

Table 24.10   Referrals to counsellors (after Waydenfield)

General Practitioners reasons	Patients perceived reasons
Marital problems	Inability to cope with a current
Other relationship	problem
difficulties	Difficulties with relationships
Situational anxiety	Sexual problem
Sexual problem	Health problems, including:
Psychosomatic problems	Headache
Violence	Backache
Depression	Stomach problem
Alcoholism	Sleep
	Depression

those applying were selected for training and only 80% of those selected completed the 2-year training programme. Additional specialised training may successfully allow marriage guidance counsellors to carry out behaviour therapy in treating sexual problems under the supervision of either the general practitioner or the psychologist.

THE PSYCHIATRIST

In the United Kingdom there is about one psychiatrist to 50 000 people. However, the range of provision is from 1:15 000 in some of the teaching centres, to more that 1:90 000 in the periphery.

Physical resources

Fundamental mistakes in planning in the 60's led to a presumption that hospital bed requirements would virtually disappear as patients were treated. More realistic assessments recognise that there are new long-term stay patients requiring in-patient care. This new group includes schizophrenics who do not respond to treatment, patients with brain damage and unstable epileptics. In addition there are the so-called 'graduate' population who reached the age of 65 as in-patients and require long-term care together with an increasingly large group of elderly with chronic organic brain syndrome (dementia).

Patients with dementia threaten to overwhelm the institutional resources available to the general practitioner. The substantial growth, of up to 40% in some regions in the population over 75 years of age between 1980 and 1990, is in no way matched by the forward planning for beds in the Health Service or in the Local Authority.

In Scotland, the Timbury Report on Services for the Elderly with Mental Disability in Scotland (1979) recommended the establishment of continuing care units as accommodation for the elderly confused. Such units would be small and retain an essentially domestic atmosphere. They further recommended that a total of 5500 new and replacement beds, including the new care units, would be required by 1987. By mid-1982 no new units had been planned. This failure poses enormous problems for many families and the general practitioner will bear the brunt of these families' frustrations.

Psychiatrists in the community

The psychiatrist outwith the academic entres has minimal junior medical support. He cannot cope with all the psychiatric or psychological problems of the community. Attempts to move into the community and provide a primary care service more akin to American or Soviet care models, may appear to be beneficial in the short term, but are likely to be less efficient in the long-term than better support and development of an effective primary network. The primary members of the network must, for their part, seek the advice of the psychiatrist, and his help in the development of overall strategies for primary care.

'Liaison psychiatry'

One area of developing psychiatric care is within the district general hospital. The general practitioner has a role to play in developing this aspect of specialist service, since he may be aware before referral of serious psychological problems or of the interplay of psychological or sociological factor with the presenting somatic illness. 'Liaison psychiatry' should help to produce a broader assessment in patients where such factors are important. This would appear to be particularly valuable in the light of epidemiological findings showing that physical and mental illness appear to cluster in some individuals. These individuals are liable to give rise to management difficulties for the physician or surgeon.

Ignoring the psychological aspects can be devastating for the patient.

> Mrs G., born 1930, joined the practice in 1976 with a bulging record envelope. On scrutinising the contents it rapidly became evident firstly that she had no problems, physical or mental, of any significance until 1966, and secondly that since that date she had had a cholecystectomy, a hysterectomy and two laparotomies. She had attended four different specialists and in one clinic, which she was still attending in 1976, she had seen no less than 14 junior doctors in the preceding 4 years. She was on seven different prescribed drugs, including three psychotropic drugs — a major tranquilliser, a hypnotic and an antidepressant. Her annual consultation rate was below average until 1966, but had gone up to 12 in 1967 and reached a peak in 1975 of 34, or nearly 10 times the average consultation rate.
>
> In 1966 a divorce for non-consummation of marriage had occurred. The enormous changes in morbidity were so closely related to that life event that coincidence seemed unlikely. In counselling the patient, her feelings on the 10 years since 1966 were explored and she came to realise that in part her physical illnesses may have been a response to that trauma. She began to accept that her 'sick' role was self-destructive.
>
> By 1979 her consultation rate was down to six per annum. Her drugs were down to one (a non-steroidal anti-inflammatory drug for arthritis) and she was attending no hospital clinics.
>
> Recently her elderly mother came to stay. It was found that she had not been outside their previous home for 4 years and had a personality very similar to that of the daughter. A smilar positive approach was taken with the mother and whilst they both remain somewhat eccentric, they appear to cope. They are now socially involved in the village and the level of use of the network is tolerable if not

always appropriate. The records showed no recognition over that 10-year period of any possible psychological element in her condition. Perhaps if a liaison psychiatrist had been available, an opinion would have been sought at any one of the stages in her progress through the various specialist (physical) clinics. The patient might have been spared some of the trauma as the Health Service would also have been spared much unnecessary work.

COMMUNITY PSYCHIATRIC NURSE

This is a relatively new role for psychiatric nurses which has developed to fill a gap in community care. In the 60's psychiatric nurses were to be found in community as an extension of hospital care of certain patients. The best examples of these were in alcoholism units and crisis intervention teams. In a few cases the complete philosophy of the hospital was to integrate back into the community. The system of care developed at Dingleton Hospital in the Scottish Borders is still one of the best models of what can be achieved. The hospital remains as a valuable resource, but the emphasis is on community care.

The community psychiatric nurse remains a member of the specialist team. She is not attached to one doctor or one primary team, but to a group of teams. She may follow up patients at home quite separately from the primary team where gaps or lack of active interest makes this necessary. However, the need does not only arise from the discrepancies in Health and Local Authority social work care for the mentally ill, but also from the special needs of certain groups of patients, especially those whose reintegration into the community will benefit from regular close monitoring and support.

The establishment of appropriate monitoring of schizophrenics on long-term depot injections or manic-depressive patients on lithium therapy in the primary setting is a possible starting point for integrating this specialist with primary care. Additional support can be offered from such a clinic for both the patient and his family (see Families of schizophrenics, p. 313).

Where nurses have been introduced to provide psychogeriatric care it has been found that their caseload quickly extends to include younger patients. Tough et al (1980) reported that their role was originally perceived as being mainly practical, for instance ensuring compliance with medication. However, an analysis of their workload showed it to be more often about assessment, psychological support for the patient, or giving advice and support to relatives.

THE CLINICAL PSYCHOLOGIST

Until recently the clinical psychologist has been based within the mental hospital. Access to the psychologist has been restricted to patients referred by psychiatrists. Despite some misgivings on the part of the psychiatrists, psychologists have now firmly established their independence as a profession. The Trethowan Report contained, amongst other recommendations, an ethical code which, if followed, should remove most of the medical profession's criticisms.

From the mid 70's, the clinical psychologist has been moving out of his hospital base. In Livingston, West Lothian, early work showed the undoubted value of the psychologist in a primary care setting. More recently the Forth Valley Health Board area has conducted a 3-year experiment in a community based clinic with direct access for general practitioners and with the psychologist working in health centres and surgeries. Jerrom et al (1982) in an initial report on the study, confirmed a number of earlier findings. The results showed that:

1. There was a clear demand for such a service.
2. The patients and general practitioners welcomed the service being based in a primary care setting.
3. There appeared to be definite benefit to a majority of patients.

Benefit was assessed by the general practitioners (Table 24.11), the psychologist, and the patients on a self-rating scale, and the changes from pre to post-treatment in a number of measures, including general health questionnaire (Table 24.12), general practitioner consultation rates (Table 24.13) and drug usage rates (Figs. 24.4 and 24.5).

The advantages of the primary care setting reviewed by Burns (1982) included accessibility, greater continuity of care, improved liaison with primary care workers, reduction of stigma, earlier involvement in treatment, facilitation of the doctor/patient relationship, improved compliance and involvement with the patient and his family. Burns also stated that he believed that work in this setting will prove to be cost effective and he also stressed the importance of training other primary care staff in behavioural concepts. For the clinical psycholog-

Table 24.11 Forth Valley Health Board Community Clinical Psychology Service: G.P. and psychiatrists patient rating outcome (Jerrom et al 1981)

'What effect has treatment had upon this patient's problem?'				
	G.P. referrals n = 261		Psychiatrist referrals n = 44	
Definite benefit	146	56%	24	54%
No change	60	23%	14	32%
Deterioration	6	2%	0	
Unable to judge	49	19%	6	14%

Table 24.12   Forth Valley Health Board Community Clinical Psychology Service: A. mean general health questionnaire scores at admission, discharge and follow-up for an unselected group of patients entering treatment in 1981. B. mean problem self-rating scores (Maximum possible score — 15) at admission, discharge and follow-up, for unselected patients entering treatment in 1981. (Jerrom et al 1981)

	Admission	Discharge	Follow-up
A			
Mean n = 38	13.2	3.3	—
Mean n = 29	11.0	—	4.2
B			
Mean n = 67	5.75	2.39	—
Mean n = 36	5.71	—	2.42

Table 24.13   Forth Valley Health Board Community Psychology Service: Mean monthly consultation rate for 6 months prior to psychological treatment, during treatment and for 6 month post-treatment. n = 177. (Jerrom et al 1981)

	Pre	During	Post
Mean monthly rate	0.744	0.498	0.479
Statistical tests on consultation data			
Pre-treatment to during treatment		t = 4.93	P .001
Pre-treatment to post treatment		t = 3.41	P .001
During treatment to post treatment		t = 0.27	N.S.

All significance levels are 2-tailed

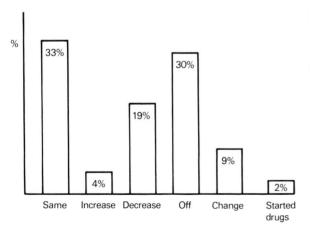

Fig. 24.4   Forth Valley Health Board Community Clinical Psychology Service; Changes in drug usage with treatment. 1. Drug use at discharge, breakdown of 97 patients using psychotropics at admission or discharge (from Jerrom et al, 1981).

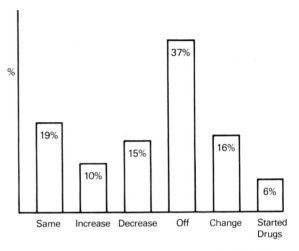

Fig. 24.5   Forth Valley Health Board Community Clinical Psychology Service; Changes in drug usage with treatment. 2. Drug use at 6 month follow-up, breakdown of 103 patients using drugs at admission or follow-up (from Jerrom et al, 1981).

ists the variety of clinical material, the challenges and the satisfaction levels appear to be high.

There has been evidence, till now anecdotal, that a younger group of patients do better with the sort of treatment offered by psychologists. The study by Jerrom et al (1982) found that those rated by the general practitioners and psychologists as unimproved were significantly older, had consulted their doctor more frequently prior to referral and tended to have had the presenting symptoms for a longer period. In addition they had a higher frequency of drug usage. This would seem to reinforce the need for early identification and referral of suitable cases.

As was stressed earlier, the chronic neurotic group will constitute a major part of the general practitioner's psychiatric workload. In assessing the strategies open to him in ameliorating or preventing the development of chronic neurosis, the general practitioner may wish to combine assessment by the clinical psychologist and treatment by a health visitor or nurse trained in behaviour therapy with social therapy from a social worker. The problems which can be referred are listed in Table 24.26, (p. 308), and the methods of behaviour therapy are considered in the section dealing with treatment strategies.

VOLUNTARY ORGANISATIONS

Self help is not always practicable or acceptable to patients or their families. However, there are many conditions where the need to discuss with others who share the same problem must be given expression. So for some patients, voluntary organisations such as those listed in

Table 24.14 provide a valuable alternative gateway to care. For some conditions it helps to remove the problem from the ambit of medical care, thus leaving the doctor to deal with specific problems which may arise in that particular patient.

Such an approach would be particularly applicable in homesexuality. The Campaign for Homosexual Equality has criticised the medical profession for its historical belief in the need to 'convert' homosexuals to heterosexuals. The profession's attitudes have changed substantially over the last 10 or 15 years and most doctors would now accept that homosexuality is not an illness, but a deviation which may produce great stress and unhappiness. The doctor's role becomes secondary to the support which may be given by other homosexuals.

STRATEGIES FOR MANAGEMENT

THE RECORDS

The importance of good records has already been stressed (see Ch. 3). The general practitioner, in managing patients with psychological problems must begin with a strategy at the time of registration. It would, of course, be excellent if both the doctor and patient had time to carry out the sort of screening programme used in the Kaiser clinics in the USA. A complete physical and mental work-up gives the physician a profile of all aspects of the new patient's health including social, leisure and work roles. Some have advocated the use of the General Health Questionnaire (GHQ), or more recently the Symptom/Sign Inventory (SSI) to establish the existence of a psychiatric disorder.

Some practices use a short questionnaire to establish a data base but most practices rely either on the records

Table 24.14   Voluntary organisations

Alcoholics Anonymous
Alanon
Anorexic Aid
Beaumont Society (for Transvestites)
Be not Anxious
Campaign for Homosexual Equality
Cruise (National Organisation for Widows and their children)
Depressives Associated (formerly Depressives Anonymous)
Gamblers Anonymous
Mental Patients Union
National Council for Alcoholism
The National Schizophrenia Fellowship
Phobics Society
Psychiatric Rehabilitation Association
Relatives of the Depressed
Richmond Fellowship
Samaritans
Scottish Association of Mental Health and Mind
The English Mental health Association

alone or on records combined with an interview with a member of the family.

Time spent at an early date examining the bulky record envelope will be time saved later, as was illustrated by the case of Mrs G. described in the section on 'Liaison psychiatry' (p. 296). After nearly 4 years as a patient the total saving by reduction in consultations and visits had reached 100 contacts when compared with the average levels of the preceding 4 years. Although her case was untypically easy, nevertheless the lack of a determined effort to actively manage this patient from the outset would have left the practice in the same morass in which the previous general practitioner had found himself inextricably sunk.

High users should always be identified. A rising consultation rate in the absence of proven pathology should quickly raise the general practitioner's index of suspicion. This rise may be masked by being spread through the family, with various children being offered for examination, or by the patient moving from doctor to doctor in a practice. One variation on this the patient who moves from trainee to trainee in training practices. A rising rate of repeat prescriptions is yet another useful warning sign.

PSYCHIATRIC DIAGNOSIS MADE BY EXCLUSION OF PHYSICAL PATHOLOGY

Most standard psychiatric texts will condemn this negative approach to diagnosis. A few general practice books will suggest that although this is quite correct, nevertheless a few tests may be needed to eliminate the possibility of physical illness. The general practitioner faced with a case of hypochondriasis, or a neurosis presenting with physical symptoms, may show through multiple investigations his fear and uncertainty of missing the physical diagnosis, thus reflecting his lack of self-confidence or worries about mental illness labelling.

Unfortunately, the response to more than simple physical investigations is a deepening adverse reaction. The patient feels that the doctor must believe that there is a physical problem or why else would these tests be carried out. An electrocardiography in cardiac neurosis may put the general practitioner's mind at rest with regard to the cardiac pathology, but it may entrench the patient's neurosis further.

Presentation

Mr J., a 45-year-old, presented with pain of a constricting nature in his chest and left arm. The pain was unpredictable and was not solely or particularly related to exercise. On inviting the patient to assess possible stress factors he identified recent promotion, the fact that his children were sitting their Higher examinations, and that his wife had just returned to full-time work. He indicated in particular that he found some of the new situations at work with which he had to deal extremely stressful and on close questioning he indicated that his pain was more likely to present in association with these situations than any other. He was a non-smoker, slim, took regular exercise, had no family history of cardiac problems and no personal history of any illness.

Alternative 1 is to carry out physical investigations. Amongst others this might include electrocardiograph and chest X-rays. The result of this approach will be to reinforce the cardiac neurosis which may well be developing.

Alternative 2 is to reassure the patient, adopting a fairly strong authoritative stance, that there is no physical problem. This is usally ineffective; the patient simply goes to another partner or sometimes obtains a full medical examination privately.

Alternative 3 is to explain the likely diagnosis, suggesting that the pain may have a psychological basis but emphasising that this does not mean that the pain is unreal; indeed the pain associated with stress or anxiety is often more unpleasant for the patient, but it is not 'heart pain'. The rationale behind this diagnosis is discussed at a level which the patient can understand.

It may not always be possible to establish why the particular physical symptoms should be occurring; in Mr H's case promotion came about through the sudden death from a coronary of his senior, a 53-year-old man.

The stresses should then be reviewed and the patient given help in adapting to his new circumstances. In this particular case Mr H. came back for a longer interview at which his increase in stress was reviewed. He was provided with a training tape in relaxation therapy which seemed to produce lasting benefits.

> Mr V., a teacher with a congenital spastic condition, was happily married with three teenage children. Following a mild viral illness his physical disabilities slowly worsened. He complained of fatigue, an increase in clonus, weakness in his lower limbs and latterly some weakness in his upper limbs. There were no major changes found on physical examination and a mental state examination demonstrated only that he was unhappy and anxious about the changes he was experiencing.

He was referred for a neurological opinion because of the subjective changes. Since he continued to maintain a strikingly high level of independent activity despite his disability, and since he showed no signs of inappropriate anxiety nor of the depressive shift characteristic of a depressive illness, a physical diagnosis seemed likely. In this case therefore a positive psychiatric diagnosis could not be reached. The neurological opinion was that this was functional overlay in a congenital spastic condition. He was referred by his general practitioner to a different unit, this time with a far more positive statement regarding the absence of new stresses and of mental ill-health. After a brief admission some physical deterioration was noted but it was still assumed to be functional in origin.

Finally he was referred to a rehabilitation unit with the request to obtain yet a further neurological opinion. On this occasion the opinion indicated that urgent decompression of the cord was required. This operation was undertaken and the subsequent report indicated that many more weeks of compression would have resulted in rapid and irreversible damage.

Of course it is not always possible for the general practitioner to know his patients so well, but no other doctor is better placed, and cases like those described above require a particularly careful assessment.

MANAGEMENT STRATEGIES

PSYCHOTHERAPY

Flash technique psychotherapy

Balint's early work was based on the hope that the doctor would give additional time to selected patients, but his major contribution came when he and his group realised that imposing upon general practice the time structure of psychiatric practice was inappropriate.

The development of what came to be called the 'Flash Technique' came when the group realised that the actual relationship between the doctor and patient was very important, even within a short consultation of 15 minutes or less. At first the main area studied was the 'detective work' being done by the doctor in ferreting out the problem. But it was soon appreciated that this rapid focussing on what *the doctor* assumed must be the problem was simply another form of what Balint had earlier called the 'apostolic function' of the doctor. Yet to achieve the sort of insights called for in what they called the 'flash technique' the doctor had to change style from convergent questioning as used in reaching most diagnoses, to an open and attentive listening style. The doctor invites the patient to focus. The patient decides what is bothering him and this is not based alone upon a list of probable problems the doctor offers for his consideration.

For example, a patient presents with asthma. The condition is worsening. The doctor may have some ideas why and in a traditional interview would offer a number of these ideas for consideration and selection. But in a Balint-style interview the patient would be invited to indicate what he thinks about his asthma and why it is worsening, if indeed the patient perceives the condition as worsening.

The term 'flash' is derived from the observation that from time to time a critical interview may take place during which there is a mutual appreciation of the nature of the problem. This can only really occur if the doctor is perceived by the patient as a friend — albeit a friend with special skills.

A 23-year-old girl whose asthma and eczema had played a dominant role in her childhood years had begun to come more often for consultation regarding her skin problem. The first interview was brief and conducted on the basis of the sympom offered. But at the second interview a fortuitous lack of pressure allowed the doctor to enquire generally how life was treating her. This produced a rather vague and general verbal response. However, the patient began to cry. The elements of an encounter of the type described by Balint were present. A moment of intense contact, an offer by the doctor to the patient to use him without anxiety. A freedom is thus given to the patient to use the offer whilst at the same time the doctor retains the freedom to observe the patient, the patient/doctor relationship and his own reactions in a disciplined way.

This patient began to talk about her desire to leave home and become independent, her fear and, up to that point, avoidance of any intimate relationships outside the family. She also revealed her feelings of disfigurement. After a pause she quite quickly moved to the observation that the current worsening of her physical condition was probably connected to these anxieties.

Over a number of further interviews, still not more than 15 minutes in length, the doctor was able to avoid the patient establishing a dependent relationship with him. He became an important resource for the patient, collaborating with her in her attempts to establish an independent adult status within the family and then in a flat with two other girls. The eczema remains but is now much more quiescent.

By no means all patients will respond as well as this and sometimes the changes achieved are questionably an improvement.

A patient, on joining the practice, was observed from her previous records to be a high user with little evident pathology. An initial interview was held inviting the patient to make observations on the historical events recorded. It was important that the patient did not see this as the doctor in effect saying 'I know you've been a proper nuisance to your last general practitioner and I'm making it clear to you that you won't get away with that behaviour here'. Rather the doctor was offering to explore a problem jointly with the patient.

In this case clear diagnoses of alcoholism and agoraphobia emerged. These conditions were subsequently controlled and treated. The patient then found a job in which she did well enough to be put forward for promotion. She remains, however, extremely anxious, though superficially this is not evident. She also now vomits five or six times daily, although this does not appear to have any particular deleterious physical effect. In terms of social functioning there is undoubtedly an improvement but the patient remains, if anything, even more deeply unhappy than when she first presented.

This brief description with examples cannot in any way do justice to Balint's work. A study of the doctor/patient relationship as suggested by Balint provides a rewarding experience for those who feel that their function, frustratingly, appears to be simply that of dispensing drugs, passing on patients to other doctors, or filling in forms.

Psychotherapy

Psychoanalysis is not a method of treatment open to the general practitioner directly or by referral within the National Health Service. Lengthy psychotherapeutic intervention on a regular and intense basis is equally beyond the scope of general practice, and is only slightly more likely to be available as a resource.

The pressure on consultation time initially led to attempts to set aside longer periods for special patients. This still has great merit as a strategy and brief or insight therapy is possible with strictly defined and limited goals (Colby 1951).

This type of therapy does not seek a total transformation of the patient, but rather seeks to help him to make a reasonable adaptation to the real world. Doctors who are interested in this type of therapy are advised to join a group, or work with an experienced psychotherapist's supervision on a limited number of cases. This type of therapy may be described as brief but it is still lengthy in general practice terms; yet the alternative to carefully reviewing the situation in a 45 minute to 1 hour session may be repeated unhelpful short interviewss.

Miss Q repeatedly attended her general practitioner with a variety of vague neurotic and depressive symptoms. The general practitioner felt unable to make a clear diagnosis and referred her to a psychiatrist for an opinion with the comment 'I hope I'm not wasting your time. It's probably just her personality but I keep feeling I'm mission something'.

Miss Q had arrived from Canada for a 2-year stay and a close friend from home joined her. She reported repeated episodes of difficulty in coping and mild depression which were getting worse both in severity and frequency. After the doctor had eliminated the formal diagnoses of depression and anxiety neurosis she was encouraged to review her present life. Her work, whilst not as satisfying or as challenging as her previous job, was described as being 'okay'. She indulged in sporting activities which she enjoyed and led an active social life. However, at this point some hesitations were detected and by focussing on this area it emerged that she had felt particularly depressed when her friend had gone into hospital for a minor and straightforward operation. She said that she realised at this point that she was very dependent upon her friend.

This observation led on to a discussion regarding the lack of any male relationship and that in turn led to the admission that she had never had a boyfriend. Indeed she was worries as she imagined in a rather non-sexual way the friend being physically close and comforting. She thought that she might have lesbian tendencies.

A review of sexual history now produced the fact that at the age of 13 she had been sexually approached by her 25-year-old uncle. She had little sexual knowledge at this time and was more curious than anything, but was upset by the experience. Since that time she had allowed no physical contact with men. Focussed discussion of her fears allowed her to begin a more appropriate adaptation to reality. She was clearly not lesbian as she had feared, and the lack of an intimate relationship was causing her current disequilibrium. Five sessions lasting a total of little more than 3 hours produced benefit with most of the previous neurotic symptoms disappearing. She remained well at 2 years follow-up.

The characteristics which a patient should have if they are to have a reasonable chance of benefit from this intensive type of therapy are listed in Table 24.15.

Supportive therapy

This is a poor term in that it implies a total absence of confrontation between therapist and patient. Certainly the objectives are even more limited than in the brief forms of psychotherapy described above.

Table 24.15 Patient characteristics for selection for psychotherapy

Not hysterical
Not obsessional
Not psychopathic
Not totally handicapped by his neurosis
Not psychotic
Not criminal
Not hypochondriacal
Not looking for a magical solution
Reasonably tolerant of frustrations
Able to judge the consequences of his actions
Positive personal qualities
Average or above in intelligence
Age 16–50
The reality of his situation is not overwhelming
He wishes for change
He has some capacity for self criticism

The goal is the restoration or sometimes the maintenance of a state of equilibrium. Conflict is not deliberately sought in the interview and critical feedback is minimised, but reality testing cannot be totally avoided.

Table 24.16 suggests the patients for whom his type of therapy may be helpful. Group A are essentially those in crisis. Group B are those where the opportunity is being taken to help recognise limitations, yet maximise any potential for development. Most of the patients in Group B will require supportive therapy over quite a long period of time, if not indefinitely. Group A on the other hand should require this only over a short period of time.

Block (1977) in his review of the role of supportive therapy, suggests that the relationship is akin to that of a child to a warm sympathetic parent. The techniques used are in accord with this view (Table 24.17). The main danger in this therapy is the development of dependency by the patient on the therapist. Dependency may come about as much through the needs of the doctor as from the needs of the patient. Supportive therapy should not be embarked upon simply because the doctor feels that he has been unable to help the patient in any other way. The doctor who infantilises his patient does him severe harm. There are a number of ways in which this substantial danger can be minimised:

1. Review with other staff involved the need to embark upon such a course of therapy. Decide which members of the network are best suited to the patient's needs.

Table 24.16 Examples of those needing supportive therapy

Group A	Group B
A child where one parent has left home	Chronic schizophrenia
Separation/divorce	Chronic affective psychosis
Redundancy	Severe personality diisorder
Bereavement/loss reaction	Bereavement/loss reaction
Serious physical illness	
Important stages in life cycle:	
puberty	
adolescence	
mid-life crisis	
old age	

Table 24.17 Techniques used in supportive psychotherapy

Active listening
Reassurance
Explanation
Persuasion
Suggestion
Encouragement
Repairing defences
Assistance in rationalising

2. Maintain a close contact between other staff members and the patient, thus preventing a solitary and isolated relationship as the only contact between the network and the patient.
3. Review the effect of therapy upon the patient with other staff.
4. Establish a limit on both the length of interview and, at least for Group A, a limit on the proposed number of sessions, and establish the objectives of the therapy jointly with the patient from the outset.
5. If dependency is beginning to develop discuss the problem and its dangers with the patient, but this should not lead to immediate termination of the contract.
6. Bring in other support such as self-help groups or other members of the team.

Group B may require a slightly different format. Sessions may be briefer, that is 10 to 20 minutes rather than 20 to 30 minutes. The intervals between sessions may be longer, monthly rather than weekly or fortnightly.

The successful outcome for Group A will be an independent patient who has come through the crises with strengthened and appropriate defences. For Group B it will be living comfortably with their problem.

Counselling

There is little difference between neutral or non-judgemental counselling and supportive psychotherapy. There is, however, a second form of counselling which is much more directive. The term 'doctor's orders' has become commonplace and the doctor continues to be expected to instruct or advise as well as to inform, explain and discuss. Being neutral or non-judgemental and helping the patient to reach an appropriate decision is probably the best approach with most patients in most instances. However, there are undoubtedly occasions where it is imperative that the doctor does not shirk from a more authoritarian role.

The non-medical counsellor may be useful in cases of anxiety, mental problems, other relationship problems and sexual problems. The need, as in supportive therapy, is to avoid dependency developing. The doctor's role may be to provide the counsellor with adequate support and advice.

The contract

This technique has already been referred to in relation to supportive therapy. There are a number of areas in which it may be useful to have a verbal or even written contract with the patient.

Type 1 — the challenge

This is a contract between the doctor and the patient, or the doctor and the spouse on the one hand and the patient on the other. It may be useful in such conditions as alcoholism, excessive gambling, unlawful sexual deviance, obesity and smoking.

> Mrs A. was identified as a high user without obvious pathology. On reviewing the situation with her to ascertain whether there were any problems she became extremely distressed and revealed that her husband was now drinking excessively. Mr A., aged 38, had a fairly high pressure job as a salesman in the whisky industry. This involved a considerable amount of drinking with customers. Recently he had found he was drinking more and faster, and that his tolerance of alcohol, which had been increasing, was showing signs of reduction. He was irritable at home and was now absent from work on occasions. His performance at work was slipping and he found that he sometimes became aggressive in social situations. He reported occasional partial amnesia after periods of drinking.

Mr A. does not believe that he has a drink problem: he has, after all, been drinking since the age of 12. He may respond to a contract of the challenge type. This will involve him not only abstaining from drink for a period of 3 weeks, but abstaining without difficulty. The doctor's side of the contract is that he will accept that the patient has not got a drink problem *at present*.

One danger here is that if Mr A. is a bout drinking type of alcoholic then this challenge may well be met and the opportunity to help will be lost.

> Mr A. came back after 5 weeks claiming that he had met his side of the contract with no difficulty. His wife, however, reported tremor and anxiety with extreme irritability in the first few days and the drinking of wine thereafter. Mr A. admits that he took wine but since he had abstained from spirits he felt that he had kept his side of the contract. A written contract stipulating all forms of alcohol would have prevented this difficulty arising.

Type 2 — the marital therapy contract

This is a contract made between spouses. As part of marital therapy a contract between the partners to establish changes in patterns of behaviour desired by the other partner can lead to the alleviation of mutual irritation and help initiate more positive mutual attitudes.

> Mr and Mrs W. had been referred for treatment because of Mrs W's loss of libido. It transpired that since the arrival of the children the marriage had not been as happy for either partner. Mrs W. had had to give up her job which she had found satisfying and Mr W. had had to work very hard to make ends meet. He had been promoted and was now quite successful.

Both partners were asked to prepare a list of three items which they would most like their spouse to do or to refrain from doing and three items which they found the most positive aspects of their spouse (Table 24.18). It became clear from the list that for both of them a major area of disharmony was related to Mr W's work pattern. Discussion then achieved a contract whereby if he knew that he was not going to be able to return home at the previously agreed time he would telephone. She, for her part, agreed to stop nagging.

Management of the children was evidently a problem for them both. This led to a more detailed look at themselves as parents and a lot of previously unspoken aggression emerged. They each felt the other's management was wrong. The resulting inconsistency and lack of mutual support led to great irritation. A more complex agreement on joint handling of the children was subsequently reached as a result of discussing this preliminary list.

The sexual problems referred to in the list arose not from fatigue as Mr W. had suggested, but because Mrs W. did not feel valued. His lack of attention to appearance was only a small part of this problem.. A mutual moratorium on sexual activity was declared for 3 weeks till the second interview. This alleviated some of the tension from the situation for them both.

The three positive points briefly were that she felt that he was generous, hard-working and a good father though she added the rider 'when he was not tired'. He felt that she was a great cook, always created a very good image as his wife in the work situation which he found a great asset, and was a good listener. Some of these points were greeted with pleased smiles by the partner at whom they were aimed and cetainly helped to create a positive atmosphere in which the other critical elements could be tolerably discussed.

The sexual problem did not completely resolve but the marriage improved and her libido increased to a level where sexual tension was not a major difficulty between them. The roles for caring about each other's feelings worked because they both genuinely wanted to make them work and didn't try to score points off each other's concessions.

Table 24.18 Critical areas in a case for marital therapy

Mrs W's list	Mr W's list
To tell me when he is going to be late back from work	Not to keep making excuses about being too tired for sex and then going out to the bingo
Take the children off my hands for a few hours during the weekend	Not to get on to me when I'm late back because of work
Take trouble to smarten up before we go out	Don't let the children climb all over me as soon as I get home

Type 3 — the family contract

Family therapy can be a very worthwhile, if time consuming, strategy, and a relatively straightforward strategy for coping with distress rather than illness is the 'family contract'.

One of the problems best suited to this approach is the stage of adolescent turmoil. This is a normal stage in which there is some rejection of parental values in favour of those of the peer group, preparatory to the child establishing independence. When the rejection of parental values is sudden and absolute and when the parents are frightened of relinquishing authority, conflict can follow. Parents may be unwilling to relax their rules and although this may seem realistic it may be because they reject the peer group values or because they themselves cannot face ageing or the loss involved in their child becoming independent. If there is added to this mixture either a passive unrebellious older child or a provocative younger child, the situation can be explosive.

The purpose of the contract in this situation is to allow any residual affection between parent and child to flourish, to allow the parents to be perceived as caring, and the child's strivings to be seen as normal or at least not 'bad'.

The rules are agreed on a basis similar to the list system in marital therapy, or alternatively may be established following the keeping of a diary in which each side lists the faults of the other.

This approach will not always work. The rigidity and self-righteousness of the parents may be so destructive that expulsion of the youngster is inevitable. Alternatively the peer group values are so unacceptable to the parents and yet adhered to so strongly by the youngster that a contract is simply not worth attempting.

Joint therapy with a counsellor, social worker or community psychiatric nurse may be useful to ensure that manipulation by individual members of the group is more readily exposed. This may also allow individual counselling as a preliminary to the establishment of a contract where difficulties are clearly going to arise.

PHARMACOTHERAPY

Every general practitioner will be aware that patients have a high expectation of receiving prescriptions. Indeed, a survey of doctors and patients carried out by Cartwright & Anderson (1977) showed that the patient's expectation of receiving a prescription at consultation had dropped since their previous study in 1964. Nevertheless, 41% of patients still expected this response from their general practitioner. A more hopeful sign in the same study was that the proportion who expected or hoped for advice or reassurance had risen from 18% in 1964 to 29% in 1977. The proportion who reported that their doctor had given them advice or reassurance at consultation had also risen from 41 to 65%.

The average general practitioner will issue about 2000 psychotropic prescriptions annually. This can amount to about 30% of his total prescriptions in any year. There is considerable evidence that compliance with prescribed psychotropic drugs is poor.

Each practitioner will wish to devise his own short list of psychotropic drugs selected from each class of drugs. There is an enormous variety of psychotropic drugs available in each class, but they have for the most part minor differences. It would be quite impracticable to discuss all the drugs available or indeed to consider in detail even the classes of drugs, but this section will consider the benzodiazepines and the antidepressants with a brief consideration of major tranquillisers in the section dealing with schizophrenia.

The benzodiazepines

In a recent review, it was suggested that more than 40 million doses of this class of drugs had been consumed by the world community since they were developed in 1960. The most common drug used is diazepam rather than the original drug, which was chlordiazepoxide. They have as a group been both effective and safe (Tables 24.19, 24.20).

However, the criticism of doctors, which is increasing, is that they over-prescribe this group of drugs. Such over-prescription probably reflects the concern and compassion which the doctor has for his patient as much as his inability to use the drug wisely.

This group of drugs should not be used in an attempt to treat unhappiness or depressive illness, nor are they helpful on the whole in treating isolated symptoms. More than a single dose given to alleviate the psychological reaction to loss or bereavement may, for example, be positively harmful. Even a single dose should not be used unless in exceptional circumstances. It is self-evident that no drug can treat material deprivation.

Table 24.19 Categories of benzodiazepines

Long-acting	Short-acting	Hypnotics
Diazepam	Oxazepam	Nitrazepam
Chlordiazepoxide	Lorazepam	Flurazepam
Medazepam	Clobazam	Temazepam
Chlorazepate		Triazolam

Table 24.20 Side effects of benzodiazpeines

Drowsiness
Ataxia (especially in the elderly)
Dizziness
Confusion (occasionally)
Dry mouth
Hypersensitivity reactions

Dependence

The Committee on Safety of Medicines has emphasised the need to use benzodiazepines for short periods only. There is a mounting body of evidence that when prescribed for less than 10 weeks, most patients experience few, if any, problems on cessation,, but a significant number, perhaps as many as a quarter, have definite withdrawal symptoms after longer use. Such patients tend to keep coming back for more and this patient-led demand makes for a high level of suspicion that dependence is developing.

Withdrawal

The symptoms of withdrawal after long-term use include severe anxiety, although this may be in part a recrudescence of the original anxiety state, trembling, poor appetite, faintness, insomnia, palpitation and, in cases where the doses have been high, depersonalisation and perceptual change. These symptoms are almost always relieved as soon as consumption of the drug is resumed.

Withdrawal of the benzodiazepines should, therefore, be attempted slowly. The patient should be warned to expect withdrawal symptoms over a period of 1 to 2 weeks. Some patients, whose somatic responses are distressing, may be helped by propranolol 80–160 mg daily in divided doses. In a few instances where withdrawal is particularly difficult, switching to either fluphenazine hydrochloride 1–2 mg daily or promazine 100–200 mg daily may be helpful.

Disinhibition

The inappropriate use of benzodiazepines in depression may well increase the likelihood of impulsive parasuicide. The possibility of releasing aggressive impulses when used in mothers with infants, in whom undiagnosed puerperal depression exists, has also been suggested as a danger.

Despite the side effects and problems listed above, the improvement in safety offered by this class of drugs over previously available drugs, such as barbiturates, is undeniable. They remain an indispensable part of a doctor's armamentarium. Some basic guidelines to be observed are suggested in Table 24.21.

Antidepressants

Tricyclic and related drugs

Although there is a marked placebo response evident on all placebo controlled trials for the treatment of depression, the tricyclic and related compounds appear to have great value. At the present time there are 17 compounds from which to choose but this choice will usually be made from a much more restricted list (Table 24.22).

Table 24.21 Guidelines for the use of benzodiazepines

1. Is the drug necessary at all?:   — YES
   If the anxiety exists sufficiently to seriously
   disrupt or handicap the individual
   If appropriate anxiety exists as a healthy and   — NO
   not overwhelming response to events and
   circumstances
2. Which drug?
   A choice must be made between a hypnotic, a long-acting or
   short-acting benzodiazepine. Long-acting hypnotics may be
   particularly problematical in the elderly.
3. Are there any contraindications relative or absolute?:
   a. machinery used
   b. driving
   c. respiratory disease
   d. elderly patients
   e. nursing mothers
   f. neuromuscular diseased patients
   g. late pregnancy
   h. closed angle glaucoma
4. How long should the drug be used for?:
   As short a time as possible and certainly not for more than 10
   weeks.

Guidelines for antidepressant prescribing

1. Is the drug necessary at all? Does a depressive illness in fact exist or is the patient showing unhappiness commensurate with his situation?

2. Which drug should be used? Is a sedating effect likely to be beneficial? If the answer is yes, then the amitriptyline group or mianserin or trazodone should be used. If the answer is no, then one of the imipramine group or nomifensine should be used.

3. Is there any history of cardiac abnormality? Is the patient elderly? *Is there a serious suicidal risk?* Have anticholinergic effects proved troublesome in the past? If the answer to any or all of these is yes, then one of the newer drugs should be used. Otherwise the appropriate older and cheaper drugs may be used (Table 24.22).

4. What dosage? In older patients and those who have previously experienced side effects, a gradual build up in medication may be used, but otherwise it is important to reach the therapeutic levels recommended by the manufacturers. There is a tendency to prescribe subtherapeutic doses.

4. How to handle a suicidal risk: the newer drugs which appear to have significantly less toxic effects are indicated. Access to the drug should be controlled either by small prescriptions of less than 1 gram, or having the drug held by a relative, the pharmacist or the doctor and only dispensing quantities well below 1 gram.

5. When should the patient take the drug? The advice on this varies according to the preparation used, but the useful general rule is that drugs with some sedative effect should probably be taken in the middle of the evening unless the sedative effect is particularly desired during the day.

Onset of action and side-effects
There is no evidence that the newer drugs are any better than the original preparations in achieving a rapid therapeutic response. It continues to be unlikely that much response will be seen in the first 10 days. Side effects, on the other hand, tend to be more pronounced early in treatment and this increases the likelihood of poor compliance.

Length of treatment
A minimum period of 3 months is advisable, yet many patients stop taking the drugs after 1 month when they feel some improvement. However, a significant number will relapse at this point. Patients in whom relapses have previously occurred may require much longer-term therapy of up to one or more years. After the first 3 months this may be at a slightly reduced dosage.

Changing the treatment
This should not be done before a trial of about 4 weeks has been given. If no response has occurred after 2 weeks it is worthwhile increasing the dose of the drug, provided

Table 24.22 Tricyclic and related antidepressants

	Sedative	Less sedative	Possibly stimulating
Older compounds	Amitriptyline Dothiepin Trimipramine	Imipramine Butriptyline Desipramine Dipenzepin Clomipramine Nortriptyline Maprotiline Iprindole	Protriptyline
'Newer' compounds	Mianserin Trazodone	Nomifensine	

that side effects have not proved troublesome.

When a change is made, a drug with a different profile should be tried. For example, if amitriptyline fails than it may be worth trying one of the newer preparations.

The elderly patient

The risks of cardiovascular toxicity occurring at therapeutic dosage levels makes the use of one of the newer antidepressants much safer. Elderly patients are prone to additional side effects, such as increased sensitivity to the drug, confusion and, in males, urinary retention.

Children

The tricyclic drugs should not be used in children under the age of 6 because of reduced tolerance although it is suggested that a dose not in excess of 2.5 mg/kg per day can be used.

Newer compounds

At present there are available three relatively new drugs as listed in Table 24.22. Although it is still too early to discuss with great certainty the role these drugs may have, they do appear to have a number of possible advantages:

1. Lack of anticholinergic effects.
2. Fewer or absent cardiovascular effects.
3. Less toxic in overdosage.
4. Well tolerated in the elderly.

These three drugs provide a useful range on the sedative scale, mianserin being the most sedative of the three, followed by trazodone. Nomifensine appears to be neutral or mildly activating. Trazodone is a completely new molecule and may, therefore, be of particular value when other antidepressants have not been successful. Nomifensine, which inhibits re-uptake at both noradrenergic and dopaminergic transmitters, may be of particular value in epileptics and patients with Parkinson's disease. Mianserin, which appears to have its effect by blocking the presynaptic noradrenergic receptors as well as increasing central noradrenergic synthesis, is already well established but may need to be used in high doses to achieve its effect.

Table 24.23 indicates contraindications to use of the older drugs.

Table 24.23 Contraindications to the use of older antidepressants

Arrhythmia
Myocardial ischaemia
Cardiac conduction defects
Abnormal ECG
Marked atherosclerosis
Other cardiovascular disease
History of severe drug reaction particularly if heart was involved

Lithium

This well established drug is used in the management of mania, hypomania and bipolar manic-depressive psychosis and recurrent endogenous depression. It has a very narrow therapeutic/toxic ratio and therefore requires particularly careful monitoring of plasma levels. The advised range of plasma levels in samples taken 12 hours after the last dose is 0.6–1.2 mmol/litre. The side effects,, which are listed in Table 24.24, may be experienced even within this therapeutic range. The weight gain, which can be excessive, can be made even worse if the lithium is used in combination with a major tranquilliser in the treatment of mania.

As can be seen from Table 24.25, which is a schedule of monitoring for lithium therapy, it is particularly necessary to examine for hypothyroidism at regular intervals.

REFERRAL

There is no possibility of the specialist services being able to manage all psychiatric patients even if referral were to be limited to those for whom a formal diagnosis could be made. Notions such as 'out reach', whereby the hospital is stretching out its services ever deeper into the community, can only be helpful in a very limited way, mainly in the rehabilitation of in-patients.

The range of referral rates in general practice is as wide for psychological problems as it is for physical ones. The rate will vary according to the perception of mental illness by the patient and his family. Stigma probably remains one of the crucial factors for not referring, though this can be minimised by the psychiatrist or other specialist workers being situated in the health centre.

Table 24.24 Side effects of lithium therapy

Short-term	Therapeutic levels Long-term	Toxic levels
Thirst/polyuria	Hypothyroidism	Serious effects occur at levels greater than
Fine tremor	Change in steroid metabolism	2 mmol/litre
Weight gain ± oedema	Change in carbohydrate metabolism	
Gastro-intestinal disturbances	Nephrogenic diabetes insipidous	

Table 24.25   Monitoring schedule for lithium therapy

All samples taken 12 hours after last dose
1. Day 3
2. Day 7
3. Day 14   More frequent intervals if levels outside
4. Day 21   therapeutic range
5. Day 28
6.
7. Monthly for 3 months
8.
9. and thereafter at 10 week intervals — but more frequently if
   a. side effects
   b. signs of toxicity
   c. intercurrent infection
Every 6 months — thyroid function tests

The attitude of the general practitioner towards psychiatric colleagues will have an effect. There is a tendency for older general practitioners to refer identified cases more frequently but the variation in rates resulting from this factor are extremely complex. Younger general practitioners perceive themselves as having a more extensive treatment and management role. An average of about one in 20 of patients presenting will be referred, but the range is from one in 10 to one in 50.

Reasons for referral

Roberts (1981) of the University of Ottowa, in a recent report on the interface between psychiatry and family medicine observed that UK general practitioners tended to refer patients who fell into the following groups:

1. Acute mania.
2. Very severe depression.
3. Geriatric patients, especially those with senile dementia and arteriosclerotic dementia.
4. Personality disorders with depression, especially non-responders.
5. Patients where it was felt that they could not work effectively with the primary therapist and where the primary therapist knew a particular psychiatrist who could help the patient. This is referred to as matching patients to psychiatrists.
6. Patients who make severe suicidal gesture.
7. Psychopaths.
8. Occasionally children.
9. Unmanageable schizophrenics.

Perhaps the most common reason for referral is the failure by the patient to respond to treatment. This would seem an appropriate reason if taken together with those cases where the condition is severe, distressing, socially disabling or disruptive, and those where the general practitioner is unable to establish a clear therapeutic plan, either because of diagnostic difficulties or lack of appropriate skills.

The general practitioner can assist the psychiatrist greatly by stating a clear reason for referral and indicating what help or advice he is seeking, in addition to any diagnosis which he may have made.

BEHAVIOUR THERAPY

This form of therapy used by clinical psychologists is based upon experimental research in the fields of learning and cognition. As we have seen in looking at models of illness, it is one of four possible approaches. It may be used alone with great effect in some conditions, or in combination with one or more sociotherapeutic, psychotherapeutic or organic physical treatments. There are a number of techniques, some general and some specific, which may be used in an individual or group setting.

The conditions most commonly referred to psychologists are general anxiety, specific phobias and sexual dysfunction. Table 24.26 is based on the first 481 referrals to the Forth Valley Health Board Community Psychology Clinic and gives a fuller picture of the variety of adult referrals. (The number of cases of sexual dysfunction referred is low because of the existence of a separate Sexual Problems Clinic.) Amongst the techniques available are:

Table 24.26   Referrals to a psychology clinic. Presenting problem as defined by psychologist in 481 consecutive cases (Jerrom et al 1981)

	% of sample
Anxiety	26
Agoraphobia	12
Depression	10
Social phobia	8
Sexual dysfunction	7
Specific phobia	7
Somatic symptoms	5
Obsessions: Ruminations	2
Headache	2
Obsessions: Rituals	2
Smoking	2
Alcoholism	2
Pain	2
Marital problems	1
Obesity	1
Insomnia	1
Temper/aggression	1
Anorexia	1
Drug abuse	1
Sexual deviation	1
Study problems	1
Family relationships	1
Other	4
Kincey categories	
Anxiety and stress	69%
Habit disorders	9%
Interpersonal social and marital	22%

Relaxation

This general technique was developed originally by Jacobson in the early 1900's. A brief description of the simplest form of this technique may be helpful.

The patient is invited to adopt a prone position and asked to ensure that he is not wearing any garments which will seriously constrict him. He is then called upon to tighten the muscles of the body. The instructor assists this process by listing sequentially the parts of the body upon which the patient is required to focus. Thus it is suggested that he should plantor flex the feet whilst curling up the toes, pressing the legs closely together, tightening the muscles of the thighs and buttocks, tightening the abdominal muscles, clenching the hands, tightening the forearm muscles, pressing the shoulders back into the couch, closing the eyes tightly, clenching the teeth and tightening the facial muscles whilst pressing the head, neck and back into the couch. The sequence of muscle movements is repeated and the patient is observed to make sure that tension is well maintained. This requires considerable effort on the part of the patient and he may begin to experience some fatigue. The period for which he is required to maintain the tension can be varied according to the observed level of fatigue, but once the patient appears to need to relax the sequence is then repeated but this time the patient is instructed to gradually relax the areas one by one. This is accompanied by suggestions to breathe deeply and slowly using not only the chest but abdominal muscles, thus increasing diaphragmatic breathing.

This very simple form of relaxation therapy can sometimes produce a light hypnotic trance state without the addition of 'distraction' which is normally employed in hypnotic induction. More complex training can be established either by direct verbal instruction or by using an instruction sheet or prepared tapes.

Systematic desensitisation

This is a widely used and effective treatment based on conditioning learning theory and is particularly effective for specific phobias. The patient and therapist construct a hierarchy of fears from the most intense and feared situation to the least frightening.

Mrs C., a 25-year-old, presented with a phobia of moths. The fear was so bad that she could not leave her flat to go down the tenement stairs. An abbreviated form of the hierarchy employed in her case was as follows:

Most feared   1. Large black moths in the dark fluttering in her hair.
              2. Small white moths fluttering round the light.
              3. Butterflies outside
              4. A canary loose in the room.
              5. A canary in a cage.
Least feared 6. Birds outside.

The patient was taught to relax and was invited to imagine the lowest item in the hierarchy. Once she remained relaxed and was able to concentrate on this item without fear the next item in the hierarchy was introduced and so on until the patient was able to imagine, concentrating hard, the most feared item in the hierarchy. Mrs C. was treated in eight sessions and the treatment remained effective for 2 years. Indeed, she described how her daughter had brought her a moth 'just to show Mummy'. Mrs C. reported that she was able to take the moth and put it out of the window.

Desensitisation along with flooding, aversion therapy, positive reinforcement and modelling are all essentially forms of exposure to the feared object or the behaviour to be changed and may be carried out either in vivo or in fantasy.

Target setting

Target setting is now the most widely used behavioural technique in the treatment of anxiety, phobias and psychosomatic conditions. The technique is derived from the hierarchy used in desensitisation, and simply involves setting specific goals which the patient will attempt to achieve by the next treatment session.

The theoretical basis for such a method is that the patient is confronting in a gradual fashion the situations and causes of his anxiety, and in the process is learning to cope with these situations and master his reactions to them. Target setting is usually combined with a self report diary technique, where the patient is asked to record all of his relevant activities in between treatment sessions, as this exercise considerably increases compliance with the treatment.

Assertive training and social skills training

Both these treatments are aimed at increasing social and relationship skills in patients who suffer from severe shyness and lack of self-confidence. Assertive training, which is American in origin, tends to focus upon situations involving conflict and emotion whilst social skills training, which is the British counterpart, deals with all aspects of social interaction.

Training involves the use of rehearsal, where the patient is asked to role play the specific social situation under analysis. He is given feedback about his performance and, if necessary, specific instructions or a demonstration as to how to make his performance more skilful. Social skills training can be done either individually or in out-patient groups, the patients most usually treated with this method being young adults or adolescents. As this style of treatment is obviously stressful for a patient suffering from shyness, it is very important that he should have a high level of motivation towards treatment if the training programme is to succeed.

Social skills training as a technique has applications in many fields outside clinical psychology and psychiatry, and is being used with increasing frequency in various institutions and as a component of various types of management and professional training courses.

Biofeedback

As the name suggests, this involves providing the patient with information regarding physiological changes in his body of which he would not normally be aware and over which he would have little or no voluntary control. It can be used in the treatment of tension headache where feedback from the frontalis muscle via an EMG may allow better relaxation. It may be helpful also in other neuromuscular conditions, such as paresis, nerve damage including Bell's palsy, hemifacial spasm and torticollis, some of which are fairly resistant to other forms of treatment.

It has been suggested that it may be of value in the treatment of migraine with feedback of the constriction of the extra-cranial blood flow. Some workers have used it in assisting the patient to control their own blood pressure. It is possible to help with general relaxation using very simple biofeedback equipment where a change in the galvanic skin response alters the pitch of the noise produced.

Stimulus control

The patient is provided with definite instructions with a view to changing his habits. Patients presenting with insomnia often report that they go to bed at a fairly set time and then toss and turn and are unable to get to sleep. The hypothesis is that this leads to a learned association between going to bed and *not* sleeping. To break this association the patient is advised to go to bed only when sleepy, not to read or listen to the radio or to use the bedroom for any other purpose except sleep. In addition, if after a period of 10–15 minutes he has not gone to sleep he should get up and do something not too stimulating. He should avoid sleeping during the day and if he does not already do so he should be advised to rise at a set time.

Flooding or implosion therapy

Instead of establishing a careful hierarchy with relaxation therapy before commencement, the patient is exposed, usually in fantasy, for a period of 45 minutes, to the maximum feared situation. Although some patients find it extremely difficult to embark on this form of treatment there seems little doubt that the levels of anxiety reduces quite quickly during each session. The reduction in the level of anxiety is increasingly maintained between sessions. Four to five sessions will often eliminate the phobia.

Aversion therapy

This technique is based upon the punishment/reward effect observed in learning theory. The event, action or thought to be eliminated is paired closely with a negative stimulus.

Early work in the treatment of alcoholism used this form of therapy. The alcoholic was required to consume alcohol whilst at the same time being given an injection to induce vomiting. Despite the strong reaction which the patient did experience, results were poor in the long-term. Treatment has also been used to help transvestites wishing to avoid cross-dressing behaviour and in the treatment of paedophilia.

Positive reinforcement

This therapy is particularly valuable where unacceptable behaviour is found to be being reinforced. The attention given to a young child when he has a tantrum may, for example, reinforce that tantrum. By avoiding the previous positive reinforcement and substituting positive reinforcement of more appropriate bits of behaviour the tantrums may be lessened or eliminated. This treatment has also been used for the treatment of anorexics where the patient has all forms of stimulus removed and any positive reinforcement is conditional upon some consumption of food with a graduated response according to the food consumption level.

Cognitive therapy

This is a term covering a number of different types of 'thinking' therapy. In the treatment of depression for example, the objective is to modify the morbid thoughts and poor self-esteem which the patient carries with him into every situation. These half conscious, often fleeting thoughts, colour every action. 'This is going to be a disaster', 'I've never been any good at this', 'No one likes me'. These sort of thoughts are recalled and questioned to see how much distortion they represent. More positive thoughts are substituted. 'I know this is usually difficult but I am finding it easier than I did before'. In this form of therapy work done with the patient is aimed at problem solving and success is then reinforced.

This is an extremely over-simplified version of a fairly complex, high structured and moderately directive form of behavioural therapy. There is some evidence that it may be as effective as pharmacotherapy, but further work needs to be done before it can be fully assessed.

Modelling

The therapist shows the patient that the particular piece of feared behaviour does not result in the expected catastrophy. In countries where snakes are more prevalent, a phobia of snakes can be seriously handicapping. The object here would be to reduce the level of fear to that appropriate to produce avoidance of dangerous snakes. The therapist will handle a live snake in front of the patient and the patient will eventually be able to handle the snake himself.

Sexual therapy

The development of Masters & Johnson of directive techniques in the treatment of sexual problems has proved to be highly successful. As with many other forms of behaviour therapy, the initial stages are aimed at relieving the anxiety and tension often found in couples with sexual difficulties. The instruction to an impotent male that he is not to have intercourse until an appropriate stage of therapy is reached can alleviate completely the performance anxiety previously experienced. Although relatively simple to learn, such techniques should not be embarked upon without adequate training. Inappropriate partial treatment can be damaging and render treatment by a specialist more difficult.

Some behavioural techniques will need further evaluation before they can replace current treatment methods, but their efficacy in areas such as specific phobias, sexual problems and general anxiety are beyond doubt. In phobias and sexual dysfunction they are the treatment method of choice. It must be emphasised that the descriptions given above are in no way adequate for a practitioner to begin therapy. They constitute a brief description which could be given to the patient if they are questioning the form of therapy to be employed.

HYPNOSIS

A workable definition of hypnosis is 'an altered state of consciousness in which changes in perception occur as uncritical responses by the subject to suggestions from an outside source or from within his own memory'.

Hypnosis has slipped in and out of fashion since its first brief but triumphant appearance in Paris under Mesmer. The traditional medical authorities reacted then with hostility and have remained unconvinced of its value. It is true that many of the claims for its efficacy by enthusiasts remain as unproven as they were at the beginning of the century. A recent review article proposed 35 conditions which could be helped significantly by hypnosis.

Table 24.27 Uses of self hypnosis (a limited list)

As an adjunct to relaxation therapy
Phobic conditions
Asthma
Pain — in terminal illness and dysmenorrhoea
Childbirth
Smoking
Obesity
Public performers

Some of the effects which can be demonstrated under moderate or deep hypnosis provide an exciting insight into the power of the mind over the body. One classic example is that of a man of average or even light physique who under hypnosis is capable of sustaining the weight of two large men seated upon his horizontal form which is supported only under his head and his feet. Table 24.27 is an uncontroversial list of conditions where the use of self-hypnosis is helpful. It will be seen that these are mainly conditions where anxiety is the predominant feature. It would not be appropriate to use it in every ante-natal case, nor in every case of asthma, and its use in smoking and obesity is probably best limited to those cases where there are additional motivating factors such as peripheral vascular or other obesity-related problems. In these latter two conditions the results are best where there is anxiety which is relieved by smoking or by eating.

Teaching the patient auto- or self-hypnosis avoids the dependency or transference problems which can be encountered. A variation of auto-hypnosis is the use of a tape recorded message for the induction and deepening of the trance state.

> Mr T., a business executive with a flying phobia, had been treated with desensitisation. This had not proved sufficiently successful to allow him to board a plane except in a state of intoxication. He proved a good hypnotic subject and after three weekly sessions (30 minutes, 20 minutes and 20 minutes) followed by two reinforcing sessions at 1- and 2-month intervals (20 minutes each) he flew without excessive alcohol and without anxiety.

> Ronald V., a 10-year-old, refused absolutely to go to the dentist despite his parents' best efforts. Treatment was now urgently required. A dentist who used hypnosis was contacted. Induction and deepening methods were jointly agreed with the doctor. After four sessions the child was able to attend the dentist where the familiarity of the previously used technique further reinforced the reduction in Ronald's anxiety. He is now able to attend the dentist without problems.

Patients in whom hypnosis should not be undertaken include children under the age of 9, patients with obsessional neurosis or marked obsessional traits, mentally handicapped and psychotic patients.

Most hypnotherapists find a success rate of about 80% in patients who are able to achieve even a light trance state. More intense use of hypnosis combined with what are called ego strengthening suggestions may be used in some chronic forms of anxiety. However, no hypnosis should be used without training. Such training can be obtained through the Medical and Dental Hypnosis Society.

SPECIFIC SYNDROMES

SCHIZOPHRENIA

Diagnois

The diagnostic criteria for schizophrenia have been tightened very considerably in the last 15 years. The previous laxity is best demonstrated by Rosenhaum et al in 1973. The authors falsified their names and vocations but otherwise maintained their previous history and presented themselves as hearing voices saying only a single word, either 'empty', 'thud' or 'hollow'. They were diagnosed on 12 separate occasions as suffering from schizophrenia and were committed to hospital for an average stay of 19 days despite offering no further symptoms at all after admission. The dilemma of the diagnosis in the United Kingdom has been highlighted by the court case of the Yorkshire Ripper; only time will tell whether he did indeed suffer from a schizophrenic illness.

The change in criteria has implications for the general practitioner. Some of his patients will have been diagnosed as schizophrenic and yet had they presented today with similar symptoms they would not be so diagnosed. Apart from the stigma which any labelling may cause, some of these patients may continue to be on long-term maintenance therapy which they do not require.

The current American criteria called DSM3 (Fox 1981) is set out in Table 24.28. The application of these criteria would exclude cases:

Table 24.28 A definition of schizophrenia (D.S.M. 3)

A PSYCHOTIC SYMPTOMS (Only one necessary)
  a. ANY DELUSION except: Persecution/Jealousy.
    i.e. Schneider first rank type including delusions of
      control. Thought
      broadcasting/insertion/withdrawal or bizarre
      delusions.
  b. DELUSIONS of a persecutory or jealousy type.
  c. AUDITORY HALLUCINATIONS must be more
    than one or two words and *not* with elated or depressed
    content.
    Commentary on behaviour or thoughts.
    Two voices discussing.
  d. FORMAL THOUGHT DISORDER Incoherence.
    Loosening of Associations. Illogical thinking. Poverty
    of content.
    ALONG WITH flat or inappropriate affect
      or delusions of any kind
      or grossly disorganised or catatonic behaviour.
+B DETERIORATION OF PREVIOUS LEVEL OF
    FUNCTION
    in work, social or self-care areas.
+C SYMPTOMS PRESENT FOR 6 MONTHS
    including active psychotic symptoms for at least a period.
+D ONSET BEFORE 45
+E NOT DUE TO AFFECTIVE DISORDER
+F NOT DUE TO ORGANIC DISORDER
    or
    MENTAL SUBNORMALITY

---

1. Where there are manifestations which have not lasted for 6 months. Thus cases with an acute onset and equally rapid resolution, which have a much better prognosis, would therefore no longer be included in the nuclear schizophrenic group.

2. Psychotic episodes of less than 2 weeks duration following psychosocial stress would now be classed as brief reactive psychoses.

3. In latent or borderline schizophrenia in which there are some of the features but not sufficient to warrant a full diagnosis. Such cases would be more akin to a schizophrenic personality type.

4. Late onset schizophrenia or paraphrenia in the elderly would also be excluded.

All these four groups have a different prognosis to that of schizophrenia as it is now defined.

Treatment

The depot tranquilliser preparations make management much easier in many cases. Neuroleptic medication either in oral form or by depot injection form can cause problems. These include:

1. Parkinsonian effects
2. Tardive dyskinesia
3. Weight gain

Of the three problems, tardive dyskinesia or bucco-linguo-masticatory syndrome, is the most difficult to treat. This condition of involuntary movements of a number of muscle groups may be due to the drugs creating an imbalance between the dopamine and acetylcholine transmitters in the basal ganglia. Unfortunately withdrawal of the phenothiazines only serves to worsen the involuntary movements. Increasing the drug produces temporary relief but Parkinsonian symptoms and involuntary movements break through again later. Drugs such as tetrabenzine are only partially effective.

Review and withdrawal of treatment

Any doubts about the original diagnosis should lead to review. The patient who has been stable and symptom-free on medication for 4 years or more will warrant a gradual withdrawal of treatment under close supervision. On the other hand, those who are unstable or have residual symptoms may well relapse upon withdrawal. Restarting the drug when such a relapse becomes evident is in almost every case accompanied by the resumption of effective control.

The schizophrenic in the community

In a recent review of all patients with this diagnosis in the author's practice (population 5350) only one of the 23 index patients was in hospital on a long-term basis. This patient is part of the small accretion in hospital of what are termed new long-stay patients. The majority of patients were found to be free of any first rank signs on maintenance therapy. However, it was evident from this review that in a majority of instances the information which was available was limited to the mental state. Little was known about the quality of life of these patients and their families.

With the development in the last three decades of effective drug management and hospital rehabilitation programmes, an increasing number of patients have been discharged from hospital. It transpired that returning them to the family setting was followed in a disturbingly high number of cases by frequent relapse and readmission. It was also found that where this pattern did not hold, a second and equally unhappy picture could be seen. This second group remained at home but spent much of their time in bed, very isolated, not joining in the family social activities and occasionally threatening violence to the family (Creer & Weing 1974). This behaviour produced a variety of reactions in the family members, ranging from depression to outright hostility, profound guilt to withdrawal from outside social contact. At best there seemed to be an unhappy and tense toleration of the situation.

There appears to be a therapeutic balance between tolerating the patient's behaviour and giving his life a structure. This supportive role will deflect the patient away from internal preoccupation and apathy but must not be too demanding. Any highly critical family member is liable to aggravate the patient's problems and may need to be distanced from him.

The assessment of the family and their likely reaction to the patient are an important part of managing his rehabilitation. The social worker may be best placed to help but the primary and secondary members of the network should jointly establish an individual management plan. This may include attendance at a day centre or participation in an enclave work scheme. An enclave work scheme is where a number of disabled people work together in an ordinary work setting.

Such a plan may involve a decision to move the patient away from his family setting to another form of sheltered accommodation. It should also look at the prevention of relapse brought on by stress since serious stressful events beyond the patient's control are likely to lead to an exacerbation of the psychosis. This may be prevented either by temporarily increasing medication or by increasing the level of supportive therapy, or both.

Depression in schizophrenia

Finally, it should not be forgotten that depression can occur in a schizophrenic illness. Some researchers have suggested that 'depression' is a commonplace feature of the illness though it is usually masked by more florid symptoms in the acute phase. The various hypotheses on the course of depression in schizophrenia remain to be proved. One hypothesis is that the neuroleptic drugs involved in treatment produce the depression. Another is that retention of insight into the bizarre quality of some of the symptoms may precipitate the depression. Whatever the cause its importance in primary care needs to be stressed because the risk of schizophrenics committing suicide has a much higher frequency than in the normal population.

DEPRESSION

Unhappiness or depressive illness?

Depression can be distinguished from unhappiness. It is crucial that this differentiation is made so that what may be a natural and healthy response should not be treated as an illness. Bereavement is one situation where many families will call upon the doctor to provide a pharmacological solution to distress when what is needed is sympathy combined with education on the normal grief reaction. Too often the bereaved patient is introduced to benzodiazepines at this point in their lives and becomes dependent upon these drugs.

A common presentation of unhappiness is where the patient indicates a sense of helplessness.

At a recent consultation Mrs M. complained that she was having increasing difficulty in coping with the situation at home. Mrs M. had recently married and was now living with her parents-in-law in a council house. Before Mrs M. and her husband had married they had both applied for housing but since they were only 16 and 18 they were awarded minimum points. Their stated *intention* to marry carried no weight.

As a result of marrying and moving into the in-laws house they gained further points because the house was now overcrowded. However, this would have qualified them only for housing in a different and poorer area. A series of 'catch 22' situations now faced the couple and created a sense of helplessness.

1. They could take a house in a socially deprived area away from their present house and work place. This would add transport costs of £12 to their weekly budget. They would then be regarded as suitably housed and could not stay on the list for an area where they both wished to be housed. Mrs M. also wanted to remain near her mother who was not in good health.

2. They could remain for a number of years where they were with increasing tensions in the family. They could have one or more children which would create more tension but would give them the necessary qualifying points.

3. They could move into rented accommodation but this would again mean that they would lose their place on the housing list.

4. Their parents could evict them and they would

then be rehoused under the appropriate Homeless Persons Act, but probably again in the poor area which they did not want.

The couple had in fact decided to remain where they were but also had decided not to act irresponsibly in starting their family under such unsuitable circumstances. Unfortunately Mr M. was then declared redundant and now Mrs M. was presenting with what she believed was depression. There was no doubt that Mrs M. was unhappy but there was no evidence of her having a depressive illness at this stage. An examination of her problems showed them to include the social problems outlined above, the increasing tensions within the family and marked difficulties in the sexual side of the marriage resulting from the inhibitions which she felt from the ever present family.

Every general practitioner has similar cases. The action here was not to prescribe a drug but to involve a social worker to look at the housing problem and the family tensions, and a marriage guidance counsellor to handle the marital stress. The doctor continued to give individual supportive therapy to Mrs M. This meant that although her expectation had been for a prescription she did not perceive the doctor's refusal as being a rejection. The doctor also avoided taking on the role of a magician who could solve all Mrs M's problems with a prescription. His role in psychotherapy was to help Mrs M. express her unhappiness not by probing at the problems but by helping the patient to explore at her own pace the various elements of her unhappiness. In addition the network combined in an advocacy role to ensure that the social elements of the case were given proper weight by the Housing Authority.

True depression

In reaching a diagnosis of depressive illness the elements which make up a true 'depressive shift' should be assessed (Table 24.29). Not only should the presence of these individual symptoms and signs be noted, but the severity of the shift in each patient should be assessed with particular attention to the extent of suicidal ideation. A treatment strategy can then be devised which may include elements of pharmacological, behavioural and social treatments.

Table 24.29 Features of depressive shift

Mood depressed
Guilt feelings, loss of self-esteem
Suicidal ideation
Loss of interest/poor concentration/short term memory problems
Lack of energy
Loss of appetite or change in appetite
Somatic and psychic anxiety features
Insomnia

Rating scales

Scales such as those of Hamilton (Table 24.30) or Beck's Inventory can be useful in assessing the severity both at initial diagnosis and in the monitoring of progress and response to treatment. It is quite feasible for a general practitioner to be trained in a few hours in the use of such scales. A self-rating version of the Hamilton Scale has been developed and work is being done to produce a computer-compatible version. This would mean that the doctor could have in front of him an objective assessment at the time of the patient's consultation.

Specialist referral

The vast majority of depressive illnesses will be treated by the general practitioner, but there are situations where a psychiatric opinion should be sought. Firstly when the overall severity rating is high, secondly where the delusional quality of the morbid thoughts is strongly psychotic and thirdly where the suicidal ideation is intense either with persistent rumination, or with serious planning, or following an attempt at suicide. Suicidal ideation must always be looked for in assessing the depressed patient. Questioning a patient about such suicidal ideation does not put the idea into his head.

Atypical presentations

Anxiety neurosis as opposed to phobic or situational anxiety rarely occurs after the age of 45. Yet somatic and psychic anxiety symptoms are amongst the most common presenting features of depression at all ages. If the doctor accepts the proferred individual symptoms he is going to miss a lot of depressive illness. Watts (1966) in analysing the presentation of depression in general practice listed the following eight most common symptoms out of the 71 which identified:

Tiredness and weakness	
Headache	50%
Anxiety and tension	
Depression	5%
Backache, insomnia	
Chest pain, dyspepsia	15%

The most striking feature of this list is that depression as the directly presenting symptom represented only 5% of the total in his study. Watts has shown that depression is also a good example of the Iceberg Phenomenon (Fig. 24.6). Presentations which may prove more difficult to diagnose include:

The smiling depression

This is found more commonly in women. The most striking feature is that the affective state is inappropriate to the circumstances of the patient. In the case described below a sense of irritation which was felt by the doctor led him to re-examine the diagnosis.

Table 24.30 Hamilton Depression Inventory

Checklist of symptoms of depressive states

Item No.	Range of Scores	Symptom	Item No.	Range of scores	Symptom
1	0–4	*Depressed Mood* Gloomy, attitude, pessimism about the future Feeling of sadness Tendency to weep Sadness, etc .... 1 Occasional weeping .... 2 Frequent weeping .... 3 Extreme symptoms 4	10	0–4	*Anxiety, psychic* Tension and irritability Worrying about minor matters Apprehensive attitude Fears
2	0–4	*Guilt* Self-reproach, feels he has let people down Ideas of guilt Present illness is a punishment Delusions of guilt Hallucinations of guilt	11	0–4	*Anxiety, somatic* Gastrointestinal, wind, indigestion Cardiovascular, palpitationss, headaches Respiratory, genito-urinary, etc.
3	0–4	*Suicide* Feels life is not worth living Wishes he were dead Suicidal ideas Attempts at suicide	12	0–2	*Somatic Symptoms, Gastrointestinal* Loss of appetite Heavy feelings in abdomen Constipation
4	0–2	*Insomnia, initial* Difficulty in falling asleep	13	0–2	*Somatic Symptoms, General* Heaviness in limbs, back, or head Diffuse backache Loss of energy and fatigability
5	0–2	*Insomnia, middle* Patients restless and disturbed during the night Waking during the night	14	0–2	*Genital Symptoms* Loss of libido Menstrual disturbances
6	0–2	*Insomnia, delayed* Waking in early hours of the morning and unable to fall asleep again	15	0–4	*Hypochondriasis* Self-absorption (bodily) Preoccupation with health Querulous attitude Hypochondriacal delusions
7	0–4	*Work and Interests* Feelings of incapacity Listlessness, indecision and vacillation Loss of interest in hobbies Decreased social activities Productivity decreased Unable to work Stopped working because of present illness only .... 4 (Absence from work after treatment or recovery may rate a lower score.)	16	0–2	*Loss of Weight*
			17	2–0	*Insight* Loss of insight .... 2 Partial or doubtful loss .... 1 No loss .... 0 (Insight must be interpreted in terms of patient's understanding and background.)
8	0–4	*Retardation* Slowness of thought, speech, and activity Apathy Stupor Slight retardation at interview .... 1 Obvious retardation at interview 2 Interview difficult .... 3 Complete stupor 4	18	0–2	*Diurnal Variation* Symptoms worse in morning or evening. (Note which it is.)
			19	0–4	*Depersonalization and Derealization* Feelings of unreality Nihilistic ideas Specify
			20	0–4	*Paranoid Symptoms* Suspicious Ideas of reference Not with a delusions of depressive reference and quality persecution Hallucinations, persecutory
9	0–2	*Agitation* Restlessness associated with anxiety	21	0–2	*Obsessional Symptoms* Obsessive thoughts and compulsions against which the patient struggles.

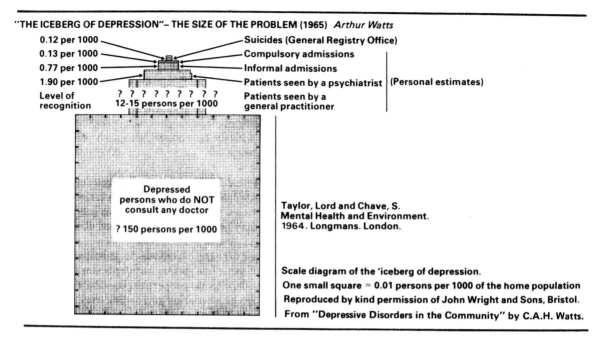

"THE ICEBERG OF DEPRESSION"— THE SIZE OF THE PROBLEM (1965) *Arthur Watts*

0.12 per 1000 ———————————————— Suicides (General Registry Office)

0.13 per 1000 ———————————————— Compulsory admissions

0.77 per 1000 ———————————————— Informal admissions

1.90 per 1000 ———————————————— Patients seen by a psychiatrist   (Personal estimates)

Level of   Patients seen by a
recognition   ? ? ? ? ? ? ? ? ?   general practitioner
              12-15 persons per 1000

Depressed
persons who do NOT
consult any doctor

? 150 persons per 1000

Taylor, Lord and Chave, S.
Mental Health and Environment.
1964. Longmans. London.

Scale diagram of the 'iceberg of depression.
One small square = 0.01 persons per 1000 of the home population
Reproduced by kind permission of John Wright and Sons, Bristol.
From "Depressive Disorders in the Community" by C.A.H. Watts.

Fig. 24.6   The iceberg of depression

Mrs B. presented with chest pain for which no obvious cause could be found. At all times in each interview she appeared both pleasant and relaxed as well as constantly smiling. She appeared very grateful for the attempts which were made to diagnose the cause of her trouble. However, when her husband had a severe attack of asthma Mrs B. intervened before the doctor reached Mr B., to enquire again about her discomfort and showed no real anxiety about her husband's state. Few of the features of the depressive shift were present but on questioning the patient revealed a previously unknown and more typical episode.

Patients such as these may present as a parasuicide and then deny all depressive features after the event. A relative's description of the real situation can be most instructive.

Dissatisfaction with appearance
This occurs most often in young women. The patient may feel that her nose is too big or that her breasts are too large or her ears stick out too much. A number of such patients are referred for plastic surgery but rarely benefit from any resulting procedures. More rarely, this presentation in late adolescence precedes a psychotic illness. The presentation as a variant of depression is fortunately rare and has much less of the delusional quality shown in a pre-psychotic state. One of the most striking delusions of disfigurement occurs in anorexia nervosa where the patient with a weight of 49 kilograms or less still believes she is fat.

Chronic pain
The most common form of this is abdominal, either epigastric or suprapubic pain. The type of pain is described as being burning or churning and is usually not accompanied by any other gastro-intestinal symptoms except for constipation. Facial or limb pain or recurrence of previously experienced organic pain in the absence of the organic pathology are further variations on this presentation. Few if any other further depressive features are present.

Marital disharmony
Here the patient, usually a woman, perceives the problem to be the marriage. This can be a projection of a depressed state. She feels that the husband has changed completely since the marriage. Marital therapy may help. However, it may prove very slow and difficult until the underlying depression is treated.

Behavioural change

Shoplifting. In older women this may be a presentation of depression, though a recent review of shoplifting suggested that only 10–15% of offenders will be suffering from a depressive illness. The most common age for shoplifters is between 10 and 18 as with much other petty crime. However, suicide in the older, and particularly in the recently widowed, shoplifter does occur, and a diagnosis of depression must clearly not be missed in these cases.

Drink problems. Where the drinking pattern changes subsequent to stress or some minor manifestation of depression, then depression should be recognised as the cause rather than the consequence of the alcohol problem.

Traffic offence. Although rare this can be the presentation of quite serious depression. Usually some depressive features may be identified preceding the offence.

Violence. Again a rare presentation of depression but must be given consideration particularly when paranoid features are present in the absence of schizophrenic symptoms.

In the elderly

Pseudodementia. This state must be distinguished from true dementia. The features are clinically similar but the prognosis is quite different. The history taken from the relatives may bring out the earlier affective change. The presentation itself will lack confabulation which is commonly present in dementia. The patient will respond to questions with answers such as 'I don't know' rather than talking round the answer. Unfortunately early dementia may be associated with depression so the distinctions are not always easy. Nevertheless the alleviation of depression is important if the patient is not to be placed inappropriately in an institution.

Hypochondriasis. This form of presentation may occur at any age but is much more frequent in the elderly. There is often a neurotic overlay and most of the symptoms of depression are present except for the central mood disturbance.

Chronic or resistant depression

The natural history of depression is that of a remitting illness, usually remission occurs after a period of between 3 and 18 months and patients who do not respond to treatment are a source of considerable anxiety to the doctor.

Since drug treatment is not effective for the first 10 to 14 days, pressure on the doctor during this period of time to 'do something' increases rapidly. However, it is not appropriate to change treatment after 2 weeks. At this juncture if there is no response the diagnosis should be rechecked and an assessment should be made of treatment compliance. It may then be necesssary to increase the dose and maintain treatment for a period of at least 4 weeks before thinking of a further change. Subtherapeutic levels of treatment are one significant cause of failure to respond.

Most double-blind trials of physical treatments have found that about 30% of patients do not respond. It is therefore important to recheck for the possibility of some other disease process such as those listed in Table 24.31.

Table 24.31 Physical illness associated with depression

Glandular fever
Continuing viral illness
Chronic infection
Hypokalaemia
Myxoedema
Cushing's disease
Vitamin B_{12} deficiency
Carcinoma—particularly intracranial or bronchial

Another possibility is that other drugs are interfering with the treatment, or are causing or maintaining the depression. Some of the drugs in this category are listed in Table 24.32.

After consideration of all these possibilities there will remain some patients who are resistant to all forms of physical and behavioural therapy. If they are already isolated and are then rejected by the doctor they can become a high suicidal risk. There are several subtle ways in which the doctor may reject. One is by reducing the amount of time allowed for consultation; another is by changing the diagnosis to that of personality disorder. The latter change carries with it the implication that the condition is now beyond the doctor's power to treat. Yet one more rejection is when the doctor refers the patient to a specialist. Such patients can only be sympathetically supported through their painful existence in the hope that the doctor's knowledge of their problems will improve or that they will spontaneously remit.

VIOLENCE AND AGGRESSION

SUICIDE AND PARASUICIDE

In a list size of 2300 patients the practitioner can expect an average of five attempted suicides annually. What has been described as an epidemic accounts for 15% of all hospital admissions. Since not all parasuicide patients are

Table 24.32 Drugs associated with depression or interacting with antidepressants

1. Hypertensive drugs
   a. Reserpine
   b. Methyl dopa
   c. Clonidine
   d. Adrenergic neurone blocking drugs
2. Oral contraceptives
3. Steroid therapy
   a. Cortisone
   b. Prednisolone
4. Anti-Parkinsonian drugs
   Levadopa
5. Neuroleptic drugs (see Schizophrenia and Depression, p. 313)
6. Appetite suppressants (usually this is on withdrawal but occurs in therapy with Fenfluramine)
7. Digoxin (usually as a toxic symptom)

admitted to hospital this figure may be low by up to one-third. After a short halt in the rate of increase of parasuicides seen in the 60's and early 70's, numbers are once again rising.

The term parasuicide was introduced to further distinguish the condition from suicide. The epidemiology of the two conditions is different although there is considerable overlap. The suicide group whose epidemiological features are shown in Table 24.33 will contain a number of parasuicide patients who were successful.

The sex ratio of females to males is now narrowing from the figure of 2:1 that was present in the 1960's to below 1.5:1. The method used is predominantly self-poisoning and mainly with minor tranquillisers although salicylates or other non-prescribed drugs are used in about a quarter of instances. Non-prescribed drugs are more common in the younger age groups and parasuicide itself is becoming more frequent in the under 16's.

Two-thirds of parasuicide patients are under 25. The precipitating factors of what is commonly an impulsive gesture include marital disharmony, alcohol problems, financial problems and unemployment.

The generalised profile of a parasuicide patient would be that of a young wife who has swallowed tranquillisers after a quarrel with her husband. She is not mentally ill but is unhappy partly because of poor housing and precarious employment, and partly because of chronic difficulties in the marriage. It is a common myth that such women have a hysteroid personality. This is not correct.

Some workers have suggested that general practitioner records should be annotated or identified in some way where there is a high risk of suicide or parasuicide. The profile of the elderly single male, or the male who has recently lost his spouse who also suffers from a chronic physical illness and has a history of depression will clearly require particular attention.

Repetition of parasuicide

Since 1 or 2% of parasuicide patients will succeed in killing themselves in the year following the original attempt, and since some 25% will repeat the attempt, it

may be helpful to know some of the predictive factors. These are listed in Table 24.34.

Considerable criticism of general practitioners has been implied in the many studies which have shown that over two-thirds of patients have seen their general practitioner within a few weeks of the attempt. Indeed, one study showed that over 40% had seen the general practitioner in the week before. Another important area of criticism is that there would appear to be significant indiscriminate prescribing as a contribution to parasuicide.

A further criticism arises from a number of studies which examined the group who did not see their general practitioners in the weeks before the event. About half of this group apparently considered seeking help from the general practitioner but did not. The most common reason given being that they thought that the general practitioner would be too busy or would not approve of being asked for help for the problems that the patient faced.

The main lesson to be drawn from most studies is that unhappiness, particularly when it is associated with social, relationship or drink problems, will not be helped by a psychotropic drug prescription. There is a great need to develop alternative strategies working with other network members in voluntary organisations such as Samaritans, Walk In Centres and Counsellors.

THE AGGRESSIVE PATIENT

Aggressive behaviour in patients is still fortunately uncommon although its management is never easy. Mentally ill patients become aggressive mainly when frightened. The differential diagnoses in violent patients are contained in Table 24.35. Management guidelines will vary depending upon the presenting circumstances but the situation should not be entered without adequate support, either from relatives, a mental health officer, nursing staff or police. This applies particularly to situations where self-violence has involved a firearm.

The main priority is to sedate the patient and this is best achieved with an injection of chlorpromazine 50–100 mg, given through clothing if necessary. In the elderly, paraldehyde may be preferred in view of the hypotensive propensities of chlorpromazine. The patient should be restrained, though in the case of the noisy drunk the

Table 24.33 Epidemiological features of suicide

Men more than women, although the figures for women are rising
Higher social and economic groups are over-represented
More often single, separated, divorced or widowed
More often socially isolated and living on their own
History of mental illness in 90% particularly depression or alcoholism
One-third to one-half will have made a previous attempt
More often older than the parasuicide group, i.e. over 50
May be associated with a chronic and particularly painful physical illness
Recent loss may have been experienced, e.g. job or spouse

Table 24.34 Predictors of repetition of parasuicide

Previous parasuicide
Prior contact with any of the psychiatric services
Evident psychopathy
Alcoholism
Not living with a relative

Table 24.35 Differential diagnosis in the violent patient

1. Alcoholic intoxication
2. Paranoid schizophrenia
3. Catatonic excitement in schizophrenia
4. Temporal lobe epilepsy
5. Post-concussional states
6. Psychopathic personality
7. Mania/hypomania
8. Premenstrual tension
9. Organic brain syndrome
10. Morbid jealousy
11. Toxic psychosis including drug abuse with heroin, amphetamine, LSD, cocaine
12. Prescribed drugs including levadopa and antidepressants

police may be more adept in handling the case, with the general practitioner playing only a supporting role.

MORBID JEALOUSY

This condition is not always associated with a clear underlying diagnosis such as schizophrenia or alcoholism Unfortunately, the paroxysm of rage, which may occur, can result in murder. Up to 12% of committed insane murderers have been found to suffer from morbid jealousy.

GLUE SNIFFERS

Adolescents are presenting more frequently with a history of glue sniffing. Fortunately most are not aggressive. However, increasing irritability, aggression and outbursts of violence occurring in a 10 to 15-year-old should make one consider glue sniffing as one of the alternative diagnoses.

ORGANIC BRAIN SYNDROME (SENILE DEMENTIA)

Following a fall, an operation, an intercurrent infection, an accidental drug overdose or a sudden change in circumstances, an old person with senile dementia may become violent in the course of developing an acute delirious state. An assault may be preceded by increasing restlessness, agitation and feelings of suspicion.

PREMENSTRUAL TENSION

It is now suggested that the small number of women who experience severe premenstrual tension can be repeatedly, and seriously, aggressive on a cyclical basis. This area needs further clarification.

BATTERED WIVES

This subject is a good example of how myths build up in medicine. There has been a growing awareness of the problem of serious or repeated physical assault upon women by the men with whom they live, but there has been little research into the phenomenon by doctors. The myths, which are not borne out by sociological research, include a picture of an inherently violent family where the wife or children may be the subject of abuse by an alcoholic or mentally-ill male. Moreover, the ill-founded attitude of the profession is to regard the woman as a bad housewife or a masochist, or being at least partially at fault due to provocation. There is no certainty about the true incidence of this form of violence in the family, but very tentative figures have suggested that between 1 and 5% of families have unstable relationships. This means that, as a social problem, it ranks below that of one-parent families.

A clearer picture of the problem has emerged from research amongst women admitted to Women's Aid refuges and those where a police record of assault is recorded. The battering tends to begin early in the marriage, usually within the first 3 years. It is commonly part of a pattern of domination of the woman by the man who may also bully her, keep her short of money and devalue and humiliate her repeatedly. The violence is usually repetitive, once or even twice weekly and often over many years.

In the early stages the woman remains in the home. After the first assault only 50% seek help and advice, usually from a relative or friend and a number of factors seem to prevent her from seeking professional help. These include a sense of shame, guilt and the feeling which pervades all marital problems that the matter is a private one which should be solved within the family. The man may reinforce her doubts about seeking help with threats.

At some point during the relationship the woman will contact the medical services in addition to social workers and police. 80% will see a doctor at some time and of this group many will have repeated contacts. The presentation to the general practitioner or to the Accident and Emergency Department is usually one of physical injury and the woman will often disguise the cause of the assault. As one doctor put it, 'there would seem to be a large number of malevolent door knobs involved'. Other presentations include vague complaints, usually perceived to be neurotic by the doctor, or 'problems with children'. In one study nearly half the general practitioners offered tranquillisers as a treatment. Drugs will not help these women. *They* are not ill.

This not uncommon problem provides a suitable subject for better co-ordination between the different groups within the network. The individual and unco-ordinated response of social worker, doctor and Women's Aid volunteer cannot provide adequate support, but together they may tackle the problem with greater effect. The general practitioner's role may start with identification of the problem. He should carefully record all evidence of physical violence, including lacerations, bruises, fractures and internal injuries. He should try to ensure that the woman will have adequate support and a group involving himself, the social worker and a volunteer from Women's Aid should meet to decide on their respective roles and to appoint a key worker. There are now over 170 temporary secure houses run by the National Federation of Women's Aid and this is a valuable resource either as a stepping stone to a new and independent life or to provide respite while the marital situation is reviewed.

A decision must be made as to whether the male should be considered an alcoholic and whether he is suffering from morbid jealousy. A further decision must be made about when to confront the male with the inappropriateness of his violence.

THE PSYCHOLOGICAL RESPONSE TO ILLNESS

Minor anxiety and depression are common as a response to physical illness but only become pathological if they are so severe as to affect recovery. The experience of illness is very subjective, no two patients responding in a similar manner, but it is possible to make some predictions about the response to illness on the basis of personality, age and premorbid attitudes.

The psychological response to illness tends to be worse in childhood, the elderly and those where there is a pre-existing mental state abnormality.

There are three specific groups whose premorbid personality traits have a significant effect upon response. Firstly the obsessional patient who finds the whole process of hospitalisation difficult and stressful. He requires any doubts to be clarified down to the last detail and his fear of giving up control can create profound distress. The second group are those who have a predominantly narcissistic outlook. Patients in this group have particular anxieties with regard to future disfigurement or dysfunction. The third group are those who have a tendency to be dependent and who may welcome and adopt the sick role as a chronic, though inappropriate, method of coping with the world.

The idiosyncratic nature of the response may be determined in part by the patient's perception of the importance of the body part affected. Disfigurement, particularly facial, may have an effect upon the individual's self-esteem far in excess of what might be expected. Even when the effect is hidden, as with a colostomy, or camouflaged with cosmetic help, the patient's image of himself can be severely disturbed.

The social circumstances in which the patient finds himself will also have an effect upon his reactions. The illness may be welcomed if it allows escape from social problems. It has been well known since the turn of the century that the possibility of litigation can enhance the sickness role, producing 'compensation neurosis'. The isolated patient is more likely to respond adversely than is the supported patient. One final aspect which may determine psychological response is that the more strange the experience for the patient the more likely it is that he is going to feel anxious. For example, in studies of intensive care units, the large amounts of equipment, as well as the serious nature of the condition, appear to have a marked stressful effect.

The most appropriate adaptation which the patient can make to illness is one which will be free from psychiatric problems. He should be able to seek and be given advice at a level which he finds appropriate. He should be able to accept this advice and comply with it, even if this means the temporary modification of his role. No patient should be made more dependent than is absolutely necessary. Once the illness has resolved he should then be able to resume his independence and individual role at a similar or better level than before.

ANXIETY REACTION

A less appropriate reaction to physical illness is severe anxiety and this appears to be maximal where there is greatest uncertainty. Studies of peptic ulceration have shown that severe anxiety at the time of first presentation is associated with a poor outcome. Similarly, patients with excessive anxiety following myocardial infarction also do less well.

A more specific form of anxiety exists where the patient is phobic regarding certain situations or procedures such as admission to hospital or injections. It is well known that some patients will indicate almost at the outset of a consultation that whatever else happens, they do not wish to go to hospital. Overcoming these anxieties may be important if resolution of the medical or surgical problem is to be achieved.

DEPRESSIVE REACTION

A number of studies have indicated that up to a quarter of medical in-patients suffer from some degree of depression, although most improve with physical recovery. The severity of the depression would appear to be closely related to the amount of perceived loss, which may be anatomical, functional or in phantasy. A few patients conceptualise illness in terms which are pathological, feeling guilt and self-blame. They tend to act passively, showing little resistance to the institutionalising process of hospitalisation. Very occasionally such patients go on to commit suicide.

In a further group, depression is associated with marked hypochondriacal features; a characteristic in the patient that can be very irritating to hospital staff. One study found that patients with such features take much longer to return to work following myocardial infarction despite the absence of cardiac pathology. Indeed, many of them adopted a role of chronic invalidism.

DENIAL

Denial, which is a common defence in many illnesses, is found in terminal illness as the most common initial response. Some patients continue to deny they are dying to the end. The size of this group is estimated to be between 20 and 30% of all those with terminal illness.

It is a source of some anxiety to many primary care workers that in seeking to establish whether the patient's defence of denial is breaking down, they may precipitate a crisis. This is an unnecessary worry since no harm will be done to the patient provided that he is offered the opportunity of discussing the anxieties which usually emerge after the denial breaks down. Indeed, it is quite common for a patient who is told and appears to accept the fact that he is dying to re-establish his denial defence mechanism if this is, for him, a necessity.

Another example of denial which can be very harmful to the patient is seen in some women with advanced breast cancer, where although they clearly must have known about the condition for some time, they fail to seek medical attention. Such form of denial is perhaps the most difficult and serious of the defences.

> Recently a 32-year-old woman, Mrs R., presented with a painless lump in her breast. She had attended the Well Woman Clinic 1 year previously and had her breasts examined and was taught self-examination. When she presented she indicated that she had been aware of the lump for 2 months. It transpired that her 44-year-old sister had had a mastectomy 2 years previously and was now terminally ill. Mrs R. had reacted to finding her own breast lump by denying the possibility that she might in time be in her sister's situation.

PREOCCUPATION

At the other end of the scale from denial there is the situation in which the patient is preoccupied with his illness. Such patients are often obsessional and difficult to manage, constantly seeking information and checking and re-checking what they have been told with other members of the team. Similar reactions can be present during childbirth.

Each doctor must find for himself the most appropriate way in which to manage these patients, but a single management strategy will not suffice. Detailed explanation of the condition, its treatment and its consequences may be required by one patient but for another this information is regarded as highly threatening. The first rule must therefore be to assess the level of information the patient requires so that his distress can be alleviated. In this respect the doctor must be guided by the nature of his patient's questions and adequate time must be allowed. One strategy that can be helpful, particularly when there is likely to be subsequent disfigurement or dysfunction, such as after mastectomy, colostomy or amputation, is to introduce the patient to someone who has already experienced the procedure, and has adjusted well to the consequences. Such counselling at an early stage can lead to the development of a clear programme of rehabilitation with more appropriate post-operative adaptation.

Whilst it is not possible to discuss every illness, a few examples will serve to illustrate the protean nature of the patient's reaction to illness.

MYOCARDIAL INFARCTION

An important part of rehabilitation after a myocardial infarction involves an assessment of the psychological reaction of both the patient and the spouse. The initial reaction may be that of denial, and at this stage this is thought to have some protective function. Since the patient is unable to do much for himself, denial may help him to avoid much of the sense of helplessness which can be a distressing component of this illness. Unfortunately, some patients go to the opposite extreme and over-extend themselves, thus creating additional risk. An early reaction found in the wives of infarct patients appears to be very close to that of the grief reaction and this may be a reaction to the loss of the 'strong husband'.

2 to 3 months following the infarction the main reactions include fatigue, depression, and in a smaller group, perhaps 25%, tension. Studies suggest that these symptoms occur almost as frequently in the spouse as in the patient. At 1 year after the original event almost a third of both patients and spouses show evidence of significant and permanent adverse psychological changes.

One aspect of rehabilitation which tends to be neglected following myocardial infarction concerns the resumption by the patient of sexual intercourse. More than one in three couples who had a previously satisfactory sexual relationship have been found to be concerned at the decline in sexual activity 1 year after the attack. Similar findings of significant deterioration in sexual relationships have been found in patients with angina. Resumption of sexual relations can be an important part of a full recovery and simple advice can help to minimise anxiety (see Table 24.36).

RECURRENT OR PERSISTENT ABDOMINAL PAIN

A study by Gomez & Dailly (1977) confirmed earlier findings that only a small percentage (15.6%) of patients referred to a general surgical outpatient department with recurrent or long-standing pain had definite organic pathology. The major group (32%) were depressed, others had chronic tension (22%) or were thought to have hysterical traits (17%). A surprisingly large number (13%) were previously unrecognised alcoholics. The authors also assessed the family and personal patterns of health and found that pain was a much more common presentation in all forms of illness in this group. 80% of such patients accepted a psychological explanation for their pain and specific treatment of the psychiatric problem. Over one-half of this group responded well to such psychological management.

MASTECTOMY

Over 3000 women in the United Kingdom each year have a mastectomy yet the psychological management of such patients has until recently been neglected. Apart from pre-operative counselling, involvement of the Mastectomy Association can provide practical help as well as support. There needs to be proper recognition of the serious levels of lasting anxiety, depression and psychosexual problems which may occur in up to 40% of such women.

In a study by Maguire et al (1978) it was reported that few women who sought help felt that they received appropriate counselling. Furthermore, less than half the disturbed group approached the general practitioner and of those who did, none asked that their psychosexual

Table 24.36 Guidance for the resumption of sexual relations after myocardial infarction and in angina

Resumption should run in parallel with general physical rehabilitation programme, i.e. except in very mild cases avoidance for only 3 to 4 weeks
Sheets should be warmed, the bedroom should be warmed
Sex should be avoided after a large meal
Sex should be avoided after a hot bath
The patient should avoid wearing constrictive clothing
A non-demand position should be used initially before intercourse
In angina take Trinitrin, if required, before intercourse

problems be discussed. Confining the follow-up to a scrutiny of the physical recovery and practical prosthesis is insufficient. The restoration of self-esteem and self-image will require more active help in many instances.

RHEUMATIC DISEASES

There are many psychological problems in chronic disabling diseases. The adaptations required to cope with pain, poor sleep, changes in social or work role and increasing dependency place a serious strain upon even the most robust personality. As one patient tearfully said recently, 'You have no idea how hard it is to bear when one has to ask one's husband to put on one's tights and shoes'. Relinquishing active participation in family life to that of an observer does not come easily to many patients. Some may become seriously depressed, and this can present as a diminished threshold to pain. Alternatively other members of the family may increasingly present with vague ill-health or behavioural problems, or with exacerbation of existing difficulties and tensions in the marriage, or between the patient and children. Elderly and isolated patients with poor control of pain are at risk of suicide. A further small but important group appear to have considerable secondary gain from their illness, playing the sick role to its greatest advantage. The early establishment of enlightened family support combined with a clear understanding of what aids and house modifications are possible can do much to prevent a deterioration in morale.

MULTIPLE SCLEROSIS

Multiple sclerosis is complicated by the fact that many patients will not be told that they have the condition until a series of attacks have occurred, or some residual disability has become evident. Doctors on the whole seem to have an unduly pessimistic view of the prognosis in this disease and so make attempts to shield the patient from reality. Yet those patients who do wish to know experience more tension and anxiety from silence. Many fear a terminal condition is being hidden from them. Patients cannot reasonably and realistically plan their lives if information is needlessly hidden from them. Plans to have children, for housing, for work and even for leisure can be affected.

> Mrs W., aged 29, presented with a third attack of weakness in the right leg combined with foot drop. Her first attack 7 years previously had been limited to retrobulbar neuritis. After recovery she was told it was a viral illness. The second attack, which she had not related to the first, presented as paraesthesia in the left leg, and again there was full recovery.

This third attack left some residual sensory and motor deficit. In the intervening 7 years she had worked hard at her career as a physical education teacher, getting promotion and postponing her family during the first few years of her marriage in order to further her career. The couple had bought a smallholding on high ground some distance from a village. Mrs W. had often extended herself to the limits of physical endurance and scorned the episodes of tiredness she had experienced over these years.

Her anger on being told that the three attacks were multiple sclerosis was not just part of the loss reaction which frequently occurs in patients diagnosed as having a long-term disabling disease. Her anger was realistic, against a profession which allowed her to prepare for and execute a life plan which was not suited to the possible prognosis. Simply to hope that she would be one of those who did not have repeated attacks was not sufficient, the profession was culpable. Diagnosis does not destroy hope. Most patients, after a period of reaction to the implications of the condition which may last up to 2 years, will adapt to a life which has much to offer.

Mrs W's parting comment after that first interview was 'thank goodness my husband is an understanding man, he married me when I already had this disease. I wouldn't really blame him if he feels as cheated as I do'.

Later reactions in multiple sclerosis include mood swings with difficulty in concentration and marked irritability, particularly if there are chronic physical changes. In the advanced stages dementia or euphoria may occur. The euphoria may mask a depression. Hostility reaction can be strong even in those with whom an open discussion of the diagnosis occurs at an early stage, but is much more severe if the diagnosis is discovered accidentally. This can occur if the patient overhears staff talking, by reading their own case notes, by opening letters sent by hand to a specialist or learning of their diagnosis from another patient.

The Multiple Sclerosis Society and its welfare officers can be of enormous help in counselling these patients.

REFERENCES

Bain D J B, Sales C M 1981 Referring children to an ENT department and prescribing psychotropic drugs to their mothers. British Medical Journal 283:585–587

Balint M 1968 The doctor, his patient and the illness, 2nd edn. Pitman, London

Balint E, Norell J S 1976 Six minutes for the patient. Tavistock Publications, London

Barber J H, Simpson R J 1978 Psychiatry — a syllabus for vocational training. Southern General Hospital, Glasgow

Bloch S 1977 Supportive psychotherapy. British Journal of Hospital Medicine 18:63–68

Burns L E 1982 The role of the clinical psychologist in primary care — an analysis of current practice. Clinical Psychology and Medicine. Plenum, London

Cartwright A, Anderson R 1981 Changes in the frequency and nature of doctor patient contacts. General Practice Revisited. Tavistock Publications, London, ch 3

Clare A 1976 Psychiatry in Dissent. Tavistock Publications, London

Colby K M 1951 A primer or psychotherapists. Ronald Press, New York

Creer C, Wing J K 1974 Schizophrenia at home. National Schizophrenia Fellowship

Crombie D L 1972 A model of the medical care system: a general systems approach. In: Hauser M M (ed) Economics of medical care. Allen and Unwin, London, p, 61–85

Fox H A 1981 The DSM III concept of schizophrenia. British Journal of Psychiatry 138:60–63

Gomez J, Dally P 1977 Attendance at outpatient surgical and medical clinics with recurrent or persistent abdominal pain. British Medical Journal 1:1451–1453

Hodgkin K 1978 Towards earlier diagnosis in primary care, 4th edn. Churchill Livingstone, Edinburgh

Horder J et al 1972 The future general practitioner. Royal College of General Practitioners, London

Howie J G R, Bigg A R 1980 Family trends in psychotropic and antibiotic prescribing in general practice. British Medical Journal 282:836–836

Ingram I M, Timbury G C, Mowbray R M 1981 Notes on psychiatry, 4th edn. Churchill Livingstone, Edinburgh

Jerrom D W A, Gerver D, Simpson R J, Pemberton D A 1981 Report to Forth Valley Health Board — Evaluation of three years experimental district community psychology clinic.

Jerrom D W A, Gerver D, Simpson R J, Pemberton D A 1982 Clinical Psychology in primarry care: issues in the evaluation of services. In: Main C J (ed) Clinical psychology and medicine. Plenum, London

Kessels W I N 1960 Psychiatric morbidity in a London practice. British Journal of Preventive and Social Medicine 14:16

Maguire G P et al 1978 Psychological reactions to mastectomy. British Medical Journal 1:963–965

Masters W H, Johnson V E 1970 Human sexual inadequacy. Little Brown, Boston.

The Mitchell Report 1976 Social work services in the Scottish Health Services, ch 3, Social work in general practice. HMSO, Edinburgh

Report from the Liaison Committee of the Royal College of Psychiatrists and the Royal College of General Practitioners — Vocational Training 1980. Journal of the Royal College of General Practitioners 30:625–627

Roberts C A 1978 The interface between psychiatry and family medicine. (Private communication)

Rowbottom R, Hey A 1978 Organisation of services for the mentally ill. Brunel Institute of Organisation and Social Studies.

Shepherd M, Clare A 1981 Psychiatric illness in general practice, 2nd edn. Oxford University Press, Oxford

Simpson R J 1981 The Team: an outmoded concept? Scottish Medicine 2

Skuse D, Dunn G 1981 Addendum to psychiatric illness in general practice, Shepherd M, Clare A 2nd edn. Oxford University Press, Oxford

Timbury G 1979 Services for the elderly with mental disability in Scotland. HMSO, Edinburgh

Tough H, Kingerlee P, Eliot P 1980 An evaluation of the psychiatric nurses in the primary care team. Journal of the Royal College of General Practitioners 30:85–89

Watts C A H 1966 Depressive disorders in the Community.
John Wright, Bristol

Watts C A H Morbidity statistics from general practice second
national study 1970–71. Studies on medical and population
subjects No. 26, HMSO, London

Waydenfield D, Waydenfield S 1980 Counsellors in a general
practice setting. Journal of the Royal College of General
Practitioners 30:671–677

Whitfield M J, Winter R D 1980 General practitioner attitudes
— Avon survey. Journal of the Royal College of General
Practitioners 30:682–686

Williams P, Clare A 1979 Social workers in primary health care
— the practitioners viewpoint. Journal of the Royal College of
General Practitioners 29:554–558

Williams P, Clare A 1979 Psychosocial disorders in general
practice. Academic Press, New York. Section 1. Goldberg D,
Blackwell B: Psychiatric illness in general practice: A detailed
study using new methods of case identification. Eastwood
M R, Trevelyan M H: Relationship between physical and
psychiatric disorder. Cooper B, Fry J, Kalton G A:
Longitudinal study of psychiatric morbidity in a general
practice population

Problems of alcohol

INTRODUCTION

There is probably no aspect of general practice medicine in which the doctor's own attitude and beliefs, and the quality of his relationship with the patient and his, or her, family are of more critical importance than in the detection and management of patients with alcohol problems. Several factors unite to provide the general practitioner with a unique opportunity to deal with alcohol-related disorders both in the individual patient and, through his role as educator, in the community at large. He has a list of patients registered with him with an opportunity to keep comprehensive records. He can, over a period of time, construct diagnoses piece by piece in physical, psychological and social dimensions. Through the primary care team he has access to the additional perspectives which community nursing staff, health visitors and social workers can provide. No one else in the community has the privilege of entering so many homes or of enquiring legitimately into aspects of behaviour as they affect health. The general practitioner is in touch with a network of statutory and non-statutory agencies which may be appropriate at various times. No one else but the family doctor has such opportunities to build relationships with so many individuals at times of stress and change.

Those who arrive eventually at the diagnosis of 'alcoholism', usually in their late 30s or early 40s but increasingly at younger ages, have travelled a road, over years, of increasing consumption, increasing harm and increasing dependence on alcohol. Most of them, if not all, have presented opportunities for intervention; opportunities when simple information, advice or constructive support might have halted their descent on a slippery slope. The aim of the general practitioner should be to prevent the pejorative title of 'alcoholic' ever being applied to one of his patients.

DEFINING THE PROBLEM

It is no longer useful to think in terms of alcoholism as a single disease entity which implies detection, diagnosis and a single treatment mode. A hundred years ago, James Miller, then Professor of Surgery at Edinburgh University wrote ... 'Drunkenness owns many a cause, and calls for many a cure. Many things have to be done, and many men are needed to do them. The principle of division of labour is fully recognised in this matter.' This view is echoed today in the acceptance of problem drinking, including the alcohol dependence syndrome, as multifactorial in cause, variable in presentation and requiring a multidisciplinary approach in management. The manifestations of problem drinking occur not only in medical dimensions, but also, and usually earlier, in social and legal dimensions. The relation of three clear cut and easily recognisable elements of drinking behaviour — intoxication, dependence and excessive consumption — to their consequences in medical, social and legal areas, makes the planning of positive and constructive strategies a necessary step. This is much more acceptable to patients who may come simply expecting to be told that they must stop drinking, which they know they cannot easily do. This approach enables the doctor to focus primarily on the problem as the central issue.

INTOXICATION

The relief of tension, anxiety, unhappiness and the feelings of benevolence engendered by drinking alcohol may strictly be regarded as 'toxic' effects brought about by the depression of various brain functions. The psychic effects felt first, and at low dosage, are the most important socially, and it is for these effects that alcohol is used by so many societies as a social lubricant. Medically speaking, however, intoxication may be defined as being significant mental and physical inco-ordination due to alcohol. It occurs, in the non-tolerant subject, at blood alcohol concentrations in excess of 40 mg% (Thorley 1980). What constitutes drunken behaviour is a matter of culture and of context. What is normal at a social gathering becomes risky in an operating theatre and criminal at the wheel of a car. In a drinking society, intoxication may be regarded as normal behaviour and only becomes problematic where the circumstances are inappropriate. Most of the problems arising from intoxication arise in the legal and social spheres and will tend to present to the general practitioner or primary care team indirectly, for example in child abuse, domestic violence or social isolation. Those suffering the acute medical effects of alcohol frequently find their way to Accident and Emergency departments with acute trauma, head injury, drug overdose or parasuicide. The 'morning-after' effects such as peripheral nerve pressure palsies, acute gastritis and hangover more commonly present in the general practitioner's surgery. Those working in small communities and rural areas will see the whole spectrum of drinking behaviour and morbidity and for this reason doctors working in such localities tend to identify more problem drinkers than their urban counterparts.

DEPENDENCE

The question of dependence on alcohol can best be considered by looking at what happens when the individual stops drinking. Those with well established physical dependence will experience withdrawal symptoms 6 to 8 hours after the last drink, the four key symptoms being tremor, nausea, sweating and disturbance of mood. Physical dependence has no threshold over which the drinker passes and thereby becomes 'hooked'. Anyone who drinks enough alcohol, often enough and over a long enough period can become physically dependent in the same way as with other drugs such as barbiturates or heroin. Edwards & Gross (1976) have enumerated the seven essential features of the dependence syndrome:

1. *Narrowing of drinking repertoire*
   Normal drinkers vary their drinking widely according to the occasion. After initially widening his scope to embrace different opportunities, the dependent drinker tends to drink more and more in the same pattern every day as the necessity of drinking to avoid withdrawal symptoms occurs.
2. *Salience of drinking behaviour*
   As dependence increases, the day's activities become related to the availability of drink. The unpleasant consequences have less and less deterrent effect.
3. *Increased tolerance of alcohol*
   Drinkers who are tolerant can achieve very high blood alcohol concentrations without apparent drunkenness: they are said to be able to 'hold their liquor'.
4. *Repeated withdrawal symptoms*
5. *Relief or avoidance of withdrawal symptoms by further drinking*
6. *Subjective awareness of a compulsion to drink*

7. *Reinstatement of the syndrome following a period of abstinence*

Few aspects of general practice medicine place greater demands on the art and skill of the consultation than does the detection and elucidation of the dependence syndrome. The medical problems arising from dependence may arise from other causes or may mimic other conditions. Tremor and sweating may suggest an anxiety state or even thyrotoxicosis. Lack of drive and early waking may suggest depression. Indeed, the patient may be drinking because he is depressed or be depressed because he is drinking. Withdrawal fits may label the patient wrongly as epileptic, with far-reaching consequences for employment. In all three examples the condition may be exacerbated by the prescription of CNS depressants which potentiate the effects of alcohol. When prescribing any psychoactive drug the doctor has a legitimate reason to introduce the topic of alcohol. This gives him the chance to explore the part that alcohol might be playing in the genesis of the problem confronting him.

When the drinker stops drinking it is not only the alcohol that he misses. His culture may expect him to be a drinker: as an abstainer he will become an outsider and lose an important part of his masculinity. Pay day and the patterns of behaviour associated with work provide potent cues to drinking, as may the ritual of preparing the drink or even of pulling the ring opener on the can. It is not by accident that this latter image appears so often in television and cinema advertising. He may mourn the loss of a favourite glass. These personal and social factors surrounding drinking may be more efficiently learned and more positively reinforce the drinking behaviour than does the relief of tension afforded by the alcohol itself. Thus non-physical or psychological dependence may be more problematic than physical dependence. It is not against the law to be alcohol dependent and the only social consequence of dependence is the stigma attached to the 'alcoholic'. Having some degree of dependence, whether physical or psychological, may be regarded as normal in a drinking society and is not necessarily productive of problems.

EXCESSIVE CONSUMPTION

Excessive consumption of alcohol is by definition problematic. A daily consumption in men of 100 g ethanol (5 pints of average beer) and in women of 60 g ethanol (3 pints of average beer) is associated with increased morbidity and mortality, and with social and legal problems. Significant liver damage may result from a daily consumption of 30 g ethanol (Thorley 1980).

Patterns of drinking may affect the type of problem. For example, Mr A. and Mr B. may both drink 5 pints of beer a day. Mr A. drinks his at one lunchtime session and so is more accident prone, less efficient at work in the afternoon and may lose his driving licence. Mr B. spreads his drinking out over the day and so avoids these short-term risks but shares with Mr A. the same long-term risks of liver disease and brain damage. It is important to realise that some people can consume large quantities of alcohol without becoming significantly intoxicated or dependent, because they have a high degree of tolerance. Simple information and advice concerning the relationship between consumption levels and physical damage may be all that such individuals require to deal with their health problem.

The medical consequences of excessive consumption are legion and are listed in standard texts. Those most commonly seen in general practice are those affecting the gastro-intestinal tract such as gastritis, peptic ulceration, gastrointestinal bleeding and alcoholic hepatitis. The social problems are those arising from the diversion of the financial and personality resources away from the family and the employer. It is much more expensive to get drunk if you have developed a high degree of tolerance. Bed-wetting is more common in the families of problem drinkers and under-attainment is more common in their children. Excessive expenditure on drink leads to debt and then homelessness, and thence to the problem of theft and vagrancy involving the law.

WHICH PATIENT

No single psychological type or personality is universally recognised as a risk of developing alcohol related problems, and there is no single biochemical marker which will identify the abnormal drinker. Heavier drinkers do tend to be found among those who use alcohol to relieve 'bad nerves', tension, restlessness or boredom. Environmental stress may invite a risk of heavy drinking; marital or business difficulties, concern over health, moving to a new town, can all generate bad feelings which the individual may cope with by resorting to alcohol. The level of consumption may rise not always to fall again when the stress is resolved, since alcohol is a drug of addiction.

ALCOHOL AND WORK

Occupation is a very potent influence on an individual's drinking and a pattern of drinking is very often learned with, or a traditional part of, various jobs. The most obvious influence will be when alcohol is available at work, at little cost as in catering and bar-tending, brewing and distilling, and people who already have alcohol problems may be attracted to such jobs simply because of the availability of alcohol (Plant 1976). The executive or sales representative with an expense account and nights to spend away from home will be vulnerable, as will the itinerant labourer, single or living away from home during the week, with nowhere but the pub to spend his evenings. Acting, journalism and the printing trades have strong traditions of heavy drinking. In general, jobs which combine flurries of activity with long periods of waiting, particularly if there is little supervision, predispose to alcohol problems.

NATURE OF NURTURE

People with drinking problems are frequently noted to have a parent, spouse or sibling with the same problem. The explanation which finds most favour lies in the potency of parenteral influence and peer group pressure but genetic factors do doubtedly play a part. Goodwin and his co-workers (1973) demonstrated that men who have an alcoholic parent but who are adopted early in life were nearly four times more likely to be alcoholic themselves than were the adopted sons of non-alcoholic parents. There is a small but increasing body of evidence confirming a genetic component.

MENTAL ILLNESS AND ALCOHOL

Psychiatric illness may predispose to the development of problem drinking. Most typically this is a depressive illness but it occurs also with anxiety states, phobias and with schizophrenia. These cases are not very significant in terms of numbers but at an individual level it is extremely rewarding to get rid of somebody's drinking problem by recognising and treating, for example, a phobia. This group of people may then, after some time, return to normal social drinking, further helping to destroy the myth of alcoholism as a lifelong 'disease'.

HELPING THE PROBLEM DRINKER

The doctors who are most effective in dealing with alcohol problems are those who are clear about their own attitudes to alcohol use, confident and secure in their ability to cope with their own drinking, in possession of a sound body of factual information about alcohol and its effects and in close contact with members of other disciplines and agencies whose help may be required. The single most critical stage in the process of helping the problem drinker is when it is first recognised that alcohol might be involved and a drinking history is taken, an assessment made and therapeutic goals agreed. If at this time, either in what he says or in the way that he says it, the doctor betrays a judgemental attitude or insecurity in his role, trust will be difficult to establish and progress will be hindered. The position of the medical profession in the 'league table' of hepatic cirrhosis would suggest that examination of our own attitudes and drinking patterns is also a matter which should concern us all.

TAKING A DRINKING HISTORY

People are sensitive about their drinking. Concentration on the relationship of drinking to the problem presented and its effect on the general health and wellbeing of the patient and his, or her, family legitimise the enquiries in the patient's eyes. It is useful and usually easier to progress backwards day by day over the preceding week eliciting the frequency, quantity and type of drink taken and score it in units of alcohol (Table 25.1). How much money is spent each week on drink? How does this relate to the total family income? Does the patient need a 'sub' from his wife before pay day? Does he have to pay off what's on the slate from the previous week? Where does he drink? When, and with whom? Many men will assert their control over their drinking by saying that they drink nothing between Sunday evening and Friday evening; but can they in fact abstain over a weekend when the cues to drink may be more frequent and stronger? Is the problem in the area of intoxication, of dependence, or is harm accumulating as a result of regular excessive consumption? What emerges is a picture of a man's (or woman's) lifestyle, of how central drink is to it, what the attitudes and responses of the family are towards the drinking behaviour and how he feels about stopping. It is then possible to draw up a short balance sheet showing the good and bad effects of his drinking and to start to plan a strategy. In the course of a consultation the linking of his problems to the known effects of alcohol by the patient himself can have a powerful therapeutic effect, when the patient may uncover further problems which he did not previously attribute to alcohol.

Assessment is incomplete without physical examination and although there maybe little to be found, the process reinforces the problem-oriented approach to the patient's health. The examination can be supplemented by any necessary special investigations. Blood should be taken for a full blood count with particular emphasis on MCV and the presence of round macrocytes in the film. The serum gamma glutamyl transpeptidase is usually elevated in excessive drinkers and although a blood alcohol level will give no indication of the degree of dependence, a level of around 150 mg% (4 mmol/l) in the absence of overt signs of intoxication is indicative of a high degree of tolerance.

PLANNING OBJECTIVES

The patient may well consult the general practitioner as a result of pressure from the spouse whose involvement is desirable not only in obtaining another perspective on the drinking behaviour, but in defining goals and in enlisting and ensuring support. Whatever the long-term objectives may be it is not unreasonable to insist that the patient abstains totally for 2 weeks and is then reviewed. If he fails it does not necessarily mean that he lacks motivation, but that the degree of dependence, physical or psychological, may be much stronger than anticipated. The results of blood tests can also be reviewed at this time.

MONITORING CONSUMPTION

The present and future implications of continuing to drink at the same level should be clearly spelled out and the patient encouraged to monitor his own consumption with the use of a diary. The target is a harm-free drinking level and though other benefits such as financial savings can be used to reinforce self-control and self-esteem, the individual should concentrate on how much alcohol he is drinking rather than on how much money he is spending.

AVOIDING INTOXICATION

The context of drinking is at least as important as the quantity that is consumed so that it is also important that the patient should recognise the particular problems which arise from his own intoxication. Anger, feelings of inferiority, guilt or frustration may precede episodes of intoxication and more appropriate ways of coping with them should be explored. Patients may find that they can control their drinking in some circumstances but yet habitually drink too much in others. Everyone who drinks should know exactly how alcohol affects him in particular and how the effects may be modified by the rate of drinking, the type of beverage and the presence of

Table 25.1 Approximate equivalents in alcohol units of common drinks (From: Good Health: The Medical Problems of Excessive Drinking, Scottish Home and Health Department)

1 Glass of wine	=	1 unit
1 Single tot of spirits	=	1 unit
1 Glass of sherry or port	=	1 unit
1 Pint of beer or lager	=	2 units
1 Can of special strength lager	=	3 units
1 Ordinary sized bottle of wine	=	6 units
1 Litre bottle of wine	=	10 units
1 Bottle of sherry	=	10 units
½ Bottle of spirits	=	15 units
1 Bottle of spirits	=	30 units

food in the stomach. Armed with such knowledge, the patient can practise different ways of drinking with the aim of recognising the features of his own intoxication and learning to stay below the level of consumption that produces it. A personal diary recording quantity and type of drink and a two or three word summary of the circumstancs and the patient's mood before drinking is invaluable.

ALCOHOL DEPENDENCE

Full assessment of the patient's problems demands a period of abstinence from alcohol. This may be achieved surprisingly easily but is likely to be short-lived unless a clearly defined strategy is agreed with the patient and a start made on the most urgent of his problems. Unless there are strong contraindications such as a previous history of withdrawal fits or delirium tremens, or a hostile home environment, detoxification can be undertaken at home. Chlormethiazole (Heminevrin) is highly effective in suppressing the symptoms of withdrawal but it is highly addictive and increasingly popular with illicit drug users. Its use therefore should be closely monitored and last no more than 6 days. A dosage of 1.5 g q.d.s. for 2 days, 1.0 g q.d.s. for 2 days and 0.5 g q.d.s. for 2 days will enable even very heavily dependent drinkers to become abstinent. A similar programme with diazepam (Valium) 10 mg q.d.s. for 3 days and gradually scaling down according to the patient's needs can be equally effective. The aim should be to have the patient off all forms of sedation and hypnotics by the end of 10–14 days at the most. It is all too easy to exchange one form of drug dependence for another. Once the patient has been detoxified in this way, problems can be confronted and drinking goals agreed. Those over the age of 45 or who have been drinking excessively for more than 10 years, or who have consistently failed to achieve harm-free drinking, should undoubtedly aim for total abstinence for life. Nevertheless, though doctor and patient may agree to differ on this goal, a marked improvement in drinking behaviour and level of problems is frequently achieved in the context of a total abstinence programme. Continuing follow-up and support is necessary with these patients in whom lapses must be accepted and analysed dispassionately.

REFERENCES

Edwards G, Gross M 1976 Alcohol dependence: provisional description of a clinical syndrome. British Medical Journal 1: 1058–1061

Goodwin D W, Schulsinger F, Hermansen L, Guze S B, Winokur G 1973 Archives of General Psychiatry 28: 238–243

Plant M 1976 Occupation and alcoholism: cause or effect. Third International Conference on Alcoholism and Drug Dependence. Liverpool, April 1976

Thorley A 1980 Medical responses to problem drinking. Medicine (3rd series) 35: 1816–1822

RECOMMENDED READING

ABC of alcohol. British Medical Journal 7 November 1981–13 February 1982

Alcohol: reducing the harm. Office of Health Economics April 1981

Grant M, Gwinner P 1979 Alcoholism in perspective. Croom Helm, London

Kendell R E 1979 Alcoholism: a medical or a political problem? British Medical Journal 1: 367–371

Murray R M, Bernadt M 1980 Early detection of alcoholism. Medicine (3rd series) 35: 1811–1815

Problems of solvent abuse

INTRODUCTION

Solvent abuse, more commonly known as glue sniffing, is not a new phenomenon. Indeed inhalation of volatile substances in order to alter psychological states, particularly mood and behaviour, dates back as far as the Delphic oracle. Many substances have been exploited by man through the centuries and no age can boast an immunity from their abuse, from the priestesses of Apollo down through the years to the 'ether frolics' of the Victorians and 'chloroform jags' of a more modern student population.

The modern habit of solvent abuse first appeared on the 20th century American scene in the 1950s, grew to large proportions in the 1960s and soon spread to involve children and adolescents in many other parts of the world. During the last decade it has become an increasingly popular pastime among young people in different parts of Britain.

SUBSTANCES AND METHODS

In understanding this problem, it is important to appreciate that many of the substances that are abused are in common domestic and industrial use. They include glues, dry-cleaning substances, hair lacquer, nail polish remover, petrol, paint-thinners and aerosols of all kinds. These substances are all readily, cheaply and legally available. When used properly these chemicals cause no trouble; concern about their toxic effects arises when they are 'misused' as a way of altering the psychological state of the abusing individual.

The methods of abuse are designed to produce a 'high' and to maintain the state of intoxication for as long as possible. In a few cases these methods are crude and simply involve inhaling the volatile chemicals directly from the tube or bottle but others are quite sophisticated and produce longer lasting effects. They include the use of plastic or polythene bags to act as dispensers, the direct discharge of aerosol can contents into the mouth or nose and the use of open fires to heat substances. Small potato crisp bags with a capacity of 500 ml are often used to dispense adhesives and they provide a good fit around the nose and mouth of the abuser. Another polythene bag is sometimes placed over the head and neck to enhance the effect and maintain intoxication for longer. The increase in effect is accompanied by increasing risk of death by suffocation. Where aerosols are sprayed direectly into the mouth or nose there is a great risk of sudden death; accidents involving severe burns are not uncommon and sometimes end fatally in circumstances where open fires are used to heat volatile chemicals.

The term 'glue-sniffing' which is used synonymously with solvent abuse or inhalant misuse is inaccurate for the following reasons:

1. It is not the glue which is inhaled but its volatile components. (As one 13-year-old said, 'you couldn't sniff glue 'cause it would get stuck in your lungs'.)
2. Many substances other than adhesives have been used.
3. The methods used have always involved intermittent deep breathing through the mouth and/or nose.

Many volatile chemicals are implicated in solvent abuse. They include toluene, trichloroethylene, tetrochloroethylene, trichloroethane and sometimes carbon tetrachloride. These substances enter the body by inhalation through the mouth and/or nose when the large surface area of the lungs provides ready and rapid access to the circulation. The onset of the effect is likely to be almost as quick as that following the intravenous injection of a drug.

THE EFFECTS

Clinically and objectively there is a great deal of similarity between acute alcoholic intoxication and solvent intoxication. There is some initial euphoria followed by depression of the central nervous system with blurring of vision, double vision, slurring of speech, inco-ordinated motor activity and eventually coma. The similarity continues with headache following the session and sometimes memory loss for events during or following it.

The differences between the two kinds of intoxication are as important as the similarities. Firstly, with solvent abuse there is extremely rapid intoxication, usually within a few minutes followed by equally rapid recovery, usually within 30 to 60 minutes of the session. Secondly, there is an extremely rapid onset of disorientation in time and space with solvent abuse. In other words, within a very short time, the sniffer no longer knows who he is, where he is or how he came to be there. Thirdly, hallucinations are a feature in 30 to 50% of sniffing sessions (Watson 1977). The hallucinations are usually visual, often frightening and frequently recurrent. They stop once the misuse of solvents stops.

When questioned about the effects on them of a sniffing session, some young people have described the 'high' as being similar to that of drinking alcohol. For others the whole experience may prove unpleasant leaving them sick and dizzy. Some say the sessions lead not only to headaches and hangovers but also to nightmares which may waken the entire household and may last some considerable time after they have abandoned the misuse of solvents.

REASONS FOR SOLVENT ABUSE

The main reasons for involvement in solvent abuse are curiosity and peer group pressure, both of which are to be expected in the young teenager. In a few cases solvent abuse provides a way of helping the individual to cope with underlying problems. In general terms, three groups of sniffers have been identified. Firstly, the experimenters whose curiosity, once aroused, has to be satisfied. Secondly, there are the peer-group or social sniffers who have to conform to the expectations of their group in order to maintain membership of it (Campbell & Watson 1978). Many of these individuals try solvent abuse as the latest fad and indulge once or twice weekly for a few weeks or months before losing interest.

There is, however, a third group which comprises a few young people who become more involved in the habit than others and who do sometimes progress to the daily use of inhalants. This group requires more and more substance as time goes on (Watson 1979a). They have become regular habitual or chronic sniffers and despite all their protestations to the contrary they find it hard if not impossible to break the habit although this may be because they have become used to the ritual or the group activity rather than to the chemical vapour itself. Whatever the reason, recovery can be a long, slow process which requires psychiatric and other medical help as well as community care. In a minority there is a progression from solvent abuse to alcohol or drug abuse (Watson 1979b). In chronic cases, there are many underlying problems of a personal, family or psychiatric nature which have to be resolved before the solvent abuse stops.

THE FEATURES OF SOLVENT ABUSE

Solvent abuse is a group activity involving young teenagers. Although wide age ranges have been reported, the majority of individuals are aged between 12 and 16 years (Oliver & Watson 1977, Watson 1978, Watson 1980). Solitary sniffing is unusual and indicates a need for an intensive investigation of the individual and family concerned. Boys outnumber girls in a ratio which varies between 2:1 depending on the area, the time and the peer groups involved. The practice is undoubtedly more common in industrialised urban areas than in rural areas. Although the publicity given to it might suggest that it appears confined to areas of deprivation, this is not the case and the practice will be encountered in a wide range of social settings.

Most of the sniffing sessions occur out of doors, many of them in isolated areas where detection is unlikely. An advantage is that sniffing in the open air may be safer than doing so in a confined space but, in the event of an emergency, help is more difficult to reach and fatalities can and do occur as a result.

Epidemiological investigations indicate that between 0.5 and 2.5% of the juvenile population is likely to be involved in solvent abuse at any one time. In the author's own studies, cases were found to cluster in certain urban areas and in specific schools within these areas; the explanation is probably the effect of peer group influences noted above (Watson 1977, Watson et al 1980). Despite these findings, solvent abuse is still a relatively small problem which has not so far reached alarming proportions. In many ways the problem is like the outbreak of an infectious disease. It appears in a community, involves a few individuals at first, then some more and then quickly disappears.

THE EFFECTS OF SOLVENTS

The direct toxic effects of solvent abuse are wide-ranging; the damage reported has included acute renal failure (Will & McLaren 1981), hepatic damage (Watson 1982), grand mal seizures (Arthur & Curnock 1982), status epilepticus (Allister et al 1981) and encephalopathy (King et al 1981). Although these consequences appear to have occurred sporadically and to have been reversible in most cases, there has been residual impairment in a few unfortunate individuals and the available evidence weighs heavily against those who wish to deny that solvent abuse can be harmful. This conclusion is further complicated, however, by the observation that direct toxic damage resulting from solvent abuse does not appear to be dose-related. In the light of current knowledge the most likely explanation is that adverse outcomes are also dependent on individual idiosyncrasy but there is an urgent need for more detailed and factual information on this topic.

The combination of intoxication, disorientation in time and space and hallucinations is a very potent and potentially dangerous one. It has led to a number of accidents, various kinds of antisocial behaviour — some of it very serious — and to deaths. The risk of accidents is a major part of the problem of solvent abuse as the following case reports illustrate:

Two boys who were having a sniffing session in a disused tunnel were trapped when the roof fell on top of them. The emergency team from the nearest hospital went out to resuscitate them and a decision had to be taken about whether or not to amputate a limb at the site of the accident. With the help of the police and other community agencies, the boys were freed from the wreckage without emergency surgery although one subsequently had the tip of a finger amputated. Both made a good recovery in hospital.

Six children and young people, ranging in age from 18 months to 19 years were in an end-gable house in a new community. The older boys were sniffing glue and became quite intoxicated and reckless. They accidentally cut into the gas supply of the house and there was an explosion. The house disappeared into rubble but the individuals all escaped unharmed.

Recently solvent abuse sessions have been associated with antisocial behaviour, some of it serious. One glue sniffing session was associated with a serious assault on a youth who died 48 hours later in hospital.

There can be no doubt that many deaths have occurred in Britain over the last decade as a direct or indirect result of solvent abuse. Watson (1979c) was able to identify reports of 45 deaths up to January, 1977 and Anderson and his colleagues (1982) reported the results of an investigation of 140 deaths which were directly or indirectly associated with solvent abuse. These deaths frequently result from multiple injuries, suffocation and the inhalation of vomit as well as from poisoning by the solvents themselves. There are, in addition, cases of sexual-masochistic hangings in which solvents are sometimes misused to enhance the asphyxiating effect. The question of whether the death was caused directly or indirectly by solvent abuse is often academic; if the individual had not been sniffing he would not have died.

CLINICAL PRESENTATION AND MANAGEMENT

General practitioners are increasingly involved in cases of solvent abuse. This is partly because of increased public and professional awareness of the hazards of the practice and partly because the first recommendation of a Working Party on solvent abuse in any area is likely to propose referral to the family doctor.

Clinically the presentation to the general practitioner may vary from a vague history from a worried mother who fears her child might be involved, through a range of unusual accidents, renal failure, jaundice and abdominal pain, fractures, burning accidents, cyanotic attacks and coma to sudden death. Others present at various stages of intoxication and some are referred by the police and social agencies on account of antisocial activities associated with the solvent abuse. These include the theft of abusing substances or a history of missing from home or staying out all night (Watson 1982).

In acute cases there are several obvious signs that solvent abuse is occurring. Varying stages of intoxication, easily recognised by all doctors, may be evident and one should remember that the period of intoxication may last following solvent abuse for anything from a few minutes to 2 hours. It is a non-specific sign however and might have been caused by alcohol or drugs. The chemical smell of the vapour from the breath is a highly specific sign and one which will not be easily missed. The smell from the breath may last up to 24 hours depending on the concentration of volatiles in the circulation.

Another obvious sign is that of glue or other substance on the face, hands and clothes of the sniffer. This is partly due to the application of the substance in a bag or on a cloth to the face itself and is partly a measure of inco-ordination. The sniffer soon stops caring about leaving tell-tale signs of his activity.

Chronic sniffers may develop 'glue-sniffers rash' which resembles acne vulgaris but which is distributed in a V shape over the chin and an inverted V shape over the bridge of the nose. It only occurs in chronic sniffers in whom the diagnosis of solvent abuse has already been made so it is of little use as a diagnostic sign. The rash is caused by the repeated application of a glue-filled bag to the nose and mouth over many months or even years. The diagnosis — if there should be any doubt — can be confirmed by asking the individual about the rash. The answer is invariably 'that's caused by the glue'. Unlike acne vulgaris, these spots disappear when the sniffing stops.

For accurate diagnosis there must be detailed attention to the history. Many people believe that the use of the phrase 'glue sniffing' or 'solvent abuse' gives sufficient information about the situation but this is not the case. The individual's involvement in the habit can and does vary from only once or twice a day to the daily use of up to 3 or 4 pints of glue or bottles of cleaning fluid, although such chronic or extreme use involves only 5 to 10% of all sniffers and the diagnosis becomes obvious as time goes on. Despite denial of heavy involvement or repeated assurances that they could stop easily this is not the case and much long-term follow-up and support will be required.

The history should include careful enquiry into details about the frequency of use, the amount used and whether or not it is a group or a solitary practice. Further useful information to be elicited would be episodes of coma, accidents, or admissions to hospital. Similarly, a careful physical examination should be carried out and a sample of venous blood sent for laboratory estimation of serum urea, electrolytes and liver function tests in order to exclude the possibility of subclinical renal or hepatic damage. A practical consideration about the taking of blood from a sniffer is that it reinforces his perception of the concern of adults for his welfare, reassures him that all is well and can sometimes serve as a deterrent to future solvent abuse.

The emergency treatment of acute intoxication consists of maintaining the airway, turning the patient to the recovery position to prevent the inhalation of vomit, monitoring levels of consciousness and speedy removal to hospital. Opening the windows to increase the supply of fresh air is of help. If respiration ceases mouth-to-mouth ventilation and external cardiac massage will be required. It should be remembered that fresh breaths of air must be taken by the doctor who will otherwise become intoxicated too.

Those who are intoxicated by solvents but who are conscious should be 'talked down' and prevented from harming themselves till they have sobered up. Sedatives should be avoided. Fresh air will facilitate excretion of solvents. The administration of coffee is not likely to facilitate recovery as most of the volatile material is excreted via the lungs.

Parents are usually alarmed for and concerned about their children's welfare so that — in the majority of cases — it is essential to explain the nature of the activity to them to make sure that they understand that solvent abuse is very likely to be only a passing phase in their child's life. They should be reassured that most individuals do not suffer damage to their organ systems and that fatalities are rare. Reassurance should also be given that any damage which does occur is likely to be mild and reversible. This reassurance however must not include an overt or tacit approval of the habit. In the case of chronic

or habitual sniffers, the family doctor is likely to seek help from a clinical psychologist, from an adolescent or forensic psychiatrist, from a social worker or from all these people in a team approach. Psychotherapy, group therapy, family therapy, social work support, rehabilitation and hypnosis have all been tried with varying degrees of success.

Any treatment programme which promotes self-esteem, improves family relationships and encourages suitable activities as an alternative to solvent abuse will increase the chance of success for the sniffer and his family. The general practitioner with his detailed knowledge of the family is ideally placed to aid the recovery process in these individuals.

REFERENCES

Allister C, Lush M, Oliver J S, Watson J M 1981 Status epilepticcus caused by solvent abuse. British Medical Journal 283: 1156

Anderson H R, Dick B, MacNair R S, Palmer J C, Ramsey J D 1982 An investigation of 140 deaths associated with volatile substance abuse in the United Kingdom (1971–1981). Human Toxicology 1: 207–221

Arthur L J H, Curnock D A 1982 Xylene-induced epilepsy following innocent glue sniffing. British Medical Journal 284: 1787

Campbell D, Watson J M 1978 A comparative study of 18 glue sniffers. Community Health 9: 207–210

King M D, Day R E, Oliver J S, Lush M, Watson J M 1981 Solvent encephalopathy. British Medical Journal 283: 663–664

Oliver J S, Watson J M 1977 Solvent sniffing 'for kicks': a review of 50 cases. Lancet i: 84–86

Watson J M 1977 Solvent abuse. M.D. Thesis, University of Glasgow

Watson J M 1978 Clinical and laboratory investigations in 132 cases of solvent abuse. Medicine, Science and the Law 18: 40–43

Waton J M 1979a Glue sniffing: two case reports. The Practitioner 222: 845–847

Watson J M 1979b Solvent abuse: a retrospective study. Community Medicine 1: 153–156

Watson J M 1979c Morbidity and mortality statistics on solvent abuse. Medicine, Science and the Law 19: 246–252

Watson J M 1980 Trends in solvent abuse. Strathclyde Police Guardian 4: 29–32

Watson J M 1982 Solvent abuse: presentation and clinical diagnosis. Human Toxicology 1: 249–256

Watson J M, Baird J, Sourindhrin I 1980 Solvent abuse: The East End Project. Strathclyde Police Guardian 4: 21–26

Will A M, McLaren A H 1981 Reversible renal damage due to glue sniffing. British Medical Journal 283: 525

Preventive care of the elderly in general practice

POPULATION TRENDS

In 1981, 5.7% of males in the United Kingdom and 11.9% of females were above retirement age. The projected population for 1991 shows a small rise in the number of elderly males (from 5.7% to 5.9%) but a small fall in the numbers of females (11.9% to 11.7%). A further small fall in these proportions is anticipated by the year 2001: to 5.5% for males and 10.9% for females. Within these proportions for both years are small but significant rises in those of 75 years and above who form the 'elderly' elderly. The average number of patients on the individual general practitioner's list in 1981 was 2000 although the number of patients registered with individual general practitioner varies considerably as do the numbers of elderly people within different urban and rural populations. The use of the 'average' general practitioner list is nevertheless a useful basis for describing both the doctor's workload and the characteristics of his practice; in 1981, the average G.P. list included 352 patients over retirement age and 112 aged more than 75 (Table 27.1).

THE CHARACTERISTICS OF ELDERLY PATIENTS

Writing in 1971 of a study in Glasgow, Isaacs identified the five dominant characteristics of elderly patients who were admitted for prolonged geriatric care; these were

immobility, incontinence, mental abnormality, falls and strokes. What is impressive about this list of disabling conditions is that each represents the end stage of a process of ill-health that must have been present, perhaps identified and treated, perhaps not, over a number of months or years.

The idea that elderly patients — in marked contrast to their younger counterparts — suffer from multifactorial problems was first expressed by Williamson and his colleagues in 1964. In this comprehensive survey of patients aged 65 years and over, the mean number of disabling conditions detected was 3.4 per patient of which half were previously unknown to the patient's general practitioner and were presumably unrecognised by the patient. An important aspect of this iceberg of unrecognised disability was that half of the identified problems were to some degree susceptible to remedial action.

The traditional model of patient care in general practice in which the doctor responded to what his patient perceived and presented as a problem is inappropriate for elderly patients. Many will have complex problems with a medical content that is likely to be both chronic and deteriorating. There are a number of reasons why elderly people may not present the problems with which they are beset. They may simply not be aware that a problem exists; problems such as increasing dyspnoea due to cardiac decompensation may be regarded as the normal and expected accompaniment of growing old or depressive illness — estimated as being present in approximately 14% of elderly people (Player et al 1971) — may be thought to be simply a reaction to loneliness. Problems of a social or environmental nature may not be considered 'proper' complaints to present to a doctor. The consequence can be that, from amongst a number of co-existing difficulties with daily living, the elderly patient will tend to present only the most pressing problem and only at a time when it becomes sufficiently serious or severe as to interfere with normal life. For those elderly who are virtually housebound, who live alone or with an equally elderly companion (estimated in 1981 as 30% of the elderly in the Strathclyde Region of Scotland) the situation can be much more serious unless medical services

Table 27.1 Number of elderly in an 'average' practice of 2000 patients (from Social Trends 1979)

		1981	1991	2001
Males	65–74 yr	78	74	70
	75–84	32	36	34
	85+	4	8	6
Females	60–74 yr	162	148	136
	75–84	62	64	62
	85+	14	22	20
Totals		352	352	328

are brought to the patient in a planned way that does not depend on patient initiative.

There are thus strong arguments for an approach to the care of the elderly in general practice which anticipates illness and its consequences. This requires a planned and co-ordinated programme which involves all members of a practice team — the doctor, the district nurse, the health visitor and the social worker. It also requires a method of ensuring that those at risk are identified and a record system that allows comprehensive baselines of the whole health of the elderly person to be constructed and maintained. An organised approach to the routine periodic assessment of the elderly allows one to intervene earlier in the process of physical, emotional or social breakdown and thus lessens the frequency with which the crisis situation occurs apparently unheralded. The general practitioner has a responsibility to the caring relatives of elderly persons which is as important in the preservation of independent living as are his duties to his patient. Little is known at present of the degree and nature of family support for elderly people, of the effects of this supportive role on the elderly and the consequences in terms of health and wellbeing for those responsible for the day by day care of old people. A comprehensive screening and assessment programme in general practice allows identification of this support — although not of its consequences — and can give warning of its impending breakdown.

THE FEATURES OF A PREVENTIVE CARE PROGRAMME

The requirements for an improved system of primary care for elderly patients can be divided into three broad areas:

1. A screening system to identify those at risk.
2. An assessment programme to provide ongoing and updated problem lists.
3. Support for both the elderly and their relatives.

METHODS OF ASSESSMENT

In essence there are four distinct though overlapping methods of assessment for elderly persons:

1. The routine and regular visit by the doctor to an old person.
2. The routine comprehensive 'physical' examination.
3. The survey of social and environmental factors relating to the elderly person.
4. A comprehensive medical, social and psychological assessment.

Many general practitioners make regular visits to their elderly patients either on their own or with the health visitor but however valuable such visits may be, they have a number of inherent drawbacks. Firstly, only those elderly patients known to the doctor or his colleagues as in need of regular visiting will be included and some — who may have greater needs — can be overlooked. This potential problem can be overcome by using the age/sex register rather than the existence of known ill-health as the means by which the visiting list is constructed. Regular visits to elderly patients at intervals of 4 weeks serve a useful social purpose but can have the same drawbacks as the surgery consultation — that only those matters which the patient believes to be appropriate are likely to be presented and discussed. A regular review of total health is possible but is less likely to be undertaken because of the pressures of time and workload.

Several studies have shown tthat a physical examination of an older person is unlikely to lead to the detection of much hitherto unknown morbidity. Currie (1974) in a comprehensive survey of the health of all patients in a group practice aged 70–72 years identified a total of 790 diseases or disabilities (3.2 per patient) of which only one-fifth were previously unknown to the practice doctors. Currie commented, 'The results of the survey were perhaps incommensurate with the effort expended since most of the unrecorded morbidity was trivial, but one case of pernicious anaemia was discovered, nine patients were referred to hospital, 20 were started on new therapy and 47 required medical advice — mainly about diets'. In the psychological assessment used by Currie and his co-workers, anxiety and overt depression frequently defeated both doctors and health visitors. In this study, Currie found that important psychiatric symptoms were present in 37 of 91 males (41%) and in 72 of 155 female patients (46%). This is a potentially fruitful area of enquiry since some improvement can be achieved in most instances of psychological ill-health. Currie's check list included the following factors: intellectual impairment, personality impairment, memory loss, confabulation, hallucinations and delusions, depression, emotional lability and anxiety. He concluded later that the inclusion of disorientation in the check list would have made it more complete.

Another approach — that of a comprehenive laboratory survey — was reported by Murray (1977). All the elderly patients in his practice were contacted and, from those who agreed to participate, blood was sent to the local hospital laboratory for the estimation of haemoglobin, serum iron and total iron binding capacity and for 18 biochemical values on autoanalysis. Urine was tested for protein and sugar and, if indicated, was cultured; 123 new diagnoses were discovered in this survey of 403 elderly patients. Approximately half were anaemia. Murray commented, 'At the end of the day, the benefits to the patient are reduced to the diagnosis of iron deficiency and megaloblastic anaemia, a single case of polymyalgia rheumatica and of hypothyroidism, urinary infection in six patients, non-clinical gout in three, diabetes in four, osteomalacia in four, and one of Paget's disease that required calcitonin. The other diagnoses tended to be academic'. The costs of this survey, excluding the doctor's time, worked out at £20 per patient at 1976 values and Murray concluded that it is 'difficult to justify the survey on a cost effective basis in addition to the low effective yield'. He concluded that of all laboratory investigations only a full blood count, blood film and an MSU analysis were of any real value.

Assessments that only include details of the social environment of the patient are of limited practical importance and there are few reports of such surveys from general practitioners. This kind of assessment is of value more in assessing unmet social needs as a means by which services to the elderly can be improved.

THE WOODSIDE SCREENING AND ASSESSMENT PROGRAMME

A comprehensive screening and assessment system has been described by Barber & Wallis (1976, 1978, 1980, 1981, 1982)) and is available in the Glasgow area and in a number of other parts of the United Kingdom. The system consists of a method of identifying those who are thought to require a comprehensive assessment, an assessment record that continues as the health visitor or geriatric visitor's working patient notes, and a problem list for the patient's medical records.

This system, together with its results in practice, is described below not so much as to define the methods that should be used in such an activity but rather to demonstrate the benefits and workload implications of this kind of approach to the preventive care of the elderly.

SCREENING OF ELDERLY PATIENTS

The initial system of screening is by means of a short (nine questions) postal questionnaire requiring simple Yes or No answers. Any affirmative answer, or non-return of the letter to the practice, is taken as indicative of the patient being in need of a comprehensive assessment. The nine questions (Table 27.2) were designed and phrased to cover known areas of potential risk to the patient's physical, psychological or social status and the 'screening letter' has been found to have a predictive value of 0.9 (a predictive value of 1 = 100% accuracy). In the lower socioeconomic population of urban practice this approach has been found to be acceptable by a high

Table 27.2 The nine questions used in the postal screening questionnaire

1. Do you live on your own?
2. Are you in the position of having *no* relative whom you can rely on for help?
3. Do you need regular help with housework or shopping?
4. Are there days when you are unable to prepare a hot meal for yourself?
5. Are you confined to your home through ill health?
6. Is there any difficulty or concern over your health, you have still to see about?
7. Do you have any problem with your eyes or eyesight?
8. Do you have any difficulty with your hearing?
9. Have you been in hospital during the past year?

proportion of elderly patients (in excess of 85%) and has repeatedly shown that approximately 75% of patients over 70 years of age have hitherto unknown or deteriorating problems of physical, psychological or social health. Following the identification of those patients who were thought to be at risk, a more comprehensive assessment is completed by the practice health visitor.

THE ASSESSMENT RECORD

The assessment record used is in three parts: the first relates to social conditions and activities of daily living; the second concerns the need for a wide range of social and ancillary services. The third is a systematic symptom enquiry (Figs. 27.1a & b, 27.2, 27.3). In each section of the record a simple numerical scoring system is used to indicate the severity of the problem. Following one or more home visits by the health visitor at which the assessment is completed, all the active problems that have been identified are entered in a specially designed problem list in the patient's medical record. The most practical means of tackling each identified problem and the member of staff who seems most appropriate to be responsible for action regarding it are then discussed by the practice and a decision is made as to the timing of subsequent assessments — which are usually after a lapse of 6, 9 or 12 months.

OUTCOME OF ASSESSMENT

The outcome of this assessment programme has been examined closely to determine its benefits to the practice population. A summary of the results of outcome in one group practice is shown in Table 27.3.

In this particular study a large number of hitherto unknown problems were discovered (6.4 per patient) of which more than half were in the area of social environment and activities of daily living. The 'improvement rate' in this first area was low — only 20% — but it rose

Medical and social

	Date	1st Assessment	Subsequent assessments				
		Code No 0–6	Code No 0–6	Code No 0–6	Code No 0–6	Code No 0–6	Code No 0–6
Household	1 34						
Caring relative	1 35						
Dependence on others	1 36						
Bereavement	1 37						
Housing problem	1 38						
Hazards (If 'yes' specify)	1 39						

a. Activities of daily living (excerpt).

Coding 0–6

34 : Household

0 Not known
1 Relative
3 Combination
5 Others
6 Alone

35 : Caring relative

0 Not known
1 Same house
3 Nearby
4 Regular visits
5 Irregular visits
6 None applicable

36 : Dependence on others

0 Not known
1 None
3 Shopping
4 Domestic care
6 Personal care

37 : Bereavement

0 Not known
1 None
3 More than 2 years
5 Less than 2 years
6 Less than 6 months

38 : Housing problem

0 Not known
1 None
3 Too many stairs
4 Poor housing
5 Other (specify)
6 Combination

39 : Hazards

0 Not known
1 None
3 Yes (specify)

b. Codes for grades of problem.

Fig. 27.1 Assessment record.

to 77% in the area of social and ancillary services and to 72% in the symptom enquiry. Overall, some remedial action could be taken in 40% of the problems detected but a further important aspect of the programme was that its ongoing nature meant that new problems were continually being detected and thus exposed to action.

EFFECTS ON WORKLOAD

The effects of the introduction of a comprehensive anticipatory care system for elderly patients was studied using a practice which had previously not been involved in any preventive programme for this population age group. The work generated by all patients of 65 years of age and over for the practice doctors, health visitor and district nurse were studied over a 4-year period. During the first 18 months the workload figures gave a baseline for the practice. During the second period of almost 12 months an additional full-time health visitor was introduced to complete the screening and assessment programme: all the problems that she discovered were handed over to the regular practice staff for further action. At the end of the intervention stage the additional health visitor withdrew and the workload generated by the elderly population was again reviewed for a futher 18 months. The results can be seen in Tables 27.4, 27.5 and 27.6 — adjusted in each phase to a 12-month period. The workload for the practice doctors, health visitor and district nurse all rose significantly during the intervention period as previously unknown problems were discovered and passed to the practice staff for subsequent action. Following the completion of the screening and assessment programme the workload for all staff fell, but most not-

Medical and social

		1st Assessment	Subsequent assessments				
	Date						

Needs
Please code:
Not known   0
No need   1
Need met   2
Need unmet   3

			1st Assessment	Subsequent assessments				
Chiropody	1	49						
Home help	1	50						
Meals on wheels	1	51						
Contacts	1	52						

Fig. 27.2 Assessment record — social and ancillary needs (excerpt).

Medical

		1st Assessment	Subsequent assessments				
	Date						

Please code
Not known   0
No symptoms   1
Known/Recorded in case notes   2
Requiring attention/not recorded   3

Gastro-intestinal

			1st Assessment	Subsequent assessments				
Indigestion/heartburn	1	60						
Abdominal pain/discomfort	1	61						
Vomiting	1	62						
Vomiting of blood	1	63						
Change in bowel habit	1	64						
Alternatively constipated/loose	1	65						
Passing blood or tarry motions	1	66						
Piles	1	67						

Fig. 27.3 Assessment record — symptom enquiry (excerpt).

Table 27.3 Results of two consecutive assessments in 100 elderly patients (mean interval between assessments 9 months)

Area of enquiry	First assessment No. of problems	Second assessment		
		Improved	Unchanged	New problems
Activities of daily living	409	80	329	39
Social Service needs	141	109	32	24
Symptom survey	91	65	26	16
Total	641	254	387	79

Table 27.4 Changes in doctor workload (source: Barber & Wallis 1982)

Doctor workload	A Pre-intervention	B Intervention	C Post-intervention	% Change C–A
No. of patients seen	72	86	56	−22
No. of patient contacts	175	214	107	−39
Surgery: Home ratio	1.7:1	1.04:1	0.6:1	
% of elderly seen	58	70	46	−12

Table 27.5 Changes in health visitors workload (source: Barber & Wallis 1982)

Health Visitor workload	A Pre-intervention	B Intervention	C Post-intervention	% Change C–A
No. of patients seen	22	49	43	+95
No. of patient contacts	130	228	229	+76
% of elderly seen	18	40	35	+17

Table 27.6 Changes in district nurse workload (source: Barber & Wallis 1982)

District Nurse workload	A Pre-intervention	B Intervention	C Post-intervention	% Change C–A
No. of patients seen	10	15	12	+20
No. of patient contacts	453	737	701	+55
% of elderly seen	8	12	10	+2

ably for the doctor; the district nurse and health visitor continued to have a greater workload than had been observed during the initial baseline 18-month period. Apart from the consideration of patient problems implied by the increased workload, a further benefit was the increased population of the elderly who were brought into contact with one or other of the practice staff.

TIME INVOLVED IN A SCREENING AND ASSESSMENT PROGRAMME

The research health visitor took careful notes of the time required for both the screening and assessment process and the additional time that was necessary for the research aspects of her work. The time required for the screening and assessment aspects of the study was 316 hours per 100 patients at risk (Table 27.7). If this time

was to be spread over the working year of 48 weeks it would involve the health visitor in approximately 7 hours each week for each 100 patients at risk.

In the average practice of 4000 patients, typically served by two general practitioners and one health visitor there would be likely to be 640 patients (16%) over the age of 65 years (Social Trends 1979). The time required for the full screening and assessment programme in this size of practice and for this age group of patients would thus be 42 hours each week: a commitment that is unrealistic in terms of manpower and priorities. It can be argued however that more benefit would be gained if only those patients of 75 years of age and over were to be included in the programme. It is the older elderly patients who are more likely to have the unreported morbidity (Williamson 1964).

The average practice of 4000 patients will include approximately 140 patients (6%) of 75 years and over. A

Table 27.7   Time required for preventive programme (source: Barber & Wallis 1982)

Activity	Hours	Hours/100 patients
Updating age/sex register	9	7
Preparing questionnaires	36	29
Preparing assessments	48	39
Visiting and assessing	216	176
Office work (problem lists etc.)	80	65
Totals	389	316
		or 7 hours/working week

screening and assessment programme for this age group would require 18 hours of health visitor time each week of they were all to be reviewed in 1 year. It is important to stress that the 18 hours of work each week however represents the *establishment* of the preventive programme; the time required in later years would be considerably reduced. Once the initial updating of the age/sex register was completed in the first year, it would be unlikely to require the same allocation of time in subsequent years. Preparation of the screening questionnaires would be required in the second and subsequent years for those who had no problems in the previous year (approximately 20%) and for those patients now reaching 75 years of age. The death rate amongst patients of 75 years of age and over is estimated to be 238 per 1000 at risk (Social Trends 1979) and on this basis, it can be assumed that 58 patients in a notional practice of 4000 patients will die each year and that 58 patients will reach their 75th birthday. Assessment records would thus only have to be prepared for those patients who were entering the programme since the same record would be used for patients previously seen. In summary, therefore, assessments would need to be completed annually on all those identified in the first year as having problems (80%) less those who die during that year and on 80% of those who reach their 75th birthday in that year. The total time required for the second year of an ongoing screening and assessment programme would thus be 505 hours or 11 hours per working week in a 48 week year (Table 27.8).

In other words, setting up a system of ongoing screening and assessment for patients aged 75 years and above in an average practice of 4000 patients with one health visitor would thus require an initial investment of 18 hours per week of health visitor time. Thereafter it would require 11 hours per week to keep the system running.

The results of this research are given in some detail to show both the potential value and the practical difficulties involved in a comprehensive screening and assessment programme. The framework that is described allows considerable variation however and can be adapted to suit the particular needs of different practices and different populations. The screening approach, for example, can use different 'at risk' criteria based on local knowledge and circumstances. The workload involved in setting up the system can be reduced by including older age groups at the start and extending the programme to

Table 27.8   Time required for preventive programme — practice of 4000 patients — 240 aged 75+ (source: Barber & Wallis 1982)

Year 1	Time required for 240 patients		861 h/year or 18 h/week
Year 2	Activity		Time required/year
	Updating age/sex register		—
	Preparing questionnaire:		
	Patients from Year 1: 20% of 240–58 who die = 36 patients		10 h
	New 75 year olds = 58 patients		17 h
	Preparing assessment records:		
	New 75 year olds only (80% of 58) = 46 patients		18 h
	Assessment visits:		
	Patients from Year 1: 80% of 240–58 who die = 145 patients		255 h
	New 75 year olds: 80% of 58 patients = 46 patients		81 h
	Office work: (problem lists, etc.) — all assessed = 191 patients		124 h
		Total	505 h or 11 h/week

the more numerous younger old people as time permits.

A regular review of the assessment record will inevitably uncover a number of areas of enquiry with which problems are associated but for which little if any improvement can be obtained. Typical of such problems may be poor or inadequate housing, hazards to health in the home, defective vision and hearing, and partial or absolute soical isolation. The work of assessment can become more productive and less time consuming if these 'non-responsive' areas of enquiry are excluded and it may then be more likely to become an ongoing part of the clinical service offered to the elderly. On the other hand, the regular documentation of apparently unmanageable problems found in *populations of elderly patients*, in contrast to the individual, can and should be of value in planning services for them and is information that can be used in support of arguments about policy changes by the local health or government authorities. This is an aspect of the activity that is worth careful consideration since the general practitioner has community responsibilities in addition to his more clearly identifiable duties towards the individual patient.

REFERENCES

Barber J H, Wallis J B 1976 Assessment of the elderly in general practice. Journal of the Royal College of General Practitioners 26: 106–114

Barber J H, Wallis J B 1978 The benefits to an elderly population of continuing geriatric assessment. Journal of the Royal College of General Practitioners 28: 428–433

Barber J H, Wallis J B 1981 Geriatric screening. Journal of the Royal College of General Practitioners 31: 57

Barber J H, Wallis J B 1982 The effects of a system of geriatric screening and assessment on general practice workload. Health Bulletin 40: 125–132

Barber J H, Wallis J B, McKeating E 1980 A postal screening questionnaire in preventive geriatric care. Journal of the Royal College of General Practitioners 30: 49–51

Currie G, Macneill, R M, Walker J G, Barnie E, Mudie E 1974 British Medical Journal, 2: 108–111

Isaacs B, Livingstone M, Neville Y 1972 Survival of the unfittest. Routledge and Kegan Paul Ltd, London

Murray T S, Young R E 1977 Laboratory survey in a geriatric population. Update 14: 191

Player D A, Irving G, Robinson R A 1971 Health Bulletin 29: 105 Social Trends 1979 HMSO, London

Strathclyde Regional Council 1980 Strathclyde Population Profiles, 1980

Williamson J et al 1964 Old people at home: their unreported needs. Lancet 1: 1117–1120

Treatment of the elderly

INTRODUCTION

Treatment in older people, as in all patients, must be based on firm and rational diagnosis. Alas, in later life this simple concept becomes even more difficult than it is in middle life for two principal reasons; firstly, the existence of multiple pathology, and secondly, the atypical presentation of disease.

Multiple pathology simply means that with increasing age we accumulate an increasing number of disease processes which affect more and more organ systems; it means, in addition, the interaction of physical, psychological, nutritional and social factors which combine to cause ill-health. The atypical presentation of disease presents major clinical problems, because many disease processes emerge with vague clinical presentations such as confusion, 'going off the feet' or 'taking to bed'. The basic rule of illness in later life is that it is unusual, asymptomatic, cryptic or insidious. The doctor is thus more dependent on help from laboratory and radiological investigations than in his care of younger patients. The situation is further complicated by the fact that the average elderly patient presents with six or seven main diagnoses, several of which are at least in part treatable, and one or two of which are critical for the patient's wellbeing. One clinical comfort in the face of this difficult clinical reality was described by Sir Ferguson Anderson as the phenomenon of unexplained spontaneous recovery — a gift which the elderly posses when placed in a therapeutic environment.

The therapeutic environment may be home, no matter how dirty or squalid, provided it is warm and that there is real care provided, the eventide home or hostel, or the hospital or nursing home. The needs of each individual vary and the precise qualities of the therapeuticenvironment appropriate to each are difficult to define. The include the provision of warmth, adequate fluid intake, loving care and the absence of any form of harmful, meddlesome interference. No elderly person should be denied proper investigation or effective drug or other therapy because of age if there is quality of life; equally no one should be needlessly subjected to unrequired therapy which carries risk.

In addition to the adverse reactions to drugs which are seen in all patients the elderly are prone to postural hypotension, hypothermia, and to confusional states. These syndromes are common and must be borne in mind when any drug is administered because they can be a consequence of any of the drugs commonly prescribed. The dosage of drugs often requires to be modified in later life and as a rule, with the exception of the antibiotics, the elderly require smaller doses than do younger people. This is alas a fact which is not always recognised in the pharmaceutical industry. Too often new drugs are released which have been evaluated in subjects who are young and fit, with the result that the dosage recommendations are excessive for the elderly. Referral to the data sheet may produce poor advice as far as this age group is concerned.

Drug metabolism is modified by age and so there is reason to be wary of slow release preparations because the transit time in the gut, and thus drug utilisation, is extremely variable. Transformation of drugs in the liver is impaired with ageing, as is renal function. When these factors are coupled with the physiological impairment of the sense of thirst, chronic dehydration can produce real hazards in everyday practice.

SPECIAL PROBLEMS — CONFUSION, PAIN, INCONTINENCE AND INSOMNIA

CONFUSION

Confusion is a symptom resulting from many different causes, and is totally non-specific. It is important to distinguish the 50–60% of confusional states which are symptomatic and reversible in their earlier stages from the remainder where the cause is not yet understood and the treatment is palliative. At the moment it is legitimate to call the latter dementia.

One of the most common causes of confusion is sensory misinterpretation. The person most likely to suffer this problem is deaf or has visual impairment — or, even worse, has both disabilities; when such a person is placed in an environment which is difficult to comprehend, confusion is almost inevitable. A typical situation is when an elderly person is taken from home late at night to a strange and often dimly-lit hospital ward and the stage is set for a confusional state of purely environmental origin.

The use and misuse of drugs leads to the second most common cause of confusion. Any drug can cause confusion in this age group, but the worst offenders are the barbiturates, the benzodiazepines and the phenothiazines. In particular, one should beware of phenobarbitone, butobarbitone and sodium amytal — and of preparations such as Aludrox SA, or Franol which include a barbiturate. Of the benzodiazepines flurazepam (Dalmane) is the worst offender because it has an extremely long half-life. Nitrazepam (Mogadon) should also be used with discretion, and in small doses (2.5 mg) for the same reason. At the time of writing, the newer drugs in this family such as temazepam (Normison) and lormetazepam (Noctamid) appear to be preferable, in doses of 10 mg and 0.5 mg respectively. Of the phenothiazines, those most frequently used are chlorpromazine (Largactil) and promazine (Sparine): both can cause postural hypotension and hypothermia. Thioridazine (Melleril) is preferable, because, in addition, the risks of jaundice and Parkinsonism are less. In a confused patient all drug therapy must be reviewed critically: in addition to the drugs named above prochlorperazine (Stemetil) and trifluoperazine (Stelazine) should be used with caution. Almost any drug may be stopped: the exceptions are the corticosteroids, drugs used for the treatment of epilepsy and the anti-Parkinsonian drugs. The latter present a special problem since many are hallucinogenic and benzhexol (Artane) is perhaps the worst offender. Great care must be used in stopping these drugs lest one precipitates a Parkinsonian crisis.

Infection is a further common cause of confusion and, since in the age group it is commonly asymptomatic, cryptic or insidious, great clinical skill is needed in diagnosis. Laboratory and radiological help is often essential to exclude chest or urinary tract infections but the rarer (although by no means uncommon) infections such as meningitis, brain abscesses and subacute bacterial endocarditis must not be forgotten. Vascular causes of confusion are also common. They include developing, continuing or completed stroke, subdural haematoma (particularly if there is a story of a recent fall) and subarachnoid haemorrhage. Cardiac insufficiency is another cause of confusion; overt cardiac failure is relatively easy to diagnose, but incipient failure presents more difficulty. Adams-Stokes attacks are not uncommon and specialist help in diagnosis and treatment is often essential.

Endocrine disease frequently presents with confusion. Thyroid, pituitary and adrenal diseases are again atypical and insidious: beware especially of apathetic thyrotoxicosis which often masquerades as depression and, again,

laboratory and specialist help are frequently needed. Electrolyte disturbance is another cause where laboratory help is imperative. Potassium, sodium, magnesium, calcium and phosphate depletion and retention all present in a manner that is indistinguishable frrom the other confusional states of old age as do blood disorders. The most common of these is anaemia due to iron folate or vitamin B_{12} deficiency. There are other, and rarer, anaemias, the leukaemias and platelet disorders in which accurate diagnosis is again the basis of rational treatment although the results in terms of improvement in the confusional state are often disappointing.

The remaining cause of confusion is dementia which has acquired the meaning of permanent loss of mind. Two main types are described — 'senile' dementia, or Alzheimer-type dementia, where loss of intellectual function is inexorably progressive, and arteriosclerotic dementia, which is characterised by episodes of remission and deterioration. Computerised axial tomography often shows the latter to be due to cortical atrophy. In the future there is little doubt that a better differentiation of these syndromes will be possible, that other treatable causes will be found, and that these terms will become obsolete. Treatment is difficult, but a short trial of one of the cerebral activators is often justified. One patient in 10 may be expected to respond within 10 days but if no response occurs the drug should be stopped. Naftidrofuryl (Praxiline — 100 mg or 200 mg thrice daily), cyclandelate (Clyclospasmol—400 mg four times a day) or co-dergocrine mesylate (Hydergine—1.5 mg three times a day) have been reported to be effective.

When a cause for confusion cannot be found symptomatic treatment is necessary. Of the phenothiazines, thioridazine is often the drug of choice and is given in a dose of 10–25 mg three or four times a day. Chlormethiazol (Heminevrin) is also of great value and does not cause postural hypotension. The dose of the capsule is 192 mg three times per day; the equivalent dose as a tablet is 250 mg or 5 ml of the syrup — these differences are a result of the different bio-availability of the three preparations.

Haloperidol (Haldol) is the drug of choice in the management of the aggressive patient and should be prescribed in the liquid form which is tasteless and without smell. This drug has replaced more aggressive therapy. The liquid is available in strengths of 2 mg/ml and 10 mg/ml and the usual dose is 0.5 mg thrice daily.

PAIN

Pain of musculo-skeletal origin, rheumatic pain, rheumatism and vague aches and pains are the lot of most older people, particularly in a cold and damp climate, and although they reduce the quality of life they are usually treatable.

The first choice of drug is aspirin. If this is tolerated it is the most effective and least expensive non-steroidal anti-inflammatory analgesic. Soluble aspirin is the preparation most used, in a dose of 600 mg up to 4-hourly, but Nu-seal aspirin and enteric-coated aspirin may be better tolerated.

Benorylate is a combination of paracetamol and aspirin which is also very effective and should be given as the suspension (the tablets are much less potent) in a dose of 5 ml, twice daily. On occasion, twice this dose may be necessary. Paracetamol is a mild analgesic without anti-inflammatory properties. It has the great value of not having unwanted effects in normal dosage which is two 500 mg tablets three or four times a day. The paediatric elixir BPC contains 120 mg of paracetamol in each 5 ml along with codeine phosphate and caffeine and is of use when tablets cannot be taken. Combinations of paracetamol with other drugs such as dextroproxyphene are difficult to justify. The author does not personally prescribe Distalgesic because of the common occurrence of confusion in older people following its administration.

Of the 80 or so non-steroidal anti-inflammatory drugs that are marketed, indomethacin is among the most potent and useful. Unfortunately, it can cause gastrointestinal bleeding when administered by any route because, once utilised, the blood-borne anti-prostaglandin effect of the drug on the gut takes place. The oral dose, taken with food in divided doses, is 50-200 mg daily. The suspension contains 25 mg per 5 ml and the suppositories contain 100 mg — they are used once at night or once night and morning.

Four other drugs in this group are used frequently. They are fenbufen (Lederfen) 600 mg at night followed by 300 mg in the morning, flurbiprofen (Froben) 150–200 mg daily in divided doses, naproxen (Naprosyn) 250–500 mg twice daily, and piroxicam (Feldene) 20 mg once a day.

Corticosteroids are not contraindicated in the elderly — indeed they are essential in the management of the acute, devastating rheumatoid arthritis which can occur for the first time in life. This disease is fatal if not treated urgently. Similarly, temporal arteritis, which may be a feature of polymyalgia rheumatica, can lead to blindness and stroke if not diagnosed and treated with steroids early.

Acute and severe medical and surgical pain
Pain of this degree occurs pre- and post-operatively, following myocardial infarction, and in renal and gall bladder disease. Pethidine is often the drug first used: unfortunately its action is unpredictable and it may make pain worse instead of relieving it. Nonetheless it is worthy of trial in a dose of 25–100 mg by mouth or by injection, depending on the size, weight and frailty of the patient. Morphine is valuable but often causes vomiting

— this can be prevented by giving cyclizine (Valoid) 50 mg by mouth, intramuscularly or intravenously up to three times a day. The injection, however, is painful. Diamorphine is the best of all the opiates and produces a feeling of happiness but it is a drug of addiction and must be used with care. The synthetic analgesics such as methadone (Physeptone), dextromoramide (Palfium) and buprenorthine (Temgesic) are all of value in some patients. Methadone is of particular value in pain which is associated with thoracic disease such as bronchogenic carcinoma. Buprenorphine is effective when given sublingually but it and dextromoramide resemble pethidine in their capacity to make pain worse in some people.

Pain and distress in the dying
Drugs play a small but important part in the care of the dying. The drugs of greatest value are diamorphine, pethidine, dextromoramide (with the reservation stated above) and oxycodone (Proladone). The last drug may be given as a suppository, a kindly route in the emaciated person. The phenothiazines should not be used to potentiate analgesics in these patients because they may deprive the dying person of self control; antidepressants also potentiate analgesics, however, and are of great value. In addition, the non-steroidal anti-inflammatory analgesics are most useful additions to the regime in the relief of pain due to bony metastases: their drawbacks are detailed above.

INSOMNIA

The most important cause of insomnia in the elderly is depression. This must be recognised, diagnosed and treated correctly. Typically the patient has difficulty in getting to sleep, wakes early in the morning and cannot get back to sleep. Simple questioning will reveal the classic symptoms of depression. This form of insomnia is best treated with the antidepressant drugs, given at bedtime. One of the safer tricyclics, quadricyclics or tetracyclics can be of use, as can L-tryptophan (Optimax). There is no advantage in the long-acting or slow release preparations. Amitriptyline (Tryptizol) is given in a dose of 10–75 mg at night, imipramine (Tofranil) in a dose of 10–25 mg thrice daily, mianserin (Bolvidon) 30 mg at night, increasing if necessary to 60 mg, nomifensine (Merital) 50 mg three times a day, and maprotiline (Ludiomil) 75 mg at night. The first two drugs can be cardiotoxic and may take up to 20 days to act. Any one of them may cause postural hypotension.

Insomnia can also result from environmental factors such as an uncomfortable bedroom or bed, noise, cold, heat or the excessive use of tea or coffee late in the day. It is very important to exclude pain as a cause of insomnia and to realise that it may not always be recognised as such by the patient because of changes in sensory awareness which can be a consequence of age. In these patients it is cruel to use any drug other than an analgesic.

If night sedation is required the barbiturates must be avoided because the changes in liver function that normally occur in ageing delay drug detoxification. Chloral hydrate is safe but unpalatable but triclofos (Tricoryl) as a tablet or syrup in a dose of 500 mg to 2.5 g is acceptable. Of the benzodiazepines, nitrazepam (Mogadon) is most often used but it has a half-life of 70-odd hours, and in a frail, light old person should be given in a dose of 2.5 mg if it is used at all. Other useful drugs are temazepam (Normison, Euhypnos) in a dose of 10 mg, and lormetazepam (Noctamid) 0.5 mg at night.

INCONTINENCE OF URINE

This is a major problem which causes embarrassment to the patient and distress to the caring person. Clinically it is important to distinguish between retention with overflow, in both sexes, and true retention although diagnosis is often difficult because the distended bladder may be hard to feel in the old. Measurement of residual bladder volume is often needed. Urinary incontinence can be divided into that occurring at night only, and that which occurs night and day. The former often responds to the use of anticholinergic drugs such as propantheline (Probanthine) 30–60 mg at night but the latter rarely responds to medical management. Rational therapy is easier when the specialist resources which enable the benefits of modern urodynamic cystometry to be brought to bear on the assessment of the problem.

When commonsense measures such as the restriction of the use of fluids at night, and of the consumption of tea and coffee have failed, and when the possibility of an excessively long action of diuretics has been ruled out, then mechanical methods must be considered. Pants and pads are of great help. There is no satisfactory female urinal, but for the male the Uridom and other forms of sheath can be of help. Catheterisation must be avoided if possible because of the risk of infection but it can be of value if the quality of life can be improved.

Retention of urine

In the male this occurs most frequently as a result of prostatism but, in both sexes, it can also be caused by venous congestion in cardiac failure, in diabetics with autonomic neuropathy, in Parkinsonism and following stroke. Drugs which cause bladder contraction are painful and dangerous; drainage using a catheter or by the suprapubic route is better.

Faecal incontinence

This distressing complaint often follows impaction and is a form of dribbling overflow when the correct treatment is disimpaction. A sane person is not incontinent of a normal stool. Diarrhoea is simply treated but the distance between living space and toilet is often difficult to change and a commode may not always be acceptable. Permanent loss of mind has as yet no treatment.

Some assistance can be given to the relatives caring for incontinent patients by an adequate supply of incontinence pads, by frequent and regular visits from the distant nurse and, in most areas, through the provision of a laundry service. This last facility can be arranged through the social work department or in some parts of the country through the local hospital geriatric service.

CONCLUSIONS

Although much of the treatment of illness in elderly patients is undramatic and may appear relatively unrewarding, it is important to realise that physical illness should be identified and treated intelligently and energetically. To consider every deterioration in health as simply the results of ageing is to do the elderly patient a disservice.

The practicalities of illness management in the elderly will frequently depend on the degree of support available to the old person. In some inner city areas the percentage of old people living alone, or with some equally elderly (and frequently equally frail) companion is in excess of 30%. The absence of support may mean that admission to hospital is arranged, not because of the severity of the illness, but to ensure that the patient can get the very necessary nursing care and supervision. A recent study in Edinburgh (Currie et al 1980) has suggested that elderly patients recovered from acute infectious illnesses more quickly and more fully when managed at home than as would have been the case in hospital. The essential 'treatment' that allowed home rather than hospital care was the early and adequate provision of a home help and the district nurse.

It must not be forgotten that the reason why many an old person can continue to live independently in the community is that regular and effective care is being provided by some friend or relative. Indeed, it may be the breakdown in the caring person's health — physical or emotional — that precipitates the need for institutional care of the old person. The doctor's responsibility should thus extend to include a concern for the carer, which on occasions will need to be more active and effective than is his contribution to the wellbeing of the elderly person.

REFERENCE

Currie C T, Burley L E, Doull C, Ravetz C, Smith R G, Wiliamson J 1980 A scheme of augmented home care for acutely and sub-acutely ill elderly patients: Report of pilot study. Age and Ageing 9:173–180

RECOMMENDED READING

Anderson Sir W F 1976 Practical management of the elderly, 3rd edn. Blackwell Scientific, Oxford

Caird F I, Judge T G 1982 Assessment of the elderly patient, 2nd edn. Pitman Medical, London

Exton-Smith A N, Caird F I 1982 Metabolic and nutritional disorders in the elderly. John Wright, Bristol

Judge T G, Caird F I 1982 Drug Treatment of the elderly patient, 2nd edn. Pitman Medical, London

Acute and chronic illness in the elderly

INTRODUCTION

Since 15% of the population of Britain is aged more than 65, it has been said that we are all geriatricians now. Do not be misled; geriatrics, like paediatrics, is a parallel system of medicine requiring a special body of knowledge, a special organisation and a special philosophy. It has to be an unhurried system and it requires an effective health team. Most illnesses have a geriatric facet and one chapter can do more than skim the surface of this rewarding discipline. The 20th century has seen dramatic changes in the age structure of society. Contrary to popular belief, man's allotted span has not been lengthened, but many more people are reaching advanced old age and are suffering the consequences. It is sobering to realise that, although the life expectancy of the newborn has doubled in the past 100 years, life expectancy at 65 has not altered and expectancy at 80 is actually less than it was in 1880. This is because we are witnessing what Isaacs (1972) has called the survival of the unfittest. Despite the advances of medical science, chronic illness remains a major feature of old age.

UNREPORTED ILLNESS

Williamson's (1964) Edinburgh survey showed that people aged 65 and over had each, on average, more than three diseases or disabilities. Half of these diseases had not been reported to the patient's doctor and most of them were treatable if not curable. The 'average' family doctor can thus expect to have about 350 elderly patients harbouring over 1000 diseases of which 500 may be unknown to him unless he can devise some system of seek and find. Unfortunately, elderly people do not use the National Health Service efficiently. Perhaps they feel threatened by appointment systems and Health Centres. Some have impaired mobility, some have impaired judgement and others, accepting illness as an inevitable consequence of old age, are reluctant to bother an overworked doctor. The problem of seeking and finding can be solved if the doctor keeps an Age/Sex Register, has a

health visitor attached to his practice, and provides her with a well thought-out but concise check list for symptom enquiry. A suggested scheme is set out in Table 29.1. Its objectives are to establish basic data, to provide a profile of environmental, social and medical hazards, and to alert the doctor to those patients who require

Table 29.1 Scheme for seeking and finding unreported illness in the elderly

HEALTH VISITOR'S CHECK LIST FOR GERIATRIC SCREENING

Introduction: Introduce yourself clearly repeating your name twice. You can use your introductory remarks later in the interview as a test of recent memory. Be careful to phrase your questions in simple language that elderly people can understand.

Basic data: Name, sex, date of birth, marital state, address, past or present occupation, caring relatives. This constitutes a test of long-term memory.

Housing and domestic: Apartments, toilet, stairs up, heating, lighting, suitability of house, hazards, adaptations required, quality of housekeeping, shopping, laundry, hygiene.

Diet: Suspect malnutrition where there is restricted mobility, housebinding, mental impairment, or less than one hot meal a day.

At risk categories: Living alone especially if lonely or showing evidence of neglect, bereavement in the previous 2 years; chronic illness or recent acute illness; housebinding; mental impairment; depression; financial hardship (real or imagined); the very old.

Dependence: Dependent on family, neighbours, home help, district nurse, social services.

Mobility: Fully mobile, out and about with difficulty, housebound, chairbound, bedbound. *Special category* — needs chiropody.

MEDICAL ASSESSMENT

General: State of health, weight excessive or falling, eyesight, hearing.

Cardiovascular and respiratory systems: Breathlessness, chest pain, cough (if sputum, purulent? blood?), ankle oedema, palpitations — check pulse rate and blood pressure.

Alimentary system: Teeth, dentures, difficulty in swallowing, indigestion, abdominal pain or heartburn, vomiting, bowel function, faecal incontinence.

Urogenital system: Urinary frequency, pain on passing urine, incontinence.

Males: Difficulty in starting micturition, weak stream, dribbling.

Females: Stress incontinence, vaginal itch, discharge or bleeding, prolapse, breast lumps, discharge from nipples.

Locomotor system: (See 'mobility' above). Pain or stiffness in joints, deformity or pain in bones, weakness or pains in muscles, intermittent claudication.

Central nervous system: Stroke, tremors or shakes, blackouts, poor balance or vertigo, fits, faints and falls, ataxia, incoordination (e.g. cannot do buttons).

Psychiatric

Mood: (affect) Anxiety, depression, labile, other.

Dementia:
  Alertness
  Short-term memory — do you remember my name?
  Long-term memory — what is your date of birth?
  Orientation in time — what day is this?
  Orientation in space — name of next street?
  Impaired intellect — can do simple arithmetic?
  Impaired personality
  Confusion, hallucinations, delusions
  Confabulation

Other mental disease
Test urine for albumin and glucose.
Take blood sample for:
  a. Full blood count
  b. Urea and electrolytes
  c. Random blood sugar
  d. Any other test the doctor considers necessary

COMMENTS

A check list for routing screening must be one which contains only essential questions. The doctor should be told of all abnormal findings and these should be noted on a report card to be incorporated into the patient's record envelope or file. Further action by the doctor or health visitor will depend on the problems identified at initial screening and the doctor's examination if it is considered necessary. From the screening exercise an At-Risk Register can be compiled for those patients requiring follow-up.

examination or attention. The commonest illnesses discovered in Williamson's survey were depression, dementia, cardiac failure, obesity, osteoarthrosis, anaemia, urinary infections, impaired vision, and deafness. As a result of examination, which need take no more than 10 minutes, an *at risk register* can be compiled of those requiring surveillance. High risk categories include:

— Living alone — particularly if there is loneliness or self neglect
— Bereavement in the previous 2 years
— Housebinding for whatever reason
— Mental impairment, especially dementia
— Chronic illness, recent hospital admission, or recent acute illness
— Extreme old age

The traditional monthly visit to the infirm elderly tends to degenerate into a script-writing social call that is soon demanded as a right by the patient. It would be far better to pay an annual visit to those on the at risk register, carrying out a methodical clinical examination, and taking a urine specimen for albumin and glucose, and blood specimens for full blood count, ESR, urea and electrolytes, and random blood sugar at the very minimum. Those few patients who require more frequent attention should be visited on an irregularly regular schedule thus avoiding offence if the rhythm is interrupted for any reason (see also Ch. 27).

WHOLE PERSON MEDICINE

Health is much more than absence of disease. Health in the elderly means having something to live for; perhaps someone to love. Health is activity of the body and the mind and this is best fostered if the environment is familiar and challenging but not threatening. Health is money, food, fluids and warmth; it is self-respect resulting in self-discipline. If any of these non-medical components is withdrawn, health may crumble. Coni et al (1977) have described the new pattern of care for the elderly as 'enablement' — that is enabling them to remain in the community while maintaining the maximum degree of independence compatible with their degree of disability. To this end a wide range of medical, social and voluntary services can be mobilised — they include community nurses, social workers, occupational therapists, home helps and housing officers. The health visitor is the acknowledged expert in co-ordinating such services and in ensuring their appropriate use.

FAILING PHYSIOLOGY

Illness in old age is set against a back-drop of failing physiology, particularly brain failure, which can be disguised by compensating mechanisms for a time but as reserve capacity deteriorates to a critical level the stage is set for a vicious circle of deterioration. Failure in one system may topple the next, and so on, in domino knock-on fashion (Fig. 29.1). Assessment is often difficult. The history has to be taken from a poor historian at slow tempo with help from relatives who must not be permitted to take over the interview. If the relative is kept within the field of vision her flitting facial expressions provide a vivid running commentary on the history and her non-verbal signals will indicate when she should be asked to fill in.

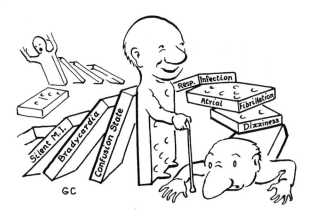

Fig. 29.1 The domino knock-on effect

POLYPHARMACY AND POOR COMPLIANCE

Multiple pathology with multiple symptoms tempt the doctor to pile prescription on prescription at the risk of drug interaction and iatrogenic disease. Failing metabolism (usually hepatic) and failing excretion (usually renal) enhance drug toxicity. Complex drug regimes confuse the patient and there is a temptation to use combination products, but the simplification that may be gained is illusory and flexibility of dosage is reduced. Only drugs suitable for the elderly should be used and they should be prescribed in an acceptable form. Although the comment may seen to be an obvious one, care must be taken to ensure that the dose is neither toxic nor inadequate. If a drug is not having the desired effect, and if non-compliance can be excluded, it should be discontinued and the patient reassessed. Compliance is helped if the drug schedule is written out in block capitals (for clarity); if it is written on a sheet of practice-headed notepaper (to lend it authority); if it can be pinned up for all to see; and if the key supporter can be persuaded to ration out each day's pills.

THE NERVOUS SYSTEM IN THE ELDERLY

DEMENTIA OR CHRONIC BRAIN FAILURE

The label 'dementia' implies chronic brain failure due to irreversible loss of cortical neurones. A neurone is an end cell: when it dies it cannot be replaced. We are born with a full complement of about 10 000 million cortical neurones each of which has between 1000 and 10 000 synapses and the permutation of possible interaction between neurones is mind-boggling. Neurones die at a fairly steady rate throughout adult life and the reserve capacity is more than 50%. A patient may therefore lose 5000 million neurones and still pass himself as 'normal'.

It is comforting to know that if neurones are lost at the usual rate dementia should not set in before the age of 120.

Senile and presenile dementia (Alzheimer's disease)

In Alzheimer's dementia the rate of death of neurones is accelerated for unknown reasons. The resulting cortical atrophy is diffuse but neurone loss is greater in the frontal, occipital and temporal lobes with greatest loss in the hippocampus. The dementia is global and the patient tends to have no insight. The earliest symptom is forgetfulness which can easily be overlooked as a normal phenomenon of ageing. Alzheimer's dementia is a fatal disease running a course of from 2 to 10 years.

Atherosclerotic or muli-infarct dementia

Atherosclerotic dementia results either from stenosis of the great vessels, or, more commonly, from multiple small vessel infarctions producing focal brain lesions. The intervening cerebral cortex is intact and the resulting dementia tends to be 'patchy'. The patient often retains insight and this can lead to profound depression. Atherosclerotic dementia is also a fatal disease which advances in step-like progression to death in about 2 years.

Symptoms

Dysmnesia

The hippocampus is selective for memory storage, and if it is damaged there will be impairment of short-term memory which is the first symptom of Alzheimer's disease. Long-term memory is a widely spread cortical function and therefore less vulnerable; old memories are the last to go.

Impaired personality

The frontal lobes subserve several peculiarly human attributes — the ability to anticipate the future, the ability to worry, and the personality. The philosophy of the man with frontal lobe atrophy is, 'I'm alright; I'll manage', and he maintains this in the face of all evidence to the contrary. Personality change is very hard to describe but easy to recognise — the character becomes a caricature, he coarsens, becomes more self-centred and less self-critical, his standards deteriorate, and his emotions become blunted or labile — flitting from laughter to weeping to rage.

Impaired intellect

There is diminished grasp of complex situations or current affairs, diminished awareness of common dangers, inability to do simple arithmetic, diminished judgement and insight, all of which add up to diminished responsibility.

Various apraxias

Many of these are parietal lobe symptoms including loss of dexterity, inability to dress or undress, speech problems, defective proprioception — which add up to a loss of efficiency in the activities of daily life.

Impaired orientation

This is probably a right parietal lobe symptom. The patient may be disorientated in *time* and so unable to name the hour, the day or the season. He may be disorientated in *space* and be liable to wander and get lost. He may be disorientated as to *person* and unable to name himself or to recognise relatives.

Confabulation

This symptom deserves special mention because it is amost pathognomonic of dementia. It is sometimes necessary to reassure distressed relatives that grannie is not telling lies: she is just explaining away her multiple incompetences with facile fibs.

Management

There is no specific therapy for dementia. The objective of management is to keep the patient in her home as long as possible while maintaining her failing skills and mobility by occupation and exercise. The key supporter must be supported and the nature of the illness must be explained in terms that will lessen resentment and rouse her compassion. Drugs should be kept to a minimum, the environment should be rendered less hostile by house modifications if these are necessary, and appropriate social services should be secured — for example, a home help, laundry facilities or an attendance allowance. The community nurse will teach the relatives to cope and will pass on some of her skills. Thioridazine (Melleril) is reputed to lessen agitation without unduly increasing confusion. Depression is sometimes present and a tricyclic amine may be necessary. If hypnotics cannot be avoided, a short-acting drug such as temazepam (Euhypnos) may be used. Long-acting benzodiazepines such as nitrazepam can cause postural hypotension, increase the confusion and impair the balance. Eventually however, disruptive behaviour, double incontinence and heavy nursing make the burden intolerable and admission to a long-term psychogeriatric hospital may be unavoidable.

CONFUSIONAL STATES

It is a grave error to diagnose 'dementia' when the illness is an organic confusional state that is due to a reversible cause. Confusion of sudden or recent onset is not dementia; it is a domino knock-on effect and the cause must be sought. This confusion has the features of delirium — it fluctuates in degree, hallucinations are common, delusions of a paranoid type are often present, and the patient tends to be noisy and restless. The following causes should be considered.

Inadequate brain perfusion

The problem may be in the *pump* — a myocardial infarction, cardiac failure, a dysrhythmia, or hypotension. It may be in the *plumbing* — a transient ischaemic incident, an arteritis, the acute phase of a cerebrovascular accident. The fault may be in the *perfusate* — anaemia, polycythaemia or anoxaemia of whatever cause.

Toxins

Drugs — neuroleptics, digoxin, steroids, alcohol, drugs for Parkinsonism, and anti-epilepsy drugs. The agent may be *metabolic* — renal or hepatic failure, thyroid imbalance, diabetes, vitamin B_{12} deficiency, and water or electrolyte imbalance. It could be an *infection*, especially pneumonia.

Stress

This can be *psychological* with anxiety or depression, or it can be some *physical* stress such as a surgical operation, urinary retention, or faecal impaction.

Organic confusional states may require hospital admission for full clinical and biochemical investigation. It is sometimes impossible to distinguish between a true dementia and a depressive pseudodementia which may be either endogenous or reactional, and a therapeutic trial of a tricyclic amine may be necessary.

FALLS, FITS AND FAINTS

Falls

About 30% of the elderly are afflicted by falls. In the young elderly the usual cause is tripping, but in the old elderly other causes predominate. The victim can usually say whether she tripped, lost her balance, had a blackout, or just fell for no apparent reason.

Tripping

This accounts for about 35% of falls in the elderly and much of it could be prevented by giving attention to hazards in the home such as poor lighting, dangerous stairs, loose mats and trailing flexes.

Syncope

Vasovagal attacks give warning and are commonly associated with stress or standing in crowded places. Cardiac dysrhythmias can cause syncope and usually give a warning except in the case of Stokes-Adams seizures. Carotid sinus syncope must be suspected if the faints occur when the patient turns her head, but such faints can also be caused by vertebrobasilar insufficiency. In postural hypotension, which accounts for 5% of falls, the incident is usually blamed on giddiness or loss of balance, but a confident diagnosis can be made if there is a drop of more then 20 in the systolic blood pressure when the patient stands upright. Since the hypotension is often iatrogenic (Caird et al 1973) suspected drugs should be discontinued. The patient should be taught to get up in stages — sit up, pause, swing legs over the edge of the bed, pause, stand up cautiously, and wait until giddiness stops before attempting to walk. Thigh-length elastic hose or support tights may be of benefit by lessening venous pooling.

Epilepsy

In the elderly, epilepsy is often non-convulsive, and will produce loss of consciousness without warning. The diagnosis cannot be made from a single incident but must be suspected if the pattern is recurrent. Post-ictal paresis (Todd's palsy) is not uncommon in the elderly and poses a diagnostic problem (Godfrey et al 1982).

Loss of balance

This usually means poor righting mechanisms and the contributory causes are multiple. In the elderly reflexes are slow, cerebellar computation sluggish, muscle and joint feedback (proprioception) defective, and awareness of the centre of gravity may be defective. The latter may be due to brain stem or frontal lobe atrophy and the tendency is to fall backwards. Muscles may be weak, there may be Parkinsonism with hypertonia and bradykinesia, joints may be stiff, eyesight poor, and attention or judgement may be at fault. When a patient thus affected is off balance he or she is unable to take corrective action quickly enough and a fall is inevitable.

Drop attacks

This phenomenon is confined almost entirely to elderly women and accounts for between 12 and 25% of falls (Sheldon 1960, Overstall et al 1977). The victim just drops to the ground with no warning and loss of consciousness. She is unable to rise because her legs are powerless and flaccid. The flaccidity may last minutes or hours during which she is unable to rise but if pressure is applied to the soles of her feet, or if she is lifted to her feet, tone may return to the legs. The fall appears to be due to a sudden interruption of the postural reflex; the cause is not known, but drop attacks are associated with cervical spondylosis and vertebrobasilar insufficiency.

Management of falls

It is important to make as accurate a diagnosis as possible and to deal with any treatable causes. The health visitor may be requested to investigate and eliminate hazards and her visit may make the elderly person more aware of her environment and its risks. Where falls are frequent or cannot be prevented an alarm system with floor level pull-cord should be considered.

STROKE ILLNESS

Cerebrovascular accidents (CVAs)

CVAs are surpassed only by ischaemic heart disease and malignancy as a cause of death. The 'average' family doctor can expect to see five new strokes a year and to have 15 completed strokes under his care. Hypertension is the most important precipitating factor and prevention begins in middle life. Traditionally strokes are classified as thrombotic, embolic and haemorrhagic, but in 50% no intracranial arterial occlusion can be demonstrated, and in such cases the cause must be extracerebral — perhaps a transient reduction in brain perfusion sufficient to cause irreversible brain damage.

Transient cerebral ischaemic accidents (TIAs)

These last less than 24 hours — commmonly 5 to 10 minutes — leaving no sequelae. Carotid TIAs usually cause transient hemiparesis: they are the sinister prognostic significance heralding a completed stroke at a later date. Vertebrobasilar TIAs are less sinister; numerous episodes can occur, and only about 20% proceed to completed stroke. They are usually associated with vertigo or balance upsets due to brain stem ischaemia.

Completed stroke

Loss of consciousness indicates a severe stroke and coma is the rule in carotid strokes: the longer the coma lasts the worse the prognosis. The paralysis is initially flaccid and there may be unilateral sensory impairment and hemianopia. There may be a history of hypertension, ischaemic heart disease, cardiac dysrhythmia, or valvular disease. Thyrotoxicosis also predisposes to carotid stroke. Silent myocardial infarction is a common extracerebral cause due to the associated hypotension, and it should be suspected if there is a tachy- or bradycardia. Where no primary cause is apparent secondary causes should be considered. A full blood count will reveal such causes as polycythaemia and thrombocythaemia — a common precursor or a reticulosis. An ESR of 100 or over may indicate a giant cell arteritis. It should be remembered that 10% of all strokes are due to tumour. The sequence of coma—recovery—coma means a haematoma. Surprisingly, papilloedema is seldom seen in strokes and this may be due to brain shrinkage in old age. Stroke on the dominant side causing right hemiplegia is usually associated with aphasia or dysphasia, and the disability may be both motor and receptive — inability to speak and inability to understand speech. In spite of the problems of communication most patients with a right hemiplegia retain their fighting spirit and motivation to regain function. Strokes affecting the non-dominant hemisphere with left hemiplegia do not result in aphasia but they do cause loss of body image on the affected side. The patient may not know where his left arm and leg are, he may deny that they are paralysed (anosognosia) or even deny that they belong to him at all. He may also have impaired spatial orientation and be unable to judge how far away objects are. These deficits can seriously interfere with rehabilitation. In addition, damage to the right hemisphere is often associated with diminished drive and motivation. Patients with right hemiplegia therefore tend to do better than those with left hemiplegia.

Management of stroke

Ideally all strokes should be admitted to a specialised stroke unit, but this is a counsel of perfection. Where admission is not possible the caring relatives will require a great deal of support including an explanation of what is going on and what they can expect and do. About 20% of stroke victims die within 2 months, 20% make a complete recovery, 20% a partial recovery, and 40% are doomed to chronic invalidism. Communication difficulties must be coped with, bladder and bowel function attended to, adequate hydration secured, pressure ulcers prevented, and the affected joints put through their full range of movement until the hoped for recovery occurs. Deep venous thrombosis, pulmonary embolism and hypostatic pneumonia are complications which can be minimised by skilful nursing. The contribution of the community nurse is important not only for carrying out the necessary procedures but also for teaching these techniques to the caring relative(s). She will also recommend or supply the equipment that will be needed. Rehabilitation, ideally supervised by a physiotherapist, should not be abandoned before 16 weeks, and this is a good stage to call on the skills of the occupational therapist who will assess the activities of daily living and advise on aids or house modifications. There is no specific drug treatment for stroke illness.

PARKINSON'S DISEASE

This is a disease of the brain stem in which the balance between dopamine and acetylcholine is upset. Dopamine is an inhibitory neurotransmitter manufactured in the substantia nigra which is transmitted via axones to receptor sites on neurones in the caudate nucleus and globus pallidus — the corpus striatum. In Parkinson's disease there is degeneration of the substantia nigra with loss of melanin production. The result is depletion of dopamine in the corpus striatum with consequent loss of inhibition. This in turn leads to excess production of the excitatory neurotransmitter acetylcholine which causes the charac-

teristic symptoms. The remedy therefore must either be dopaminergic or anticholinergic. In the average practice there may be five cases of Parkinson's disease. Diagnosis is often instant based on facies, posture and gait: the expression mask-like, the neck, hips, elbows and knees flexed, the trunk rigid, the arms adducted and failing to swing, the gait anteropulsive with short rapid steps. Turning is difficult and poor righting mechanisms lead to frequent falls. The classical symptom of resting tremor of pill-rolling type is often absent in the elderly but, in addition to lead pipe rigidity, cog-wheeling may be detected. Tremor is a great source of embarrassment — the patient is distressed when his teacup rattles in the saucer and he may shun company. The mask-line facies is due to a mixture of spasticity and bradykinesia; there is difficulty in initiating any movement, in rising from a chair, speaking, chewing, and sometimes even swallowing. The latter may be due to dopamine depletion in the nucleus of the vagus nerve. Hyperreflexia is present in 40% of patients and may be associated with extensor plantar responses not necessarily due to pyramidal tract damage. Drooling of saliva may be present.

Differential diagnosis of Parkinson's disease

Parkinsonian symptoms may be induced by drugs which block dopamine receptors in the basal nuclei. The main culprits are phenothiazines such as chlorpromazine (Largactil) and prochlorperazine (Stemetil). Haloperidol (Serenace) and metoclopramide (Maxolon) may also induce Parkinsonism. Antherosclerosis may cause Parkinsonism but the spastic arteriopath who just happens to have a somatic tremor must not be misdiagnosed as Parkinson's disease. The arteriopath will probably give a history of minor CVAs and he may have incipient dementia or a language disorder. Typically his gait is wide-based with irregular little steps (marche à petits pas) and frequent freezing to the ground (magnetic ataxia), a picture very different from the gait of true Parkinson's disease.

Treatment of Parkinson's disease

Levodopa has displaced the anticholinergics as the drug of choice. It restores the deficient neurotransmitter and is prescribed in a combined tablet containing levodopa plus a decarboxylase inhibitor permitting smaller dosage and reduction in side effects. Sinemet 110 contains levodopa 100 mg with carbidopa 10 mg. Madopar contains levodopa 100 mg with benserazide. The rule is to begin with the smallest effective dose, perhaps levodopa 100 mg daily in divided doses, increasing if necessary up to 1.0 g daily. Control can usually be maintained for 2 to 3 years after which a slow decrease in effectiveness can be expected. A troublesome problem at this stage is the 'on-off' phenomenon in which control fluctuates unpredictably. Symptoms are well controlled in the 'on' periods but control is lost in the 'off' periods which can last more than 2 hours during which the patient may be incapacitated by spasticity and akinesia. Another limiting factor is the high incidence of side effects which include confusion, hallucinations, depression, dyskinesia, tachydysrhythmias and postural hypotension.

Levodopa is contraindicated in the presence of dementia, ischaemic heart disease, glaucoma and prostatism. Anticholinergic drugs are synergistic to levodopa in Parkinson's disease. Orphenadrine (Disipal) 50 mg three times daily, benzhexol (Artane) 2 mg thrice daily, or benztropine mesylate (Cogentin) 2 mg twice a day may be used. If these measures fail, symptom control is sometimes regained by prescribing bromocriptine (Parlodel) 2.5–10 mg daily in divided doses. The drug is very expensive and can produce side effects similar to those of levodopa. It should perhaps be prescribed under Consultant advice. The terminal stages of Parkinson's disease are very distressing to the patient and skilled nursing is necessary with judicious use of antidepressive drugs.

PSYCHIATRIC ILLNESS IN THE ELDERLY

The elderly constitute a psychologically vulnerable group. The doctor is only too aware of those elderly patients whose psychiatric problems have nuisance value; those with neurotic personality (about 15%), the paranoid, the depressives with hypochondriasis, the 'difficult' dements, and a proportion of the alcoholics. The patient's premorbid personality may cast light on the diagnosis. Depression, for example, is commoner in persons who, when younger, were obsessional, rigid and conscientious but introverted and unable to display aggression (Pitt 1974). Depression in old age is twice as common as dementia which it can mimic so closely that a therapeutic trial of an antidepressant may be the only way to distinguish them. Masked depression is also common, the patient displaying the multiple concomitant symptoms, such as tiredness, anorexia, weight loss, early morning insomnia, poor concentration, etc. but denying that she is depressed. The true nature of the illness will be missed if the wrong questions are asked. Paraphrenia is an illness peculiar to old age affecting between 1–4% of those over 65. The patient is often deaf; she is lucid but delusional; her premorbid personality was probably distant, detached, eccentric and prickly. Over the years she builds up suspicions about her neighbours which turn into delusions or hallucinatory voices, and these are usually restricted to the people next door or upstairs. Intellect is unimpaired but there is no insight. The response to trifluoperazine (Stelazine) in dosage of up to 5 mg thrice daily is usually excellent.

CARDIOVASCULAR DISEASE IN THE ELDERLY

Atherosclerosis is by far the commonest cause of death in the elderly and results in enormous morbidity from ischaemic heart disease, peripheral vascular disease, strokes, renal failure, etc. Elimination of this one disease would add 10 good years to the expectancy of life at all ages.

Myocardial infarction

Acute myocardial infarction is often painless in the elderly and the classical picture of severe central chest pain is seen in only 20%. Pain may be minimal, atypical or absent, and the 'silent' myocardial infarction may present as dyspnoea, confusion, syncope, a TIA or CVA, a dysrhythmia, vomiting or just weakness. The diagnosis is made on suspicion confirmed in due course by elevated transaminases or characteristic ECG changes. If the patient has persistent pain, has tachy- or bradydysrhythmia, cardiac failure, or has nobody to look after him, he should be admitted to hospital. If there is adequate home support and no complications, the patient may be treated at home but should be mobilised after 24 hours to minimise the risk of deep venous thrombosis and invalidism.

Congestive cardiac failure (CCF)

This means right ventricular failure with, almost inevitably, a degree of left-sided failure as well. The diagnosis is rewarding because drug treatment on conventional lines is very effective. Conversely the diagnosis can be dangerous when it is wrongly made and the patient is exposed to inappropriate therapy. A common error is to misdiagnose CCF on the evidence of breathlessness with ankle oedema — symptoms for which there are multiple alternative causes. The diagnosis should only be made confidently if five diagnostic signs can be demonstrated (Caird & Judge 1974). The signs are:

1. Dyspnoea
2. Bilateral symmetrical ankle oedema
3. Elevation of pressure in the *right* jugular vein
4. Bilateral basal rales
5. Enlargement of the liver

If one sign is absent the diagnosis is unlikely. Subclinical LVF, demonstrable radiographically, may of course be present in the absence of rales. Raised jugular venous pressure on the left side is commonly due to elevation of the aortic arch obstructing venous return in the left innominate vein during expiration: elevation is only significant if it occurs on the right side. Depression of the diaphragm due to emphysema may render a normal liver palpable well below the right costal margin and this also can be confirmed by chest X-ray.

Atrial fibrilliation (AF)

If ectopic heart beats are excluded, atrial fibrillation is the commonest cardiac arrhythmia of the elderly. Rapid atrial fibrillation of sudden onset must be suspected to be the knock-on effect of some disturbance in another organ system, such as pneumonia, thyrotoxicosis or trauma. In young persons AF tends to be self-perpetuating arrhythmia but in the elderly, reversion to sinus rhythm is remarkably common provided the precipitating cause is transient. *Slow atrial fibrillation* is a variety peculiar to old age in which the onset is insidious with no clinical evidence of heart disease other than the irregular pulse. The ventricular rate is slow, presumably because of a conduction defect. Provided there is no cardiac failure, no treatment is required and digitalis is contraindicated because it could precipitate a complete heart block.

Digitalis therapy in the elderly

Digitalis excretion is determined largely by the glomerular filtration rate. If renal function is normal or near-normal with a serum urea below 12 mmol/l, the loading dose of digoxin should be 500 μg and the maintenance dose 250 μg daily. If impaired renal function is present (evidenced by a serum urea above 12 mmol/l) the loading dose should be 250 μg and the maintenance dose 125 μg daily. Many elderly patients are receiving only 62.5 μg of digoxin (one tablet of Lanoxin PG) which is below the therapeutic level and unlikely to be effective. Dall (1970) has shown that, once heart failure has been controlled, digoxin can be withdrawn in nearly three-quarters of elderly patients without any clinical deterioration. The toxicity of digoxin is enhanced by hypokalaemia which is usually a consequence of taking diuretics without potassium supplement. Other causes of hypokalaemia are diarrhoea, vomiting, purgative abuse, subnutrition, gastrointestinal neoplasm and chronic pyelonephritis. If digoxin is ineffective in controlling rapid AF in the elderly one should suspect non-compliance, or hypokalaemia, or thyrotoxicosis — and remember that digoxin itself can cause tachydysrhythmias including fibrillation. Blood specimens should be taken for serum digoxin level, urea and electrolytes, and thyroid function tests. Digoxin should be discontinued while the situation is being reviewed.

Hypertension

In primitive societies blood pressure tends not to rise with age: in Westernised societies it does. Elderly people with blood pressure in excess of 180/110 are at greater risk of cardiovascular morbidity and mortality. Unfortunately, treatment is likely to be beneficial only if given before the hypertension has damaged the target organs. To reduce blood pressure in a patient with atherosclerotic renal failure or completed stroke is to risk a further reduction in perfusion which could aggravate the organ failure. This rule does not apply when the heart or the retina are the damaged organs. Indeed, evidence of cardiac stress is the main indication for antihypertensive therapy in the elderly. Assessment is essentially the same as in yonger patients but the search for treatable causes is less likely to be rewarding. Examination should concentrate on evidence of left ventricular hypertrophy or left heart failure. Triple rhythm in a stressed heart is highly likely to be significant. The presence of angina should not affect the decision since it is not aggravated by lowering the blood pressure. Treatment, also, is the same as in younger patients except that the pressure must be reduced slowly — a sudden lowering of pressure could reduce organ perfusion to disaster level. The objective should be a diastolic pressure of around 100 mg mmHg if this can be achieved without side effects.

Peripheral vascular disease

Gradual narrowing of the arteries to the lower limbs is much more common than sudden dramatic infarction. The presenting symptom, intermittent claudication, may or may not be of sinister import; 25% get better, 50% remain fairly static, and 25% get worse. The occurrence of rest pain or the appearance of necrotic ulcers are the warnings of impending gangrene. Patients with intermittent claudication should be encouraged to walk to the point of pain or even walk 'through' the pain because muscle ischaemia is a powerful enhancer of collateral circulation. Some patients learn to walk long distances by adopting a flat-footed trick gait which lessens the workload of the calf muscles. Despite the blandishments of advertisers vasodilator drugs are usually of little benefit. Lumbar sympathectomy will often improve limb temperature but is less effective for ischaemic pain. The chances of improvement are much lessened by smoking, and tobacco addicts should be left in no doubt as to the dangers of nicotine.

The abdominal aorta, if atherosclerotic, is often very prominent due to displacement across the ridge of the spine and it may be mistakenly diagnosed as an aneurysm. The thickness should be estimated by gripping the aorta between finger and thumb while making allowance for the thickness of the abdominal wall. A normal aorta does not feel more than 2.5 cm thick; an aneurysm may be more than 4 cm thick. If a bruit is heard over the pulsating swelling and can be traced down to the common iliac and femoral arteries, an aneurysm must be presumed (Caird & Judge 1974).

Thrombophlebitis of superficial veins needs no treatment other than the application of a crepe bandage, but deep venous thrombosis (DVT) must always be regarded as potentially serious. It may be symptomless or present as pain and swelling in the calf accompanied by oedema. The main sequelae of DVT are pulmonary embolism, permanent obstruction of venous return from the affected leg leading to superficial varices, pigmentation and stasis ulcers. Prevention is the best treatment and this involves an awareness of the risks of any illness leading to recumbency or chairbinding; this applies particularly to strokes and surgical operations. Mobilisation is the best prophylactic. Ideally all patients with DVT should be admitted to hospital for intravenous heparin infusion followed by anticoagulation with warfarin under strict monitoring. If this is not possible the patient may be treated at home, provided with a below knee elastic stocking, and instructed to elevate the leg whenever he sits down. The latter advice is usually ignored unless the rationale is well and vehemently explained. Phenylbutazone 100 mg thrice daily will relieve the pain and may help to resolve the thrombus.

RESPIRATORY ILLNESS IN THE ELDERLY

Chronic bronchitis

Much of the respiratory morbidity of old age is due to air pollution by industry or by cigarettes, both of which are eminently preventable. A history of smoking must rouse suspicion of chronic bronchitis which affects about 25% of elderly males. Many of them deny coughing but admit to producing a morning spit, and the appearace of the sputum is the single most important physical sign of their respiratory disease. A purulent sputum in a patient with a weak cough spells danger. Physical signs have the same meaning as in youth: bronchial breathing suggests consolidation, rales usually mean alveolar exudate, medium crepitations suggest bronchitis or fibrosis, and coarse crepitations suggest bronchiectasis. One must be aware that tracheal displacement may be due to dorsal scoliosis. Breathlessness in old age can be very hard to interpret. It may merely indicate debility or anxiety, but a cardiac cause is usually indicated if there is orthopnoea, nocturnal dyspnoea or Cheyne-Stokes respiration. Strange to relate, dyspnoea is frequently replaced by fatigue in the elderly cardiac patient; apparently effort can induce exhaustion before it results in breathlessness. Digital clubbing is a much misinterpreted sign: it is unlikely to be due to chronic bronchitis and should strongly suggest bronchial carcinoma. Two variants of chronic bronchitis are worthy of mention.

The blue bloater

Although late onset asthma of old age is a well recognised entity, the wheezy old man whose chronic airways obstruction owes as much as to secretions as to bronchospasm is much commoner. Both verge on patchy pneuomnia and cor pulmonale. He presents with cyanosis, pulmonary hypertension, right heart failure and polycythaemia.

The pink puffer

At the opposite end of the bronchitis spectrum is the patient whose predominant lesion is emphysema. He tends to be underweight. He looks pale because his pulmonary artery tension is normal but he is in danger of death from respiratory failure. He has usually learned the trick of ventilating his alveoli by exhaling through pursed lips — hence the name 'pink puffer'.

Pulmonary tuberculosis in the elderly

Tuberculosis in Britain has declined much less in the elderly than it has in the young and most cases are due to reactivation of old 'healed' lesions. Miliary tuberculosis is not uncommon in the elderly, especially those receiving steroids. Onset is insidious with non-specific malaise, weight loss and intermittent fever. The chest X-ray will be clear and diagnosis depends on the suspicion of an alert clinician backed up by culture of laryngeal swabs. Choroidal tubercles are, of course, pathognomonic but rarely seen and even more rarely recognised as such.

Carcinoma of the bronchus

By the time this neoplasm is diagnosed it may already have spread to lymph nodes, bones, brain, liver or skin. It is one of the great imitators and its guises include general pruritus and proximal myopathy. Of the three common presenting symptoms — cough, chest, pain and hemoptysis — only the latter is likely to bring the patient quickly to the doctor. A high level of suspicion is necessary if the diagnosis is not to be missed. Digital clubbing of recent onset should arouse such suspicion. Unfortunately palliation is usually all that can be offered.

GASTRO-INTESTINAL ILLNESS IN THE ELDERLY

Gastro-intestinal problems in the elderly tend to be clustered at either end of the gut. 95% are edentulous and 12% of those supplied with dentures never use them. Dysphagia is common and should always be taken seriously. A barium meal will demonstrate carcinoma, strictures, diverticula, spasm or achalasia. A glossy tongue and an iron deficiency anaemia will point to Plummer-Vinson syndrome. Dysphagia in patients who have no evidence of physical obstruction may be due to neuromuscular dysfunction such as occurs in the pseudobulbar palsy of patients with bilateral stroke. Neuromuscular dysphagia also occurs in Parkinson's disease. Hiatus hernia with or without reflux oesophagitis is common: so is peptic ulcer which may be silent; and either condition can lead to chronic blood loss with iron deficiency anaemia. Sudden massive bleeding may produce knock-on effects in other systems such as renal failure, myocardial infarction or stroke.

Constipation and diarrhoea

Constipation is merely a symptom requiring an diagnosis and *habit constipation* is the commonest variety — the result of ignoring the 'call to stool'. Contributory causes include anything which makes the patient reluctant to go to the toilet — be it the apathy of dementia, depression or hypothyroidism, be it immobility or just painful piles. The cure may be the re-education of the lazy bowel and its equally lazy owner. *Low residue diet* is the next commonest cause and its cure should be dietetic. If the patient proves ineducable or refuses to take dietary fibre (such as bran, one tablespoonful daily), bulking agents like sterculia (Normacol), psyllium (Metamucil) or ispaghula (Isogel) may be necessary. For hard constipation, faecal softeners such as dicotyl sodium sulphosuccinate (Dioctyl-Forte) will help to retain moisture in the stool and softeners are sometimes combined with an anthracene purgative such as danthron (in Normax and Dorbanex). Fluid intake is important — neither bulking agents nor faecal softeners are likely to work in a dehydrated patient. Irritant purgatives, formerly so popular, should not be used regularly, and preference should be given to laxatives which stimulate peristalsis by acting on the intramural nerve plexuses; these include senna glycosides (Senokot) or bisacodyl (Dulcolax tablets or suppositories). Even these may, with prolonged usage, damage the myenteric plexuses.

Bowel habits are well established by middle age and any change in bowel habit should arouse suspicion of organic disease. Alternating constipation and diarrhoea in a younger patient would immediately alert the doctor to the possibility of carcinoma of the colon. Although carcinoma of the colon is common in the elderly, the cause is much more likely to be diverticulitis, faecal impaction with *spurious diarrhoea*, or purgative abuse by a costive patient. Rectal examination to exclude faecal impaction is essential. If the rectum is empty the next procedure should be sigmoidoscopy since 75% of large bowel growths are accessible to direct inspection. A barium enema is more useful for demonstrating diverticular disease. Diarrhoea in the elderly must never be treated with antidiarrhoeal agents until a rectal examination has been done. The diarrhoea may turn out to be constipation with liquid faeces bypassing the impacted faecal mass and trickling uncontrolled through the anus. Treatment usually requires digital evacuation followed by daily enemas and it may well take a week to clear the obstructed colon. *Soft* faecal impaction occurs in feeble patients taking bulking agents, especially if their fluid intake is inadequate, and this also will require daily enemas. Rectal examination will show that the bowel is loaded to the anus with soft faeces and the underclothing will probably be soiled.

Hepatic disease and jaundice in the elderly

Painless jaundice in an elderly patient is an indication for admission to hospital. The jaundice is usually obstructive, and usually due to gall-stones but neoplasm is also common. Hepatocellular jaundice due to alcoholic cirrhosis is not uncommon, an occasional case of chlopromazine jaundice may be seen, but viral hepatitis is uncommon in patients over 65. Mild haemolytic jaundice may occur in pernicious anaemia, pulmonary embolism and septicaemia. Liver function tests can be difficult to interpret in the elderly and Consultant advice may be necessary.

UROGENITAL DISEASE

Urinary incontinence

7% of men and 11% of women over 65 complain in varying degree of urinary incontinence. By far the commonest cause is the *uninhibited neurogenic bladder*, the result of atrophy of the bladder control centre in the cortex of the frontal lobe. It is therefore part of the spectrum of dementia. The patient feels the urge to pass urine but is unable to inhibit the reflexes mediated by the sacral segment of the cord (Brocklehurst 1978). Unless she can reach the toilet or commode within 2 minutes she will lose control and wet herself. The problem, sometimes called 'urge incontinence' is often compounded by immobility. Drugs are of little value but the problem can be managed by toiletting the patient every 2 hours throughout the day and by using incontinence pads at night, or as a last resort by inserting an indwelling catheter. Urinary incontinence may also be due to diuretics, sedatives, recumbency, faecal impaction, and in men, prostatic obstruction with overflow. Stress incontinence is usually due to inadequate pelvic floor support following childbirth but the history sometimes goes back to childhood. A gynaecological opinion will be needed. In all cases a midstream specimen of urine should be taken for culture but infection is usually the result of incontinence rather than its cause, and eradication of infection seldom improves control.

IMMOBILITY IN THE ELDERLY

More than 50% of the elderly will admit to some degree of difficulty in getting about due to pains in their joints, bones or muscles. Osteoarthritis can be demonstrated in 80%, rheumatoid arthritis arising in old age for the first time is not uncommon, and metabolic bone disease contributes to impaired mobility.

Osteomalacia

Osteomalacia affects about 4% of the elderly and can develop insidiously in housebound patients. The cause is lack of vitamin D or its metabolites due to subnutrition, malabsorption, hepatic disease, renal disease, drugs such as anticonvulsants, or lack of sunshine. Vitamin D is a group of fat soluble steroids which are metabolised in skin, liver and kidneys with eventual conversion into 1,25-dihydroxy-cholecalciferol (1,25-DHCC) which is the most active form of vitamin D and promotes absorption of calcium from the bowel, reabsorption of calcium from the renal tubules, and with the help of parathormone mobilises calcium from the bones. When serum calcium is too low parathormone switches on and (helped by calcitonin) acts on the osteoclasts with resorption of bone. Vitamin D deficiency must be suspected in all housebold elderly persons, particularly those with intellectual impairment who are living alone. The symptoms are loss of height, backache, bone tenderness, and muscle weakness. The latter may be general or take the form of a *proximal myopathy* affecting shoulder girdle muscles and the glutei. This causes difficulty in rising from chairs or climbing stairs and produces the characteristic waddling myopathic gait. X-rays are usually unhelpful unless by chance Looser's zones are demonstrated. The diagnosis is strongly supported if the alkaline phosphatase is high but the serum calcium and phosphate are low. Treatment with calcium and vitamin D tablets BPC, one tablet thrice daily is given until clinical and biochemical improvement occurs and maintenance therapy consists of one tablet daily. Progress should be monitored by checking serum calcium, phosphorus and alkaline phosphatase initially at monthly intervals and annually thereafter. Millard & Hastie's review (1978) is excellent.

Osteoporosis

Body bone mass increases until the age of 50 and then declines, slowly in men, but more rapidly in women. Oestrogen deprivation in women leads to a bone calcium loss of about 1% per annum, but in some women the loss is more rapid resulting in osteoporosis. There is no practical way of detecting the rapid calcium losers. The process is hastened by hyperthyroidism, scurvy, neoplasia, steroids and immobility. There are no symptoms and the disease presents by chance or by the occurrence of a fractured wrist or neck of femur, or a crushed vertebra: X-ray examination will confirm the reduction in bone density. There is no specific treatment, and oestrogen replacement therapy is not without its dangers. Support corsets should be avoided if at all possible because they hasten vertebral decalcification. Backache of sudden onset in an old woman should rouse suspicion of vertebral collapse due to osteoporosis.

Paget's disease

This is an idiopathic disease in which osteoblastic and osteoclastic activity leads to areas of dense bone or rarification respectively. Lesions tend to occur in pelvis, skull, long bones or spine, but many patients have no symptoms and the diagnosis is made by chance on an X-ray taken for other reasons or by routine biochemistry revealing an elevated serum alkaline phosphatase with *normal* serum calcium and phosphorus levels. Some patients have bone pains, some develop deformities, and pathological fractures may occur. Affected bones may be thickened or feel abnormally warm due to increased vascularity; indeed the hyperaemia in the bone acts like an arterio-venous shunt and can lead to high output cardiac failure. The only effective treatment is calcitonin which is so expensive that it must be reserved for the few patients suffering intolerable pain or who are developing deafness due to compression of the auditory nerve.

HYPOTHERMIA

Only 0.5% of elderly people are hypothermic in cold weather but 10% are on the borderline. Impaired thermoregulation is evidenced by failure to shiver when cold or to sweat when hot. Hypothermia is associated with hypothyroidism, dementia, diabetes, alcohol and neuroleptic drugs. Clinically the patient is very cold even in places that are usually warm such as the axilla. The face is pale and puffy, the voice is husky. If the rectal temperature is below 32°C the patient will be stuporose; if it falls below 27°C she will be comatose. There is muscular hypertonia with hyporeflexia — an odd combination. Breathing is slow and shallow and bradycardia or slow atrial fibrillation may be present. Common complications are bronchopneumonia and acute pancreatitis with no clinical signs and they may be missed if chest X-ray and serum amylase are not done routinely. Hospital admission is essential.

REFERENCES

Brocklehurst J C 1978 The investigation and management of incontinence. In: Isaacs B (ed) Recent advances in geriatric medicine — 1. Churchill Livingstone, Edinburgh, ch 2, p 30

Caird F I, Andrews G R, Kennedy R D 1973 Effect of posture on blood pressure in the elderly. British Heart Journal 35:527

Caird F I, Judge T G 1974 Assessment of the elderly patient. Pitman, London, ch 5, p 38–42

Coni N, Davison W, Webster S 1977 Lecture notes on geriatrics. Blackwell, Oxford, ch 2, p 11

Dall J L C 1970 Maintenance digoxin in elderly patients. British Medical Journal i:705

Isaacs B, Livingstone M, Neville Y 1972 Survival of the unfittest. Routledge & Kegan Paul, London

Godfrey J W, Roberts M A, Caird F I 1982 Epileptic seizures in the elderly. Age and Ageing 11:29

Millard P H, Hastie I R 1978 Bone disorders in old age. In: Isaacs B (ed) Recent advances in geriatric medicine — 1. Churchill Livingstone, Edinburgh. ch 5, p 73

Overstall P W, Innes F J, Exton-Smith A N, Johnson A L 1977 Falls in the elderly related to postural imbalance. British Medical Journal i: 261

Pitt B 1974 Psychogeriatrics. Churchill Livingstone, Edinburgh, ch 7, p 46

Sheldon J H 1960 On the natural history of falls in old age. British Medical Journal ii: 1685

Williamson J, Stokoe I H, Gray S, Fisher M, Smith A, McGee A, Stephenson S 1964 Old people at home: their unreported needs. Lancet i: 1117

Brain failure in the elderly

INTRODUCTION

In almost all developed countries, the 20th century has been characterised by an ageing population and a reduction in the proportion of those who are economically active, changes which are mainly due to the lowered fertility and reduced infant mortality rates early in the century rather than to improvements in the medical care of the elderly. At the end of the 19th century 5% of the population of England and Wales were over the age of 65 years (Brandon 1979) in contrast to the present day when the proportion of elderly in the population is around 16% with indications that this figure will continue to rise until the end of the present century. Approximately 25% of the elderly population are over 75 years of age with the bias of an excess of women over men increasing progressively with age. It is estimated that by 1996 the number of those aged 75 years or more will have increased by nearly a quarter although beyond that year the elderly population is expected to decline as a result of the low birth rates of the 1930's.

Community surveys (Kay et al 1964) have shown that 5% of the population aged over 65 suffered from senile dementia. This percentage can rise to as high as 40% for those aged over 75 years. Other organic brain syndromes account for a further 5% whilst functional psychoses and neuroses, and personality disorders account for 5 and 10% respectively. In the same year Strömgrens (1964) studied an island population and showed that 78% of that population aged over 75 years presented with a psychiatric problem during the study period. Dementia accounted for 56% of this total, psychosis being the only other major category which amounted to 10%.

The elderly are major users of the Health Service in Britain, occupying one-half of the adult beds in the National Health Service at any one time, 49% of all psychiatric beds and 70% of the registered disabled (Age Concern 1977). The annual cost per person in the United Kingdom as far as health care is concerned runs at £507 for males aged over 75 years and £625 for each female (Social Trends 1982). These figures compare with averages for all ages of £126 for males and £146 for females.

In general practice patients over 65 years take up 40% of all consultations (Royal College of General Practitioners 1974). The consultation rate for the 65–74 age group is 3.7 per year, increasing to 4.5 for those aged 75 and over compared with a rate of three for the population as a whole. These figures are further increased when one looks at the consultation rates for senile and presenile dementias. The annual consulting rate for males aged between 64 and 70 is 2.9 whilst the rate for females is 8.4. When the comparison is made for those aged 75 and over the rate for males is 22.6 and for females 31.4. The ratio of surgery consultations to home visits for the 65–74 age group is 2:1 and 0.6:1 for the older group. As the average practice contains 350 persons over the age of 65 this gives a total of 1400 consultations per annum.

This increased workload is a reflection of the morbidity of the population group. It has been shown by Williamson et al (1964) that patients over the age of 70 years have on average three disabling conditions, half of which are unknown to their family doctor and of these half are treatable. It is difficult to separate physical disability from social functioning especially in the elderly and Akhtar (1973) has shown that major disability, defined as the inability to live an independent existence, increases continuously beyond 70 years of age. The state of being able to live at home only with assistance increases in prevalence from 12% in the 65–69 age group to over 80% in those over 85 years old. The percentage of diagnoses contributing to disability were:

Urological	48
Cardio-respiratory	38
Joint disease	24
Functional psychiatric	22
Obesity	16
Visual impairment	11
Other	8

Where self-care was not possible the term 'dependence' was used and was found in 7% of those under 65 and in 25% of those above that age. Of these 93% had a neurological disorder.

PRESENTATION

Elderly patients can suffer from a variety of assaults on the brain which can produce varying forms of organic brain reaction. It is therefore important to consider the different types of response which can be encountered so that potentially treatable conditions can be appropriately managed. There is considerable ambiguity of terminology in this field but it can be broken down into two broad categories of acute or sub-acute organic reactions and chronic organic reactions which will embrace the dementing disorders mentioned below.

Diagnostically the first task is to distinguish between the acute and chronic brain syndrome and this is usually done on the basis of the history and mode of onset. A history of short duration, acute onset or clear association with physical illness is strongly suggestive of an acute reaction. These two groups are illustrated in Tables 30.1 and 30.2, which indicate the most probable causes of organic brain reactions in the elderly. Transient acute brain reactions may develop in association with almost every known condition and since in the elderly single causes are uncommon the search should not be discontinued when a single possible cause has been identified. In a variable proportion of cases no organic cause will be found and it is then possible that an environmental stress has produced an acute brain reaction in an elderly person with a diminished coping reserve.

In considering chronic brain syndromes the term dementia is too well-established to be entirely discarded, although this should be confined to the syndrome consisting of global impairment of intellect, memory and personality without impairment of consciousness. A clear distinction must be made between the clinical syndrome which may have many causes and the so-called primary dementias which are specific disease entities characterised by progressive and widespread brain degeneration.

While the syndrome of dementia has many causes, both cerebral and extracerebral, prominent among them are certain intrinsic degenerative diseases of the brain occurring in middle or late life which have acquired the title of dementia as signifying specific disease entities. Dementia is an acquired impairment of intellect and memory from an organic cause which is often accompanied by changes in personality, mood and behaviour. The condition is of a chronic nature, is usually progressive and is irreversible. The primary dementias include senile dementia and the presenile dementias such as Alzheimer's disease, Pick's disease, Huntington's chorea and Creutzfeldt-Jacob disease. The presenile dementias by definition are those dementing processes which occur before the age of 65. While senile dementia and arteriosclerotic dementia are by far the commonest, one of the most frequent errors in diagnosis is that of pseudodementia, depression or drug intoxication and these possibilities

Table 30.1 Causes of acute organic reactions (from Lishman 1978)

Degenerative	Presenile or senile dementias complicated by infection, anoxia, etc.
Space occupying lesions	Cerebral tumour, subdural haematoma, abscess
Trauma	Acute post-traumatic psychosis
Infection	Encephalitis, meningitis, subacute meningovascular syphilis Streptococcal infection, septicaemia, pneumonia, influenza
Vascular	Acute cerebral thrombosis or embolism, transient ischaemic attack, hypertensive encephalopathy
Epileptic	Seizure, post-ictal states
Metabolic	Uraemia, liver disease, electrolyte disturbance, remote effects of carcinoma, porphyria
Endocrine	Thyroid disease, Addisonian crises, diabetic pre-coma, hypoglycaemia, hypo- and hyperparathyroidism
Toxic	Alcohol — Wernicke's encephalopath delirium tremens Drugs — barbiturates (including withdrawal)
Anoxia	Bronchopneumonia, congestive cardiac failure
Vitamin lack	Thiamine, B$_{12}$ and folic acid deficiency

Table 30.2 Causes of chronic organic reactions (from Lishman 1978)

Degenerative	Senile dementia, arteriosclerotic dementia, Alzheimer's, Pick's, Huntington's, Creutzfeldt-Jakob, normal pressure hydrocephalus, Parkinson's
Space occupying lesions	Cerebral tumour, subdural haematoma
Trauma	Post-traumatic dementia
Infection	General paresis, chronic meningo-vascular syphilis, subacute and chronic encephalitis
Vascular	Cerebral arteriosclerosis
Epileptic	'Epileptic dementia'
Metabolic	Uraemia, liver disease, remote effects of carcinoma, hypo- and hyperparathyroidism
Endocrine	Myxoedema, Addison's disease, hypoglycaemia
Toxic	Alcoholic dementia and Korsakoff psychosis. Chronic barbiturate intoxication
Anoxia	Anaemia, congestive cardiac failure, chronic pulmonary disease
Vitamin lack	Thiamine, nicotiniic acid, B$_{12}$, folic acid

should always be borne in mind when considering such a diagnosis in an elderly patient.

SENILE DEMENTIA

The dementias of old age may rest on a parenchymatous

or an arteriosclerotic basis. The parenchymatous form which is usually referred to as senile dementia is by far the commonest primary dementing illness and accounts for a large part of the increased incidence of mental disorder of those who survive to old age. Despite the close neurological similarities between senile dementia and the normal ageing process, it has become clear that there are marked genetic determinants for the appearance of the disease. Larsson et al (1963) studied the incidence of the disease in first degree relatives of 377 cases of senile dementia. They found that the risk of developing dementia was about four times that of corresponding age groups in the general population and was not simply due to the longevity of certain families. The authors concluded that a dominant chromosomal gene was probably responsible. Other workers (Nielsen 1970, Jarvik et al 1974) have reported loss of chromosomal material in patients with senile dementia. It would therefore appear that there are good reasons for considering a genetic linkage although the precise mechanism is still in some doubt. Patients suffering from senile dementia have a shrunken brain with narrowed gyri and widened sulci, often with a thickening of the leptomeninges over the convexity. The ventricles are dilated, the cortical ribbon narrowed and the sub-cortical grey matter reduced in size. While the neurons are seen microscopically to have decreased both in number and size, with an increase in astrocytes, the senile plaques which can be seen are specific markers of senile dementia. Found within the brain alongside these plaques are fibrous tangles called Alzheimer's neurofibropillary degeneration. Roth (1971) demonstrated a relationship between the clinical and psychometric observations during life and quantitative measures of the neuropathological changes after death. Non-dementing elderly subjects frequently showed senile plaques in the cortex and neurofibrillary changes within the hippocampi. In the absence of dementia the outfall of cells was also seen but quantitative estimates of the number of plaques or severity of neurofibrillary changes correlated very highly with scores of intellectual personality impairment.

The onset of the condition is gradual and normally takes place over a year or more. Loss of recent memory is usually the first finding followed by deterioration in other intellectual functions, emotional lability and personality change. Delusions and hallucinations can occur in advanced cases. In patients with senile dementia, insight is usually absent and the patient normally comes to medical attention because relatives or neighbours notice the failing memory, confusion or complete inability to cope with basic self-care.

A differential diagnosis must be made between a tumour, arteriosclerotic psychosis and Alzheimer's disease. In arteriosclerotic psychosis the course is usually more acute and the illness remits and fluctuates. Neuro-

logical signs and symptoms occur sooner or later but there is preservation of personality until the later stages. In Alzheimer's disease the illness occurs in an earlier age group and there is a discrepancy between the degree of physical and mental ageing.

ARTERIOSCLEROTIC DEMENTIA

Vascular disease is responsible for dementia through the occurrence of multiple small or large cerebral infarcts most of which are due to thromboembolism from the extracranial arteries and the heart rather than to inadequacy of the cerebral vasculature. Peripheral or retinal arteriosclerosis often bears little relationship to the state of the cerebral vasculature and although the presence of hypertension is a more reliable guide it can be similarly misleading.

Arteriosclerotic dementia is slightly more common in males than females and usually begins after the seventh decade of life although it is occasionally seen in patients in their early 40's. The clinical picture is characterised by a variable course with an abrupt step-like progression. The patient exhibits loss of memory and intellectual deterioration with affective changes. However, insight and personality are better retained than in those suffering from senile dementia. In patients where the onset is more gradual, variable symptoms, including personality change, may precede the impairment of memory or intellect. There may also be somatic symptoms such as headache, dizziness, tinnitus or syncopy although psychological symptoms such as anxiety, depression or hypochondriacal self-concern may be the main complaint for some considerable time.

The distinction between arteriosclerotic and senile dementia, which is often unclear during life, has also been debated in terms of neuropathology. There are, however, a number of distinguishing clinical features to assist in the differential diagnosis. The diagnosis of arteriosclerotic dementia is favoured by its sudden onset and its step-like progression which can leave transient or permanent neurological deficits. Psychological deficits tend to be patchy with good preservation of insight and personality. Arteriosclerotic dementia is also frequently associated with hypertension and seizures, with somatic complaints featuring more often in the history. On neurological examination there is both gross and subtle evidence of focal cerebral dysfunction and occasionally evidence of arteriosclerosis can be found elsewhere in the body. Senile dementia on the other hand shows a smoother, more gradual progression with a global disintegration of all functions. There is less tendency to mood liability, depression or anxiety. Other disease entities which must be excluded in the differential diagnosis include cerebral tumour and presenile dementia. Subdural haematoma should also be considered as a possible cause for the patient's symptoms.

OTHER FORMS OF DEMENTIA

ALZHEIMER'S DISEASE

This is the commonest of the presenile dementias and usually has an onset between the ages of 40 and 60 years with women affected at least twice as often as men. The disease tends to run a steadily progressive course without remission or fluctuation to the patient's death some 2 to 5 years after onset. Although the pathology of this condition is similar to that found in senile dementia there would appear to be no genetic linkage between the two conditions. Patients with Down's syndrome, however, who survive to middle age are particularly liable to develop Alzheimer's disease.

The onset of the disease is usually insidious and cannot be dated with precision. Memory disturbance is the firt symptom which is followed by rapid intellectual deterioration with symptoms involving parietal lobe dysfunction. These include such features as dysphasia, apraxia, agnosia and acalcula. These are often accompanied by extrapyramidal signs. Patients in the terminal phase suffer from severe dementia with marked neurological abnormalities.

PICK'S DISEASE

This condition is much rarer than Alzheimer's disease and the ratio of Alzheimer's to Pick's disease is 100:1. The onset is between the ages of 50 and 60 with women again being affected twice as often as men. In this condition however there is a strong suggestion of a hereditary pattern with transmission by a dominant autosomal gene being considered responsible. The clinical picture in the early stages is dominated by frontal lobe damage with blunting of emotion, diminution of drive and general coarsening of the character. This is accompanied by a complete loss of insight. Although memory and intellectual functions may be comparatively well preserved in the early stages the patient gradually loses all spontaneity of thought and behaviour and becomes inert, apathetic or acts in a repetitive, disinhibited fashion. Dysphagia, apraxia, agnosia and extrapyramidal symptoms are sometimes present and death tends to occur 2 to 10 years after onset.

NORMOTENSIVE HYDROCEPHALUS

This unusual condition, which was first described by

Adams et al (1965), affects patients who show dementing symptoms in association with an obstructive communicating hydrocephalus with normal cerebrospinal pressure.

Disturbance of gait may be the presenting symptom when the patient walks slowly on a broad base in a stiff-legged, shuffling fashion. This is accompanied, over several weeks or months, by progressive memory impairment with physical and mental slowness. Although social competence may be maintained, insight is limited or absent from an early stage.

Urinary incontinence appears only when the other symptoms are well established, while faecal incontinence is very unusual. The patient does not complain of a headache and papilloedema does not occur.

Surprisingly few precipitating causes can be elicited although some patients may have an antecedent history of subarachnoid haemorrhage, head injury or meningitis. Tumours are even more unusual causes of this condition.

Fortunately this is one form of dementia which can be treated, although the outcome is unpredictable, by insertion of a ventriculo-canal shunt.

CRETUZFELDT-JAKOB'S DISEASE

This is an extrremely rare form of presenile dementia whose onset may occur at any age but is most frequently seen between the ages of 30 and 50. Men and women are equally affected. The condition is one of the four spongiform encephalopathies, the others being Kuru, scrapie and transmissible mink encephalopathy. A viral cause is suspected because some cases have developed following surgery with infected instruments and it can also be experimentally transmitted to monkeys. Dementia and diverse neurological abnormalities develop simultaneously and very rapidly, leading to death within 2 years. Although the danger of cross infection exists, it appears to be of a very low order and should not exclude the taking of sensible precautions, particularly avoiding the percutaneous innoculation of blood. Any such accident should be rigorously treated with the affected area being immediately treated with thorough washing followed by the application of an alcoholic iodine solution. This may usefully be followed by prophylactic treatment with amantadine.

HUNTINGTON'S CHOREA

This is a rare form of inherited presenile dementia which is important because of its genetic aspects. It affects 5 per 100 000 of the population with a regional variation. Although onset can occur at any age it is most typically between the ages of 35 and 45 with men and women being affected equally. An autosomal dominant gene is the principal cause of the condition and so gives rise to 50% of the children of an affected parent developing the condition. Unfortunately because of its late onset many patients have already had their children by the time the disease is first diagnosed.

Choreiform movements and dementia are the most characteristic symptoms but there may be any type of psychiatric abnormality. While the disease can progress without a variation of the presenting symptoms the average survival time is 15 years. The choreiform movements can be treated with phenothiazines or tetrabenzine and any psychiatric symptoms present should be treated with the appropriate drug management.

PARKINSON'S DISEASE

This may be associated with a dementing process and many patients with a primary dementing disorder show the Parkinsonian syndrome. This picture is quite independent of any side-effects produced by psychotropic medication.

PSEUDODEMENTIAS

Pseudodementias incorporate a number of conditions in which the clinical picture resembles organic dementia but in which there is little evidence of physical disease. While the distinction from organic dementia can sometimes be difficult it is important to try to establish a difference between the pseudodementias and the primary dementias. Although they are considered below under separate headings the dividing line between the various forms is in fact far from clear.

The Ganser syndrome
This is an unusual condition in which the patient exhibits some disturbance of consciousness, characteristically gives approximate answers to any questions and has a subsequent complete amnesia for the episode after recovery. The condition is usually found in association with other psychiatric disorders, often occurring in the context of organic brain disease but may be present with a functional psychotic illness. The disorder would appear to rest principally on a complex psychogenic basis in which hysterical mechanisms are largely responsible.

Hysterical pseudodementia
Hysterical pseudodementia is probably the least difficult form of pseudodementia to differentiate from true organic dementia: since it is mostly seen in persons of limited intellectual capacity. The patient tends to be mute or responds with monosyllabic replies and is frequently in-

coherent. He often appears disorientated and performs very badly on simple tests of cognitive function; however careful observation usually reveals that the patient is inconsistent or self-contradictory in his behaviour. Since these patients are usually suggestible the level of their performance is readily influenced by the way in which they are handled. Patients with hysterical pseudodementia often have a past history of severe personality instability and occasionally one of hysterical conversion reactions.

Simulated dementia
This is an extremely rare condition which involves the entirely conscious simulation of dementia by the patient. In the majority of these cases once they have been discovered the patient's very obvious motivation can be easily determined. However in the initial stages of assessment the concealment may be effective enough to cause confusion for the examining physician for some time.

Depressive pseudodementia
This is perhaps the commonest form of pseudodementia and can easily lead to a mistaken diagnosis. When this occurs the outcome is extremely unfortunate because the cause of the patient's dementing symptoms is readily treatable. Confusion can easily arises because, when a depressive illness occurs in the elderly, it does so in a person whose neuronal reserves are already reduced, thus bringing the level of functioning below a critical threshold. However possibly the commonest cause is related to the general psychomotor retardation which accompanies depression with the associated withdrawal of interest and attention from the environment. The patient becomes slow to grasp essentials, his thinking is laboured and his general behaviour becomes slipshod and inefficient. As a result he may show faulty orientation, poor short-term memory and a defective knowledge of current events. The impression of dementia can be strengthened by the patient's loss of weight and his decrepit appearance due to self-neglect.

In the differentiation between dementia and depressive illness the onset of endogenous depression is normally acute and recent, whereas a dementing process is a slow, insidious disease. The depressed patient will often communicate a sense of distress and tests of cognitive function may be inconsistent. Whenever a diagnosis of depressive pseudodementia is suspected it is best managed by an appropriate antidepressant, preferably one which has least cardiotoxic activity.

ASSESSMENT

A patient suspected of suffering from organic brain disease should be carefully examined not only to establish an appropriate baseline of performance so that future comparisons can be made but also to exclude remediable conditions.

HISTORY

There are several important aspects to history-taking in patients suffering from suspected dementia and it will often be found that the best historian is either a neighbour, a home help or other members of the family. A detailed history may for instance reveal a family history of Huntington's chorea or there may be an antecedent history of a head injury which could lead to a diagnosis of subdural haematoma. Other relevant features are the presence of epileptic seizures, the patient's dietary and alcohol intake and a comprehensive drug history.

MENTAL ASSESSMENT

In the assessment of the patient the presence, duration, nature and severity of brain failure frequently depends on observations made by family or neighbours and considerable reliance has to be placed on the opinions of these unqualified observers. There are however several formal tests which can be carried out to assist in defining the degree of brain failure present as well as in establishing an important baseline to allow assessments of the effects of management. Whilst attaching a numerical value to the patient's degree of brain failure may be very appealing as it tends to give a rather crisp and precise indication of how the individual is functioning, it can be rather misleading and should be used with some degree of caution. An example of an assessment form is shown in Table 30.3 and this is scored by the patient who gives one full mark for an accurate answer, and half a mark for an approximate answer. Gray & Isaacs (1979) indicate three forms of assessment procedures which can also be of value. These are summarised below.

Newspaper test
The patient is asked to describe a picture in a newspaper or to read a paragraph of news and to repeat the gist of what has been seen or read. Although the performance of this test is influenced by the patient's intelligence and educational level it should be possible to determine any changes from what could be reasonably expected for a person in that social setting.

Digit reversal test
The patient is given a three digit number, for example 739 and asked to repeat it and then to say the number backwards. If this is successful the whole procedure is repeated with a four digit number. Normally old people should have no difficulty in reversing a four digit number

---

Table 30.3 Assessment form

Name:
Date of birth:
Address:

Reason for consultation:
Patient questions: Score
1. What is your full name   ☐
2. What is the name of this place   ☐
3. What day is it today?   ☐
4. What month is it?   ☐
5. What year it is?   ☐
6. What age are you?   ☐
7. In what year were you born?   ☐
8. What time is it?   ☐
9. How long have you been in here?   ☐
                                                                         Total ☐

Learn and remember for 2 minutes
    Mrs Jean Black, 12, West Street, Bathgate
    a. Score number of trials to learn   ☐
        Abandon at 5.   Score as minus 1, 2, 3, etc.
    b. Score 2-minute recall as words out of 7   ☐
                                                                         Total ☐

Clinical impression: *Good* *Mild* *Severe*
                                    2   1   0
Memory
Habits/incontinence/eating
General behaviour/dressing/communication

while patients with brain failure are of tne unable to perform this with a three digit number.

Set-test

The patient is asked to state all the different colours they can remember which is continued until his stock of knowledge is exhausted and he begins to repeat himself or becomes anecdotal. The test can be repeated with names of animals, fruits and towns. The patient is allowed a maximum score of 10 in each part of the test. Although many factors can influence the score, old people with normal cerebral function should be able to score 25 or more and those with brain failure 15 or less.

EXAMINATION

Although it can be difficult to carry out a comprehensive physical examination in the confines of a domestic setting it is important to exclude any physical causes of organic brain disorder. Particular attention must be paid to the cardiovascular and respiratory systems, and of course a neurological examination should be as complete as possible.

INVESTIGATIONS

In both senile and presenile dementia there are no specific abnormalities to be found in the blood, urine or on X-ray examination. Any investigations carried out therefore principally directed at detecting remediable medical conditions or uncovering systematic disorders which may be complicating the clinical picture. A list of suggested investigations which could be carried out in a community setting are indicated in Table 30.4.

MANAGEMENT

The dementias are the most compelling problem con-

Table 30.4 Investigations

Haematology	Full blood count
	ESR
	B_{12} and Folic acid
Biochemistry	Urea and electrolytes
	Liver function tests
	Calcium and Phosphorus
	Blood sugar (random)
	Thyroid function tests
Bacteriology	MSSU
	Glucose
Serology	WR
Cardiovascular	ECG
Radiology	Chest X-ray

fronting the medical services today and this quiet epidemic (British Medical Journal 1978) affects every branch of the Health and Social Services. The DHSS (1972) recommends the provision of 2.5–3.0 beds plus 2 to 3 day places per 1000 of the population aged 65 and over to deal with elderly patients with severe dementia but not suffering from other significant physical disease or illness. Patients with dementia, whether mild or severe, and who are also suffering from other significant physical disease or illness are intended to be managed within the recommended provision of 10 beds and 2 day places per 1000 population aged 65 and over in the normal geriatric services. Furthermore, 25 residential places per 1000 elderly people has been the figure suggested to Local Authorities as a reasonable provision provided there is also sufficient development of domiciliary and day care support. It is also inttended that three of the 25 places should be designated for the elderly mentally ill either in special elderly mentally infirm homes or in old people's homes. However, even if this level of provision is eventually achieved the majority of demented patients will remain within the community and will require the constant attention of the practice staff.

It is with this background that the general practitioner, who is responsible for many elderly patients suffering from organic brain failure, must make use of all the social resources which he is able to muster as the patient is liable to remain within the community for a longer period of time than would necessarily appear desirable. Fortunately over the past 20 years both central and local governments favoured a rapid expansion of such services in order to keep elderly patients in their own homes as this was thought to be the best and cheapest way of caring for them. As a consequence there are a wide variety of facilities, aids and services which are designed to help the practitioner maintain and care for these people within the community.

NURSING AND ANCILLARY HELP

The attachment of community nurses and health visitors to the practice and the availability of age/sex registers gives the practitioner an opportunity to organise the surveillance and identification of early manifestations of mental illness within his practice population. Unfortunately, although the health visitor is increasingly involved with the care and screening of the elderly the greatest proportion of her caseload is with children below the age of 5.

District nurses spend a far greater percentage of their time looking after the elderly, and workload figures (Social Trends 1982) show that those aged under 5 occupy 5% of the caseload, those aged between 5 and 64 years old represent 52% and those aged 65 and over 43%. It is hardly surprisingly that of the workload of the chiropody services only 8% are patients aged under 65 with the remaining 92% being aged 65 and above.

HOME HELP SERVICE

The home help service is probably the most important single community service run by the Social Service Department. The number of home helps in England rose from 20 000 to 88 065 between 1959 and 1976 (DHSS 1977). The number of patients attended in the United Kingdom by the Home Help Services is illustrated in Table 30.5 (Regional Trends 1982). Home helps carry out cleaning, washing and shopping duties as well as helping the patient with her personal toilet. They may also collect bills, pay bills, collect pensions and medical prescriptions. Unfortunately the mentally infirm patient is not always willing to accept a home help and a great deal of patience and tact may be necessary to reduce this resistance. The home help however is more than simply a cleaner, she can act as a vital link between the social services and the primary care team and can often provide valuable information about the patient's progress, or deterioration.

MEALS-ON-WHEELS

This service, pioneered by the WRVS, provides a basic element in the community support programme and is now under the auspices of either the Local Authority Social Work Department or of volunteer agencies with or without its financial support. Meals are either served in the patient's home or in lunch clubs which provide company as well as food. Lunch clubs are particularly popular in Scotland.

VISITING SERVICES

This service consists of welfare assistants or volunteers who visit elderly patients to provide information about benefits that they are entitled to under the Social Services Act. In addition they provide company to many an elderly and isolated person.

Table 30.5 Home help services, year ending 31st March 1980 (per 1000 households)

	All cases	Aged 65+	Aged below 65
England	47.7	158.0	7.4
Wales	49.3	162.1	8.3
Scotland	50.7	130.7	8.5
Northern Ireland	54.5	209.7	—

SOCIAL AID

Under this title is a wide variety of physical aids which can be provided by the Local Authority to assist patients suffering from some form of associated physical disease.

LAUNDRY

In cases of extreme need the bed linen and a free laundry service is provided for elderly patients by Local Authorities or by volunteer groups. This service however is only available in a few areas but it is of particular help to those who are looking after incontinent patients.

NIGHT WATCH SERVICE

Social Service departments and the Red Cross sometimes provide persons to watch over patients at night. The staff are not trained nurses but do provide important relief for families who are caring for confused elderly relatives.

DAY CENTRES AND CLUBS

Local Authorities in Great Britain provide over 300 day centres for the elderly while volunteer organisations run several thousand social clubs. The Local Authority can also offer facilities within residential homes. These centres help to prevent loneliness and provide a place for old people to meet each other, receive care and attention whilst the caring relative is at work.

The management and containment of the patient within the home can often be accomplished and maintained by making appropriate use of some or all of the above services.

MEDICAL TREATMENT

The drugs which are advocated for the treatment of brain failure fall into three broad areas. There are the 'pure' vasodilators, the cerebral vasodilators, which are said to have an additional effect on cerebral metabolism, and the drugs that modify neuronal metabolism but have no vasodilator effect.

The first group includes cyclandalate, isoxusprine, papaverine hydrochloride and cinnarizine.

Cyclandelate
Cyclandelate has a direct action on smooth muscle. While several clinical trials have shown its superiority to placebo not all have been double-blind and only two appear to have been carried out in a general practice

population. Blackmore (1970) reported an open study on 353 elderly patients and showed a gradual improvement using a variety of scales. Judge, Urquhart & Blackmore (1973) carried out a study on healthy volunteers in a group practice. They had a high default rate (from 114 patients starting only 54 completed the study) and found that they were unable to use the data collected from the male patients (23). The female patients treated with the active drug however did show an improvement over those on placebo as judged by intelligence tests and Ravens Coloured Progressive Matrices. Rao et al (1977) showed a significant improvement in the treated group in a double-blind study but also showed improvement with placebo over time on some of the rating scales used. Other authors feel that the case for cyclandelate has yet to be fully made.

Isoxsuprine

This is a beta anti-adrenergic stimulant which, according to Yesavage et al (1979) has only had five inconclusive trials between 1958 and 1979. One large open trial in general practice which examined 500 elderly patients (Guyer 1977) showed some improvement, particularly in the area of anxiety, memory, communication and orientation in 28% of the patients studied. Only 2.5% showed deterioration.

Papaverine

Papaverine is a non-specific smooth muscle relaxant which received a similar dismissal from Yesavage.

Cinnarizine

This drug is a piperazine vasodilator which has yet to undergo specific trials for cerebral arteriosclerosis. It has been shown to have some peripheral vasodilator effects.

The drugs with mixed effect include dihydroergotoxine mysylate, naftidrofuryl and pentifylline.

Dihydroergotoxine mysylate

This is a preparation consisting of three hydrogenated alkaloids of ergot. It acts by alpha blockade and animal studies have shown that it increases the activities of enzymes of intermediary metabolism within the ganglian cells. Its side effects include sinus bradycardia and hypotension while prolonged use of the drug may lead to vascular insufficiency and gangrene of the fingers and toes.

Naftidrofuryl

This acts in a variety of ways by increasing the cerebral concentration of ATP and reducing lactic acid. It is also shown to have a protective action against hypoxia which is a known cause of a reduction in cerebral catecholamines.

Pentifylline

This drug is structurally related to caffeine and may increase cerebral glucose uptake. More work is required to be carried out before this drug's use can be fully assessed.

The third group of drugs include meclofenoxate and pyritinol hydrochloride. The former drug reduces the brain's requirements for oxygen while the latter, which is a derivative of pyridoxine, is claimed to improve cerebral metabolism, glucose uptake and blood flow.

A variety of other agents have been suggested to try to improve other cerebral functions such as protein synthesis, and ribonucleic acid and magnesium pemoline have been suggested. There has also been a suggestion that vasoconstrictors may be useful in the management of cerebral arteriosclerosis with the idea that they may increase cerebral blood flow particularly to localised ischaemic areas.

There have however been a variety of objections raised to the use of drugs, and vasodilators in particular, in the management of dementia. The arguments against them have been well summarised by Sathananthan & Gershon (1975):

1. Does cerebral arteriosclerosis cause dementia?
2. If cerebral arteriosclerosis causes dementia:
   a) can the calibre of the cerebral blood vessels be altered?
   b) if the calibre could be increased will ischaemic areas in the brain obtain an increased blood flow?
   c) if there is an increase in blood flow to the ischaemic areas of the brain can ischaemic areas make use of it?

It is interesting to postulate that although Roth has established a relationship between senile plaques and dementia there has not been a similar relationship established between cerebral arteriosclerosis and the clinical picture. In view of this it may well be possible that the management of brain failure in the elderly with vasodilators will be reconsidered.

LEGAL ASPECTS

When dealing with the patient who is suffering from irreversible brain failure there are a wide variety of legal aspects which may well require consideration or attention by the individual practitioner.

Power of attorney

This is a document which grants a person or persons the power to act on another's behalf. It may be limited to one specific transaction or it may be an unfettered authority to allow the person's affairs to be administered by another.

Court of protection

If it is the considered opinion that the elderly patient is not capable of granting a Power of Attorney to another person because of his inability to think rationally then an application to the Court of Protection under Part VIII of the Mental Health Act 1959 for Receivership or Management Order can be made. This has the advantage that the patient's affairs can be managed by a professional person who will be unable to sell any assets without the prior consent of the Court of Protection. Applications for this may be made directly to the Court of Protection either by a relative or social worker or a solicitor. The address of the Court of Protection is 25, Store Street, London EC1E 7PB (Tel. No. 01-636-6877).

Compulsory removal of persons needing care and attention

Section 47 of the National Assistance Act (1948) as amended by the National Assistance (Amendment) Act (1951) gives certain powers to community physicians to arrange for the removal of persons requiring care and attention who are:

1. Suffering from a serious chronic disease or when elderly, are infirm or physically incapacitated and are living in insanitary conditions.
2. Unable to provide proper care and attention for themselves or are not receiving it from another person.

After the community physician has satisfied himself in writing that the above holds true application can be made to a Court of Summary Justice for such an order. The Court can then order the person's removal to a suitable hospital or other place and their subsequent detention there.

The Mental Health Act

The relevant acts are the Mental Health Act (1959) in England and Wales, the Mental Health (Scotland) Act (1960) and the Mental Health Act (Northern Ireland) (1961). Their importance in psychogeriatrics is principally restricted to emergency admission and is intended to facilitate the admission of reluctant patients rather than persuade reluctant consultants to accept a patient.

In England and Wales the appropriate section of the Act is Section 29. The applicant must have seen the patient personally within a period of 3 days, ending with the date of the application. The patient must be admitted to hospital within a period of 3 days, beginning with the date on which they were examined or the date of application, whichever is the earlier. The admission lasts for 3 days.

Section 31 of the Act applies to Scotland and is similar to the English Act with a proviso that, when practicable, the medical practitioner involved shall seek the consent of a relative or Mental Health Officer. The period of detention lasts for 7 days.

REFERENCES

Adams R P, Fisher C R, Harkin S, Ojemann R G, Sweet W H 1965 Symptomatic occult hydrocephalus with 'normal' cerebrospinal fluid pressure: a treatable syndrome. New England Journal of Medicine 273: 117–126

Age Concern 1977 Profiles of the elderly, Vols 1–4. Age Concern, london.

Akhtar A J, Broe J A, Crombie A, McLean W M R, Andrews G R, Caird F I 1973 Disability and dependence in the elderly at home. Age and Ageing 2: 102–111

Blackmore C R 1970 Impprovement in certain aspects of behaviour of elderly patients treated by cyclandelate. Assessment in Cerebrovascular Insufficiency, Wurzburg

Brandon S 1979 The organic psychiatry of old age. In: Granville-Grossman K (ed) Recent advances in clinical psychiatry — 3 Churchill Livingstone, Edinburgh, ch 4, p 135

British Medical Journal 1978 Leading article, Vasodilators in senile dementia. British Medical Journal 511–512

Department of Health and Social Security 1972. Services for mental illness related to old age. HM(72) 71. HMSO, London

Department of Health and Social Security 1977 Health and personal social services. Statistics for England. HMSO, London

Gray B, Isaacs B 1979 Care of the elderly mentally infirm. Tavistock Publications, London

Guyer B M 1977 The management of cerebrovascular disease with isoxsuprine resinate. Clinical Trials Journal 14: 159–162

Jarvik L F, Yen F S, Goldstein F 1974 Chromosomes and mental status. Archives of General Psychiatry 30: 186–190

Judge T G, Urquhart A, Blackmore C B 1973 Cyclandelate and mental functions: a double-blind cross-over trial in normal elderly subjects. Age and Ageing 2: 121–124

Kay D W K, Beumish P, Roth M 1964 Old age mental disorders in Newcastle-upon-Tyne. I. A study of prevalence. British Journal of Psychiatry 126: 423–430

Larsson T, Sjogren T, Jacobson G 1963 Senile dementia: a clinical, sociomedical and genetic study. Acta Psychiatrica Scandinavica, Supplement 167: 1–259

Lishman A W 1978 Organic psychiatry. Blackwell Scientific Publications, Oxford

Nielsen J 1970 Chromosomes in senile, presenile and arteriosclerotic dementia. Journal of Gerontology 25: 312–315

Rao D B, Georgiev E L, Paul P P, Guzman A B 1977 Cyclandelate in the treatment of senile mental changes: a double-blind evaluation. Journal of the American Geriatrics Society 25: 548–551

Regional Trends 1982 Central Statistical Office. HMSO, London

Roth M 1971 Classification and aetiology in mental disorders of old age: some recent developments. In: Kay D W K, Walk A (eds) Recent developments in psychogeriatrics, British Journal of Psychiatry Special Publication No. 6. Headley Brothers, Ashford, Kent

Royal College of General Practitioners 1974 Morbidity statistics from general practice. Second National Study 1970–71. HMSO, London

Sathananthan G L, Gershon S 1975 Cerebral vasodilators: a review. In: Gerson S, Raskin A (eds) Aging. Raven Press, New York, Vol 2, ch 7, p 155

Social Trends 1982 Central Statistical Office. HMSO, London

Stromgren E 1964 Recent studies on the prevalence of mental disorders in the aged. In: Hansen P (ed) Age with a future, Proceedings of the Sixth International Congress of Gerontology, Munksgaard, Copenhagen

Williamson J et al 1964 Old people at home, their unreported needs. Lancet i: 1117–1120

Yesavage J A, Tinklenberg J R, Hollister L E, Berger P A 1979 Vasodilators in senile dementia. Archives of General Psychiatry 36: 220–224

Terminal care and bereavement

TERMINAL CARE

No matter how many individuals are involved in the care of a terminally ill patient the principal professional 'care givers' are the General Practitioner and his nursing associates in the Primary Health Care Team. The fact that many different hospital specialists may also be involved, often using high technology, far from lessening the role of the general practitioner actually makes his responsibility even greater. However, unless he recognises this, he may find his role eroded and lose a unique opportunity to serve his patient in a way no hospital specialist can do.

THE CHALLENGE TO THE G.P.

1. To ensure continuity of care.
2. To supervise co-ordination of care.
3. To demonstrate communication between all concerned.
4. To safeguard character of care.

... each intimately inter-related.

CONTINUITY OF CARE

The uniqueness of his role is nowhere better illustrated than in his responsibility for initial diagnosis and in continuing care even whilst the patient attends many different hospital departments, during the relapses and remissions of the illness, through the patient's final illness and with the family who remain on his list for years to come. Failure to accept this challenge can lead to a patient falling between many colleagues, each an expert in his own field, but understandably responsible for action and intervention for limited periods in the course of the illness. The initial care given and the consultants selected to provide the specialist help may affect not only the patient himself but the members of his family for a generation or more.

CO-ORDINATION OF CARE

The more professionals that are required the greater is the general practitioner's responsibility to act as co-ordinator, yet many shrink from this task. Admittedly much of the diagnostic and therapeutic activity may take place in hospital but, with his knowledge of the patient, his personality and his family, no-one is better placed than the general practitioner to ensure optimum use of hospital, community, social work and voluntary agencies for the overall good of the whole family.

He may for example feel the need for domiciliary consultations or the involvement of a specialist Home Care Service or the assistance of a social worker and is usually better placed than anyone else to decide on the critical timing for each. He may elect to cancel what he regards as unnecessary follow-up visits to a clinic when another consultant has become the key figure at that stage, or even advise against a suggested new course of action when it does not appear to him to be in the best interest of his patient. This is his right and, provided his acts are supported by well-founded reasons, and good communications, hospital colleagues should respect it. In the same way he must demonstrate co-ordination within his own team so that partners and nurses respect his plan of co-ordinated care. Only in this way can a terminally-ill patient be confident that all are working together with shared information, common aims and mutual confidence and respect.

COMMUNICATION

Experience shows that most patients regard the general practitioner as the one ultimately responsible and respected for accurate information on their illness at any stage. Not only must he supply basic clinical information to a consultant when referring the patient but he must, either in the original letter or subsequently, fill in the whole picture of his patient's background, his personality, his family, his knowledge of the condition, and be prepared to keep that information updated so long as any other colleagues are sharing in the care. It is inexcusable for a general practitioner to know something which might affect the management and not share this with colleagues. Interdepartmental letters will usually contain all the diagnostic, pathological and pharmacological details available but only the general practitioner can report on the patient's changing attitude and expectations, the anxieties shared with his general practitioner and the kaleidoscopic picture of his social problems. If the general practitioner gains a reputation for painstakingly detailed reports he may expect — he may demand — equally valuable reports from hospital colleagues. Here one thinks particularly of what the patient has been told, what he asked and what he seemed to understand, what further action is contemplated and whose responsibility it will be. Nothing less will suffice.

CHARACTER OF CARE

We cannot talk of the quality of terminal care without respecting the *quality of life*. The need to stand back and look at this is ever more pressing with the development and employment of high technology medicine with its cytotoxics, immunotherapy, transplantations and sophisticated surgical procedures. Whether they can maintain or enhance the quality of life of the patient (and ultimately only the patient himself can try to define that quality) is a problem for all the professionals involved. However the general practitioner will usually find himself as the final arbiter on behalf of the patient.

He must discipline himself, whatever others may be doing, to define when cure is no longer a reasonable objective and care and palliation become the goals. Having done that he will set the example to all in providing care for the whole patient — physical, emotional, social and spiritual — with all his energies devoted to maximum symptom relief, contentment and fulfilment, and the patient's remaining months or years spent *living* rather than dying!

THE PLANNING OF TERMINAL CARE

In planning the care the doctor will consider where it should be offered and whether it is reasonable, for all concerned, to aim for both care and death at home. He will have to decide (because no-one else will) when terminal care should start because on this decision will depend whether any further active treatment is given or whether all energies should be devoted to palliation. This decision will also govern whether he should encourage or even permit further investigations whose results may have little or no bearing on later management. Planning cannot be done without forethought being given, in con-

sultation with all the other members of the team, to the locus for terminal care.

LOCUS OF CARE

In considering the place for terminal care the doctor has to remember that much as patients *seem* to spend a large part of their final year in hospital in fact more than 90% is spent at home where inevitably more problems arise: 85% of bedsores, 89% of double incontinence and 95% of all other symptoms.

Rarely can a decision be made in advance about whether the patient should die in hospital, hospice or at home but the readiness of a hospital to re-admit can be ascertained, the attitude of patient and family explored, the availability of such specialist support as a MacMillan Home Care Service based in a hospice ascertained, and the resources (emotional, social and economic) of the family studied. The good general practitioner will know his own limitations as well as his strengths and not attempt to provide terminal care which, on some occasions, will demand more than he is able or willing to provide. One thinks of the particular problems of dying children, young men with disseminated carcinoma suffering intractable pain but wanting to die near their young family, a grieving relative with a history of psychiatric illness or personality disorder, or a patient vehemently denying the reality of his condition — each demands the highest standards of professional care married to the most sensitive compassion.

PRINCIPLES OF CARE

The principles of good terminal care are easily stated, difficult to practice and often never attempted!

The first is intelligent anticipation of likely problems and their solutions. The increasingly frail patient may need a commode or walking aid; the dyspnoeic a backrest or Delta pillow; the incontinent a catheter or incontinence appliances; the opiate user a laxative; the anorectic good oral hygiene and an antifungal agent. All can be foreseen and prepared for. There can be no excuse for the doctor being caught unawares or the practice nurse called in so late that bedsores have already developed.

The second principle is that good terminal care is always a team exercise involving every member of the practice, the family and — importantly — the patient! The third, almost too self-evident to mention, is that it is total care respecting the patient's physical, emotional, social and spiritual needs. A neglect of any one of these is certain to be detrimental.

The fourth principle, and one difficult to learn, is that good terminal care is problem *not* pathology based. No

Table 31.1   The principal symptoms in terminal illness

	All cases (%)	Cancer (%)
Pain	66	87
Insomnia	49	69
Anorexia	48	76
Dyspnoea	45	47
Depression	36	45
Confusion	36	36
Vomiting and nausea	30	54
Double incontinence	24	36
Bed sores	16	24
Bad smells	15	26
Urinary incontinence	8	38
Faecal incontinence	4	37
Others	25	31

longer do symptoms have much diagnostic significance nor are they likely to alter the basic diagnosis. Each is a window on the patient's suffering, a picture of the burdens he must suffer, yet each is usually capable of being relieved if the doctor can discipline himself to see the patient as being as interesting and challenging as he was when he first presented to the surgery, months or years before.

THE PROBLEMS OF CARE

The problems of the patient include the commonest symptoms encountered (Table 31.1) and those distresses, said to be 50% again, borne in silence as the doctor is thought not to be interested in them or they are thought to be too trivial to mention. It cannot be said too often that, when caring for the dying, nothing is trivial.

COMMON PROBLEMS IN TERMINAL CARE

PAIN

The importance of pain as a problem cannot be exaggerated. Failure to control pain undermines any good work being done for the patient. Energetic and successful pain control makes all else in terminal care much easier.

Failure usually results from:

1. Inaccurate assessment of its cause, type and intensity. The longer a patient has suffered pain the less dramatically will he describe it, and the more sceptical will he become of anyone taking it seriously or being able or keen to relieve it. In the dying patient 'pain not reported' does not mean 'pain not present'.
2. The use of inappropriate analgesics and drug combinations.
3. A reluctance to use palliative radiotherapy, chemotherapy, neurolytic procedures and even neurosurgery where indicated.

4. 'prn' prescribing rather than attempting to prevent pain breakthrough by advising the patient to take each dose at intervals based on the known period of efficacy of each drug (Table 31.2).
5. Inadequate attention to factors capable of raising the pain threshold (Table 31.3).

An analgesic check-list is useful (Table 31.4) and can be employed for all patients, irrespective of their pathology. Starting with mild strength analgesics (Table 31.5) the doctor can change to stronger ones according to the grade of pain (Table 31.6). He should not hesitate to employ narcotics, if they seem appropriate, from an early stage in terminal care knowing that addiction is no longer a problem and that no other group of drugs is so likely to relieve severe pain and, without unnecessary sedation, produce the anxiolytic and euphoric effect that such patients need.

Experience confirms that pneumonia is rarely 'the old man's friend' until the final days of life and judicious use of antibiotics will do much, not only for cellulitis, respiratory and urinary infection, and secondary chest infection, but to relieve associated pain and discomfort. In the same way the good general practitioner will employ his highest skills in counselling and supporting the patient who is depressed, but will not hesitate to use antidepressant drugs to raise the pain threshold.

Table 31.2   Analgesics: duration of effectiveness

	Effectiveness (hours)
Dextromoramide (Palfium)	2
Pethidine	3
Morphine	4
Diamorphine (Heroin)	4
Devorphanol (Dromoran)	6
Dipipanol (Diconal)	6
Papaveretum (Omnopon)	6
Phenazocine (Narphen)	6
Nefopam (Acupan)	6
Buprenorphine (Temgesic)	8
Methadone (Physeptone)	8
Morphine (Duromorph)	12

Table 31.3   Raising pain threshold

Physical	Emotional	Spiritual
Symptom relief	Empathy	Understanding
Sleep	Understanding	Companionship
Rest	Diverson	Prayer
Improved	Mood elevation	
appearance		
Environment		
	±	
	Antidepressants	
	Anxiolytics	

Table 31.4 Terminal care: pain control

Drugs	Analgesics
	Antibiotics
	Cytotoxics
	Antidepressants
	Tranquillisers
Radiotherapy (Especially for bone pain)	
Nerve blocks	Local anaesthetic
	5–10% Phenol in oil
	Alcohol
	Cryoprobe
Neurosurgery	Cordotomy
	Rhizotomy
	Electrode implant
	Myelotomy
Hypophysectomy	Surgical
	Vitrium
	Phenol Ablation
	Alcohol
Barbotage	
Acupuncture	
Hypnotherapy	

Table 31.5 Analgesics: relative strengths

Mild	Salicylates
	Paracetamol
	Dextropropoxyphene (Distalgesic, Doloxene)
	Pentazocine (Fortral)
	Mefanamic acid (Ponstan)
	Phenylbutazone
	Codeine (Codis)
Moderate	Pethidine
	Dipipanone (Diconal)
	Dihydrocodeine (DF 118)
	Nefopam (Acupan)
	Buphrenorphine (Temgesic)
Strong	Dextromoramide (Palfium)
	Methadone (Physeptone)
	Phenazocine (Narphen)
	Levorphanol (Dromoran)
	Papaveretum (Omnopon)
	Morphine
	Diamorphine (Heroin)

Table 31.6 Grading of pain

1. Relieved by occasional mild strength analgesics
2. Relieved by regular mild strength and analgesics
3. Relieved by regular middle strength analgesics
4. Relieved by regular strong (narcotic) analgesics
5. Not relieved by regular strong analgesics

Where pain is unilateral and confined to a few dermatomes nerve blocks should be considered and the assistance of an anaesthetist or Hospice colleague should be sought. Where disseminated carcinoma is producing the pain, whether or not the procedure called for is a hormone ablatant, Phenol hypophysectomy should be considered.

In *all* patients with bone secondaries and primary bladder cancer a prostaglandin biosynthetase inhibitor should be given; in nerve compression a steroid and in the headache of cerebral metastases high dose dexamethasone (10–16 mg a day) with a simple non-steroidal anti-inflammatory agent should be prescribed rather than an opiate. Injections should not be used unless the sublingual and rectal routes are inappropriate (Tables 31.7 and 31.8).

Whereas in hospital it is usually easier to order injections (though it is seldom recognised that both morphine and diamorphine must be given 3-hourly by this route) it is seldom possible for the doctor or practice nurse to visit so frequently. There is thus a need to consider alternative routes, such as the use of a syringe driver, a transcutaneous nerve stimulator (TCNS), or the insertion of an epidural cannula for low dose morphine. The doctor trained in hospital medicine with its twice-daily ward rounds must remind himself of the half-life of each drug prescribed in order to plan his analgesia-monitoring visits to the patient at home. For example, he should revisit 36 hours after starting methodone and be aware of its cumulative effect, but will expect to revisit the following day when using morphine. The exceptionally long life of diazepam (and indeed many of the benzodiazepines) will necessitate twice-weekly visits even in early terminal care planning. The newcomer to general practice will notice how anxiety plays an even greater role in lowering pain threshold than in the hospital setting where the patient is surrounded by medical and nursing staff constantly on hand rather than the strained relative who may have been sworn to silence, secrecy or deception when the diagnosis was first made.

CONSTIPATION

This has been found to be a problem in not less than 8% of patients and is known to be the principal cause of

Table 31.7 Analgesics — sub-lingual administration

Dextromoramide (Palfium)	5, 10 mg
Phenazocine (Narphen)	5 mg
Diamorphine (Hypodermic Tab: Roche)	10 mg
Buprenorphine (Temgesic)	0.2 mg

Table 31.8 Analgesics: Rectal administration

	Effect rectal oral	
Morphine (15, 30, 6 mg)	2 : 3	
Dextromoramide (Palfium) (10 mg)	2 : 3	
Oxycodone (Proladone) (30 mg) =	20 mg oral Morphine	

vomiting in the dying patient: it thus cannot be ignored. When caused by a predominantly 'invalid food' diet, poor fluid intake and relative immobility, little can be done to prevent it and certainly not a 'high bulk' diet which is rarely acceptable to the patient. When constipation is a consequence of an opiate, antidepressant, anxiolytic (especially diazepam) or anticholinergic therapy it is essential to prescribe an appropriate laxative and to examine the patient regularly for signs of faecal impaction. (Asking if the bowels have moved is no quarantee of *adequate* bowel emptying.)

It is important to prescribe a laxative acceptable to the patient and capable of working when the colonic neuromusculature is paralyzed by opiates. Faecal expanders will only produce increased colonic distension and drugs designed to enhance peristalsis will be ineffective. It is better to prescribe a laxative such as Duphalac, Dorbanex Forte, Dioctyl Forte or Laxoberol.

If impaction has occurred before starting this regime it is almost useless to work 'from the top' — rather empty the rectum with arachis oil enemata daily for 2 days followed by a Fletcher enema and then start on oral laxatives.

Newcomers to general practice will soon learn to respect the advice of the experienced community nurse but they must not, as so often happens in hospital, leave the problem of constipation to her — she is not trained in rectal or abdominal examinations nor in the selection of the appropriate laxative.

DIARRHOEA

This problem, present in no more than 6% of terminally ill patients, is mentioned only as a necessary reminder that it should be considered as spurious until proved otherwise and resort should not automatically be made to a constipating agent. A different matter is steatorrhoea which is as troublesome for relatives as to the patient because of the difficulty in flushing the stool away and cleaning the lavatory pan. There is also a commonly held, though reluctantly admitted, fear that cancer is excreted in the stools thus endangering other members of the household.

ANOREXIA

Attention to anorexia is a means of helping the relatives more than the patient since the former so often feel their efforts to encourage the patient to eat are in vain. In 75% of patients the cause of anorexia is oral candidiasis, so easily controlled with Nystatin provided dentures are removed when the treatment is given and cleaned nightly in 0.2% chlorhexidine.

With enthusiastic attention to the problem, a readiness to advise on special foods, with attention being given to such basic principles, such as that all drinks should be ice cold, the mouth kept clean with sucked pineapple slices, sips of iced sherry before meals, and the use of prednisolone 5 mg t.i.d., most patients regain much of their appetite.

DYSPNOEA

Though close on 50% of men and 25% of women suffer severe dyspnoea in a terminal illness less than 1% die in respiratory distress. This does not change the fact that every patient with any degree of dyspnoea fears death from suffocation, and here, more than anywhere, there is a place for the most positive, understanding support and appreciation of this fear, coupled with skill in prescribing.

Patients with bronchogenic carcinoma should be encouraged to spend the day (and even the night) in a reclining chair and should not be propped up as would a patient with a chronic obstructive airways disease. Regular examination of the chest should be completed to exclude pleural effusion, chest infection, cardiac failure and treatable anaemia (probably the only indication for blood transfusion in terminal care). Thereafter the patient should be given low dose morphine (for example 2.5 mg 4-hourly in solution) since no other drug will be as effective in relieving tachypnoea. The skilled used of an opiate is markedly more effective than the anxiolytic effect of a benzodiazepine. Rarely is oxygen called for, unless for the usual strict clinical indications, but a fan playing near the patient's face will achieve admirably good results.

NAUSEA AND VOMITING

Experience proves that whilst vomiting is relatively easy to control, nausea (particularly with ovarian tumours) can be intractable. Contrary to outdated teaching the opiates only produce nausea (in less than 50% of patients) during the first 4 days of use and when the dose is increased.

Having excluded opiates as the cause, faecal impaction, subacute obstruction (itself usually exacerbated by constipation), hypercalcaemia and unexpressed anxiety and fear should be considered.

The most effective drugs for nausea and vomiting are not the antihistamines and phenothiazines (either too sedative or liable to produce extrapyramidal effects). Haloperidol (0.5 mg q.i.d.), metochlopramide (10 mg q.i.d.) or a 6-day course of high dose methylprednisolone (Solu-Medrone 250 mg daily) are more effective treatments.

Some relief can also be achieved by prescribing ice cold drinks and ice-lollipops, a regular small intake of alcohol, and enthusiastic attention to bowel function.

PRURITUS

Unless the cause of pruritus is obstructive jaundice, when cholestyramine (1 sachet b.d.) may help, there is no specific remedy and the use of antihistamines may sedate a patient who insists (as most dying patients do) on remaining alert and 'in control'. It is better to use sodium bicarbonate washes as required, haloperidol (0.5 mg q.i.d.), chlorpromazine suppository (100 mg) at night and the avoidance of nylon clothing.

HICCUPS

Having excluded dyspepsia, hiatus hernia and upper abdominal distension elevating the diaphragm (for all of which metoclopramide may be effective) diaphragmatic pleurisy and uraemia, the possible treatments include regular chlorpromazine (25 mg t.i.d.), haloperidol (0.5 mg q.i.d.) or occasional hyoscine hydrobromide (400 micrograms). In the intractable case a phrenic crush block should be considered.

ANXIETY AND DEPRESSION

It cannot be strongly enough stated that a policy of caring, openness and honesty with the patient, at all times, will do more to prevent or alleviate anxiety and panic than any anxiolytic drug. Dying patients fear the unknown more than the known and every effort to dispel unfounded fears and demonstrate an ability to make even dying a bearable experience will never be wasted.

Similarly it is important to recognise the difference between 'misery' and 'depressive state' and to resort to tricyclics only for true depression or when seeking to elevate the pain threshold.

The dying patient fears any symptom whose significance has not been explained, catastrophies whose likelihood can usually be prevented, isolation which can be guarded against if the sensitive doctor is capable of sharing himself and strengthening the family to do likewise, and the loss of control and autonomy which need not be inevitable features of dying.

No chapter on the care of the dying would be complete without reference to the question of 'what to tell'! Each entrant to general practice comes to appreciate that the central issues are not in fact 'what to tell' but 'when to tell', 'whom to tell', 'how to tell', and 'who should tell'. No doctor can avoid this issue and, coming as many do

from hospital practice, may be upset by patients being left with a false diagnosis yet have gleaned everything from other sources and by other means, desperately trying to present a brave face and maintain a conspiracy of silence with relatives who, having been fully informed, have been given no guidance on what next to do with their painful, fateful knowledge.

Experience with thousands of such patients has convinced the writer that no-one is better placed than the family doctor gradually, often over many meetings, to infuse the full facts to the patient as well as the relatives. He, above all, must accept this responsibility whatever may be the views of his consultant colleagues, if the bond between him and the patient is to be maintained, strengthened and used in the last remaining years or months. Mutual trust and respect, which should be the hallmarks of good general practice, cannot be built on deception or silence whether well intentioned or urged by relatives who, whether they admit it or not, are equally concerned about their own grief and profound sense of inadequacy at this time. A policy of openness — not harsh, insensitive frankness — undoubtedly leads to reduced physical suffering and emotional distress, spiritual preparedness and improved relationships with family members who will learn they have a general practitioner whom they can trust when trouble strikes them.

BEREAVEMENT

Profoundly distressing as the death of a loved one may be, bereavement itself must be understood as one of life's major experiences, producing morbidity and even mortality, as well as social upheavals with lifelong implications. Abundant evidence testifies that it cannot be regarded as 'usually physiological' or 'something we all have to come through' as is so often stated. In the 12 months subsequent to the death there is an increased incidence of both physical and emotional illness and, statistically proven for widowers, a much increased mortality rate. Separate but related are the changes in social status (particularly for widows who can expect sympathy, unsolicited sexual approaches and social taboo against re-marrying), economic security and the whole pattern of life when a spouse has died.

General practitioners and their colleagues in the Primary Health Care Team must be aware of the factors affecting bereavement, the times of danger, possible ways of mitigating some of the suffering, and be constantly on their guard lest they follow the trend in modern society of ignoring a person's silent grief on the false assumption that he or she seems to be coping because they are not consulting the doctor.

The care of the bereaved can be planned, performed and monitored scientifically as well as compassionately

FACTORS AFFECTING GRIEF OUTCOME

1. Time to prepare for the deceased's death.
2. Griever's sense of usefulness in caring for the deceased.
3. Griever's perception of personal support received.
4. Previous personality and health.
5. Quality of relationship with the deceased.

Sudden, unexpected death produces the profoundest emotional shock and subsequent grief reaction whereas time spent caring for the cancer patient will lessen the reaction. Every immediate relative of someone dying unexpectedly must be regarded as 'at risk' and the general practitioner must plan accordingly.

The more more 'useful' a relative can be made to feel the less will be the grief. The modern tendency is to hospitalise all seriously ill and dying patients in the mistaken belief that they need such facilities and that most relatives are unwilling or unable to care for them at home. This view has important implications for the grievers who may thus be deprived of an opportunity to demonstrate their love and devotion to the patient.

Several studies have shown that the grievers' perception of the support given to them is more important than the amount of support actually given. Some of this is probably more easily ascertained by a health visitor or clergyman than by the general practitioner and obviously is related to the previous personality and relationship with the deceased.

Contrary to what might be expected patients with extrovert personalities usually suffer the worst reactive depression but, predictably, those with dependent personalities who have leaned heavily on the one they have now lost will intuitively seek someone else on whom to depend. These are features of which a general practitioner should already be aware and for which he should be able to prepare. The person with an inflexible, obsessional personality will find adapting to a new way of life especially difficult and may fail to appreciate that most people cope with grief in the same way that they have coped with any other episodes of loss whether of a job, status, or popularity. It is important to realise that intellectual prowess may bear no relationship to emotional maturity and stability.

PREDICTION OF GRIEF OUTCOME

The following questions should be asked when preparing a plan of bereavement support or counselling by the practice staff:

1. Was the death expected and if so did it take the form expected by the bereaved?

2. Does the bereaved feel that he or she was enabled to do everything they wanted to do for the deceased and that what they did was appreciated by the patient and recognised by the professional attendants?
3. What is the personality type of the bereaved and what pattern of behaviour at a time of loss can be expected?
4. Have the bereaved been given adequate opportunity to ventilate even the most secret and unpleasant emotions they feel about the patient, his care, his attendants and themselves?

It is essential to appreciate that most, if not all, grievers will need to ventilate anger against some well meaning medical or nursing colleague, against God or even against the patient for being so inconsiderate as to die when he did. It is equally important that the doctor does not defend, retaliate or attempt to rationalise, but instead he should permit an uninhibited outpouring. Some relatives may need to express relief or even happiness at the end of an unsatisfactory relationship but may feel unable to contravene the socially accepted grieving pattern.

FEATURES OF GRIEF

More than 50% of bereaved persons experience many of the symptoms suffered by the deceased during the first months after the loss, and inevitably suspect that they are to suffer a similar fate. This is particularly the case in cardiac and malignant disease with such symptoms as palpitation, breathlessness, chest tightness, weight loss, anorexia, dyspepsia and dysphagia. In spite of their denial, and any professional confidence in the impact of health education, most lay men retain a sneaking fear that cancer is communicable.

The only way to deal with these symptoms, often reported with reluctance and embarrassment, is to conduct a thorough examination and the relevant investigations in as understanding a manner as possible no matter how unlikely it is that anything organic will be found. Superficial, perfunctory or cursory examinations at the time of reporting of each new symptom will mean a heightening of anxiety or may encourage the fear of neuroticism and inadequacy.

90% of bereaved persons suffer a disturbed sleep pattern in the first 6 months, with frequent wakening, vivid dreams involving the deceased and bouts of profound misery (not to be confused with a true depressive state) at night. More than 50% will have auditory or visual hallucinations of the dead person behaving exactly as he did in life. Fewer than 10% will report this for fear of being declared psychotic. An explanation of these phenomena in advance reinforcing that this is a normal aspect of bereavement saves much sadness and silent fear.

STAGES OF GRIEF

Though seen in a more complete form after a protracted death as in cancer, respiratory or neurological disease several 'stages' are seen in most grieving people. It would be wrong however to expect a steady progression from one stage to another or that the dying patient always goes through the stages outlined by Kubler-Ross.

It is generally accepted that there are 5 main stages in bereavement:

1. Period of relief
2. Period of relaxing
3. Period of resenting
4. Period of remembering
5. Period of repairing

RELIEF

This follows immediately on the death and usually lasts no more than days. It is characterised by happiness for the deceased ('thank goodness he will have no more suffering'), coupled with personal relief ('I couldn't have coped with much more' or 'I wouldn't have wanted him to be a cripple'). There is much expressed gratitude for the care givers, especially for the general practitioner and a pervading sense of unreality and numbness ('I can't take it in' or 'I don't feel like crying').

Visits by the doctor or health visitor may be appreciated at the time but are soon completely forgotten in this period of stunned insensibility. Hypnotics, usually demanded by relatives rather than by the remaining spouse, seldom if ever work but may be a token of the doctor's continuing role (see p. 378).

RELAXING

This follows the funeral and usually lasts only as long as near relatives remain with the widow(er). This seems to be about 3 weeks at the most but creates a sense of support aand acceptance and shared pain. These weeks are usually preoccupied with practical problems related to wills, possessions or insurance claims but the ready assistance of family and the minister prevent the impact of loneliness being felt until nearer the time for their departure.

Nevertheless this is a time when precipitate decisions may be made about selling a house, emigrating or moving in with a daughter. Inappropriate advice is often given to get rid of every visible reminder of the deceased, but such mementos as photographs, letters and trophies should be kept and treasured for the time when the world, but not the widow, seems to have forgotten he ever existed.

RESENTING

This dates from the time of departure of the family and lasts anything from 3 to 4 months coinciding, it will be noted, with the end of 'acceptable grief' in modern society. There is a profound sense not only of loneliness but 'aloneness', of insecurity and self pity with much criticism both of self ('I should never have left him that night') and of professional helpers ('The doctor could have got here much sooner')

The suffering is heightened by friends describing how well she looks and by an increasing incidence of symptoms so similar to those experienced in the final illness by the deceased; symptoms that are not often mentioned to the doctor for fear of genuine pathology being found or of neurosis being suspected. The good outward appearance of health and coping leads to invitations to resume social and church activities. The pain however is felt not when in company but when returning to an empty house.

Business matters loom large, accounts have to be paid without advice from a spouse and the commonest question asked is, 'how on earth will I cope?'

It is frequently reported by the grievers that the 3-month mark is noteworthy for the way friends and neighbours go out of their way to avoid casual meetings, crossing to the other side of the street rather than stopping to ask how she is.

REMEMBERING

This may start at 3 months and continue at least for a further 12 or 15 months, with constant reminiscing and reliving of events before the death coupled by a conscious effort to recapture the happy emotions of the past. No longer is it so painful to speak of the death and seldom, unless it is becoming pathological or the patient has a personality disorder, is there much recrimination. Great efforts will be made to create only the happiest memories even if the marriage was not, in fact, a happy one. This is the time of the visual and auditory hallucinations already referred to and the time (around 7 months) of most breakdowns.

REPAIRING

The patient begins to make a deliberate effort to make a fresh start, shown by positive and rational thinking and a careful appraisal of his or her resources and skills. New interests, hobbies and friendships are cultivated and at each consultation with the G.P. some new evidence of this can usually be elicited. This is not to say that anniversaries, particularly birthdays, Christmas and the date of the death, are not extremely painful and often ignored completely by other family members and even by the doctor. It is a stage characterised by the expression 'life must go on'.

BEREAVEMENT SUPPORT BY THE DOCTOR

The following guidelines may assist:

1. Visit as soon after the death as possible to remind the patient of your continuing support and concern. The visit will be a short one.
2. Visit again, and allocate sufficient time, at a time when the relatives plan to leave and be positive in advice, emphatic in advising against precipitate action and reassuring about your concern for his or her own health.
3. Book a visit or a consultation for 3 months and conduct a careful physical examination, giving the patient the opportunity to express and deep fears and suppressed emotions. Take pains to explain the features of 'normal' grief because no-one else will!
4. Find an opportunity for a further consultation 6 months later when the world accepts her 'everything is fine' appearance but experience shows that she is most at risk.
5. Keep a diary of dates of deaths of paients on your list for planned follow-up for the first year. Contrary to what may be thought, the number is not unmanageable!
6. Make use of CRUSE or any other bereavement service in your area no matter how enthusiastic are the members of your team about bereavement support.

Remember that grief is like a surgical wound — painful and ugly at first, gradually fading but still easily damaged and hurt, never disappearing and always a permanent reminder of a time of profound pain, shock, change and fear.

Time does not heal — it only makes the scar less visible to onlookers!

PRESCRIBING IN BEREAVEMENT

Considerable pressures are often brought to bear on the doctor to prescribe antidepressants or sedatives for the bereaved, not so much by the patient herself as by well-meaning relatives. Failure or reluctance to do so is seen as uncaring or as professional callousness but experience shows that such drugs will only help if used for the same strict clinical indications, and with the same caution, as at any other time. That is to say, hypnotics should be prescribed only when there is good evidence of a grossly disturbed sleep pattern, and even then in as low a dose as possible and for the shortest possible time. Antidepressants will be totally ineffective unless the classical features of a psychiatric depressive state are present. This is a time when, all too easily, a sedative taking habit may be induced, a patient started on the long-term use of a tranquilliser such as diazepam (Valium), or a patient may turn to alcohol. It is a time when barbiturates seem to offer distinct advantages yet must be withheld at all costs.

If a sedative is thought desirable, immediately after the death or when the family have dispersed leaving the griever alone and hopeless, it should be a benzodiazpeine with a short half life (Ativan or Normison) or dichloral-phenazone (Welldorm); nitrazepam (Mogadon) is contraindicated because its long half-life produces mental blurring the next day, and occasionally hallucinations.

When depressive features are present it is useful to prescribe a sustained release tricyclic, taken at night, such as amitriptyline (Lentizol) or trimipramine (Surmontil). Repeat prescriptions must not be made available for any of these drugs without a consultation. This rule affords an excellent opportunity to see and support the patient in a way which is infinitely superior to any prescription. Strict instructions should be given that 'sleeping tablets' and 'tranquillisers' are not to be accepted from family or friends.

It cannot be stated strongly enough that, profoundly painful as bereavement is, its course is rarely altered by pharmacological means.

RECOMMENDED READING

Terminal care
Barton D 1977 Dying and death: A clinical guide for care-givers. Williams and Wilkins Co, Baltimore
Lipton S 1979 Relief of Pain in Clinical Practice. Blackwell Scientific Publications, OXford
Martinson I M 1976 Home care for the dying child. Appleton-Century Crofts, New York
Saunders C M (ed) 1978 The management of terminal illness. Edward Arnold, London
Thomson I (ed) 1979 Dilemmas of dying. Edinburgh University Press, Edinburgh
Twycross R G, Ventafridda V 1980 The continuing care of terminal cancer patient. Pergamon Press, Oxford

Bereavement
Lewis C S 1961 A grief observed. Faber and Faber Ltd, London
Lindemann E   Beyond grief: Studies in crisis intervention. Jason Aronson, New York
Parkes C M 1976 Bereavement. Pelican Books, London
Speck P 1978 Loss and grief in medicine. Balliere Tindall, London

Index